Diet Therapy in Advanced Practice Nursing: Nutrition Prescriptions for Improved Patient Outcomes

Katie Ferraro, MPH, RD, CDE
Assistant Clinical Professor, Nutrition
University of California San Francisco
School of Nursing
San Francisco, California

Cheryl Haas Winter, MS RD, MS APRN, CDE, BC-ADM, FNP-BC
Family Nurse Practitioner
DiabetesAmerica & DiabeteSteps Rx
Houston, Texas

D1202987

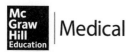 Medical

New York   Chicago   San Francisco   Athens   London   Madrid
Mexico City   New Delhi   Seoul   Singapore   Sydney   Toronto

Diet Therapy in Advanced Practice Nursing: Nutrition Prescriptions for Improved Patient Outcomes

1 2 3 4 5 6 7 8 9 0   DOC/DOC   18 17 16 15 14 13

ISBN 978-0-07-177148-1
MHID 0-07-177148-4

This book was set in Times by Thomson Digital.
The editors were Andrew Moyer and Christie Naglieri.
The production supervisor was Catherine H. Saggese.
Project management was provided by Garima Sharma, Thomson Digital.
Cover credit: Michelle Del Guercio.
RR Donnelley was printer and binder.

This book is printed on acid-free paper.

Library of Congress Cataloging-in-Publication Data

Ferraro, Katie.
  Diet therapy in advanced practice nursing: nutrition prescriptions for improved patient outcomes / Katie Ferraro, Cheryl Haas Winter.
    p. ; cm.
  Includes bibliographical references and index.
  Summary: "The first book to cover diet nutrition therapy as it pertains to advanced practice nursing, Diet Therapy in Advanced Practice Nursing: Nutrition Prescriptions for Improved Patient Outcomes is a concise compilation of best nutrition practices for specific disease states. The authors are both Registered Dietitians and Certified Diabetes Educators, and Cheryl Haas Winter is also an Advanced Practice Registered Nurse. Features - Organized by disease states, Focuses on nutrition-related prevention and therapeutic strategies for disease states, Valuable to both students and licensed practitioners"—Provided by publisher.
  ISBN-13: 978-0-07-177148-1 (pbk.)
  ISBN-10: 0-07-177148-4 (pbk.)
  I. Winter, Cheryl. II. Title.
  [DNLM: 1. Diet Therapy—nursing. 2. Advanced Practice Nursing—standards. 3. Nutritional Physiological Phenomena. 4. Practice Guidelines as Topic. WB 400]
  RM217
  615.8'54—dc23
                                                          2013008980

Diet Therapy in Advanced Practice Nursing: Nutrition Prescriptions for Improved Patient Outcomes

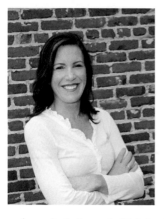

Katie Ferraro, MPH, RD, CDE is a Registered Dietitian, Certified Diabetes Educator and nutrition consultant based in San Diego, California. Specializing in nutrition communications and curriculum development, Katie's approach to primary care nutrition is, "If you can't beat 'em... teach 'em!" She is an Assistant Clinical Professor of Nutrition in the graduate schools of nursing at the University of California San Francisco and the University of San Diego. Katie obtained her undergraduate degree in Dietetics from Texas Christian University and Master of Public Health in Public Health Nutrition from the University of California, Berkeley. She is a former Peace Corps Volunteer (Nepal) and an avid traveler and intrepid taster of new foods. You can find Katie online at www.ingrainhealth.com.

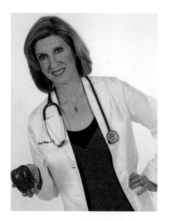

Cheryl Haas Winter, MS RD, MS APRN, CDE, BC-ADM, FNP-BC is a masters-prepared registered dietitian and masters-prepared advanced practice registered nurse, who is board-certified as a family nurse practitioner. Cheryl has been passionate about the powers of food and nutrition since high school, which is why she first became a registered dietitian. Believing food and nutrition to be the best medicine for prevention and treatment of disease eventually led her to become a registered nurse, and then family nurse practitioner, so that her patients were sure to be prescribed necessary medical nutrition therapy. Being focused on preventing and treating obesity and diabetes, Cheryl also became board-certified in advanced diabetes management, and practices as a diabetes specialist healthcare provider in the Houston, Texas markets at DiabetesAmerica. Additionally, she is a weight-management specialist and certified diabetes educator/consultant with her own company, http://DiabeteStepsRx.com.

Dedication

As a long-time nutrition educator of advanced practice nurses, this book is written for and dedicated to you. While I do not share your advanced practice nursing scope of practice, I certainly do honor and admire the unfailing dedication and compassion you show to your patients. I know the realities of your practice: you are short on time, working in settings that are strapped for cash, and with patient populations whose needs often appear endless. This book is for you, a small and humble attempt to educate your patients about the importance of food and nutrition.

Despite much discussion and data about the importance of prevention, we live and work in a healthcare environment that favors pills and procedures over sourcing the real roots of problems. For so many of our patients, food and nutrition issues are at the core of poor health; but they are also part of the cure for the prevention and treatment of many conditions. In a healthcare setting such as ours, where insurance companies don't blink to pay $25,000 for bariatric surgery, but nothing for preventive nutrition counseling with a registered dietitian, I applaud the work that you do in helping to educate patients about the importance and real impact that food and nutrition can have on health.

My co-author Cheryl Haas Winter and I believe that all patients should have a right to evidence-based diet therapies that can most positively impact their health outcomes. We hope that you will find the nutrition information and diet therapy guidelines in this book to be valuable resources in providing your patients with the most current and scientifically proven approaches to using food as medicine.

Katie Ferraro, MPH, RD, CDE

Like Katie, I am very passionate about the importance of food and nutrition in the treatment and prevention of disease. However, being a generation older than Katie, during my infancy as a registered dietitian, I was part of a medically oriented healthcare system designed to treat illness with drugs and medicine, not with food and nutrition. I often struggled with convincing my fellow colleagues about the benefits of incorporating medical nutrition therapy in the patient's medical treatment in order to improve their outcomes. Unfortunately, as far as many of these colleagues were concerned, I was just the lady from the hospital kitchen, a stigma that registered dietitians still have to contend with to this day. I also discovered, during this early part of my nutrition career, that treating illness medically was more lucrative than preventing illness. For example, still today, our healthcare system would rather pay to amputate a diabetic limb instead of paying for nutrition and diabetes education that could prevent it. Frustrated by this model, but ever so passionate about the importance of medical nutrition therapy, led me to join the medical profession as a nurse and then nurse practitioner, where I felt that I could better make a difference for my patients and be in a position to be able to prescribe this very important and necessary treatment: medical nutrition therapy.

During my nursing training, I also discovered that there was next to no "nutrition" education provided to student nurses or student nurse practitioners, so it became clear to me why I struggled as a young, passionate registered dietitian in a medically oriented healthcare system. Like medical schools, nursing programs were also practically void of nutrition courses, so why would these healthcare professionals prioritize nutrition therapy? How crazy is it that doctors and nurses, the most instrumental part of the healthcare team, lack the knowledge and skills for this most valuable medical treatment: nutrition?

No matter what healthcare profession you are in, we all know that "knowledge is power." Isn't that what we tell our patients? I am thrilled to be part of this "knowledge is power" movement along with Katie Ferraro to educate my fellow nurses and nurse practitioners, because I know that this is an incredible group of caring and dedicated healthcare professionals, who like me, love their patients, and only want the best for them. For me, I dedicate "Diet Therapy in Advanced Practice Nursing: Nutrition Prescriptions for Improved Patient Outcomes," to all my fellow nurses and nurse practitioners who love and care for their patients.

Cheryl Haas Winter, MS RD, MS APRN, CDE, BC-ADM, FNP-BC

Contents

1. Diet by Design: Healthy Meal Planning 1

2. Face-to-Face: Nutrition Screening,
   Assessment, and Counseling Techniques. 33

3. Finding Your Weigh: Mastering Weight Management 113

4. From Infants to Ancients:
   Nutrition Throughout the Lifecycle 168

5. Matters of the Heart: Nutrition and
   Cardiovascular Disease. 251

6. A Not-So-Sweet Metabolic Disruption:
   Diabetes Mellitus. 289

7. A Pain in the Gut: Nutrition in
   Gastrointestinal Disorders. 361

8. Blood and Bones: Nutrition in Musculoskeletal
   Disorders, Rheumatic Disease, and Anemias 421

9. Nutrition in Hepatobiliary, Pancreatic,
   and Kidney Disease 453

10. Skin, Surgery, and Stress: Nutrition in
    Metabolic Stress, Cancer, and HIV/AIDS 493

11. When Food Won't Do: Nutrition Support 523

12. Nutrition as a Complementary and Alternative Medicine. . . . 555

Appendix A. 599

Appendix B. 619

Appendix C. 624

Appendix D 632

Index 635

1

Diet by Design:
Healthy Meal Planning

Humans have been debating the basis of a balanced diet since time immemorial. Adam and Eve deliberated over the apple in the Garden of Eden. Greek and Roman philosophers disagreed about the hot and cold health attributes ascribed to different foods. And even today, we cannot make up our minds about butter or margarine: which one really *is* better for you? Despite our differences, we can all agree on one thing, that as sure as the sun will rise, we will at some point in our near future feel hungry. And when that hunger hits, what are we supposed to eat? The next section of this book will help you unravel some of the mysteries about healthy meal planning.

Government Guidelines for Good Nutrition

This book is written with the assumption that you, the reader, have a generally good grasp of basic nutrition science. The book does not cover introductory nutrition topics in great detail, but rather focuses on the evidence-based guidelines and practices that are recommended for the prevention, management, and treatment of a variety of disease states. In this book, the terms *kilocalorie* (kcal) and *calorie* (cal) have been used interchangeably. Calories are units of heat energy, and the term *energy* will also be used to mean calories. If a patient suggests he is taking a B-complex vitamin supplement because it "gives him energy," unless he experiences a placebo-derived invigorating rush from ingesting the capsule, he clearly misunderstands the concept of energy. Although vitamins do serve as important precursors for unlocking the energy (calories) in the foods we eat, the vitamins themselves do not contain energy, as they do not yield calories. One kilocalorie is equal to 4.184 kilojoules (kJ), and a kilocalorie is defined as the quantity of heat necessary to raise the temperature of 1 kilogram of water by 1 degree Celsius.[1]

■ Pyramids, Plates, and Portions

The United States Department of Agriculture (USDA) has had a heavy hand in recommending healthy nutrition guidelines for over 100 years. The first government dietary guide was a Farmers' Bulletin written by the USDA's initial director of the Office of Experiment Stations, W.O. Atwater, published in 1894. Despite the fact that vitamins and minerals had yet to be discovered, Atwater's cautionary words resonate even today:

> *Unless care is exercised in selecting food, a diet may result which is one-sided or badly balanced—that is, one in which either*

1

protein or fuel ingredients (carbohydrate and fat) are provided in excess.... The evils of overeating may not be felt at once, but sooner or later they are sure to appear—perhaps in an excessive amount of fatty tissue, perhaps in general debility, perhaps in actual disease.[2]

In 1916, nutritionist Caroline Hunt wrote the USDA's first guide *Food for Young Children.* She categorized foods as belonging to one of five groups: milk and meat, cereals, vegetables and fruits, sugars and sugary foods, and fats and fatty foods.[3] In 1917, Hunt and W.O. Atwater's daughter Helen teamed up, putting out *How to Select Foods*, using these same food groups, with information targeted to the larger, general public.[4]

US dietary guidance in the 1930s was driven largely by economic limitations related to the Great Depression. The 1940s saw the advent of the Recommended Dietary Allowances (RDAs), a set of specific recommended intakes of calories and nine essential nutrients: protein, iron, calcium, vitamins A and D, thiamin, riboflavin, niacin, and vitamin C.[5] In 1943, the USDA went on to release the *Basic Seven* food guide, which, during wartime, helped families handle rationing and limited supplies. The USDA put forth their next adaptation in 1956, and this version was commonly referred to as the "Basic Four," as it grouped foods into one of four food groups: milk, meat, fruits and vegetables, and grains. These four food groups, with their focus on obtaining adequate nutrients (as opposed to avoiding excess), were used extensively as the widespread basis of nutrition education for the next 20 years.

Nutrition education in the 1970s underwent a sea change with regard to how public nutrition messages were conveyed. Evidence mounted that dietary components consumed in excess (calories, fat, saturated fat, cholesterol, and sodium) were jeopardizing Americans' health. In 1977, the Senate Select Committee on Nutrition and Human Needs published the *Dietary Goals for the United States*, marking a discernible food messaging departure. Whereas the previous emphasis had been on obtaining *enough* nutrition, the tide was now turning toward caution against consuming *too much*.[6] The year 1980 saw the publication of the first edition of *Nutrition and Your Health: Dietary Guidelines for Americans.* After the 1980 release, subsequent revisions of the Dietary Guidelines for Americans trended toward suggesting numerical targets, such as eating less than 30% of calories from fat, and eating less than 10% of calories from saturated fat.[5] To this day, the Dietary Guidelines for Americans (DGAs) are revised jointly by the USDA and the United States Department of Health and Human Services (DHHS) every 5 years.

A desire to create a nationally recognizable and visually appealing nutrition teaching tool led to the design and eventual release of the 1992 *Food Guide Pyramid.* The 1992 pyramid emphasized variety among food groups that were separated into different categories and levels of the pyramid. The pyramid intended to convey proportionality through

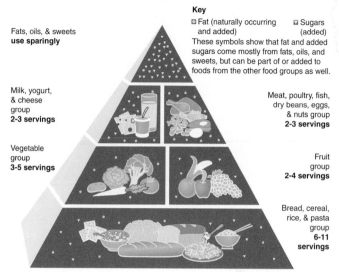

Figure 1–1. 1992 food guide pyramid. (Data from US Department of Agriculture. http://www.nal.usda.gov/fnic/Fpyr/fgpyramid.tif. Accessed January 2, 2013.)

different sizes of the pyramid food groups and in accompanying text that stated the number of daily servings to be consumed. The tip of the pyramid was intended to indicate moderation, showing that sugars and added fat should be used sparingly (Figure 1–1).

Despite its ubiquitous presence on virtually all packaged and pro-cessed foods sold in the United States for over a decade, the 1992 pyramid was ultimately considered a failed experiment. During the period from the pyramid's 1992 rollout to its eventual demise in 2005, Americans' weight and waistlines expanded dramatically, with body mass index (BMI) increasing every year during that period.[7] Although most Americans could recognize, to some degree, what the pyramid was trying to convey, very few people were actually using it to drive healthy food choices.[8] The much-maligned pyramid was criticized for its lack of portion size information, failure to differentiate between whole grains and refined grains, lumping of high-fat animal proteins in with healthier or leaner protein sources, disregard for statements about the benefits of healthy fats, failure to mention the benefits of exercise or impact of alcohol in the diet, as well as an overemphasis on dairy.

In conjunction with the 2005 revision of the *Dietary Guidelines for Americans*, the USDA replaced the 1992 *Food Guide Pyramid* with its updated pyramid, called MyPyramid. The MyPyramid tool was designed to be simple, and to drive traffic to the USDA's MyPyramid.

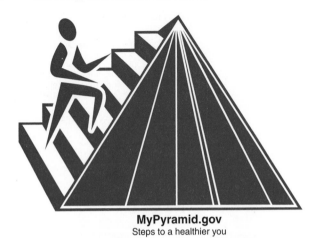

MyPyramid.gov
Steps to a healthier you

Figure 1–2. MyPyramid. (Data from US Department of Agriculture. MyPyramid. gov Website. Washington, DC. MyPlate Graphic Resources Website. http://www .choosemyplate.gov/print-materials-ordering/graphic-resources.html. Accessed January 2, 2013.)

gov website, where more detailed information on calorie patterns for various age groups and life stages (eg, pregnancy, preschoolers, and adolescents) could be accessed. In this version of the pyramid, different colored bands in the pyramid represented the various food groups. The narrowing width of the bands as they approached the tip of the pyramid indicated moderation and proportionality. Activity was represented by the person climbing the stairs, while the "Steps to a Healthier You" tagline stood for gradual improvement. The MyPyramid.gov url indicated personalization (Figure 1–2).

Five years later, for the 2010 edition of the *Dietary Guidelines for Americans,* the USDA scrapped its pyramid approach altogether, this time in favor of a plate called MyPlate. The MyPlate tool, ChooseMyPlate.gov website, and accompanying consumer messages promote a simplified approach to meal planning: make half your plate fruits and vegetables and balance the remainder of your meal with whole grains, lean protein, and low-fat dairy (Figure 1–3).

■ Dietary Guidelines for Americans, 2010

The *Dietary Guidelines for Americans, 2010* were released in June 2011 and serve as the federal government's "evidence-based nutritional guidance to promote health, reduce the risk of chronic diseases, and reduce the prevalence of overweight and obesity through improved nutrition and physical activity."[9] The guidelines include 23 key recommendations for the general population and six additional recommendations for specific population groups, such as pregnant women and older Americans. Table 1–1 contains the *Dietary Guidelines for Americans, 2010* selected

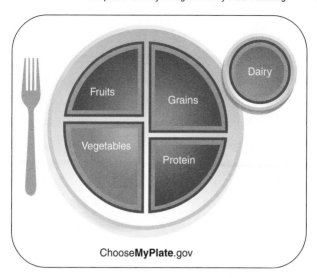

Figure 1–3. MyPlate. (Data from US Department of Agriculture. ChooseMyPlate.gov Website. Washington, DC. MyPlate Graphic Resources Website. http://www.choosemyplate.gov/print-materials-ordering/graphic-resources.html. Accessed January 2, 2013.)

messages for consumers, and Table 1–2 contains the *Dietary Guidelines for Americans, 2010* key recommendations.[10,11]

■ Healthy People 2020

Healthy People is a US DHHS initiative that serves to provide evidence-based, 10-year national objectives for improving the health of all Americans. Healthy People 2020 tracks over 1200 objectives organized

Table 1–1. Dietary guidelines for Americans, 2010 selected messages for consumers.

Balancing calories
Enjoy your food, but eat less.
Avoid oversized portions.
Foods to increase
Make half your plate fruits and vegetables.
Make at least half your grains whole grains.
Switch to fat-free or low-fat (1%) milk.
Foods to reduce
Compare sodium in foods such as soup, bread, and frozen meals—choose the foods with lower numbers.
Drink water instead of sugary drinks.

Data from US Department of Agriculture, 2011.

Table 1–2. Dietary guidelines for Americans, 2010 key recommendations.

Balancing calories to manage weight
  Prevent and/or reduce overweight and obesity through improved eating and physical activity behaviors.
  Control total calorie intake to manage body weight. For people who are overweight or obese, this will mean consuming fewer calories from foods and beverages.
  Increase physical activity and reduce time spent in sedentary behaviors.
  Maintain appropriate calorie balance during each stage of life—childhood, adolescence, adulthood, pregnancy and breastfeeding, and older age.

Foods and food components to reduce
  Reduce daily sodium to less than 2300 mg and further reduce intake to 1500 mg among persons who are aged 51 and older and those of any age who are African American or have hypertension, diabetes, or chronic kidney disease. The 1500 mg recommendation applies to about half of the US population, including children, and the majority of adults.
  Consume less than 10% of calories from saturated fatty acids by replacing them with monounsaturated and polyunsaturated fatty acids.
  Consume less than 300 mg per day of dietary cholesterol.
  Keep *trans* fatty acid consumption as low as possible by limiting foods that contain synthetic sources of *trans* fats, such as partially hydrogenated oils, and by limiting other solid fats.
  Reduce the intake of calories from solid fats and added sugars.
  Limit the consumption of foods that contain refined grains, especially refined grain foods that contain solid fats, added sugars, and sodium.
  If alcohol is consumed, it should be consumed in moderation—up to one drink per day for women and two drinks per day for men—and only by adults of legal drinking age.

Foods and nutrients to increase
  Individuals should meet the following recommendations as part of a healthy eating pattern while staying within their calorie needs:
  Increase vegetable and fruit intake.
  Eat a variety of vegetables, especially dark-green and red and orange vegetables and beans and peas.
  Consume at least half of all grains as whole grains. Increase whole-grain intake by replacing refined grains with whole grains.
  Increase intake of fat-free or low-fat milk and milk products, such as milk, yogurt, cheese, or fortified soy beverages.
  Choose a variety of protein foods, which include seafood, lean meat and poultry, eggs, beans and peas, soy products, and unsalted nuts and seeds.
  Increase the amount and variety of seafood consumed by choosing seafood in place of some meat and poultry.
  Replace protein foods that are higher in solid fats with choices that are lower in solid fats and calories and/or sources of oils.

(Continued)

Table 1–2. Dietary guidelines for Americans, 2010 key recommendations. (*Continued*)

Use oils to replace solid fats where possible.

Choose foods that provide more potassium, dietary fiber, calcium, and vitamin D, which are nutrients of concern in American diets. These foods include vegetables, fruits, whole grains, and milk and milk products.

Recommendations for specific population groups

Women capable of becoming pregnant

- Choose foods that supply heme iron, which is more readily absorbed by the body, additional iron sources, and enhancers of iron absorption such as vitamin C-rich foods.
- Consume 400 mcg per day of synthetic folic acid (from fortified foods and/or supplements) in addition to food forms of folate from a varied diet.

Women who are pregnant or breastfeeding

- Consume 8–12 ounces of seafood per week from a variety of seafood types.
- Due to their high methyl mercury content, limit white (albacore) tuna to 6 ounces per week and do not eat the following four types of fish: tilefish, shark, swordfish, and king mackerel.
- If pregnant, take an iron supplement as recommended by an obstetrician or other healthcare provider.

Individuals aged 50 years and older

Consume foods fortified with vitamin B_{12}, such as fortified cereals, or dietary supplements.

Data from US Department of Agriculture and US Department of Health and Human Services, 2011.

into 42 topic areas, each covering an important public health target. The goal of the Nutrition and Weight Status area of Healthy People 2020 is to "promote health and reduce chronic disease risk through the consumption of healthful diets and achievement and maintenance of healthy body weights." Further objectives seek to increase household food security and to eliminate hunger, encouraging Americans with a healthful diet to:

- Consume a variety of nutrient-dense foods within and across the food groups, especially whole grains, fruits, vegetables, low-fat or fat-free milk or milk products, and lean meats and other protein sources
- Limit the intake of saturated and *trans* fats, cholesterol, added sugars, sodium (salt), and alcohol
- Limit caloric intake to meet caloric needs

Table 1–3 further outlines the Nutrition and Weight Status objectives of Healthy People 2020 and more information can be found at http://www.healthypeople.gov.[12]

Table 1–3. Healthy People 2020 nutrition and weight status objectives.

Healthier food access

NWS-1: Increase the number of States with nutrition standards for foods and beverages provided to preschool-aged children in child care.

NWS-2: Increase the proportion of school districts that require schools to make fruits or vegetables available whenever other food is offered or sold.

NWS-3: Increase the number of States that have State-level policies that incentivize food retail outlets to provide foods that are encouraged by the Dietary Guidelines for Americans.

NWS-4: Increase the proportion of Americans who have access to a food retail outlet that sells a variety of foods that are encouraged by the Dietary Guidelines for Americans.

Health care and worksite settings

NWS-5: Increase the proportion of primary care physicians who regularly measure the body mass index of their patients.

NWS-6: Increase the proportion of physician office visits that include counseling or education related to nutrition or weight.

NWS-7: Increase the proportion of worksites that offer nutrition or weight management classes or counseling.

Weight status

NWS-8: Increase the proportion of adults who are at a healthy weight.

NWS-9: Reduce the proportion of adults who are obese.

NWS-10: Reduce the proportion of children and adolescents who are considered obese.

NWS-11: Prevent inappropriate weight gain in youth and adults.

Food insecurity

NWS-12: Eliminate very low food security among children.

NWS-13: Reduce household food insecurity and in so doing reduce hunger.

Food and nutrient consumptions

NWS-14: Increase the contribution of fruits to the diets of the population aged 2 years and older.

NWS-15: Increase the variety and contribution of vegetables to the diets of the population aged 2 years and older.

NWS-16: Increase the contribution of whole grains to the diets of the population aged 2 years and older.

NWS-17: Reduce consumption of calories from solid fats and added sugars in the population aged 2 years and older.

NWS-18: Reduce consumption of saturated fat in the population aged 2 years and older.

NWS-19: Reduce consumption of sodium in the population aged 2 years and older.

NWS-20: Increase consumption of calcium in the population aged 2 years and older.

Iron deficiency

NWS-21: Reduce iron deficiency among young children and females of childbearing age.

NWS-22: Reduce iron deficiency among pregnant females.

Data from US Department of Health and Human Services, 2010.

■ The Food Label

While the Nutrition Facts panel on the packaging of nearly all of the foods and beverages may now seem like a familiar standard, things were not always this way. The Nutrition Labeling and Education Act of 1990 (NLEA) mandated that nutrition information be displayed on almost all packaged and processed food sold in the United States. The law, implemented in 1994, required manufacturers to use a standardized Nutrition Facts panel displayed on food packaging to disclose the amounts of certain nutrients in the product. The law also gave the US Food and Drug Administration (FDA) the authority to regulate nutrient content claims. As a concession to food manufacturers, a limited number of health claims (eg, low fat, fat-free, low sodium) were permitted by the FDA.

The Nutrition Facts panel (required under the 1990 legislation) lists the serving size, servings per container, and amount of calories per serving. It contains information about nutrients to limit (total fat, saturated fat, *trans* fat, cholesterol, and sodium) and nutrients to get enough of (dietary fiber, vitamin A, vitamin C, calcium, and iron). The percent Daily Value (%DV) column tells you what percent of your daily recommended allotment of particular nutrients one serving size provides. Although the information on the food label is given for a daily 2000 calorie level diet, the bottom of the expanded food label also includes nutrient-specific information and daily recommendations for both a 2000 and a 2500 calorie diet. Figure 1–4 explains how to use the Nutrition Facts label, and Table 1–4 outlines the daily values for each nutrient.[13]

■ Dietary Reference Intakes

In the United States, the Food and Nutrition Board of the Institute of Medicine originally developed and periodically revises the dietary reference intakes (DRIs). The DRIs contain a variety of energy (calorie) and nutrient intake standards for Americans. While the DRIs encompass a number of terms and standards, the most familiar DRI is the recommended dietary allowance, (RDA). The RDA is an amount of a nutrient that meets the nutrient needs of 98% of individuals in a given age and gender group. In the event that there is not enough scientific data to set an RDA for a particular nutrient, the DRI committee establishes an adequate intake (AI) level for that nutrient. In addition to the RDAs and AIs, nutrition scientists have also established tolerable upper intake levels (ULs), also called upper levels, for some nutrients. The UL is the highest average amount of a nutrient for a given age and gender group that is unlikely to be harmful or pose a toxicity threat when consumed daily. There are not ULs for all nutrients, but for those that have ULs, consumers are advised not to consume that nutrient in levels above the UL. Practitioners should be aware of the DRIs in order to make nutrient and energy intake recommendations for patients of different age and gender groups, and to advise patients about potential

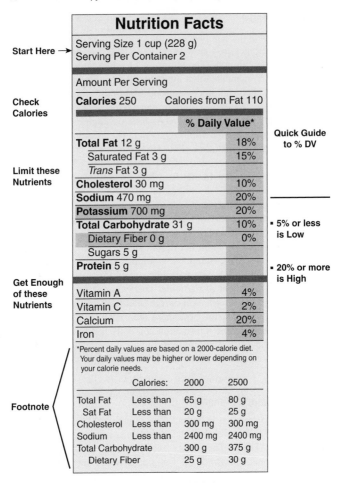

Figure 1–4. How to use the nutrition facts label.

safety concerns of supplements consumed in very high doses. Appendix A contains the DRI tables, and you can find an interactive DRI for Healthcare Professionals tool online at: http://fnic.nal.usda.gov/fnic/interactiveDRI/.

Menu Planning Basics

What goes on a person's plate is certainly a personal matter. While our palates and food preferences may differ, there are a few basic tenets to healthy meal planning that most patient and client groups should follow.

Table 1–4. Daily values (DVs) used on the food label for a 2000-calorie diet.

Food Component	Daily Value (DV)
Total fat	65 g
Saturated fat	20 g
Cholesterol	300 mg
Sodium	2400 mg
Potassium	3500 mg
Total carbohydrate	300 g
Dietary fiber	25 g
Vitamin A	5000 IU
Vitamin C	60 mg
Calcium	1000 mg
Iron	18 mg

Data from US Food and Drug Administration, 2011.

Note, however, that specific medical conditions and disease states may require diet modifications, and that nutrient recommendations vary based on age and gender groups.

■ Build Food Group Foundations

While the four basic food groups are no longer a primary method of teaching nutrition in the United States, most healthful meal plans and guides still classify foods and beverages according to their primary nutrients and natural origins. The following sections on grains, dairy products, fruits, vegetables, and protein-rich foods summarize key concepts about each of the groups that may be useful to practitioners in clinical and community settings. Appendix B contains the USDA Food Patterns for 12 different calorie levels.

Grains

Grains are starchy foods made from wheat, rice, oats, cornmeal, barley, or other cereal grain products. These include foods such as bread, pasta, cereals, tortillas, and a variety of different whole grains such as quinoa, spelt, and millet. In general, a serving of grains is equivalent to one ounce, roughly the size of one slice of a 100-calorie bread. One cup of cooked rice or pasta is roughly two ounces, or two grain servings. Corn is technically a grain, although it is often grouped with vegetables

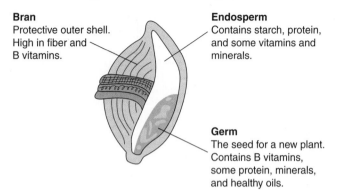

Bran
Protective outer shell.
High in fiber and
B vitamins.

Endosperm
Contains starch, protein,
and some vitamins and
minerals.

Germ
The seed for a new plant.
Contains B vitamins,
some protein, minerals,
and healthy oils.

Figure 1–5. Anatomy of a whole grain.

(or high-starch vegetables), whereas cornmeal and popcorn tend to be grouped with grains.

Grains can also be classified as being either whole grains or refined grains. Whole grains are primarily unprocessed and include all components of the grain kernel—the bran, germ, and endosperm (see Figure 1–5). The consensus among nutrition professionals is that the general public will benefit from increasing whole-grain intake and reducing refined-grain intake. Refined grains include foods such as white flour, white bread, white rice, and degermed cornmeal. Table 1–5 gives some examples of whole grains. The *Dietary Guidelines for Americans, 2010* recommends making at least half of your grains whole. Because Americans are increasingly relying on foods prepared outside of the home (roughly 50 cents of every food dollar is spent on foods prepared outside the home), a practical application of the "make half

Table 1–5. List of some whole grains.

Examples of Whole Grains		
Amaranth	Kamut®	Sorghum/milo
Barley	Millet	Spelt
Buckwheat	Oats	Teff
Bulgur	Quinoa	Triticale
Corn	Rice	Wheat
Farro	Rye	Wild rice

Data from Whole Grains Council.

your grains whole" recommendation is to advise people to try to eat only whole grains at home, assuming anything they will be eating outside the home is most likely to be refined.

Whole grain, minimally processed foods not only have more fiber than do their refined counterparts, but also have higher levels of other vitamins and minerals that are not replaced during enrichment. Enriched flours are from grains—usually wheat—that have been stripped of the bran and germ, leaving only the less nutritious endosperm remaining in the flour. In the United States, refined flours must be enriched with prescribed amounts of iron, thiamin, niacin, riboflavin, and folic acid (the synthetic form of folate). They may also be enriched with fiber, which is naturally occurring in the bran, but removed during the processing of refined grains. Consumers should be encouraged to look for grain products that contain the word "whole" in the first ingredient in the ingredients list, and to avoid or minimize those that say "enriched." Table 1–6 contains the USDA recommendations for daily grain food intake for different age and gender groups.

Dairy Foods

Dairy foods include calcium-containing products such as fluid milk and milk products, yogurt, and hard cheese. Dairy foods that are made from milk, but that have little or no calcium, such as cream cheese, butter,

Table 1–6. USDA-recommended grain food intake levels.

		Daily Recommendation	Daily Minimum Amount of Whole Grains
Children	2–3 years old	3 ounce equivalents	1½ ounce equivalents
	4–8 years old	5 ounce equivalents	2½ ounce equivalents
Girls	9–13 years old	5 ounce equivalents	3 ounce equivalents
	14–18 years old	6 ounce equivalents	3 ounce equivalents
Boys	9–13 years old	6 ounce equivalents	3 ounce equivalents
	14–18 years old	8 ounce equivalents	4 ounce equivalents
Women	19–30 years old	6 ounce equivalents	3 ounce equivalents
	31–50 years old	6 ounce equivalents	3 ounce equivalents
	51+ years old	5 ounce equivalents	3 ounce equivalents
Men	19–30 years old	8 ounce equivalents	4 ounce equivalents
	31–50 years old	7 ounce equivalents	3½ ounce equivalents
	51+ years old	6 ounce equivalents	3 ounce equivalents

Data from US Department of Agriculture.

and cream, are not considered part of the dairy group. Calcium-fortified soy beverages (soymilk) are also part of the dairy group. Despite their micronutrient and protein contributions, full-fat dairy foods tend to be high in calories, fat, and saturated fat. Most dietary recommendations include choosing fat-free (skim, nonfat) or low-fat (1%) dairy foods. Whole milk is 3.25% fat by weight, and reduced fat is 2%. Making the switch from full-fat dairy foods to reduced-fat 2%, low-fat 1%, or nonfat milk, cheese, and yogurt is an easy, yet significantly impactful, way to reduce saturated fat and cholesterol intake. Saturated fat elevates LDL cholesterol levels, and those on a 2000 calorie per day diet should aim to eat less than 20 grams of saturated fat per day. A one-ounce serving of regular, full-fat cheese (the size of a domino or a slice of prepackaged processed American cheese) or a cup of whole milk has 5 grams of saturated fat. Although four servings of those full-fat dairy foods per day would help you reach your recommended calcium levels, it also provides 100% of the recommended amount of saturated fat, essentially leaving no room for any other saturated fats in the diet that day. Replacing one full-fat dairy serving with a low-fat equivalent reduces the saturated fat to 1.5 grams per serving. Four servings of a low-fat dairy equivalent per day totals only 6 grams of saturated fat at the end of the day, compared to the 20 grams obtained with the full-fat alternatives.

The USDA considers a standard serving of dairy to be one cup of fluid milk, yogurt, or soymilk, 1½ ounces of natural cheese, or two ounces of processed cheese. Each of these equate to roughly 300 mg of calcium per serving. Flavored milks and sugar-sweetened yogurts should be avoided or limited as they contain high amounts of added sugars or empty calories. Because lactose intolerance is a condition that occurs commonly in adulthood and disproportionately in some ethnic and racial populations, many individuals must achieve their recommended calcium intake through the consumption of calcium-fortified foods, calcium supplements, or nondairy calcium-containing foods.[14] Chapter 7 contains more information on lactose intolerance. Table 1–7 lists dairy foods and calcium-fortified soy beverages that are equivalent to a one cup of milk serving. Note that although ice cream is listed, the amount of calories and fat in the 1½ cups of ice cream required to obtain the equivalent amount of calcium you get in one cup of milk would be significantly higher than the calories and fat found in milk. All dairy foods are indeed *not* created equal!

Fruits

Any fruit or 100% fruit juice counts as part of the USDA's fruit group. Fruit can be in the fresh, canned, frozen, dried, whole, cut-up, or pureed forms. Many dried fruit foods have added sugars, so check the ingredient list and avoid any dried fruit that has sugar or sucrose in the ingredients list. A standard serving of fruit is one cup of fruit or 100% fruit juice, or one-half cup of dried fruit, such as apricots or raisins. Frozen

Table 1–7. USDA one-cup dairy serving sizes.

	Amount That Counts as a Cup in the Dairy Group	Common Portions and Cup Equivalents
Milk (choose fat-free or low-fat milk)	1 cup milk ½ cup evaporated milk	
Yogurt (choose fat-free or low-fat yogurt)	1 regular container (8 fluid ounces) 1 cup yogurt	1 small container (6 ounces = ¾ cup)
Cheese (choose reduced-fat or low-fat cheeses)	1½ ounces hard cheese (cheddar, mozzarella, Swiss, and Parmesan) ½ cup shredded cheese 2 ounces processed cheese (American) ½ cup ricotta cheese 2 cups cottage cheese	1 slice of hard cheese is equivalent to ½ cup milk 1 slice processed cheese is equivalent to ⅓ cup milk ½ cup cottage cheese is equivalent to ¼ cup milk
Milk-based desserts (choose fat-free or low-fat types)	1 cup pudding made with milk 1 cup frozen yogurt 1½ cups ice cream	1 scoop ice cream is equivalent to ½ cup milk
Soymilk (soy beverage)	1 cup calcium-fortified soymilk	

Data from US Department of Agriculture.

fruits are a good option when fresh fruit is not available year-round; however, some frozen fruits may contain added sugars.

Although 100% fruit juice is included in the fruit group, most patients and clients will benefit from avoiding fruit juices, instead sticking to whole, fresh fruit whenever possible. Fruit juice is a concentrated source of calories, and while 100% fruit juice is helpful for those who have difficulty meeting calorie needs, the lower-calorie and higher-fiber benefits of eating intact versus juiced fruits is beneficial for the majority of the general public. One small orange has roughly 50 calories and 3 grams of fiber. To make one cup of fresh squeezed orange juice, three or four oranges would have to be juiced, thus tripling or quadrupling the calories in the juice as compared to the fruit, not to mention discarding the valuable dietary fiber as part of the pulp remnants. The dietary fiber in whole, intact fruit promotes satiety, may protect against heart disease and certain types of cancer, and minimizes blood glucose spikes. Additionally, fresh fruit is a valuable source of water, vitamins, minerals, and phytochemicals. For most patient populations, your best advice about fruit will likely be, "Eat your fruit, and don't drink it."

Consumers—and particularly those with diabetes—are often confused about fruit because it contains fructose, a form of simple carbohydrate or fruit sugar. Fructose is sweeter than common table sugar, and is the sweetest of all sugars.[15] When included as a component of high-fructose corn syrup (HFCS) in sweetened drinks and other foods, fructose can contribute unnecessary or empty calories and promote unwanted weight gain. The wise practitioner will quickly allay any consumer or client fears about fruit by pointing out the obvious differences between fruit and fructose-sweetened processed foods and drinks. Encourage people, including those with diabetes, to eat fruit as a between-meal snack, and instruct clients to aim for two or three servings of fruit per day. With roughly 3–5 grams of fiber per serving, two to three servings of fruit can help most individuals reach about one-third to one-half of their daily fiber needs. Table 1–8 contains some commonly eaten fruits to recommend for people who are looking to increase their fruit variety and intake.

Protein Foods

The protein foods group includes all foods made from meat, poultry, seafood, eggs, beans and peas, processed soy products, nuts, and seeds. In addition to being part of the protein group, beans and peas are also part of the vegetable group given their plant-based origin. In the USDA food plan, protein foods are listed in one ounce equivalents; Table 1–9 lists the amount of different protein foods that count as a one ounce equivalent. Because meat and other animal foods can be high in calories, total fat and saturated fat, and cholesterol, a general heart-healthy recommendation is to focus on lean sources of protein and to

Table 1–8. Commonly eaten fruits.

Apples	Grapes	Nectarines	Pineapple
Apricots	Kiwi fruit	Oranges	Plums
Bananas	Lemons	Peaches	Prunes
Cherries	Limes	Pears	Raisins
Grapefruit	Mangoes	Papaya	Tangerines
Berries: strawberries, blueberries, raspberries, and blackberries			
Melons: cantaloupe, honeydew, and watermelon			

Data from US Department of Agriculture.

Table 1–9. One ounce equivalents in the protein foods group.

	Amount that Counts as 1 ounce Equivalents in the Protein Foods Group	Common Portions and Ounce Equivalents
Meats	1 ounce cooked lean beef 1 ounce cooked lean pork or ham	1 small steak (eye of round, filet) = 3½–4 ounce equivalents 1 small lean hamburger = 2–3 ounce equivalents
Poultry	1 ounce cooked chicken or turkey, without skin 1 sandwich slice of turkey (4½ × 2½ × ⅛″)	1 small chicken breast half = 3 ounce equivalents ½ Cornish game hen = 4 ounce equivalents
Seafood	1 ounce cooked fish or shellfish	1 can of tuna, drained = 3–4 ounce equivalents 1 salmon steak = 4–6 ounce equivalents 1 small trout = 3 ounce equivalents
Eggs	1 egg	3 egg whites = 2 ounce equivalents 3 egg yolks = 1 ounce equivalent
Nuts and seeds	½ ounce of nuts (12 almonds, 24 pistachios, 7 walnut halves) ½ ounce of seeds (pumpkin, sunflower or squash seeds, hulled, roasted) 1 tablespoon of peanut butter or almond butter	1 ounce of nuts or seeds = 2 ounce equivalents
Beans and peas	¼ cup of cooked beans (such as black, kidney, pinto, or white beans) ¼ cup of cooked peas (such as chickpeas, cowpeas, lentils, or split peas) ¼ cup of baked beans, refried beans ¼ cup (about 2 ounces) of tofu 1 oz. tempeh, cooked ¼ cup roasted soybeans 1 falafel patty (2¼″, 4 oz) 2 Tablespoons hummus	1 cup split pea soup = 2 ounce equivalents 1 cup lentil soup = 2 ounce equivalents 1 cup bean soup = 2 ounce equivalents 1 soy or bean burger patty = 2 ounce equivalents

Data from US Department of Agriculture.

Table 1–10. Seafood guidelines for pregnant or breastfeeding women.

Consume 8-12 ounces of seafood per week from a variety of seafood types (including tuna)
Limit white (albacore) tuna to 6 ounces per week
Avoid tilefish, shark, swordfish, and king mackerel

Data from US Department of Agriculture.

limit high-fat protein foods. Regular milk, bacon, sausages, and hot dogs are examples of high-fat protein foods. Low-fat cottage cheese, the white (breast) meat of turkey and chicken are very lean meats; whereas ground beef that is not more than 15% fat by weight and tuna are examples of lean meats. Although Western cultures traditionally make meat the center of the meal plate, there is an increasing focus on reducing meat portions such that they comprise no more than one-quarter of the plate.

Many public health and nutrition organizations are increasingly adopting an "eat more seafood" stance when it comes to protein foods. Fish and shellfish are low in total and saturated fat, and rich in omega-3 fatty acids. In its "Foods and Nutrients to Increase" messaging, the *Dietary Guidelines for Americans, 2010* encourages individuals to "increase the amount and variety of seafood consumed by choosing seafood in place of some meat and poultry." Women who are pregnant or breastfeeding can safely consume 8–12 ounces of seafood per week from a variety of seafood types. These women are advised to limit white (albacore) tuna to six ounces per week and to avoid the large, predator-type fish including tilefish, shark, swordfish, and king mackerel due to their higher methyl mercury content (see Table 1–10). For the rest of the population (the nonpregnant and nonbreastfeeding), the benefits of consuming more fish and seafood far outweigh any likely detriments or concerns about potential mercury intake.

■ Monitor Frequency of Food Consumption

For many medical conditions, particularly diabetes, hypoglycemia, and obesity or weight control, small frequent meals are most advisable for meal patterning purposes. The rationale behind this recommendation is that consuming small, frequent meals helps to taper hunger and prevent subsequent overeating. For individuals with diabetes, this frequent meal patterning also optimizes glycemic control. While there are certainly other factors beyond hunger that contribute to overeating and weight gain, frequent, calorie-controlled meals and snacks are a useful way for many people to meet their calorie and nutrient targets without feeling deprived. The Academy of Nutrition and Dietetics

Evidence Analysis Library states that there is fair evidence supporting this notion:

> *Several studies show that consumption of four to five meals or snacks per day is associated with reduced or no obesity risk, while three or fewer and six or more meals or snacks per day may result in increased risk of obesity, depending on gender. Higher eating frequency is related to lower total daily energy intake and body weights in men, but in women the data is less conclusive* (Evidence Grade II—fair).[16]

■ Promote Variety in Diet

A balanced diet is one that contains a variety of foods. Despite efforts of the fad diet industry to convince us otherwise, there is no one single food or food group with adequate nutriture to sustain human life. While it may take a twist of the imagination to find ways to incorporate doughnuts and regular soda into a healthy meal plan for an individual looking to lose weight, it can be done, and there is no "one-size-fits-all" approach to meal planning that is guaranteed to work. A good mantra to keep in mind when helping patients and clients plan meals is "All foods can fit in moderation." Promoting foods as taboo or off-limits only serves to increase their desirability and to promote a feeling of failure if the individual gives into consumption. On the other hand, promoting reasonable portions and small intakes of desirable foods on occasion and in moderation can help avoid cravings and promotes feelings of satiety and satisfaction.

When faced with a medical, health, or weight condition that necessitates a change in diet, human nature is such that individuals automatically focus on the foods they cannot eat. "I have high blood pressure, I can't eat salty foods." "I have elevated LDL cholesterol levels, I can't eat meat anymore." "I have celiac disease, I can't eat bread", or "I have diabetes, I can't eat fruit." (The last one being a fallacy, but one you no doubt encounter regularly in nutrition counseling for diabetes.) If you notice that the "can'ts" are starting to stack up in your patients' vocabulary, turn the tide and encourage individuals with special dietary needs to embrace all of the new foods that they *can* eat. For example, a person with high blood pressure will benefit from increased potassium intake from fruits and vegetables. Someone with elevated LDL cholesterol levels might enjoy trying out new lean sources of animal protein, or even embrace a semivegetarian lifestyle. For clients with celiac disease, there is ample opportunity to embrace gluten-free whole grains. And fruit is certainly an important part of a well-balanced meal plan for diabetes.

Colors count when it comes to healthy meal planning. Have clients keep food records and use these records as talking points when discussing the color palate of typical meals and snacks. The colors or pigments in various plant-based foods often serve as indicators of their nutritional values. For example, the orange pigment in carrots is a derivative of vitamin A; thus, seeing the orange color indicates carrots are an excellent source of this nutrient. When looking at your clients' meal records, take note of the colors. Are the foods that are commonly consumed mostly brown and white in color? A brightly colored plate generally indicates more nutritious foods (with the obvious exclusion of artificially colored processed high-fat and high-sugar junk foods). Encourage your clients to set attainable and quantifiable color goals, like aiming for two different brightly colored fruit or vegetable servings per meal, or three different colored fruit servings per day. One study found that a highly varied diet in elderly nursing home residents was associated with better nutritional status when assessed by nutrient intake, and biochemical and body composition measures.[17] So when it comes to meal planning, get out of your every day rut and promote colorful variety to help ensure adequate nutrient intake and to promote overall health. Table 1–11 contains tips for improving your meals with fruits and vegetables.[18]

- ## Control Portion Size

There is not one predominant factor that is solely responsible for the rapid rise in overweight and obesity over the past three decades. But if you *had* to pick one precipitating part, the calorie culprit, it would probably have to be portion size. The growing size of commonly consumed amounts of foods and beverages is sometimes referred to as "Portion Distortion." Whereas the average American family in 1970 spent just 26% of every food dollar on meals purchased away from home, that number climbed to nearly half of every food dollar spent in 2010.[19,20] To compound this issue, the foods we are consuming outside of the home are increasingly further removed from what our plates *should* look like. Think about the last restaurant meal you had. Did half of the plate consist of lower-calorie fruits and vegetables, with the rest divided between whole grains and low-fat protein sources? Probably not. And because energy expenditure levels—in the form of exercise—have not increased much since the 1980s, we are left with the reality that portions are certainly part of the problem.[21]

Casual dining and fast food restaurants have routinely increased the sizes of the portions of food they serve, along with calories and fat. It is no longer shocking to see menu items with more than 1000 calories per entrée and a full day's worth of fat, saturated fat, and sodium. And that is in one meal! Young and Nestle cite 147 new large-size portions introduced from 2000 to 2009 by the top fast-food chains, including an 850-calorie Angus Third Pounder from McDonald's, a 1300-calorie Triple Baconator burger from Wendy's, and a 1000-calorie Quad Stacker sandwich from Burger King.[22] Given this, it is no wonder that as the size of portions has increased, so has the intake of calories per capita per day, and the percentage of overweight and obese individuals.

While it is one thing to bemoan the increasing size (and decreasing prices) of nutrient-poor foods, it is another to offer real and meaningful

Table 1–11. Ten tips to improve your meals with vegetables and fruits.

Fire up the grill!
Use the grill to cook vegetables and fruits
Grill mushrooms, carrots, peppers, or potatoes on a kabob skewer
Brush or spray veggies with canola or olive oil to prevent sticking and drying out
Try grilled fruits such as peaches, pineapple, or mangoes for added flavor to a cookout

Expand your casserole flavors
Mix vegetables like sautéed onions, peas, pinto beans, or tomatoes into your favorite dish

Flavor-full Italian foods
Add extra vegetables to your pasta dishes
Slip some peppers, spinach, red beans, onions, or tomatoes into your traditional tomato sauce

Spice up your salads
Toss in shredded carrots, strawberries, orange segments, or berries to your standard salads
Mix up your greens by adding spinach, watercress, and cabbage to different types of lettuce

Try fruit from the salad bar
Use sliced fruit on a salad bar as your go-to dessert when dining out
Fruits help you avoid baked desserts that are high in calories while satisfying your sweet tooth

Stir-fry something new
Stir-fry veggies such as broccoli, carrots, sugar snap peas, mushrooms, or green beans for a "quick-and-easy" addition to any meal

Switch up your sandwiches
Vegetables make a great addition to sandwiches or wraps
Add sprouts, cucumbers, avocadoes, lettuce, or tomatoes to your everyday sandwich

Bulk up baked goods
Add apples, bananas, blueberries, or pears to your favorite muffin and cobbler recipes

Smoothie central
Blend strawberries, blueberries, raspberries, and frozen bananas with milk or soy milk and ice
Use fresh or frozen fruit and have for breakfast, snack, or a small portion for dessert

Liven up an omelet
Boost color and flavor of your omelet with vegetables
Chop, sauté, and add vegetables such as mushrooms, spinach, onion, or bell peppers and add to egg as it cooks

Data from US Department of Agriculture, 2011.

counters to this public health threat. Proposed solutions to the portion size problem involve education and public health campaigns aimed at individuals (such as calorie counts displayed clearly next to menu items), uniform and reality-based serving-size standards, price incentives for smaller portions, and possibly even limits on portion sizes in food-service establishments.[22] Industry does respond to consumer feedback. McDonald's phased out their extra-large Super Size portions following unwanted publicity garnered by the award-winning documentary "Super Size Me."[23] Just as no one issue is solely responsible for rising obesity rates, there is likely not going to be one solution to resetting our portion distortion.

Teaching patients and clients what healthy portions *should* look like, and having open and honest discussions about why they *don't* look that way, is something practitioners can do to elicit change. Focusing on the energy density and relatively lower calorie content of fruits and vegetables, while eschewing large servings of high-calorie and high-fat grain and protein foods, is a good start. Using common household measurements (eg, measuring cups and teaspoons and tablespoons), food scales, and easily recognizable equivalent converters (eg, 3 oz is equivalent to a deck of cards) can help teach individuals about appropriate portioning. Keep a set of dishes, a plate, cup, measuring spoons, bowl, coffee mug, and juice and wine glasses in your office. Use food models or real food and drinks to ask clients to show you what their typical portions look like, and use that as a starting point to assess their calorie intake. In addition, focus on beverages: get patients with weight-control issues to cut out or severely limit all calories from beverages, with the exception of nonfat or low-fat milk or calcium-fortified milk alternatives (Figure 1–6).

- ■ Reduce Energy Density

Manipulation of both portion size and the energy density of foods has influential effects on total energy intake in adults and children.[24] Energy density refers to the available energy per unit weight—essentially, the amount of calories in a given weight of food.[25] The water and macronutrient content of a food determines the food's energy density. Fat, which contains 9 kilocalories per gram by weight, is the most energy dense of the macronutrients, with protein and carbohydrate each contributing 4 kilocalories per gram. Theoretically, a person adopting a lower-fat diet should lose weight due to the reduction in calories or energy. Realistically however, if the fat in the diet is replaced with an equal number of calories from carbohydrate- or protein-rich foods, total caloric intake stays constant, prohibiting weight loss. This was the phenomenon seen with the low-fat diet craze of the 1990s. American consumers gobbled up low-fat brownies, fat-free cookies, and reduced-fat cakes and crackers, but US rates of overweight and obesity increased during this period. Why? The fat in the diet was

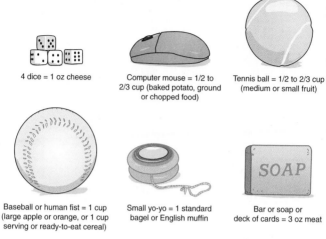

4 dice = 1 oz cheese

Computer mouse = 1/2 to 2/3 cup (baked potato, ground or chopped food)

Tennis ball = 1/2 to 2/3 cup (medium or small fruit)

Baseball or human fist = 1 cup (large apple or orange, or 1 cup serving or ready-to-eat cereal)

Small yo-yo = 1 standard bagel or English muffin

Bar or soap or deck of cards = 3 oz meat

Figure 1–6. Estimating portion sizes.

replaced with an equal, if not greater, amount of calories from refined grain products and carbohydrate. Holding all other things constant, any reduction in fat calories was immediately replaced—and, in this case, surpassed—by calories from refined carbohydrate. An important lesson learned from the 1990s was that a low-fat diet does not make a low-fat person!

In addition to a food's macronutrient composition, water content greatly affects energy density. Water has the greatest influence on density as it adds significant weight without adding calories. Low-energy-dense foods are those that contain less energy relative to their weight, whereas high-energy-dense foods are those with more energy relative to weight. In recent years, Rolls and colleagues have extensively studied the effect of energy density on satiety and weight. They found that reducing the energy density of foods by increasing water content or lowering the proportion of fat and/or sugar can lead to reductions in overall energy intake.[26] One such mechanism for lowering energy density while increasing satiety is to consume a food low in energy density at the start of a meal, what is often referred to as a "preload." One study demonstrated that lowering the energy density of a milk-based preload by increasing its water content (and in turn, its total volume) led to a demonstrated reduction in energy intake.[27] Other low-energy-density foods, such as soup, have been shown to significantly reduce energy intake at the meal when consumed prior to the meal as a preload.[28-31] Interestingly however, Rolls has shown that drinking water along with food has not been shown to have the same effect on satiety as does including water into a food in order to lower the food's energy density.[32]

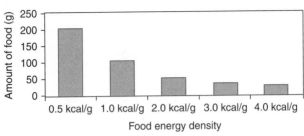

Examples: ½ cup spaghetti with tomato sauce
             1½ oranges
             1 fried egg
             ¼ cup raisins
             3 large pretzel rods

Figure 1–7. 100-calorie portions of foods differing in energy density (kcal/g) (Data from Centers for Disease Control, 2011.)

Figure 1–7 shows the different energy densities of a variety of foods.[33] Table 1–12 provides tips on how to lower energy while promoting satiety for weight management.[33]

- ■ Limit Empty Calories

When planning meals, another approach for improving overall dietary intake is to eliminate sources of empty calories. Empty calories come from solid fats and/or added sugars that contribute energy but few or no nutrients to dietary intake. Research has shown that nearly 40% of the calories consumed by US children aged 2–18 years come from empty calories, with sugar-sweetened beverages contributing 10% of all total energy. Most of these empty calories are provided by six sources: soda, fruit drinks, dairy desserts, grain desserts, pizza, and whole milk. (Table 1–13).[34]

Those who want to reduce overall caloric intake to promote weight loss or weight maintenance should be encouraged to eat—not drink— their calories. There are data indicating that calories from beverages

Table 1–12. Tips for lowering energy density.

Prepare fruits, vegetables, and other foods without added fat and sugar
Add vegetables to main dishes such as omelets, lasagna, pizza, chili, soups, and other hot dishes
Choose meats and cheese that are lower in fat or reduced fat
Eat an appetizer low in energy density such as a 100-calorie serving of soup or a green salad
Keep energy-dense snacks such as fruits and vegetables close at hand
Quench thirst with water and other low or no-calorie beverages

Data from Centers for Disease Control, 2011.

Table 1-13. Half of empty calories consumed by kids aged 2-18 years come from just six sources.

Soda
Fruit drinks
Dairy desserts
Grain desserts
Pizza
Whole milk

Data from Reedy and Krebs-Smith, 2010.

consumed with a meal add overall energy intake to the meal, without necessarily affecting the feelings of satiety.[35] In other words, you consume calories from sweetened beverages that your body does not necessarily register in the same way that it does calories from solid foods. Elimination of sugar-sweetened beverages is a first-line approach to cutting out excess or empty calories. Other positive changes that can be made involve swapping foods with few or no empty calories for those that contain greater quantities of empty calories. Table 1–14 provides examples of foods with empty calories and those with few or no empty calories. There is certainly room for some—although not a lot—of empty calories in a well-balanced diet. The USDA recommends that an adult

Table 1-14. Foods with some empty calories compared to those with few or no empty calories.

Foods Containing Some Empty Calories	Foods Containing Few or No Empty Calories
Sweetened applesauce—contains added sugars	Unsweetened applesauce
Regular ground beef (25% fat/75% lean)—contains solid fats	Extra lean ground beef (5% fat/95% lean)
Fried chicken—contains solid fats from frying and skin	Baked skinless chicken breast
Sugar-sweetened cereals—contain added sugars	Unsweetened cereals or unsweetened oatmeal
Whole milk—contains solid fats	Fat-free (skim or nonfat) milk

Data from US Department of Agriculture.

following a 2000-calorie diet limit his empty calories (also referred to as discretionary calories) to no more than 260 empty calories per day. For those who want to include dessert, additional fats, or alcohol in their daily diet, tracking and documenting these empty calories and conscientiously limiting them to roughly 250 calories per day is wise. Examples of 250 calories worth of empty calories include one cup of ice cream, 10 ounces of wine, or 2½ tablespoons of butter. Those who eat out at restaurants frequently may find it more difficult to control and minimize empty or discretionary calorie intake than those who eat at home. Preparing food at home gives you ultimate control over the amount of empty calories that you choose to add to your meals and snacks. This is especially true when compared to eating out, which are situations when those choices are made for you, and will almost always result in caloric intake of foods and ingredients that will easily surpass the 250 discretionary calorie budget. Those who are not regularly engaging in physical activity are encouraged to be the most vigilant and mindful about empty calories, as they do not have the benefit of energy expenditure working to help counteract this unnecessary energy source. Table 1–15

Table 1–15. Empty calories: how many can I have?

Age and Gender	Estimated Calories for Those Who Are Not Physically Active	
	Total Daily Calorie Needs	Daily Limit for Empty Calories
Children 2–3 years	1000 calories	135
Children 4–8 years	1200–1400 calories	120
Girls 9–13 years	1600 calories	120
Boys 9–13 years	1800 calories	160
Girls 14–18 years	1800 calories	160
Boys 14–18 years	2200 calories	265
Females 19–30 years	2000 calories	260
Males 19–30 years	2400 calories	330
Females 31–50 years	1800 calories	160
Males 31–50 years	2200 calories	265
Females 51+ years	1600 calories	120
Males 51+ years	2000 calories	260

Data from US Department of Agriculture.

contains the USDA recommendations for maximum empty calories for different calorie levels of varying age and gender groups of physically inactive people.

Meal Planning and Tracking Tools and Guides

Prior to the digital ages, individual meal planning was a tedious task fraught with pencils, paper, graphs, and charts. Adding up calories, calculating nutrients, and portioning food servings were time-consuming tasks, which often resulted in bland meal plans that were more mathematically inspired than culinary derived. With the proliferation of the internet, the era of powerful web-based meal planning tools has arrived. Inventive meal planning websites easily calculate, track, and create meal, and snack patterns to meet a host of lifestyles and palate preferences.

■ Self-Monitoring

Patients and clients are increasingly involved in electronically documenting and tracking many aspects of their own lives, healthcare, and diet. By one estimate, 60% of adults in the United States are currently tracking their weight, diet, or exercise routine. One-third of American adults track some other health indicator or symptom such as blood pressure, sleep patterns, or blood sugar.[36] Self-monitoring is an important aspect of successful weight loss and weight maintenance.[37,38] The following contains a list of helpful web-based tools for meal planning as well as diet and exercise tracking.

ChooseMyPlate SuperTracker

SuperTracker is the USDA and ChooseMyPlate.gov's accompanying meal planning and tracking program. It is a no-cost web-based program that helps plan, analyze, and track diet and physical activity. Patients may use the program to set personal calorie goals, and with an extensive database of more than 8000 foods and beverages, compare the nutritional content of foods side by side. SuperTracker is available at: https://www.supertracker.usda.gov/.

ChooseMyPlate for Moms

The USDA's ChooseMyPlate.gov website has a separate section called "Health & Nutrition Information for Pregnant & Breastfeeding Women." Pregnant women can enter their information to generate a personalized meal plan during the various stages of pregnancy and breastfeeding. The site is available at: www.choosemyplate.gov/pregnancy-breastfeeding.html.

USDA Nutrient Database

The USDA Nutrient Database is a useful tool for those who may want to do their own individual menu planning or who are looking for reliable nutrition information for foods that do not feature a Nutrition Facts panel (eg, fresh fruits and vegetables, various types of meat, fish, and poultry). The USDA National Nutrient Database for Standard Reference has nutrient information for over 8000 foods and is available at: http://ndb.nal.usda.gov/.

NIH Menu Planner

The National Heart, Lung and Blood Institute Menus and Menu Planner website has a variety of reduced-calorie menus available at: http://www.nhlbi.nih.gov/health/public/heart/obesity/lose_wt/sampmenu.htm. The site provides 1200 and 1600 calorie level menus for traditional American, Asian-American, Southern, Mexican-American, and lacto-ovo vegetarian cuisines. You can track food groups, calories, and nutrients consumed from foods at the NHLBI's Interactive Menu Planner page at: http://hp2010.nhlbihin.net/menuplanner/menu.cgi.

Nutrihand

Nutrihand is an interactive menu planning and tracking program used by healthcare professionals to help patients and clients plan meals and meat nutrition and exercise goals. The program is subscription-based and can be built into your practice or clinic's existing website to help establish a personalized approach to health management and meal planning. Nutrihand is accessible at: http://www.nutrihand.com.

■ Additional Web-based Tools

FDA—Raw Fruits Poster, Nutrition Facts: http://www.fda.gov/Food/GuidanceRegulation/GuidanceDocumentsRegulatoryInformation/LabelingNutrition/ucm063482.htm

FDA—Raw Vegetables Poster, Nutrition Facts: http://www.fda.gov/Food/IngredientsPackagingLabeling/LabelingNutrition/FoodLabelingGuidanceRegulatoryInformation/InformationforRestaurantsRetailEstablishments/ucm114222.htm

FDA—Cooked Seafood (Purchased Raw), Nutrition Facts: http://www.fda.gov/Food/IngredientsPackagingLabeling/LabelingNutrition/FoodLabelingGuidanceRegulatoryInformation/InformationforRestaurantsRetailEstablishments/ucm114223.htm

NHLBI—Portion Distortion Information and Quiz: http://hp2010.nhlbihin.net/portion/

USDA SNAP-ED Recipe Finder: http://recipefinder.nal.usda.gov/

USDA Ground Beef Calculator: http://ndb.nal.usda.gov/ndb/beef/show

NHLBI Deliciously Healthy Eating Recipes: http://hp2010.nhlbihin.net/healthyeating/Default.aspx?AspxAutoDetectCookieSupport=1

USDA—What's in Season? (Fruits and Vegetables): http://healthymeals.nal.usda.gov/features-month/whats-season

NHLBI—Lower-Calorie, Lower Fat Alternative Foods: http://www.nhlbi.nih.gov/health/public/heart/obesity/lose_wt/lcal_fat.htm

NHLBI—Your Guide to Lowering Your Blood Pressure with DASH (also see Chapter 5 for more DASH diet information): http://www.nhlbi.nih.gov/health/public/heart/hbp/dash/index.htm

Fruits & Veggies More Matters—Healthy Meal Planning: http://www.fruitsandveggiesmorematters.org/healthy-meal-planning-with-fruits-and-vegetables

MedlinePlus—Diabetes and Meal Planning Interactive Tutorial: http://www.nlm.nih.gov/medlineplus/tutorials/diabetesmealplanning/htm/index.htm

American Diabetes Association—MyFoodAdvisor (also see Chapter 6 for more diabetes meal planning information): http://tracker.diabetes.org/

Weight Control Information Network–Just Enough for You (About Food Portions): http://win.niddk.nih.gov/publications/just_enough.htm

DHHS—A Healthier You Healthy Shopping List: http://www.health.gov/dietaryguidelines/dga2005/healthieryou/html/shopping_list.html

NHLBI—Shopping Tips: http://www.nhlbi.nih.gov/health/public/heart/obesity/lose_wt/shopping.htm

References

1. Hargrove J. History of the calorie in nutrition. J Nutr 2006;136(12): 2957–2961.

2. Atwater W. Principles of Nutrition and Nutritive Value of Food. No. 142, US Department of Agriculture, Farmers' Bulletin 1902.

3. Hunt C. Food for Young Children. No. 717, US Department of Agriculture, Farmers' Bulletin 1916.

4. Hunt C, Atwater H. How to Select Foods. No. 808, US Department of Agriculture, Farmer's Bulletin 1917.

5. Davis C, Saltos E. Dietary recomenndations and how they have changed over time. 1999. In: Frazao E. America's Eating Habits: Changes and Consequences. US Department of Agriculture. Vols. AIB-750, p. 35.

6. US Senate. Dietary Goals for the United States. 2nd ed. Select Committee on Nutrition and Human Needs 1977.

7. Truong K, Sturm R. Weight gain trends across sociodemographic groups in the United States. Am J Public Health 2005;95(9):1602–1606.

8. Britten P, Haven J, Davis C. Consumer research for development of educational messages for the mypyramid food guidance system. J Nutr Educ Behav 2006;38:S108–S123.

9. US Department of Agriculture. ChooseMyPlate.gov. June 2011. Retrieved from: MyPlate Information for Health Care Professionals January 2, 2013. http://www.choosemyplate.gov/information-healthcare-professionals.html

10. US Department of Agriculture. (n.d.). ChooseMyPlate.gov. Retrieved January 2, 2012, from Dairy: What Counts as a Cup in the Dairy Group: http://www.choosemyplate.gov/food-groups/dairy-counts.html; US Department of Agriculture. (n.d.). ChooseMyPlate.gov. Retrieved January 2, 2013, from Grains—How Many Grain Foods are Needed: http://www.choosemyplate.gov/food-groups/grains_amount_table.html; US Department of Agriculture. (n.d.). ChooseMyPlate.gov. Retrieved

January 2, 2013, from Fruits—What Foods are in the Fruit Group?: http://www.choosemyplate.gov/food-groups/fruits.html; US Department of Agriculture. (n.d.). ChooseMyPlate.gov. Retrieved January 2, 2013, from What are Empty Calories?: http://www.choosemyplate.gov/weight-management-calories/calories/empty-calories.html; US Department of Agriculture. (n.d.). ChooseMyPlate.gov. Retrieved January 2, 2013, from Protein Foods—What Counts as an Ounce Equivalent in the Protein Foods Group?: http://www.choosemyplate.gov/food-groups/protein-foods-counts.html; US Department of Agriculture. (n.d.). ChooseMyPlate. Gov. Retrieved January 2, 2013, from Empty Calories: How Many Can I have: http://www.choosemyplate.gov/weight-management-calories/calories/empty-calories-amount.html; US Department of Agriculture. (June, 2011). ChooseMyPlate.gov. Retrieved January 2, 2013, from MyPlate Information for Health Care Professionals: http://www.choosemyplate.gov/information-healthcare-professionals.html; US Department of Agriculture. (June, 2011). ChooseMyPlate.gov. Retrieved January 2, 2013, from 10 Tips Nutrition Series—Liven up your meals with vegetables and fruits: http://www.choosemyplate.gov/healthy-eating-tips/ten-tips.html; US Department of Agriculture. (January 31, 2011). Dietary Guidelines for Americans, 2010. Retrieved January 2, 2013, from USDA Press Release: http://www.cnpp.usda.gov/dgas2010-policydocument.htm; US Department of Agriculture. (July 5, 2012). Economic Research Service. Retrieved January 2, 2013, from Food Dollar Series: http://www.ers.usda.gov/data-products/food-dollar-series.aspx

11. US Department of Health and Human Services. Healthy people. December 2, 2010. Retrieved from: Nutrition and Weight Status Objectives January 2, 2013. http://www.healthypeople.gov/2020/topicsobjectives2020/objectiveslist.aspx?topicId=29

12. US Food and Drug Administration. Guidance for industry: a food labeling guide. May 23, 2011. Retrieved from: 14. Appendix F: Calculate the Percent Daily Value for the Appropriate Nutrients January 2, 2013. http://www.fda.gov/Food/GuidanceComplianceRegulatoryInformation/GuidanceDocuments/FoodLabelingNutrition/FoodLabelingGuide/ucm064928.htm

13. Whole Grains Council. (n.d.). Whole grains 101. Retrieved from: Whole Grains A to Z January 2, 2013. http://www.wholegrainscouncil.org/whole-grains-101/whole-grains-a-to-z

14. National Digestive Diseases Information Clearinghouse. Lactose intolerance. April 23, 2012. Retrieved from: Digestive Diseases A-Z List of Toipcs and Titles January 31, 2013. http://www.digestive.niddk.nih.gov/ddiseases/pubs/lactoseintolerance/#risk

15. Bray G, Nielsen S, Popkin B. Consumption of high-fructose corn syrup in beverages may play a role in the epidemic of obesity. Am J Clin Nutr 2004;79:537–543.

16. Academy of Nutrition and Dietetics. How effective (in terms of client adherence and weight and loss maintenance) is a regular meal and snack pattern? 2005. Retrieved from: Evidence Analysis Library. http://www.andevidencelibrary.com

17. Bernstein M, Tucker K, Ryan N, O'Neill E, Clements K, Nelson M, et al. Higher dietary variety is associated with better nutritional status in frail elderly people. J Am Diet Assoc 2002;102(8):1096–1104.

18. US Department of Agriculture. ChooseMyPlate.gov. June 2011. Retrieved from: 10 Tips Nutrition Series—Liven Up Your Meals with Vegetables and Fruits January 2, 2013. http://www.choosemyplate.gov/healthy-eating-tips/ten-tips.html

19. Lin B, Frazao E, Guthrie J. Away-from-home foods increasingly important to quality of American diet. 1999. Agriculture Information Bulletin (749).

20. US Department of Agriculture. Economic research service. July 5, 2012. Retrieved from: Food Dollar Series January 2, 2013. http://www.ers.usda .gov/data-products/food-dollar-series.aspx

21. Centers for Disease Control. Physical activity trends—US, 1990-1990. MMWR Morb Mortal Wkly Rep 2001;50:16–169.

22. Young L, Nestle M. Reducing portion sizes to prevent obesity—a call to action. Am J Prev Med 2012;43(5):565–568.

23. Associated Press. McDonald's phasing out supersize fries, drinks. March 3, 2004. Retrieved from: NBCNews.com January 31, 2013. http://www .nbcnews.com/id/4433307/ns/business-us_business/t/mcdonalds-phasing-out-supersize-fries-drinks/#.UQsqKOhYvFE

24. Kral T, Rolls B. Energy density and portion size: their independent and combined effects on energy intake. Physiol Behav 2004;82:131–138.

25. Drewnowski A. Obesity and the food environment: dietary energy density and diet costs. Am J Prev Med 2004;27 (suppl 3):154–162.

26. Rolls B. Plenary Lecture 1 Dietary strategies for the prevention and treatment of obesity. Proc Nutr Soc 2010;69(1):70–79.

27. Rolls B, Castellanos V, Halford J, Kilara A, Panyam D, Pelkman C, et al. Volume of food consumed affects satiety in men. Am J Clin Nutr 1998;67:1170–1177.

28. Kissileff H, Gruss L, Thornton J, Jordan H. The satiating efficiency of foods. Physiol Behav 1984;32(2):319–332.

29. Himaya A, Louis-Sylvestre J. The effect of soup on satiation. Appetite 1998;30:199–210.

30. Rolls BF, Guthrie J, Laster L. Effects of temperature and mode of presentation of juice on hunger, thirst and food intake in humans. Appetite 1990;15(3):199–208.

31. Flood J, Rolls B. Soup preloads in a variety of forms reduce meal energy intake. Appetite 2007;49:626–634.

32. Rolls BJ, Bell EA, Thorwart ML. Water incorporated into a food but not served with a food decreases energy intake in lean women. Am J Clin Nutr 1999;70:448–455.

33. Centers for Disease Control. Resources for health professionals. March 11, 2011. Retrieved from: Low-Energy-Dense Foods and Weight Management: Cutting Calories While Controlling Hunger January 2, 2013. http://www .cdc.gov/nutrition/professionals/researchtopractice/index.html

34. Reedy J, Krebs-Smith S. Dietary sources of energy, solid fats, and added sugars among children and adolescents in the United States. J Am Diet Assoc 2010;110(10):1477–1484.

35. DellaValle D, Roe L, Rolls B. Does the consumption of caloric and non-caloric beverages with a meal affect energy intake. Appetite 2005;44(2): 187–193.

36. University of California, San Francisco. UCSF news center. October 5, 2012. Retrieved from: Self-Tracking May Become Key Element of Personalized Medicine January 2, 2012. http://www.ucsf.edu/news/2012/10/12913/self-tracking-may-become-key-element-personalized-medicine

37. Butryn M, Phelan S, Hill J, Wing R. Consistent self-monitoring of weight: a key component of successful weight loss maintenance. Obesity 2007;15(12):3091–3096.

38. Wing R, Phelan S. Long-term weight loss maintenance. Am J Clin Nutr 2005;82(suppl 1):222S–225S.

2

Face-to-Face: Nutrition Screening, Assessment, and Counseling Techniques

Introduction to Nutrition Assessment and Counseling

Preparing yourself to address someone else's eating habits can be a daunting task. As a practitioner and student of medicine, you likely acknowledge and understand the relationship between diet and disease; however, translating this knowledge into practical applications and making meaningful nutrition recommendations for patients and clients presents a real challenge that unfortunately too few practitioners are willing to undertake. This chapter will help you identify nutrition-related health issues, assess an individual's nutrition status, and design meaningful interventions to help your patients and clients achieve their maximum health potential using food and nutrition.

▪ Incorporating Nutrition in Primary Care

The way we eat is highly complex and personal. From the outset, choosing certain foods, and not choosing others, may seem like a mundane part of our daily routine. But, in reality, the food choices we make today shape our health outcomes of tomorrow. In the US, the leading causes of preventable death are smoking, high blood pressure, and obesity. Together, these three causes, all which are modifiable, account for over one million premature deaths each year. According to one analysis, obesity alone has been found to be the cause of 216,000 annual premature deaths in the United States.[1] Obesity statistics are, by their very nature, ominous. But, take a look at that last statistic a little more closely: nearly *one quarter of a million people* in the United States die unnecessarily each year because of their weight status. And because weight status is so heavily affected by food intake, understanding and promoting good nutrition is tantamount to preventing early death. What, then, is the role that primary care practitioners should play in this arena? The answer—like most things related to "good nutrition"—is not simple.

The dearth of nutrition education in medical and primary care curricula is well established and is certainly lamentable. Only 25% of accredited medical schools in the United States offer their students a dedicated nutrition class. And only 27% of those institutions meet the minimum 25 hours of nutrition education recommended by the National Academy of Sciences. Despite the public's increasing interest in nutrition and society's coincident and ironically spiking obesity rates, these medical nutrition education numbers are actually on the decline.[2] As the general population grows, the more we need practitioners educated in nutrition, the less likely we are to be actually getting them. With approximately two-thirds of the American adult population being overweight or obese, and the majority of our primary care providers having never taken a nutrition course, the gaping knowledge deficit about diet and disease becomes more pronounced. One analysis of more than 10,000 patient visits found that the odds of receiving counseling for diet and nutrition, exercise, or weight loss from a physician actually declined by 22% from the period of 1995/1996 to 2001/2002.[3]

Why do primary care practitioners shy away from educating patients about the relationship between their food choices and health status? There are a myriad of reasons, or perhaps excuses in today's healthcare environment. Among them, time constraints, scarcity of training resources, lack of reimbursement for nutrition counseling, questionable nutrition intervention studies, patient noncompliance, and even practitioners' own weight insecurities may all contribute. Recall the story of Dr. Terry Bennett in New Hampshire, whose patient filed a complaint with the state Board of Medicine after he told her she was obese and that it was hurting her health.[4] Even fear of litigation can limit one's willingness to talk about weight.

But it turns out that even talking about weight can jumpstart positive behaviors. One recent study looked at the effect on overweight and obese people of being told by a physician that they were overweight. Those who were overweight (BMI of 25 or greater) or obese (BMI of 30 or greater) had an increased likelihood to have attempted to lose weight in the previous year, if their doctor had told them that they were overweight. The problem was, only 45.2% of individuals with a BMI of 25 or greater and 66.4% of those with a BMI of 30 or greater reported being told by a physician that they were overweight.[5] Without making light, we are essentially ignoring the elephant in the room.

Perhaps, above all of these reasons, it is a lack of confidence in nutrition counseling techniques that is the most likely culprit paralyzing even the best of practitioners' intentions. In one survey of over 500 American physicians, 36% said they were knowledgeable about weight management techniques, but only 3% were confident that those counseling techniques succeed in their practice.[6] And it's not just American primary care providers (PCPs). In Canada, 82.3% of physicians surveyed in one study reported their formal nutrition training in medical school to be inadequate, and nearly all of those physicians surveyed identified a lack of time and compensation as the largest barriers to providing nutrition guidance.[7] European healthcare professionals do not fare well either, with numerous studies concluding that knowledge about the prevention and treatment of malnutrition is poor.[8-10]

There are less data regarding the nutrition education and nutrition counseling competency of advanced practice nurses. Of the top ten Family Nurse Practitioner and top 16 Adult Nurse Practitioner graduate school programs ranked by US News & World Report in 2011, only

1 of the 16 different schools offers a stand-alone nutrition course.[11] While nutrition is no doubt included as part of other classes within the advanced practice nursing curriculum, the inattention to the importance of directly addressing nutrition-related concerns and the system-wide lack of development of nutrition counseling skills for practitioners are concerning. The problem is not limited to advanced practice nurses, as all PCPs are likely undertrained with regards to addressing nutrition- and weight-related problems. And these limitations also spill over into the territory of herbal and dietary supplements.

Patients and clients are increasingly turning to the use of and asking about the effectiveness and safety of dietary supplements and herbal remedies. One recent study analyzed physicians', APNs', pharmacists', and dietitians' knowledge, attitudes, and practices of herbs and other dietary supplements. The average score on knowledge was 10 out of 20 points, confidence was 4 out of 10 possible points, and average communication score was 1.4 out of 4 possible points.[12] Essentially, we are about halfway there when it comes to knowing what we need to know for safe and effective implementation of these nontraditional therapies. (See Chapter 12 for more information about nutrition as a complementary and alternative medicine and therapy.)

In today's healthcare environment, practitioners do not have the luxury of spending a leisurely hour or two with each patient, carefully combing through their food intake patterns and gently broaching the topics of weight, nutrition, and health. Our breakneck pace requires multitasking, prioritizing, and triaging. When it comes to talking nutrition, our modus operandi is more likely to be *reactive* than it is *proactive*. Think about a single mother who brings her sick infant along with his healthy older brother to a clinic appointment. The mom is concerned about her baby getting better, and she is not likely to focus on her sedentary, video-game playing, overweight school-age son with prediabetes and high blood pressure who happens to be munching on potato chips while in the clinic.

It is understandable that not every patient encounter presents an appropriate time to discuss nutrition; however, practitioners can learn to recognize nutrition-teaching moments, screen for nutrition risk, implement brief assessment tools, and identify and refer to other community nutrition resources that will help those patients who need education, information, and assistance. Increasingly, the majority of our patients need these resources. Ignoring their needs is not a viable option. It is up to the front-line practitioners to make nutrition a priority and to bridge the knowledge gap about diet and disease for our patients and clients.

Determining Nutrition Risk

Before you can work on solving a problem, you must first identify the problem, but only after you determine that a problem even exists. Determining nutritional risk involves examining a host of factors that may be negatively impacting nutrition status. While inadequate nutrient intake is the likeliest cause of unbalanced nutritional health, practitioners must consider a number of possible underlying contributors that may be precipitating poor dietary intake. To effectively paint a patient's nutrition picture, the practitioner should ask questions and consider inputs aside from mere food intake. There are other social factors, such as socioeconomic status, lifestyle choices, work patterns, family structures, living environments, co-morbidities, and physical capabilities that all impact food choices. While this list may seem overwhelming, the good news is that you have food on your side. People like to talk about food. No matter what your culture, socioeconomic status, geographic location, or disease state, you must eat in order to live. And because everybody eats, you will always have some common ground upon which to develop rapport as you seek to learn more about your patient's nutrition profile.

Individuals who live and work outside of the healthcare spectrum may be intimidated by many of the constructs that you, an advanced practice nurse, represent: medication, surgery, disease, confusing medical terminology…the list goes on. But talking about food, appetite, diet, and nutrition can be an effective approach for disarming a patient and for developing rapport. While many institutions implement formal nutrition screening protocols, you may also consider the value of and start employing less formal, more conversational approaches to identifying nutrition risk. Use your professional judgment, and if the situation allows, let your patients know you are going to ask them a few questions to learn a little bit about their current health status. Ask some nonjudgmental questions: What time do you get up today? Did you have anything to eat or drink today before you got here? Oh, eggs? I love eggs. How did you prepare your eggs? Where did you purchase that milkshake? Do you always have milkshakes for lunch? You say you skip dinner most days after work, what are your reasons for skipping dinner sometimes on the weekdays? In addition to these medications, what, if any, dietary supplements, vitamins, minerals, or herbs do you regularly take?

After quick and careful questioning, what sounds like casual banter to the patient will actually reveal significant details about nutrition status to you, the practitioner. Table 2–1 contains a list of topics for questions to consider asking patients as you seek to reveal nutrition risk factors in both informal screening and formal assessment environments.[13]

Nutrition Care Process

The Nutrition Care Process (NCP) is the model and framework for the critical thinking process that is used by nutrition and dietetics professionals as they craft their approach to nutrition care. While traditionally used by Registered Dietitians (RDs), the NCP is represented by a simple

Table 2-1. Questions for consideration in determining nutrition risk.

Medical history	Previous surgeries, trauma, and illnesses
Family medical history	Predisposition for genetic conditions, diseases
Anthropometric data	Height, weight, usual weight, weight one year ago, goal weight, last time you were at stated goal weight, waist circumference or pant size, and noticeable differences in how clothes fit
Laboratory data	Blood sugar checks, blood pressure readings, lipid panel, liver function tests, and kidney function tests
Clinical features	Alterations in taste, smell, difficulty chewing or swallowing, skin changes, pressure ulcers, and neuropathy
Gastrointestinal	Constipation, gas, diarrhea, nausea, vomiting, belching, and intolerances to food
Food and cultural Preferences	Food allergies, religious food rules or fasting observance, perceived health of certain foods, and use of dietary supplements
Medication	Doses, types, schedule, consume with or without food, and possible GI upset related to medications
Living environment	Access to food, frequency of food purchases, and presence of food preparation or storage appliances such as hot plate, refrigerator
Physical capabilities	Able to open cans, jars, packages, and travel to stores, engage in physical activity
Food environment	What types of stores shopping at: liquor stores, pharmacies, traditional grocery stores, reliant on others to bring in food, or home delivered meal service
Psychological and cognitive status	Depression, obsessiveness

Data from Academy of Nutrition and Dietetics, 2012; Nelms M and Habash D, 2011.

schematic that is helpful for all disciplines and healthcare professionals who may be involved or participating in the nutrition care of a patient, client, or resident. The NCP contains four steps: Nutrition Assessment, Nutrition Diagnosis, Nutrition Intervention, Monitoring and Evaluation. While the RD on the healthcare team is the most qualified individual to determine the Nutrition Diagnosis, advanced practice nurses often

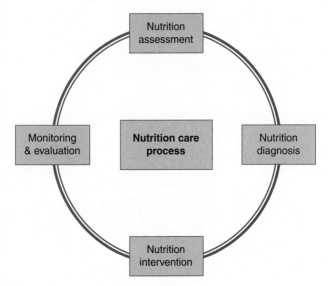

Figure 2-1. The nutrition care process (NCP).

play a vital role in conducting Nutrition Assessment, implementing Nutrition Interventions, and participating in the ongoing Monitoring and Evaluation steps (Figure 2–1).

Nutrition Screening

Nutrition screening is the first step in the larger realm of Nutrition Assessment. The foundation of nutrition contact begins with nutrition screening. Nutrition screening is a process defined as "identifying characteristics known to be associated with nutrition problems with the purpose of identifying individuals who are malnourished or at nutritional risk".[14] The American Society for Parenteral and Enteral Nutrition (ASPEN) states that screening is done "to determine if a detailed nutrition assessment is indicated".[15] While nutrition screening is part of the Nutrition Care Process that is conducted by RDs, the screening component is often implemented by other disciplines, and rightly so. Nutrition screening is integral to comprehensive care in the inpatient, outpatient, clinic, and long-term care settings. In the outpatient environment, practitioners often find themselves screening for nutritional status that is the effect of overnutrition or excessive intake of particular nutrients, which, in most cases, is related to the intake of excessive calories. In the hospital setting, malnutrition may affect between 25% and 50% of the patient population with an even greater number who are likely to be *at risk* for malnutrition.[16-19] Despite the reality that cases of malnutrition certainly exist, we seem to be missing a great deal of them. A number of studies indicate that between one-half to two-thirds of patients with malnutrition, including elderly patients, go unrecognized.[19-21]

Screening provides us with a nutrition snapshot. Just as testing an individual's blood sugar level only tells us what is going on at *that moment*, that blood sugar is still a helpful piece of data as it is indicative of what may be a larger problem at hand. Patients present not as one particular disease state or condition, but as a sum of their parts. Due to the complexity of interconnected disease states, nutrition screening can help practitioners "pick their battles," and screening helps us decide where to start when it comes to food and nutrition education. While it is generally accepted that nutrition screening is an important first step in the care process, there are limited numbers of validated nutrition screening tools available for use in general practice.[22] Effective nutrition screeners are those that can be quickly completed by any member of the healthcare team. In addition to their user friendliness, other characteristics of an effective screener include simplicity, efficiency, reliability, low cost to implement, and low burden to the subject; they should also exhibit acceptable levels of sensitivity, specificity, and both positive and negative predictive values.[14] Figure 2-2 demonstrates how nutrition screening sets the stage for nutrition care in a nutrition care algorithm.[23]

The types of screening tools available, and the way that they are used, vary among institutions. Height and weight are routinely used in nutrition screening, as are questions about recent and historical weight fluctuations. Other screener considerations include questions about diet, such as food allergies and food preferences, and possible difficulties chewing or swallowing. Screeners may also look for alterations in appetite and bowel regularity, and they should consider medical diagnoses and available laboratory data. Screeners may also include age-appropriate questions (eg, teenage nutrition vs. geriatric nutrition) and information about pregnancy, if relevant. It is important to note that while screeners may capture a host of parameters related to nutrition status, only changes in weight and decreased appetite and food intake have been validated as accurate gauges of nutrition status (Table 2-2).[24]

Who is at the highest risk for malnutrition or altered nutrition status? Those who are underweight, who have a history of poor nutrient or energy intake, conditions that promote nutrient loss, hypermetabolic states, alcohol or drug abusers and those of low socioeconomic status, the elderly, and isolated people with minimal access to food. Table 2-3 summarizes who is at high nutrition risk.[25]

When Do You Screen for Nutrition Risk?

The Joint Commission on the Accreditation of Healthcare Organizations (JCAHO) mandates that nutrition screening take place within 24 hours of admission to an acute care center.[26] In the outpatient environment, screening is done upon intake or at first contact.

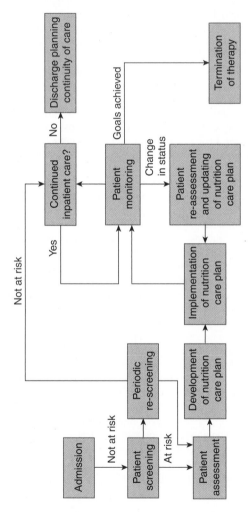

Figure 2-2. Nutrition care algorithm. (Data from Ukleja et al., 2010.)

Table 2-2. Nutrition screener considerations by category.

Anthropometrics	Height, weight, head circumference, and weight fluctuations
Diet	Food preferences, allergies, and changes in appetite
Physiological	Difficulties chewing or swallowing, bowel regularity, nausea, and vomiting
Medical	Medical diagnosis, laboratory data

Screening Using Anthropometric Data

Anthropometry is the study of the measurement of the human body. Anthropometric measurements include metrics such as height, weight, or head circumference. Height is assessed using a stadiometer. Length refers to the measurement of infants and children who are 2 years or younger or those 24–36 months who are not able to stand without assistance, or who measure less than 30 inches while lying down.[27] Growth charts used for children age 0–36 months use recumbent length, whereas stature is used for those age 2–20 years.[28]

Table 2-3. Identifying nutrition risk.

Underweight	**Adults:** BMI <18.5 and recent significant, unintentional weight loss of 5 lbs or 5% in 1 month, 7.5% in 3 months of 10% in 6 months **Pediatrics:** BMI-for-age <5th percentile
Poor intake	Anorexia, food avoidance behavior (eg, psychiatric condition) or those who have been NPO for a period of 5 days or more
Nutrient loss	From malabsorption, bariatric surgery, enteric fistulas, renal dialysis, wounds, burns, vomiting, and diarrhea
Hypermetabolic states	Trauma, sepsis, fever, and burns
Abuse	Alcohol abuse, drug abuse or medications with antinutrient or catabolic properties (eg, steroids, antimetabolites such as methotrexate), immunosuppressants, and antitumor agents
Social situation	Elderly (eg, 80 years or older), isolated living conditions, low income, or depression

Data from Heimburger, 2012 and Academy of Nutrition and Dietetics, 2012.

- ## BMI and Body Weight

For screening purposes, weight and body mass index (BMI) are the two most important indicators of nutrition status.[29] Scales that are used for obtaining body weight should be calibrated regularly. An individual's BMI determines his or her weight category. BMI is measured in kg/m², and a BMI of <18.5 is classified as underweight, 18.5–24.9 is normal or healthy weight, 25–29.9 is overweight and >30 is obese. There are limitations to using the BMI; most notably that it does not make accommodations for differences in gender, age, body type, disease state, or race/ethnicity. Note that BMI is not a direct measure of lean body mass or body fat mass. In fact, BMI is thought to overestimate fat in athletes who have a muscular build, and it is also likely to underestimate body fat in elderly who may have lost muscle mass.[30] Despite these limitations, BMI is commonly used as the default measurement for linking weight and health in practice, policy, and research because it is easy to calculate. It is also cheap, as obtaining height and weight requires minimal equipment and training (Table 2–4).

- ## Other Equations and Measurements

Although body weight is the most notable metric used to link anthropometrics and health, there are other measurements that are useful in assessing nutrition status. Mid upper arm circumference (MUAC) measured in centimeters, triceps skinfold thickness (TSF) measured in millimeters, and arm muscle circumference (AMC) in centimeters are used in screening and assessment. Skinfold thickness is a helpful indicator for estimating body fat stores, since approximately half of body fat is stored in the subcutaneous region. A triceps skinfold thickness of less than 3 mm indicates nearly complete exhaustion of fat stores.[25] Midarm muscle circumferences (MAMC) can also be obtained, and this equation incorporates TSF measurements.

MAMC is: MAMC (cm) = midarm circumference (cm) − [0.314 x TSF (mm)]

Table 2–4. BMI weight categories for adults.

BMI (kg/m²)	Weight Category
Underweight	<18.5
Normal	18.5–24.9
Overweight	25–29.9
Obesity	30.0–34.9 (Obesity Class I)
	35–39.9 (Obesity Class II)
	40+ (Extreme Obesity, Morbid Obesity, or Obesity Class III)

Table 2–5 outlines the relationship between triceps skinfold thickness levels and calorie reserves in men and women.[31]

Obtaining accurate measurements requires proper measurement techniques. The CDC's National Health and Nutrition Examination Survey (NHANES) website has a series of videos on obtaining anthropometric measurements available at: http://www.cdc.gov/nchs/nhanes/nhanes3/anthropometric_videos.htm. If body weight is not available or cannot be obtained, there are equations that can be used to estimate body weight from a combination of other anthropometric measurements such as knee height (KH), MAC, calf circumference (CC), and subscapular skinfold thickness (SSF) (Table 2–6).[32]

Table 2–5. Triceps skinfold measurements and MAMC in adults.

Reference Value (%)	Males (mm)	Females (mm)	Nutrition Status
Triceps skinfold thickness			
100	12.5	16.5	
90	11	15	
80	10	13	Reflects adequate nutrition status
70	9	11.5	
60	7.5	10	
50	6	8	
40	5	6.5	Reflects moderately depleted/borderline nutrition status
30	4	5	
20	2.5	3	Severely depleted
Midarm muscle circumference			
100	25.5	23	
90	23	21	Reflects adequate nutrition status
80	20	18.5	
70	18	16	Reflects moderately depleted/borderline
60	15	14	
50	12.5	11.5	Severely depleted
40	10	9	

Data from Heimburger, 2006.

Table 2-6. Anthropometric measures for estimating body weight (for use in persons 65 years or older).

Equation	Standard Error of the Estimate
Females	
Weight = (MAC × 1.63) + (CC × 1.43) − 37.46	±4.96 kg
Weight = (MAC × 0.92) + (CC × 1.50) + (SSF × 0.42) − 26.19	±4.21 kg
Weight = (MAC × 0.98) + (CC × 1.27) + (SSF × 0.40)	±3.80 kg
Males	
Weight = (MAC × 2.31) + (CC × 1.50) − 50.10	±5.37 kg
Weight = (MAC × 1.92) + (CC × 1.44) + (SSF X 0.26) − 39.97	±5.34 kg
Weight = (MAC × 1.73) + (CC × 0.98) + (SSF × 0.37) + (KH × 1.16) − 81.69	±4.48 kg

Data from Chumlea et al., 1988.

■ Ideal Body Weight

Once you have braved the waters of broaching the topic of weight and health, patients will likely challenge your assertions with, "Alright then, how much *should* I weigh?" In other words, "What is my *ideal* body weight?" The hair on the back of your neck should be standing up, as right off the bat, the use of the word "ideal" when discussing body weight is controversial. Ideal body weight estimations simply cannot accommodate all of the variations that make up who we are and what impacts our weight status: genetics, age, race, gender, activity level, disease state, time of the day, week, month, etc. It is not realistic to think we are inspiring our clientele by urging them to work toward an unattainable and rather arbitrarily set "ideal" weight. When a 300-pound person visits your office, it does you or him no good to report that his "ideal" weight is half of what he currently weighs! A more enlightened approach would be to discuss a "healthy" weight, linking the relationship between his weight and health.

As a healthcare provider, you are acutely aware of the link between health and weight. Just as a patient who is a quantum physicist would not expect you to understand the Quantum Theory, you should not automatically assume that your patients know that their weight affects their health. You may find that many patients are actually surprised to learn that type 2 diabetes does not "have" to run in their family, and that improvements in diet and lifestyle *can* lower blood pressure as effectively as medication. Sometimes the greatest thing you can do for your patients is to get them thinking about the role that diet plays on health, perhaps nudging their movement from the precontemplation to the contemplation stage of change, part of a behavior change model discussed later in this chapter.

Despite the limitations of the BMI, it does do one thing pretty well: predict early mortality in outlying BMI values. While health and nutrition professionals may dither about the degree to which weight affects health, it is well established that high weight for height and very low weight for height increase the risk of early mortality.[33-35] However, most of our patients are *not* at the very high or very low extremes of the BMI spectrum. They fall somewhere in the middle, and in general practice, more often closer to the high end. And because excess fatness does increase the risk for a cascade of chronic diseases, gradual weight loss toward a healthy body weight is advisable for most overweight and obese people. (At least it's never been shown to be a harmful approach!)

With the understanding that there is no "right" weight for every person, use of ideal or healthy body weights still does have a limited place in clinical practice. Ideal body weight (IBW) can be quickly and easily determined using the Hamwi equation. In females, the Hamwi equation allows 100 pounds for 5 feet of height with an additional 5 pounds for every inch over 5 feet. In males, it is 106 pounds for 5 feet of height with an additional 6 pounds for every inch over 5 feet of height. In this way, IBW for a 5'8" female is 140 pounds [100 + (8 × 5)], and for a 5'8" male, the IBW is 154 pounds [106 + (8 × 6)].

An accommodation factor of ±10% is added to the IBW equation in order to produce an ideal body weight range (IBWR). For the 5'8" (68") female, her IBWR is 126–154 pounds (140 ± 10%) and for the 5'8" (68") male, his IBWR is 139–169 pounds (154 ± 10%). Although it lacks scientific reference, when estimating IBW for individuals under 5 feet of height, some practitioners adjust this equation and subtract 2.5 pounds for every inch under 5 feet in females or 3 pounds for every inch under 5 feet in males. Other adjustments include subtracting 5–10% from IBW in paraplegics and 10–15% from IBW in quadriplegics (Table 2–7).[36]

One way in which the IBW equation is useful is in broaching the topics of weight gain or weight loss. It is generally accepted in nutrition

Table 2-7. Determining ideal body weight (IBW) using the Hamwi equation.

Females	Males
100 pounds for 5 feet of height + 5 pounds for every inch over 5 feet	106 pounds for 5 feet of height + 6 pounds for every inch over 5 feet
If under 5 feet of height subtract 2.5 pounds for every inch under 5 feet	If under 5 feet of height subtract 3 pounds for every inch under 5 feet
Paraplegic	**Quadriplegic**
Subtract 5–10% from IBW	Subtract 10–15% from IBW

Table 2–8. Underweight and significant weight change criteria.

Underweight using BMI	
BMI <18.5 indicates underweight	
Significant weight loss using % UBW	
Time Period	% Weight Change
>2% weight loss	In 1 week
>5% weight loss	In 1 month
>7.5% weight loss	In 3 months
>10% weight loss	In 6 months

Data from Academy of Nutrition and Dietetics, 2012.

practice that individuals who are at or above 125% of their IBW would benefit from weight loss and those who are 85% or below their IBW are underweight and would benefit from weight gain. As with all weight-related issues, there are exceptions to these rules, but they are presented as a general rule of thumb to help initiate discussions about weight using objective measurements related to the calculated IBW.

Questioning about weight status and weight history is also useful as it sheds light on recent or habitual food intake. Calculating percent of usual body weight (UBW) aids in determining whether percent body weight loss or gain is significant or not. To determine percent of usual body weight, use the equation: %UBW = (actual weight ÷ usual weight) × 100. Significant weight loss is defined as loss of >2% in 1 week, >5% in 1 month, >7.5% in 3 months, or >10% in 6 months.[13] In addition to significant weight change, a BMI of <18.5 meets criteria for underweight and warrants further nutrition assessment (Table 2–8).[13]

There is no shortage of reasons why an individual may be underweight or have sustained recent and significant weight loss. Underconsumption of energy (calories), overexertion of activity, malabsorptive diseases, previously unresolved malnutrition, metabolic aberrations, and emotional stressors or mental illness may all contribute to unintentional weight loss.[13] Practitioners can help identify contributing factors by questioning the patient and family members, reviewing the medical history, and analyzing recent dietary intake patterns.

Screening Based on Recent Dietary Intake

Measuring dietary intake is perhaps the most commonly used approach for the indirect measurement of nutrition status. Dietary assessment and nutrient analysis tools range from simple to the complex. Among the most commonly used dietary intake screening tools is the 24-hour recall.[28] Using this tool, a well-trained interviewer is able to quickly elicit important nutrition and health data based on food and beverage intake patterns. In the 24-hour recall method, respondents are questioned in detail regarding all foods and drinks consumed in the preceding 24 hours. Information about food preparation methods, portion sizes, location of eating events, and even emotions and feelings associated with the intake may be included. Figure 2–3 shows a sample 24-hour food recall form.

For national-level surveys, including What We Eat in America—the dietary interview component of the National Health and Nutrition Examination Survey (NHANES), the USDA employs the automated

24-Hour Food Recall Form

Write in all food & beverage consumed over a 24-hour period

Your Name: _____   Date that food was recorded: _____

Time	Food or beverage	Amount eaten

Figure 2–3. Sample 24-hour recall form.

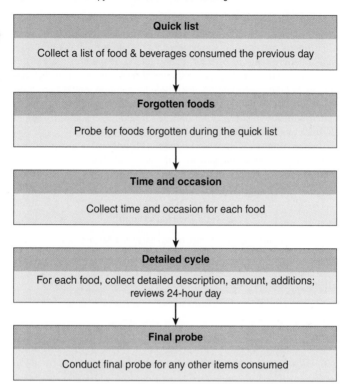

Figure 2-4. USDA automated multiple-pass method for 24-hour dietary recalls.

multiple-pass method (AMPM) for collecting 24-hour dietary recalls. AMPM is a computerized method that is administered by an interviewer and conducted either in person or by telephone.[37] This method is designed to enhance the quality of dietary recall data and makes use of a validated five-step approach that is frequently adapted for use in other healthcare environments.[38] Figure 2–4 outlines the five steps in the multiple-pass approach.

Other rapid dietary intake tools include food records or food diaries. These are kept by the respondent and brought to the practitioner for review. Practitioners may request that a new patient or client fill out a food record or food diary for a set number of days and bring the completed record(s) to the first appointment. While any variation of total days of food records can be requested (eg, 1, 3, or 5 days), it may be helpful to start by requesting 3 days of intake record-keeping: two weekdays and one weekend day, based on the assumption that individual food and beverage intake on the weekends may be quite different from that of the weekdays. Once the completed records have been received, the practitioner reviews the intake and then calculates to identify areas of possible over- or undernutrition. Even without detailed data analysis, a quick review of a client's 3-day food record can be very telling, and can set the stage for conversation regarding diet. Does the patient regularly skip meals? Why are all of the foods on the record brown or white in color? Are the majority of meals coming from a fast food outlet? Are the stated portion sizes realistic and reflective of actual intake? Food records do not tell the whole story, but they certainly can help establish a starting point with regards to the status of an individual's current intake.

There are limitations to self-kept records, including under-reporting in areas such as binge-eating and alcohol consumption or over-reporting of foods perceived to be healthy.[28] Due to time constraints in the initial screening period, brief dietary intake assessment methods such as the 24-hour dietary recall or brief questioning about diet history are preferred over more thorough and lengthy methods. More detailed methods of obtaining dietary intake are covered later in the chapter under Assessment.

Screening with Biochemical Tests

There is no single laboratory test that will accurately detect "malnutrition." Rather, practitioners should utilize a host of laboratory data to illustrate an individual's nutrition status. Iron studies, plasma proteins, renal function tests, plasma lipids, liver function tests, blood glucose, and complete blood counts are useful for elucidating components of nutrient status. While these tests can indicate certain conditions when considered alone, in combination, they may paint a broader picture of adequate or inadequate nutrition status. Serum albumin is the most readily available and abundant of the visceral proteins. The normal range for albumin is 3.5–5.0 g/dL, where 2.8–3.5 g/dL indicates compromised protein status and possible kwashiorkor is suspected at levels <2.8 g/dL. Low albumin is associated with compromised protein intake, and albumin will most always be low in chronic malnutrition, although its long 21-day half-life and its fluctuations related to hydration status make it a less-than-reliable indicator. Prealbumin (also called transthyretin), with its 2 ½-day half-life, is a better indicator of acute malnutrition and more accurately reflects recent dietary protein intake. The normal range for prealbumin is generally >18 mg/dL, with 10–15 mg/dL indicating mild protein depletion and 5–10 mg/dL for severe protein depletion.[25] Prealbumin levels tend to fluctuate depending on fluid status and inflammation, so low values alone are not sufficient to diagnose malnutrition. Further discussion of laboratory tests for nutritional assessment is included in the Nutrition Assessment section of this chapter.

Examples of Screeners

There are a variety of types and iterations of nutrition screeners available. While most screeners consider similar parameters (weight loss, intake, appetite, and BMI) and can be completed quickly, clinicians are encouraged to consider the availability of published data regarding their particular choice of screeners' reliability and validity. In 2009, the American Dietetic Association (now the Academy of Nutrition and Dietetics) published an Evidence Analysis Library (EAL) conclusion statement regarding the reliability and validity of nutrition screeners commonly used in the hospital and ambulatory care settings. Eleven tools were identified, and only one screener, the Malnutrition Screening Tool, received a Grade I, indicating acceptable reliability and validity with regards to identifying malnutrition in both the inpatient and ambulatory care.[39]

- ■ Malnutrition Screening Tool (MST)

The Malnutrition Screening Tool for Hospital Patients by Ferguson et al. is a quick screener that questions unintentional weight loss and reduced appetite. A score of two or more on this tool indicates that the patient is at risk for malnutrition (Table 2–9).[24]

Table 2-9. Rapid nutrition screen for hospitalized patients: a malnutrition screening tool.

Malnutrition Screening Tool (MST) for Hospitalized Patients	
Have you lost weight recently without trying?	
No	0
Unsure	2
If yes, how much weight (kilograms) have you lost?	
1-5	1
6-10	2
11-15	3
>15	4
Unsure	2
Have you been eating poorly because of a decreased appetite?	
No	0
Yes	1
Total[a]	

[a]Score of 2 or more indicates patient is at risk for malnutrition.
Data from Ferguson et al., 1999.

- Malnutrition Universal Screening Tool (MUST)

Screeners may also utilize information about a patient's BMI and/
or severity of illness. The Malnutrition Universal Screening Tool
(MUST) has been validated and shows relative sensitivity and
specificity (but not reliability) for use in the acute-care environment
(Table 2–10).[22,39]

- Short Nutritional Assessment Questionnaire (SNAQ)

Short questionnaires can also shed light on potential nutrition
problems or nutrition risk. The Short Nutritional Assessment
Questionnaire (SNAQ) by Kruizenga et al. is another validated and
cost-effective hospital screening tool for malnutrition. Utilization of
the SNAQ has been shown to improve recognition of malnutrition
from 50% of cases to 80% of cases upon admission to the hospital
(Table 2–11).[19,40]

Table 2–10. Malnutrition universal screening tool (MUST).

	Score
Step 1:Obtain BMI (kg/m²)[a]	
BMI >20 = 0	
BMI 18.5–20.0 = 1	
BMI <18.5 = 2	
Step 2: Obtain weight loss score (unplanned weight loss in 3-6 months)	
Wt loss <5% = 0	
Wt loss 5–10% = 1	
Wt loss >10% = 2	
Step 3: Acute disease effect score	
Add score of 2 if there has been or is likely to be no nutritional intake for >5 days	
Risk level	Total score
0	Low
1	Medium
>2	High

[a]If height and weight are unavailable, alternative measurements and subjective criteria may be used. To learn more visit: http://www.bapen.org.uk/
Data from Stratton et al., 2006.

Table 2–11. Short nutritional assessment questionnaire (SNAQ).

Question	Score
Did you lose weight unintentionally? • More than 6 kg in the last 6 months • More than 3 kg in the last month	3 2
Did you experience a decreased appetite over the past month?	1
Did you use supplemental drinks or tube feeding over the past month?	1
Risk level	Total score
Well nourished, no intervention	0 or 1 points
Moderately malnourished, nutrition intervention warranted	2 points
Severely malnourished, nutrition intervention & dietitian treatment	3 points

Data from Kruizenga et al., 2005.

- **Mini Nutrition Assessment (MNA®)**

The Mini Nutrition Assessment, developed by the Nestle Nutrition Institute is "a validated nutrition screening and assessment tool that can identify geriatric patients age 65 and above who are malnourished or at risk of malnutrition".[41] MNA was developed over 20 years ago and is the most well-researched nutrition screening tool for elderly people. The Mini Nutritional Assessment short-form (MNA®SF) refers to the shorter six-question form of the original, full, 18-item Mini Nutrition Assessment (MNA). In the revised short-form, if BMI is not available, calf circumference may be substituted and has been validated as an appropriate alternative.[42] The MNA is available in almost 30 languages. A new self-MNA has been developed to be used by adults 65 years of age and older or their caregivers. To learn more and to download the interactive forms and assessment tools, visit: http://www.mna-elderly.com/mna_forms.html. Figure 2–5 demonstrates the MNA®SF.

- **DETERMINE Nutrition Checklist**

The DETERMINE Nutrition Checklist was developed by the Nutrition Screening Initiative, a project of the American Academy of Family Physicians, the American Dietetic Association (now the Academy of Nutrition and Dietetics), and the National Council on the Aging, Inc.

Mini Nutritional Assessment
MNA®

Nestlé
Nutrition Institute

Last name:		First name:		
Sex:	Age:	Weight, kg:	Height, cm:	Date:

Complete the screen by filling in the boxes with the appropriate numbers. Total the numbers for the final screening score.

Screening

A Has food intake declined over the past 3 months due to loss of appetite, digestive problems, chewing or swallowing difficulties?

0 = severe decrease in food intake
1 = moderate decrease in food intake
2 = no decrease in food intake ☐

B Weight loss during the last 3 months

0 = weight loss greater than 3 kg (6.6 lbs)
1 = does not know
2 = weight loss between 1 and 3 kg (2.2 and 6.6 lbs)
3 = no weight loss ☐

C Mobility

0 = bed or chair bound
1 = able to get out of bed / chair but does not go out
2 = goes out ☐

D Has suffered psychological stress or acute disease in the past 3 months?

0 = yes   2 = no ☐

E Neuropsychological problems

0 = severe dementia or depression
1 = mild dementia
2 = no psychological problems ☐

F1 Body Mass Index (BMI) (weight in kg) / (height in m^2)

0 = BMI less than 19
1 = BMI 19 to less than 21
2 = BMI 21 to less than 23
3 = BMI 23 or greater ☐

IF BMI IS NOT AVAILABLE, REPLACE QUESTION F1 WITH QUESTION F2.
DO NOT ANSWER QUESTION F2 IF QUESTION F1 IS ALREADY COMPLETED.

F2 Calf circumference (CC) in cm

0 = CC less than 31
3 = CC 31 or greater ☐

Screening score (max. 14 points)

12 - 14 points: Normal nutritional status
8 - 11 points: At risk of malnutrition
0 - 7 points: Malnourished ☐☐

References
1. Vellas B, Villars H, Abellan G, *et al.* Overview of the MNA® - Its History and Challenges. *J Nutr Health Aging.* 2006;**10**:456-465.
2. Rubenstein LZ, Harker JO, Salva A, Guigoz Y, Vellas B. Screening for Undernutrition in Geriatric Practice: Developing the Short-Form Mini Nutritional Assessment (MNA-SF). *J. Geront.* 2001; **56A**: M366-377
3. Guigoz Y. The Mini-Nutritional Assessment (MNA®) Review of the Literature - What does it tell us? *J Nutr Health Aging.* 2006; **10**:466-487.
4. Kaiser MJ, Bauer JM, Ramsch C, et al. Validation of the Mini Nutritional Assessment Short-Form (MNA®-SF): A practical tool for identification of nutritional status. *J Nutr Health Aging.* 2009; **13**:782-788.
® Société des Produits Nestlé, S.A., Vevey, Switzerland, Trademark Owners © Nestlé, 1994, Revision 2009. N67200 12/99 10M
For more information: www.mna-elderly.com

Figure 2–5. Mini nutritional assessment (MNA). (Data from Nestle Nutrition Institute.)

The checklist can be quickly completed by healthcare practitioners, or families and friends, to identify nutrition risk in the elderly. The DETERMINE acronym stands for the warning signs of malnutrition in elderly that involve: Disease, Eating poorly, Tooth loss/mouth pain, Economic hardship, Reduced social contact, Multiple medicines, Involuntary weight loss/gain, Needs assistance in self-care, and Elder years above age 80. Figure 2–6 shows the components and scoring of the DETERMINE nutrition checklist.

- ■ Subjective Global Assessment

Subjective Global Assessment (SGA, Figure 2–7) is a nutrition screening tool that analyzes five components of a patient's history in relation to nutrition requirements: weight change, changes in dietary intake, GI symptoms, functional capacity, and disease. SGA helps to determine whether a patient is well nourished, moderately malnourished or suspected of malnutrition, or severely malnourished. SGA was developed and refined in the mid- to late-1980s as a comprehensive assessment tool to address nutrition status by observing clinical criteria versus using anthropometric and laboratory values, which require time and labor to gather.[43] The SGA is subjective in that it does not provide a concrete

The warning signs of poor nutritional health are often overlooked. Use this checklist to find out if you or someone you know is at nutritional risk.

Determine Your Nutritional Health

Read the statements below. Circle the number in the yes column for those that apply to you or someone you know. For each yes answer, score the number in the box. Total your nutritional score.

	YES
I have an illness or condition that made me change the kind and /or amount of food I eat.	2
I eat fewer than two meals per day.	3
I eat few fruits or vegetables, or milk products.	2
I have three or more drinks of beer, liquor, or wine almost every day.	2
I have tooth or mouth problems that make it hard for me to eat.	2
I don't always have enough money to buy the food I need.	4
I eat alone most of the time.	1
I take three or more different prescribed or over-the-counter drugs a day.	1
Without wanting to, I have lost or gained 10 pounds in the last six months.	2
I am not always physically able to shop, cook, and/or feed myself.	2
TOTAL	

Total your nutritional score. If it's --

0–2   **Good!** Recheck your nutritional score in 6 months.

3–5   **You are at moderate nutritional risk.** See what can be done to improve your eating habits and lifestyle. Your office on aging, senior nutrition program, senior citizens center, or health department can help. Recheck your nutritional score in 3 months.

6 or mor e   **You are at high nutritional risk.** Bring this checklist the next time you see your doctor, dietitian or other qualified health or social service professional. Talk with them about any problems you may have. Ask for help to improve your nutritional health.

Remember that warning signs suggest risk, but do not represent diagnosis of any condition. Turn the page to learn more about the Warning Signs of poor nutritional health.

Figure 2-6. DETERMINE your health checklist.

The Nutrition Checklist is based on the warning signs described below. Use the word DETERMINE to remind you of the warning signs.

Disease

Any disease, illness, or chronic condition that causes you to change the way you eat, or makes it hard for you to eat, puts your nutritional health at risk. Four out of five adults have chronic diseases that are affected by diet. Confusion or memory loss that keeps getting worse is estimated to affect one out of five or more of older adults. This can make it hard to remember what, when or if you've eaten. Feeling sad or depressed, which happens to about one in eight older adults, can cause big changes in appetite, digestion, energy level, weight, and well-being.

Eating Poorly

Eating too little and eating too much both lead to poor health. Eating the same foods day after day or not eating fruit, vegetables, and milk products daily will also cause poor nutritional health. One in five adults skips meals daily. Only 13% of adults eat the minimum amount of fruits and vegetables needed. One in four older adults drinks too much alcohol. Many health problems become worse if you drink more than one or two alcoholic beverages per day.

Tooth Loss/Mouth Pain

A healthy mouth, teeth and gums are needed to eat. Missing, loose or rotten teeth or dentures, which don't fit well or cause mouth sores make it hard to eat.

Economic Hardship

As many as 40% of older Americans have incomes of less than $6,000 per year. Having less-- or choosing to spend less--than $25-$30 per week for food makes it very hard to get the foods you need to stay healthy.

Reduced Social Contact

One-third of all older people live alone. Being with people daily has a positive effect on morale, well-being, and eating.

Multiple Medicines

Many older Americans must take medicines for health problems. Almost one half of older Americans take multiple medicines daily. Growing old may change the way we respond to drugs. The more medicines you take, the greater chance for side effects such as increased or decreased appetite, change in taste, constipation, weakness, drowsiness, diarrhea, nausea and others. Vitamins or minerals when taken in large doses act like drugs and can cause harm. Alert your doctor to everything you take.

Involuntary Weight Loss/Gain

Losing or gaining a lot of weight when you are not trying to do so is an important warning sign that must not be ignored. Being overweight or underweight also increases your chance of poor health.

Needs Assistance in Self Care

Although most older people are able to eat, one of every five has trouble walking, shopping, buying and cooking food, especially as they get older.

Elder Years Above Age 80

Most older people lead full and productive lives. But as age increases, risk of frailty and health problems increase. Checking you nutritional health regularly makes good sense.

Figure 2–6. DETERMINE your health checklist. (*Continued*)

"score" or "risk number", but relies on clinical interpretation of the SGA ratings.[44]

Electronic Screeners, Calculators, and Tools

When time is tight, a quick online screener can shed light on a previously unrecognized problem for a patient. These screeners do not provide full in-depth assessments, but rather are helpful third-party tools for broaching food and diet topics. The Block Food Frequency Questionnaire (FFQ), developed by Dr. Gladys Block, can be adapted as a screener to question about sodium, fat, sugar, fruit and vegetable,

Features of the Subjective Global Assessment (SGA)

(Select appropriate category with a checkmark, or enter numerical value where indicated by '#')

A. History
   1. Weight change
      Overall loss in past 6 months: amount = #_____ kg; % loss = #
      _____
      Change in past 2 weeks _____ increase
      _____ no change
      _____ decrease
   2. Dietary intake change (relative to normal)
      _____ No change
      _____ Change _____ duration = # _____
      weeks
      _____ type: _____ suboptimal diet, _____ full
      liquid diet
      _____ hypocaloric liquids, _____
      starvation
   3. Gastrointestinal symptoms (that persisted for >2 weeks)
      _____ none, _____ nausea, _____ vomiting,
      _____diarrhea, _____anorexia
   4. Functional capacity
      _____ No dysfunction (eg, full capacity)
      _____ Dysfunction _____ duration = # _____ weeks
      _____ type: _____ working
      suboptimally
      _____ ambulatory
      _____ bedridden.
   5. Disease and its relation to nutritional requirements.
      Primary diagnosis (specify)
      _____
      Metabolic demand (stress): _____ No stress, _____ Low stress
      _____ Moderate stress, _____ High stress

B. Physical (for each trait specify: 0 = normal, 1 + = mild, 2 + = moderate, 3 + = severe)
   # _____ loss of subcutaneous fat (triceps, chest)
   # _____ muscle wasting (quadriceps, deltoids)
   # _____ ankle edema
   # _____ sacral edema
   # _____ ascites

C. SGA rating (select one)
   _____ A = well nourished
   _____ B = moderately (or suspected of being) malnourished
   _____ C = severely malnourished.

Figure 2–7. Subjective global assessment form. (Data from Detsky et al., 1987.)

calcium, folic acid, soy foods, and a host of other tailored nutrient intake patterns. Preset or custom screeners can be designed, purchased, and implemented for use in various healthcare or research settings in both paper and electronic format. Consider using the free online Fat Intake Screener and Fruit/Vegetable/Fiber Screener, both of which are based on Block's longer FFQ, to initiate conversations with your patients about their current intake levels. Table 2–12 contains a list of links for these and other free online nutrition and health screeners,

Table 2–12. Web resource for nutrition screeners.

Block fat intake screener from NutritionQuest	http://www.nutritionquest.com/wellness/free-assessment-tools-for-individuals/fat-intake-screener/
Block fruit, vegetable, and fiber screener from NutritionQuest	http://nutritionquest.com/wellness/free-assessment-tools-for-individuals/fruit-vegetable-fiber-screener/
Supplemental nutrition assistance program (SNAP, formerly food stamps) prescreening eligibility tool from USDA	http://www.snap-step1.usda.gov/fns/
Type 2 diabetes risk test from American Diabetes Association	http://www.diabetes.org/diabetes-basics/prevention/diabetes-risk-test/
Heart attack risk calculator from American Heart Association	https://www.heart.org/gglRisk/locale/en_US/index.html?gtype=health
Get moving! calculator from Calorie Control Council	http://www.caloriecontrol.org/healthy-weight-tool-kit/lighten-up-and-get-moving
Diet history questionnaire II from National Cancer Institute	http://riskfactor.cancer.gov/dhq2/
Interactive DRIs for healthcare professionals from USDA	http://fnic.nal.usda.gov/fnic/interactiveDRI/
Basal energy expenditure: Harris-Benedict equation calculator from Cornell University	http://www-users.med.cornell.edu/~spon/picu/calc/beecalc.htm
Body mass index calculator from DHHS	http://www.nhlbisupport.com/bmi/bmicalc.htm

(Continued)

Table 2-12. Web resource for nutrition screeners. *(Continued)*

BMI calculator for child and teen from CDC	http://apps.nccd.cdc.gov/dnpabmi/
Ground beef calculator from USDA	http://ndb.nal.usda.gov/ndb/beef/show
Food buying guide calculator for child nutrition programs	http://fbg.nfsmi.org/
Children's healthy eating calculator from Baylor College of Medicine	http://www.bcm.edu/cnrc/healthyeatingcalculator/eatingCal.html
Online calcium quiz from Dairy Council of California	http://www.healthyeating.org/Healthy-Eating/Healthy-Eating-Tools/Calcium-Quiz.aspx?Referer=dairycouncilofca
Portion distortion quizzes from NHLBI	http://hp2010.nhlbihin.net/portion/index.htm
Rate your restaurant diet quiz from CSPI	http://www.cspinet.org/nah/quiz/index.html
Saturated fat IQ quiz from HealthyFridge.org	http://www.healthyfridge.org/satfat.html
Serving size surprise game from Aetna	http://www.intelihealth.com/IH/ihtIH/WSIHW000/24479/20760/227175.html?d=dmtContent
Alcohol calorie calculator from NIAAA	http://rethinkingdrinking.niaaa.nih.gov/toolsresources/caloriecalculator.asp
Ten-year probability of fracture with BMD: WHO fracture risk assessment tool (FRAX)	http://www.shef.ac.uk/FRAX/tool.jsp
Body weight simulator from NIDDK/NIH	http://bwsimulator.niddk.nih.gov/

calculators, and games. Most take less than 5 minutes to complete and they can provide valuable insight on areas for improvement in dietary patterning.

Nutrition Assessment

It is important to understand the difference between nutrition screening and nutrition assessment. Effective nutrition screeners are characterized as being simple, quick, and inexpensive to use, with a wide range of patient applications. At the same time they should be reliant on routine tests and data that are available upon admission.[24] Nutrition assessment is more complex than screening, and it incorporates a comprehensive, detailed look at anthropometric, biochemical, clinical, and dietary intake data, along with physical examination, to determine who is malnourished.[13] Those determined to be at risk for malnutrition are identified by a screen, then should be referred to a dietitian for further in-depth assessment and for confirmation of diagnosis. Nutrition assessment seeks to identify specific nutrition risk or risks and to clear the presence of malnutrition. Assessments might lead to implementation of therapies that help improve nutrition status, or they may set the stage for rescreening (Table 2–13 and Figure 2–8).[13,15,45]

Table 2–13. The differences between screening and assessment.

Screening	Assessment
Quickly captures glimpse of individual's health status, identifying those who are already malnourished or who are at risk for becoming so	Provides opportunity for an in-depth look at many contributing factors
Evaluates for the presence of a particular nutrition problem	Defines the nature of that particular nutrition problem, determines diagnosis, and guides treatment recommendations
Uses standardized screening instruments readily available upon admission	May require more specific equipment, data, or material for thorough analysis
Outcome may be as simple as "yes" or "no"	Provides detailed insight into relationship between nutrition and health status

Data from Center for Substance Abuse Treatment, 2009; Ferguson et al., 1999; Academy of Nutrition and Dietetics, 2012.

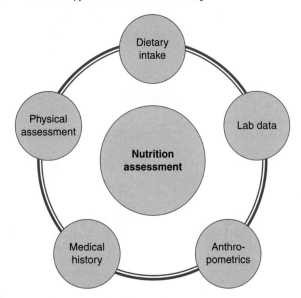

Figure 2–8. The components of nutrition assessment.

Diagnosing Malnutrition

Currently, there are no established or mutually agreed upon criteria for the diagnosis or management of adult malnutrition, also called undernutrition.[13] Estimated prevalence rates of adult malnutrition vary widely from 15 to 60%.[46] In the absence of definitive parameters that define adult malnutrition, the Academy of Nutrition and Dietetics and the American Society for Parenteral and Enteral Nutrition have put forth a consensus statement recommending the following six criteria for diagnosis:

- Insufficient energy intake
- Weight loss
- Loss of muscle mass
- Loss of subcutaneous fat
- Localized or generalized fluid accumulation that may sometimes mask weight loss
- Diminished functional status as measured by hand grip strength

Table 2–14 contains the current ICD-9-CM criteria for diagnosing malnutrition. While laboratory data including albumin, prealbumin, and C-reactive protein have traditionally been used in the assessment and diagnosis of malnutrition, recent scientific findings indicate that these lab values are not useful in diagnosing malnutrition, but that they are helpful markers of inflammation, which contributes to the malnourished state.[13,47-49]

Table 2–14. Diagnosing malnutrition.

Diagnosis and Description (ICD-9-CM Code) for Malnutrition-Associated Conditions	
Kwashiorkor: Nutritional edema with dyspigmentation of skin and hair (260.0)	• Normal anthropometrics: weight >90% of standard weight for height • Depressed visceral protein concentrations: serum albumin <3.0 g/dL, transferrin <180 mg/dL • Caused by acute energy and protein deficiency or reflecting a metabolic response to injury • Characterized by edema, catabolism of muscle tissue, weakness, neurological changes, loss of vigor secondary infections, stunted growth in children, and changes in hair
Nutritional marasmus: Nutritional atrophy; severe, chronic calorie deficiency; and severe malnutrition (261.0)	• Depressed anthropometrics: weight <80% of standard weight for height, and/or a weight loss of >10% of usual weight in last 6 months with muscle wasting • Relative preservation of visceral proteins: serum albumin >3.0 g/dL • Caused by chronically deficient energy intake • Characterized by catabolism of fat and muscle tissue, lethargy, generalized weakness, and weight loss
Other severe protein-calorie malnutrition: Nutritional edema without mention of dyspigmentation of skin and hair (262.0)	• Depressed anthropometrics: weight <60% of standard weight for height, and/or a weight loss of >10% of usual weight in last 6 months with muscle wasting • Depressed visceral protein concentration: serum albumin <3.0 g/dL • Occurs when a marasmic patient is exposed to stress (eg, trauma, surgery, or acute illness) • Characterized by combined symptoms of marasmus and kwashiorkor, a high risk of infection, and poor wound healing
Malnutrition of moderate degree (263.0)	• Depressed anthropometrics: weight 60–75% of standard weight for height • Relative preservation of visceral proteins: serum albumin 3.0–3.5 g/dL
Malnutrition of mild degree (263.1)	• Depressed anthropometrics: weight 75–90% of standard weight for height • Preservation of visceral proteins: serum albumin 3.5–5.0 g/dL
Other protein-calorie malnutrition (263.8)	

(Continued)

Table 2–14. Diagnosing malnutrition. (*Continued*)

Diagnosis and Description (ICD-9-CM Code) for Malnutrition-Associated Conditions	
Other and unspecified postsurgical nonabsorption (hypoglycemia, malnutrition following gastrointestinal surgery (579.3)	
Abnormal loss of weight and underweight (783.2)	
Loss of weight (783.21)	
Underweight (783.22)	

Data from World Health Organization, 1975; Academy of Nutrition and Dietetics, 2012.

Laboratory Data

■ Serum Proteins

Protein status is most commonly associated with nutrition assessment because, unlike carbohydrate and fat, protein is not readily stored by the body. Protein status can be evaluated by looking at somatic protein (found within the skeletal muscle) and visceral protein (that which is circulating or located in the organs of the viscera). Serum proteins that reflect nutritional status include albumin, transferrin, prealbumin, retinol-binding protein (RBP), insulin-like growth factor-1 (IGF-1), and fibronectin. Of these, albumin, prealbumin, and transferrin are most often considered. While decreased albumin and prealbumin levels have traditionally been used as indicators of prolonged and acute protein and energy restriction, emerging evidence suggests they better reflect severity of the inflammatory response rather than poor nutritional status.[47,50,51] A recent evidence analysis conclusion statement analyzed reduction and/or change in serum albumin and prealbumin along with weight loss in prolonged protein energy restriction, nonmalabsorptive gastric partitioning bariatric surgery, anorexia nervosa, calorie-restricted diets, low-calorie diets, starvation, and nitrogen balance. The evidence indicates that these acute-phase proteins were not predictably or consistently altered with weight loss, calorie restriction, or nitrogen balance.[52]

Albumin

Albumin is the most abundant of the serum proteins. The half-life of albumin is 21 days, thus making it useful when identifying chronic (as opposed to acute) undernutrition. Serum albumin concentrations tend to be low in protein energy malnutrition and the acute catabolic phase of an injury, and they are elevated in positive protein balance.[25,28] As with all serum proteins, albumin is influenced by hydration status and may be artificially high in dehydrated persons and low with over-hydration. The normal range for albumin is 3.5–5.0 g/dL.

Prealbumin

Because of its relatively short half-life of 2–3 days, prealbumin is a more sensitive marker of recent protein intake than albumin. Prealbumin is also called transthyretin and thyroxine-binding prealbumin. With reinitiation of adequate protein and energy intake, prealbumin levels quickly return to normal levels, although that does not necessarily indicate that malnutrition has been resolved. The normal range for prealbumin is 18–40 mg/dL, with 10–15 mg/dL indicating mild protein depletion and 5–10 mg/dL severe protein depletion.[25] Table 2–15 stratifies nutrition risk level by prealbumin value.[53]

Transferrin

Transferrin is responsible for the transport of iron in the plasma and its transport to bone marrow. It too has a shorter half-life than albumin and is also considered a more accurate indicator of recent intake than is albumin. While transferrin can be measured directly, it is more commonly measured indirectly from the total iron-binding capacity (TIBC). Hepatic synthesis and plasma transferrin levels are increased in iron deficiency, while levels are lower in chronic infections and acute catabolic states (Lee & Nieman, 2007). The normal value for transferrin is 2.3 g/L.

▪ Vitamin and Mineral Status

Given that there rarely exists adequate physical manifestations evident with vitamin and mineral deficiencies, the use of laboratory data to help identify such shortages is extremely helpful in the clinical setting.

Table 2–15. Prealbumin and nutrition risk.

Prealbumin Level	Nutrition Risk Level
<5.0 mg/dL	Poor prognosis
5.0–10.9 mg/dL	Significant nutrition risk indicating aggressive nutrition support
11.0–15.0 mg/dL	Increased nutrition risk warranting biweekly monitoring of prealbumin
15.0–35.0 mg/dL	Reduced or no nutrition risk

Data from Bernstein et al., 1995.

Table 2-16. Selected reference blood cell values for adults.

Lab Value	Males	Females
Hemoglobin[a]	140–180 (g/L of blood)	120–160 (g/L of blood)
Hematocrit	40–54%	37–47%
Mean corpuscular volume	80–100 (fL)	80–100 (fL)

[a]Reference values are for white men and women; reference values for black men and women are 5–10 g/L lower.

Data from Ravel, 1989.

Iron Status

Iron deficiency is the most common micronutrient deficiency around the world.[54] Despite its prevalence in the developing world, iron deficiency is also strikingly present in developed nations. Chapter 8 covers iron deficiency, iron deficiency anemia, and other anemias along with their recommended therapies for prevention and treatment. Anemia refers to a hemoglobin level that is less than normal for people in a given age and gender group. Hemoglobin is the iron-containing molecule that carries oxygen and is located in the red blood cells. Normal ranges are 140–180 g/L (14–18/dL) for men and 120–160 g/l (12–16 g/dL) for women. On an average, hemoglobin levels are 5–10 g/L less in black men and women than in white men and women for most age groups.[55]

Hematocrit is the percentage of red blood cells that make up the whole volume of whole blood. Normal ranges for hematocrit are 40–54% for males and 37–47% for females. Hemoglobin and hematocrit are used in the diagnosis of anemia, but because they do not become abnormal until the latter stages of iron deficiency, they are less useful in detecting early stages of iron deficiency. Other laboratory indicators of iron status include transferrin, serum iron, total iron-binding capacity, erythrocyte protoporphyrin, mean corpuscular hemoglobin, and mean corpuscular volume. Table 2–16 outlines reference laboratory values for adults in iron studies, and Table 2–17 covers other laboratory tests for nutrition assessment.[25,31,55]

Dietary Data

The 24-hour recall and food record techniques discussed earlier in the chapter (under Nutrition Screening) are methods for uncovering potential deficits in nutrient intake. However, these methods have limitations in that they may not be entirely reflective of usual dietary intake, and the information derived from the recall or food record is subject to bias. If the practitioner obtaining the information is not well trained in dietary questioning or if

Table 2–17. Laboratory tests for nutritional assessment.

Test	Normal Values	Nutrition Implication	Function	Notes
Albumin	(3.5–5.5 g/dL)	• 2.8–3.5 compromised protein status • <2.8 possible kwashiorkor • Increasing value shows positive protein balance	Regulates oncotic pressure in plasma	High in dehydration or infusion of albumin, fresh frozen plasma, or whole blood Low (common) infection, trauma, burns, CHF, fluid overload, and liver disease Low (uncommon) nephrotic syndrome, zinc deficiency, and bacterial stasis/overgrowth of small intestine
Serum prealbumin, also called transthyretin	(20–40 mg/dL; lower in prepubertal children)	• 10–15 mg/dL: mild protein depletion • 5–10 mg/dl: moderate protein depletion • <5 mg/dl: severe protein depletion	Carrier for retinol-binding protein; carries T3 and some T4	Similar to that of albumin
Serum total iron-binding capacity (TIBC)	240–450 mcg/dl	• <200: compromised protein status, possible kwashiorkor • Increasing values reflect positive protein balance	Measures ability of the blood to bind transferrin with iron	High with iron deficiency and reasons similar to that of low albumin
Prothrombin time	12.0–15.5 seconds	• Prolongation: vitamin K deficiency		High with iron deficiency Prolonged with anticoagulant therapy (warfarin) and severe liver disease

(Continued)

Table 2-17. Laboratory tests for nutritional assessment. (*Continued*)

Test	Normal Values	Nutrition Implication	Function	Notes
Serum creatinine	(0.6-1.6 mg/dL)	• <0.6: muscle wasting due to prolonged energy deficit	Reflects muscle mass	High despite muscle wasting in renal failure and severe dehydration
24-hour urinary creatinine	500-1200 mg/d (standardized for height and sex)			Low with muscle wasting due to prolonged energy deficit May be normal despite malnutrition if >24 h collection or with decreasing serum creatinine May be normal, despite malnutrition with decreasing serum creatinine May also be low if incomplete urine collection, increasing serum creatinine, and neuromuscular wasting
24-hour urinary urea nitrogen (UUN)	<5 g/d (depends on level of protein intake)	• Determine level of catabolism (as long as protein intake is ≥10 g below calculated protein loss or <20 g total, but at least 100 g carbohydrate is provided) • 5-10 g/d = mild catabolism or normal fed state • 10-15 g/d = moderate catabolism • >15 g/d = severe catabolism		

		• Protein balance = protein intake − protein loss where protein loss (protein catabolic rate) = [24-h UUN (g) + 4] × 6.25 • Adjustments required in burn patients and others with large nonurinary nitrogen losses and in patients with fluctuating BUN levels (eg, renal failure)	
Blood urea nitrogen (BUN)	8–23 mg/dL	<8: possibly inadequate protein intake 12–23: possibly adequate protein intake >23: possibly excessive protein intake	Urea nitrogen is the byproduct of protein breakdown	If serum creatinine is normal, use BUN If serum creatinine is elevated, use BUN/creatinine ratio (normal range is essentially the same as for BUN) Low with severe liver disease, anabolic state, and syndrome of inappropriate antidiuretic hormone High despite poor protein intake with renal failure (use BUN/creatinine ratio), CHF, and GI hemorrhage

Adapted from Heimburger, 2006; Heimburger, 2012.

the client is not accurately recording food and beverage intake, the data will be skewed. Other methods for assessing dietary and nutrient intake include food frequency questionnaires, calorie counts, and electronic resources such as the USDA's SuperTracker and the Interactive DRI for Healthcare Professionals. Before you can assess the adequacy of a patient's diet, you must first compare their baseline intake to their nutritional needs.

■ Estimating Energy Needs

Estimating a patient's energy, or total caloric, needs can be done through the use of equipment or by performing calculations. The use of equipment, such as a metabolic cart, is considered the most accurate means of estimating energy needs; thus, you will often find metabolic carts in research laboratories or in sophisticated clinics and hospitals. Metabolic carts are utilized when performing indirect calorimetry, the gold-standard for estimating resting energy requirements. During indirect calorimetry, a metabolic cart measures the amount of heat energy produced by an individual by determining the amount of oxygen consumed and the quantity of carbon dioxide eliminated. Because indirect calorimetry is costly and not widely available in all healthcare settings, predictive equations have been developed to help estimate energy expenditure and to calculate energy needs. The predictive equations covered in the next section are used for the adult population and are not appropriate for pregnant women or children.

Harris-Benedict Equation

The Harris-Benedict equation has traditionally been the most widely used equation for estimating energy requirements. It determines resting metabolic rate (RMR) that is then multiplied by an activity factor (AF) and injury factor (IF). The Harris-Benedict equation has been found to predict RMR within 10% of measured RMR in 69% of individuals for which it is applied. If not entirely accurate—which no predictive equation is—the Harris-Benedict equation is significantly more likely to overestimate energy needs (27% of the time) than it is to underestimate (4%).[39]

The Harris-Benedict Equation

Men: Resting metabolic rate (RMR) = 66.47 + 13.75(W*) +
5(H) − 6.76(A)
Women: RMR = 655.1 + 9.56 (W) + 1.7 (H) − 4.7 (A)

*Equation uses weight (W) in kilograms, height (H) in centimeters, and age (A) in years. Activity and injury factors are covered in Chapter 10.

Mifflin-St. Jeor

According to an evidence analysis conducted by the Academy of Nutrition and Dietetics, "the Mifflin-St. Jeor equation was found to be the most reliable, predicting REE within 10% of measured in more nonobese and obese individuals than any other equation." It was also found to have the most narrow error range.[52]

Table 2–18. Calories per kg estimation method for determining calorie needs.

To lose weight	20-25 calories per kg body weight
To maintain weight	25-30 calories per kg body weight
To gain weight	30-35 calories per kg body weight

Mifflin-St. Jeor Equation

Men: RMR = (9.99 × weight) + (6.25 × height) − (4.92 × age) + 5
Women: RMR = (9.99 × weight) + (6.25 × height) −
(4.92 × age) − 161

*Equation uses weight in kilograms height in centimeters, and age in years.

Calories per kg Estimation Method

Another method of estimating energy needs is based on using a set number of calories per kg of body weight. The calories per kg method—although not scientifically validated—produces results that are close to those of the validated equations above in an easier-to-use format. The calories per kg method states that, in order to maintain weight, multiply kg of body weight by 25–30 calories per kg. To gain weight, multiply kg of body weight by 30–35 calories per kg. And to lose weight, multiply kg of body weight by 20–25 calories per kg (Table 2–18).

Depending upon activity level and starting body weight, especially in the very overweight and obese, this ratio of calories to kilogram of body weight method may not produce entirely accurate results. It is, however, a good starting point for estimating calorie needs, which are often quite different than what the individual is actually eating. For individuals >125% IBW, some practitioners use an adjusted body weight (ABW) to obtain a lower weight from which to estimate caloric needs. The adjusted body weight also has not been validated as an accurate measure, yet it is widely used in practice. The equation for determining adjusted body weight is listed in Table 2–19. For individuals >125%, obtain ABW in kilograms and then multiply by 20–25 cal/kg or 25–30 cal/kg (depending on professional interpretation of calorie needs). Chapters 3 and 10 contain more information about determining energy needs.

Table 2–19. Adjusted body weight equation for use in individuals >125% ideal body weight.

Determining Adjusted Body Weight (ABW) for use in Individuals >125%
ABW: [(actual body weight – ideal body weight) × 0.25] + ideal body weight

- ## Estimating Macronutrient Needs

The Dietary Reference Intakes (DRIs) introduced in Chapter 1 also set parameters for the established acceptable macronutrient distribution ranges (AMDRs) that provide detail on how distribution of total calories should look in a well-balanced diet. The AMDRs set an upper and lower range for percent of calories from the three essential macronutrients: carbohydrate, fat, and protein. Practitioners can use the AMDR to recommend grams of carbohydrate, fat, and protein for individuals' diets. The AMDR can then be compared against current dietary intakes of patients and clients or to make recommendations about how much of each macronutrient to consume.

The AMDRs, and the scientific data from which they are derived, state that the majority of calories in a well-balanced diet should come from carbohydrate (45–65% of calories in an adult diet), with less calories coming from fat and protein (20–35% and 10–35%, respectively). The AMDRs are outlined in Table 2–20 and require the practitioner to know the energy density of each macronutrient: 1 gram of carbohydrate contains 4 calories, 1 gram of fat contains 9 calories, and 1 gram of protein contains 4 calories.[56]

There are no significant data to set forth a DRI for fat. In addition to the AMDR for fat of 20–35% of calories, other fat-related guidelines recommend a diet of <35% calories from fat, equating to no more than 65 grams per day total fat when following a 2,000-calorie diet. For protein, the dietary reference intake for healthy adults is 0.8 g/kg body weight; however, certain medical conditions require an increase or decrease in protein compared to this level. Table 2–21 further outlines the DRIs for water, carbohydrate, fiber, and protein for different age and gender groups. (See Appendix A for more DRI information).

- ## Estimating Micronutrient Needs

As with the macronutrients, the amount of micronutrients (vitamins and minerals) required by individuals varies by age and gender group. Appendix A contains the DRIs for vitamins and minerals, as well as the Tolerable Upper Intake Level (UL) for these micronutrients.

Table 2–20. AMDR for macronutrients.

Macronutrient	Macronutrient Distribution Range (percent of energy/calories)		
	Children, 1-3 years	Children, 4-18 years	Adults >18 years
Carbohydrate	45–65%	45–65%	45–65%
Fat	30–40%	25–35%	20–35%
Protein	5–20%	10–30%	10–35%

Data from National Research Council, 2005.

Table 2–21. DRIs for water, carbohydrate, dietary fiber, fat, and protein.

	Total Water (L/d)[a]	Carbohydrate (g/d)	Total Fiber (g/d)	Fat (g/d)	Protein (g/d)[b]
Infants					
0–6 mo	0.7*	60*	ND[c]	31*	9.1*
6–12 mo	0.8*	95*	ND	30*	11.0
Children					
1–3 y	1.3*	130	19*	ND	13
4–8 y	1.7*	130	25*	ND	19
Males					
9–13 y	2.4*	130	31*	ND	34
14–18 y	3.3*	130	38*	ND	52
19–30 y	3.7*	130	38*	ND	56
31–50 y	3.7*	130	38*	ND	56
51–70 y	3.7*	130	30*	ND	56
>70 y	3.7*	130	30*	ND	56
Females					
9–13 y	2.1*	130	26*	ND	34
14–18 y	2.3*	130	26*	ND	46
19–30 y	2.7*	130	25*	ND	46
31–50 y	2.7*	130	25*	ND	46
51–70 y	2.7*	130	21*	ND	46
>70 y	2.7*	130	21*	ND	46
Pregnancy					
14–18 y	3.0*	175	28*	ND	71
19–30 y	3.0*	175	28*	ND	71
31–50 y	3.0*	175	28*	ND	71
Lactation					
14–18 y	3.8*	210	29*	ND	71
19–30 y	3.8*	210	29*	ND	71
31–50 y	3.8*	210	29*	ND	71

ND, Not determined.

*Values marked by asterisk (*) indicate Adequate Intake (AI) values; an AI is set when there is not enough data to determine a Recommended Dietary Allowance (RDA) value. The RDA is the average daily dietary intake level; sufficient to meet the nutrient requirements of nearly all (97–98%) of healthy individuals in a group. The AI is believed to cover the needs of all healthy individuals in the group, but lack of data or uncertainty in the data prevents being able to specify with confidence the percentage of individuals covered by this intake.

[a]Total water includes all water contained in food, beverages, and drinking water.

[b]Based on gram protein per kg of body weight for the reference body weight; eg, for adults 0.8 g/kg body weight for the reference body weight.

Data from National Research Council, 2005.

As covered in Chapter 1, the DRI values are what an individual should aim to consume each day, whereas the UL is the highest level of daily nutrient intake that is likely to pose no risk of adverse health effects to almost all individuals in the general population. While people should aim to meet the DRIs for each vitamin and mineral, they should avoid exceeding the UL as it presents an increased risk for vitamin and mineral toxicity. Individuals rarely can achieve greater-than-UL intakes of vitamins and minerals through food consumption, but using high doses of dietary supplements can easily lead a person to surpass the UL.

■ Food Frequency

Food frequency tools such as a Food Frequency Questionnaire (FFQ) employ a retrospective approach to quantify how often during a set period of time (eg, day, week, month, or year) a type of food or food group is consumed. FFQs are used commonly in large epidemiologic studies that explore the link between diet and health as well as in national household-level surveys such as the National Health and Nutrition Examination Survey (NHANES). FFQs can also be tailored for use in the clinic, office, or community setting, and they can be configured to probe for information about certain nutrients or dietary components (eg, calcium, caffeine, soy, or fiber intake). The foods in an FFQ are grouped together because of similar nutrient profiles. The respondent answers questions about how frequently certain foods or types of foods are consumed, and the results are then either scanned or coded to reveal dietary intake patterns. When compared to other dietary intake assessment methods, FFQs are relatively cost-effective, easy to complete, and require minimal oversight, since they can be completed without an accompanying note-taker. As with all dietary assessment methods, there are limitations, including errors in self-reporting and self-recall, as well as inevitable shifts in consumption during injury and illness that may not always be representative of usual, healthy intake.

■ Calorie Counts

Calorie counts are used to track actual caloric intake in an institution-alized setting. They may be requested in the inpatient or long-term care environment and require cooperation from and participation of multiple disciplines. Calorie counts are usually 3 days in length, and they are used to determine whether a patient or resident is meeting his or her estimated nutrition needs with p.o. intake. The means by which calories are recorded vary by institution, but generally, nursing assistants observe and document the total amount or percentages of foods and beverages consumed at each meal and snack for 3 days. The RD or other trained nutrition professional analyzes the recorded intake and equates that to calories per day based on known quantities of foods served in the institution. A 3-day calorie intake average is determined, and the medical team then analyzes if nutrient goals are being met. Calorie counts are helpful for justifying which patients or residents may benefit from enteral nutrition or for weaning those who are receiving enteral nutrition off of tube feeding and back on to p.o. meals.

■ SuperTracker

The USDA's SuperTracker is a free, web-based program that helps individuals plan, track, and analyze dietary intake and physical activity. SuperTracker allows users to search and compare foods, track foods and compare them to nutrition targets, record physical activity and track progress, manage weight, set food- and beverage-related goals, and use reports to follow progress over time. The food, nutrient, and activity goals and materials in SuperTracker are aligned with the Dietary Guidelines for Americans, and the program provides personalized nutrition and physical activity plans for users. While the web-based aspects of SuperTracker contribute to its robust capabilities, it may also be a drawback for those patients, clients, or clinical settings with limited internet access. Learn more about SuperTracker at: https://www.supertracker.usda.gov/.

■ Interactive DRI for Healthcare Professionals

The Interactive DRI for Healthcare Professionals is a web-based tool used to calculate daily nutrient recommendations for dietary planning. The tool is based on the Dietary Reference Intakes (DRIs), developed by the National Academy of Science's Institute on Medicine. The practitioner enters the client's gender, age, height, weight, and activity level, and then generates a detailed report of individual calorie and nutrient needs based on the DRI for that age/gender group. Useful applications of this tool include establishing minimum daily carbohydrate needs for people with diabetes, explaining baseline dietary fiber recommendations, comparing current versus recommended calcium intake, or explaining how increased physical activity affects individual energy needs. You can access the interactive DRI tool at: http://fnic .nal.usda.gov/fnic/interactiveDRI/. The DRI tables are available in Appendix A.

Nutrition-Focused Physical Assessment

Nutrition-Focused Physical Assessment (NFPA) is defined as, "findings from an evaluation of body systems, muscle and subcutaneous fat wasting, oral health, suck, swallow/breathe ability, appetite, and affect".[57] NFPA is a focused assessment that reviews selected parts of the body and body systems, looking at overall appearance, vital signs, skin, GI system, nerves and cognition, cardiopulmonary system, extremities including muscles and bones, and HEENT (head, eyes, ears, notes, and throat).[58] There are four classic techniques of physical examination

Table 2–22. Techniques of physical examination.

Physical Examination Technique	Description and Use in NFPA
Inspection	• General observation of details of appearance, behavior, and movements including facial expression, mood, conditioning, and skin color • In the focused observation, uses senses of sight, smell, and hearing; most frequently used technique
Palpation	• Tactile examination to feel pulsations and vibrations; assessment of body structures, including texture, size, temperature, tenderness, and mobility • NFPA assesses for edema, skin warmth, texture, tenderness, etc
Percussion	• Assessment of sounds to determine body organ borders, shape, and position • Not always used in nutrition-focused physical examination
Auscultation	• Use of the naked ear or a stethoscope to listen to body sounds • NFPA sounds include heart and lung sounds, bowel sounds, and blood vessels

Data from Hammond, 1996; Litchford, 2012.

(detailed in Table 2–22): inspection, palpation, percussion, and auscultation. The two techniques that are most commonly employed in NFPA are inspection and palpation.[59]

■ Body System Alterations and Nutrient Status

The following is a list of ways in which results of physical examination may shed light on nutrition status (Litchford, 2012):

Vital Signs:

- Hypotension and lower than usual blood pressure may be indicative of dehydration.
- Abnormal heart rate due to tachycardia, bradycardia, or arrhythmias can impair eating and lead to inadequate intake and involuntary weight loss.
- Target heart rates can shed light on physical fitness; the maximum age-related heart rate zone for men is 220 minus chronological age and for women 226 minus chronological age (when monitoring physical activity intensity, a person's target heart rate should be 50–70% of this maximum heart rate).[60]
- Oxygen saturation of 95% or greater is needed for wound healing; abnormal respiration that causes shortness of breath or

reliance on supplemental oxygen can lead to fatigue that impairs food and nutrient intake.

- Abnormal body temperatures indicate changes in health status that can lead to decreased appetite and intake.

Physical Strength:

- Hand grip strength—measured using a dynamometer and classified by manufacturers standards of excellent, good, average, fair, and poor performance—presents the strongest correlation between muscle mass and nutrition status.[61,62]

Changes in Skin:

Pressure ulcers are covered in Chapter 10. Table 2–23 outlines risk factors that increase risk for skin breakdown and pressure ulcers.

- Russell's sign (raw areas on knuckles seen in those who self-induce vomiting), inflamed or sore throat, swollen salivary glands, decayed tooth enamel, GERD, laxative abuse, and abnormal lab tests are all indicative of bulimia nervosa.
- Acanthosis nigricans (presence of dark, thick, and velvety skin in body folds and creases) is a reliable indicator of early metabolic syndrome, and insulin resistance in children and in adults is seen alongside conditions such as insulin resistance, metabolic

Table 2–23. Factors associated with increased risk for skin breakdown.

Advanced age
Low weight for height (low BMI) and low body weight (usually <85% IBW)
Bedbound or chairbound and/or alteration of intact skin with both excessively dry or moist skin
Inadequate dietary protein intake
Inflammation evidenced by low albumin or prealbumin
Compromised immune status evidenced by decreased total lymphocyte count
Presence of nutritional anemias, diabetes, cardiovascular instability/norepinephrine use, low BP, ankle brachial index, and oxygen use
Increased difficulty with self-feeding
Inadequate food intake
Requires assistance for 7 or more activities of daily living

Data from Litchford, 2012; European Pressure Ulcer Advisory Panel and National Pressure Ulcer Advisory Panel, 2009; Bergstrom et al., 2005.

syndrome, hypertension, dyslipidemia, Addison's disease, hypothyroidism, growth hormone therapy, and disorders of the pituitary gland.[58,63]

- Yellow and orange tints to skin can be indicative of overconsumption of beta-carotene from either food (dark orange and yellow fruits and vegetables) or dietary supplements.
- Light colored or pale conjunctivae or skin color may indicate nutritional anemia.
- Flushing of skin can be caused by high doses of supplemental niacin.
- Copper deficiencies—which can form as a result of oversupplementation with zinc or malabsorption associated with surgical weight loss—result in physical signs such as numbness in lower extremities, poor wound healing, and abnormal gait patterns.[58,64,65]

Changes in Hair and Nails:

- Hair loss can be triggered by stress related to major illness, polycystic ovary syndrome, thyroid disease and rapid weight loss, and inadequate protein, iron, zinc, and biotin following surgical weight loss procedure.[58]
- Bleeding nails may indicate malnutrition and give insight into potential deficiencies in magnesium, calcium, iron, zinc, sodium, and copper.[66]
- The presence of spoon-shaped, concave nails is called koilonychias and is common in children, usually resolving with aging; persistent koilonychias into adulthood may be caused by iron deficiency, diabetes mellitus, protein deficiency, or Raynaud's disease. Test for koilonychia using the water drop test: place a drop of water on the nail—if it does not slide off, the nail is flattened from early spooning.[67]
- Thin, brittle nails are seen in severe malnutrition, metabolic bone disease, and thyroid disorders.[67]

Hydration:

- With dehydration, hemoconcentration leads to elevated lab values of transferrin, sodium, BUN, creatinine, BUN:creatinine ratio, hemoglobin, and hematocrit.
- In overhydration or fluid accumulation, albumin, transferrin, and sodium levels are all decreased.[13]
- Physical signs of dehydration include dry and scaly skin, cracked lips, cracking around sides of mouth (cheilosis), and dry mucous membranes around lips, mouth, and tongue; tongue may be sunken in appearance.[58]
- Dehydration is apparent with poor skin turgor, evidenced when pinched skin does not spring back into place but stays in pinched position and sags back slowly.[68]
- Urine color is a good indicator of hydration status: the closer to clear or yellow the urine is, the more well hydrated a person is;

dark yellow or orange color and foul-smelling urine indicates dehydration.

Gastrointestinal Tract Cues:

- Loosened or "clicking" dentures may represent changes in mouth structure that accompany aging and can negatively impact intake and promote unintentional weight fluctuation.
- During abdominal examination, look for the "Six F's" of abdominal distention that explain possible etiology: fluid (ascites), fat (obesity), flatulence (gas), fetus (pregnancy), feces (constipation), and full-sized tumor (abnormal lesion).
- Hypoactive bowel sounds may be suggestive of ileus, peritonitis, or dysfunctional or nonfunctional gut following surgery and may indicate need for nutrition support via vein (TPN) if gut is not functional.

Bone Health:

- Reduced height and presence of kyphosis (curvature of the spine) indicates osteoporosis.
- Bowed legs in children indicate rickets and inadequate vitamin D and/or calcium intake or utilization.[58,69]

■ Vitamin- and Mineral-Specific Clues During NFPA

See Tables 2–24 to 2–27.

Nutrition Counseling Tips and Techniques

Nutrition counseling is defined as "a supportive process to set priorities, establish goals, and create individualized action plans that acknowledge and foster responsibility for self-care".[39] Maintaining objectivity and supporting behavior change are essential tools for nutrition counseling success. There are a number of personal characteristics and theoretical approaches that can facilitate positive behavior changes in those clients and patients who are actively engaged in nutrition counseling.

■ Characteristics of Effective Counseling

What are the characteristics of an effective counselor? Unfortunately, there is no hard and fast answer to this question. Your approach to providing nutrition information is much like that of your general patient interactions: highly personalized and individualized. You may be able to have a light-hearted, off-the-cuff conversation about sodium and potassium intake with one patient who has hypertension, while another may require a more calculated and directed message delivered in a serious and respectful tone. There is no "one-size-fits-all" approach when it comes to nutrition counseling. The directions you can take a patient with regards to your methods of imparting nutrition knowledge are truly limitless. While this may at first seem overwhelming, it may be helpful

Table 2-24. Fat-soluble vitamins, deficiency and toxicity.

Fat-Soluble Vitamin	Deficiency	Toxicity	Notes
Vitamin A	• Early signs of deficiency include changes in eyes, skin, hair, nails, and pruritus (itching), and chronic dry eye (not medication related) • Worsening deficiency leads to conjunctival xerosis, corneal xerosis, impaired night vision, xerophthalmia, and difficulty adjusting from light to dark environments (nyctalopia) • Cutaneous changes: dry skin, dermatitis, goose flesh (follicular hyperkeratosis), dry hair, and brittle nails • Advancing deficiency: Bitot's spots on sclera, hardened and scarred cornea, and permanent blindness	• Yellow-orange hue to skin from excess beta-carotene; usually harmless • Excess preformed vitamin A called hypervitaminosis A causes hypercalcemia, impaired bone remodeling, bone abnormalities, and decreased bone mass • High-dose vitamin A supplementation causes birth defects in pregnant women; pregnant women should not take preformed vitamin A supplements	• Deficiency is rare in developed countries, common in developing countries • Lab tests for deficiency include serum retinol, retinol-binding protein, zinc, and CBC • Beta-carotene not known to be teratogenic or cause reproductive toxicity • UL is 3,000 mcg RAE (10,000 IU) vitamin A and applies to products from animal sources and supplements only—not beta-carotene from plants
Vitamin D	• Same as risk factors for osteoporosis: kyphosis, reduction in height, and bone malformations/rickets/osteomalacia • Prolonged exclusive breastfeeding without supplemental vitamin D or adequate sunlight exposure can cause deficiency • Others at risk: older adults, limited sun exposure, dark skin, fat malabsorption, obese, or those status postgastric bypass surgery	• Toxicity symptoms: muscle weakness, apathy, headache, anorexia, irritability, nausea vomiting, bone pain, proteinuria, azotemia, declining kidney function, metastatic calcifications, hypertension, and cardiac arrhythmias	• Toxicity is unlikely from food sources; exception is high-dose consumption of cod liver oil • Upper Limit (UL) for vitamin D is 100 mcg (4,000 IU) per day • Lab test of 25(OH)D >150 ng/mL (>375 nmol/L) and serum calcium >11 mg/dL indicate vitamin D overload

Vitamin E	• Causes hemolytic anemia • Symptoms: hyporeflexia, ataxia, limitation in upward gaze, and profound muscle weakness • Severe deficiency: total blindness, cardiac arrhythmia, and dementia	• Acute toxicity: anorexia, polyuria, nausea, gastric distress, abdominal cramps, diarrhea, headache, fatigue, bruises easily, prolonged prothrombin time, muscle weakness, and creatinuria • Chronic toxicity: as above plus suppression of antioxidants, hemorrhagic stroke • Taking large doses with Coumadin can increase bleeding risk	• Deficiency is rare in developed countries because vitamin E prevalent in plant oils and oil/fat intake is high in these parts of the world • UL is 1,000 mg/d for adults • High-dose supplement does not protect against heart attacks, strokes, unstable angina, or death from CVD
Vitamin K	• Ecchymosis, petechiae, hematomas, menorrhagia, hematuria, bleeding gums, and blood loss at surgical and puncture sites • Elevated serum prothrombin time (PT) and activated partial thromboplastin time (apt)—may have high PT and normal apt level	• N/A	• Deficiency seen in alcoholics, malnourished, and long-term TPN reliance • No UL has been set

Data from National Institutes of Health Office of Dietary Supplements, 2011; Litchford, 2012.

Table 2–25. Water-soluble vitamins, deficiency and toxicity.

Water-Soluble Vitamin	Deficiency	Toxicity	Notes
Thiamin	• Deficiency disease called beriberi • Symptoms (early): fatigue, vomiting; (later) neurologic signs, ataxia, burning pain, progressive mental decline, memory loss, delusions, hallucinations, and psychosis • Similar changes to that are seen with vitamin B12 deficiency • CV symptoms: tachycardia, chest pain, heart failure, and hypotension • GI symptoms: anorexia, abdominal discomfort	• Rare but has been seen in those on TPN receiving 100× recommended intake levels • Symptoms: tachycardia, hypotension, cardiac dysrhythmia, headache, anaphylaxis, vasodilation, weakness, and convulsions	• Absorbed in jejunum • Beriberi—seen in LT peritoneal dialysis w/o replacement, starvation, alcoholism, s/p bariatric surgery, or IV infusion with high glucose content • Lab assessment not usually available • Can measure thiamin diphosphate in whole blood; pyruvate level >1mg/dL is indicative of deficiency as is erythrocyte transketolase activity of <0.017 u/dL • No UL established
Niacin	• Deficiency disease called pellagra • Pellagra characterized by 4 D's: dermatitis, diarrhea, dementia, and death • Primary deficiency can be caused by low intake or eating foods with niacin bound up (eg. maize not treated with alkali) • Secondary deficiency can be due to diarrhea, cirrhosis, and alcoholism • Symptoms (early): darkly pigmented rash on light-exposed areas of skin, burning in GI system; (later) nausea, vomiting, bloody diarrhea, neurologic symptoms, and death	• Causes niacin flush: flushing of skin on face, arms, chest, pruritus, nausea, and vomiting • Increases blood sugar • Causes peptic ulcers • Can lead to skin rashes	• Absorbed in stomach and small intestine • Dietary tryptophan can convert to meet niacin needs, if niacin intake inadequate • UL: 35 mg/day for adults

| Folate | Symptoms (early): fatigue, weakness, headaches, difficulty concentrating, palpitations, diarrhea, red tongue with soreness, yellow pallor; (later) pancytopenia, symptomatic megaloblastic anemia, high MCV and ferritin with low hemoglobin, serum iron, and hematocrit • Dx by confirming low serum folate, low erythrocyte folate, and high plasma homocysteine • Rule out vitamin B12 deficiency before diagnosing folate deficiency—normal methylmalonic acid (MMA) level differentiates folate deficiency from B12 as MM levels are high in B12 deficiency but not in folate deficiency | • High doses of folic acid intake can mask B12 deficiency • Folate toxicity from food unlikely • Folate toxicity from supplements or fortified foods also low because body stores of folate are low | • Absorbed in duodenum and proximal jejunum • Folic acid is synthetic form of folate found in supplements and fortified foods • UL is 1,000 mcg per day, but applies to synthetic forms from supplements, fortified foods, or combination of both |
| Vitamin B6 | • Dietary deficiency rare • Secondary deficiency from malnutrition, malabsorption, alcoholism, use of anticonvulsants, or isoniazid • Symptoms: peripheral neuropathy, anemia, depression, confusion, EEG abnormalities, and seizures • Causes pellagra-like condition with seborrheic dermatitis, glossitis, and cheilosis | • Megadose (>500 mg/day) erroneously recommended to treat carpal tunnel and premenstrual syndromes; unproven • Can cause peripheral neuropathy | • Fasting pyridoxal 5'-phosphate blood test indicates vitamin B6 nutrition status • UL is 100 mg/day for adults |

(Continued)

Table 2–25. Water-soluble vitamins, deficiency and toxicity. *(Continued)*

Water-Soluble Vitamin	Deficiency	Toxicity	Notes
Vitamin B12	• Possible in vegans as vitamin B12 sources are all animal foods • Caused by pernicious anemia and inadequate absorption and intake • Can be caused by surgical procedures, bacterial overgrowth and pancreatitis, and Zollinger-Ellison syndrome • Symptoms are "insidious and vague"; include weakness, sore tongue, paresthesia with anorexia, and weight loss in about ½ patients • Lemon-yellow waxy pallor, premature hair whitening, loss of sense of touch, stiffness in arms and legs, and tachycardia • May have red patches or soreness on tongue, change in taste, constipation, and diarrhea • Neurologic symptoms: paresthesias, weakness, clumsiness, unsteady gait, memory loss, irritability, and personality changes • "Megaloblastic madness": less common, delusions, hallucinations, outbursts, and paranoid schizophrenic behavior	• None reported	• B12 absorption reduced by omeprazole, lansoprazole, Tagamet, Pepcid, Zantac, cholestyramine, chloramphenicol, neomycin, colchicine, and metformin • Low B12 marked by low levels of hemoglobin, hematocrit, erythrocyte counts, lymphocyte and platelet counts, reticulocyte count, and serum vitamin B12 • Indirect bilirubin level may be high in deficiency as is serum iron, MCV, ferritin, methylmalonic acid, homocysteine, lactic dehydrogenase, and antiparietal cell antibodies • No UL established

| Biotin | • Seen in prolonged TPN without biotin supplementation
• Seen in very high raw egg white consumption—protein in egg white avidin binds biotin; avidin is denatured when egg white is cooked
• Symptoms confined to GI tract, skin, hair, CNS, and peripheral nervous system
• First signs: dry skin, skin lesions, fine and brittle hair, and alopecia
• Advanced: neurological symptoms, depression, somnolence, myalgias, hyperesthesias, paresthesias, nausea, vomiting, and anorexia | • None reported | • Long-term use of phenytoin, primidone, and carbamazepine can lead to biotin deficiency
• Hair loss after bariatric surgery can be related to biotin deficiency
• No UL established |

Data from National Institutes of Health Office of Dietary Supplements, 2011; Litchford, 2012.

Table 2-26. Selected minerals, deficiency and toxicity.

Mineral (Element)	Deficiency	Toxicity	Notes
Iodine	• Marked by goiter (can be seen in toxicity too) • See Table 2-27 for signs and symptoms of thyroid dysfunction	• Marked by goiter (can be seen in deficiency too)	• UL is 1,100 mcg/day for adults
Zinc	• Common in areas with malnutrition, causes growth retardation, impairs immune function, and loss of appetite • Severe cases: impairs glucose tolerance, diarrhea, alopecia, stomatitis, acrodermatitis enteropathica, paronychia, nystagmus, night blindness, blepharitis, delayed sexual maturation, impotence, hypogonadism in males, weight loss, delayed wound-healing, abnormalities in taste, and impaired concentration • Increased risk with advanced age, celiac disease, Crohn's disease, short bowel syndrome, AIDS enteropathy, ileostomy, chronic diarrhea, enteric fistula output, chronic liver disease, cirrhosis, nephritic syndrome, diabetes, alcoholism, trauma, burns, sickle cell anemia, and high alcohol intake • Losses seen with large wounds, diarrhea, and after sleeve gastrectomy weight loss surgery	• High doses cause nausea, vomiting, anorexia, abdominal cramping, diarrhea, and headaches • High doses can impair copper status, alter iron function, lead to incurable anemia, impair immune function, and lower HDL	• UL is 40 mg/day for adults • Body cannot store zinc • Medication use that promotes loss of zinc: penicillamine, diuretics, diethylenetriamine pentaacetate, and valproate • Do not take calcium supplements with zinc supplements because of lowered absorption of both

Data from National Institute of Health Office of Dietary Supplements, 2011; Litchford, 2012.

Table 2–27. Signs and symptoms of dysfunction.

Hyperthyroidism Symptoms	Hypothyroidism Symptoms
Unexplained weight loss	Unexplained weight gain, puffy face
Tremors, nervousness, restlessness, anxiety	Taste & smell alterations
Heat intolerance	Cold intolerance
Rapid heart rate, tremors	Slowed heart rate
Fatigue	Fatigue
Diarrhea, frequent bowel movements	Constipation
Difficulty concentrating	Depression
Exophthalmos (protruding eyes)	Joint and muscle pain
Increased appetite	Hashimoto's: fullness in throat
Goiter	Goiter, hoarse voice
Thinning hair and hair loss	Thinning hair, brittle nails
Increased sweat production	Reduced sweat production
Edema	Elevated triglycerides and cholesterol
Menstrual irregularities	Menstrual irregularities, infertility

Data from Litchford, 2012.

http://www.nlm.nih.gov/medlineplus/ency/article/000356.htm.

http://www.endocrine.niddk.nih.gov/pubs/hypothyroidism/

to note that while there is no one right way to provide nutrition counseling, it also means that there is really no one wrong way to do the same!

In one study that looked at the personal characteristics of effective counselors, ten expert counselors were questioned about 22 personality characteristics that could be attributable to effective counselors. The experts ranked empathy, acceptance, and warmth as the most important characteristics, while the least important traits included resourcefulness, sympathy, and sociability.[70]

■ Empathy

To express empathy means that you are identifying with and understanding the other person's feelings, beliefs, and point of view. Essentially, expressing empathy is not just about putting yourself in another person's shoes, but also forcing yourself to shift perspective.[71] Take the example of organic foods. While you might personally extol the environmental and ethical reasons behind increasing organic food intake, if your client

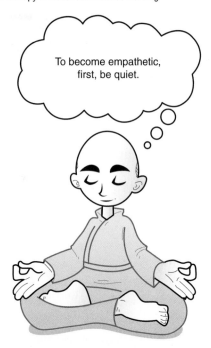

Figure 2–9. An empathetic person is a good listener.

has a minimal, fixed income and cites financial reasons behind his or her limited fruit and vegetable intake, are you being empathetic when you tout organics? Probably not. In this situation, the empathetic thing would be to first ask yourself, "If I were this client, why would I not be eating more fruits and vegetables?" If the answer is, "Because I don't think I can afford them," then a recommendation to buy the most expensive tier of fruits and vegetables would be inappropriate. An empathetic counselor listens patiently, processes the information internally, and seeks to truly understand the other person's perspective before responding.

To become empathetic, first, be quiet. Listen to your client and process what he or she is saying. Too often we are so excited to share what we know about the benefits of this and the drawbacks of that, that we end up imparting information before truly understanding the issue at hand (Figure 2–9). Lastly, when considering empathy, Murphy and Dillon caution interviewers not to confuse empathy with sympathy, saying, "Empathy is not sympathy. Sympathy is what I feel toward you; empathy is what I feel as you."[71]

■ Supportiveness

While it is often unlikely that you can fix someone else's problems, letting that person know that you are there to support him or her can help the individual work toward solutions of their own. One way you can offer support is to provide information about what others in a similar situation have done. Consider referring people who are interested in weight loss to the National Weight Control Registry (NWCR). The NWCR was established in 1994 by researchers from Brown Medical School and the University of Colorado. It tracks people who have lost 30 pounds and kept that weight off for at least one year or more. Researchers then analyze what the more than 10,000 people enrolled in the registry have in common, and how their exercise and eating patterns influence or have influenced their successful weight loss. Motivated clients may find inspiration and strength in the researchers' findings. For example, 78% of the successful losers eat breakfast every day and 90% exercise, on average, at least 1 hour per day. Learn more at http://www.nwcr.ws/.

▪ Warmth

The renowned Dallas Cowboys football coach Jimmy Johnson once said, "The only thing worse than a coach or CEO who doesn't care about his people is one who pretends to care. People can spot a phony every time." Your clients know exactly when you don't care; but they also know and respond positively when you *do* care. When you sit down to talk about food, nutrition, or weight—or any sensitive topic for that matter—don't be a phony. Leave your attitude, judgments, and preconceived notions at the door. Think about where people are coming from, and learn where they are going.

Take the case of an overweight client named Rose. Rose is 250 pounds, and she has type 2 diabetes. If you were to meet Rose in your clinic waiting room, you might think, "Wow, Rose is huge, and I bet her blood sugar is through the roof." But what you don't know is that just a year ago, Rose weighed over 350 pounds, and she had been hospitalized multiple times for diabetic ketoacidosis. A perceptive intern in the emergency department recognized Rose as having been admitted multiple times for the same diagnosis. Upon discharge the intern initiated a casual discussion with Rose about an outpatient diabetes clinic that she might consider to help her lose weight, improve her glycemic control, and ultimately eliminate the need for her to endure the recurrent, expensive, and stressful hospital admissions. The intern stressed that he was concerned for Rose's well-being and recommended the clinic as a means to help her out. Rose reacted positively to the intern's warmth and concern for her well-being, and she eventually enrolled in the diabetes self-management program. She has been working with the clinic's diabetes educators on gradually losing weight, improving her diet, and increasing her exercise capacity. Rose is not at her goal, but she is getting there, and all it took was the warmth of a concerned healthcare practitioner to redirect her path from a downward health spiral into a more healthful direction. Now that you know Rose's story, do you see her in a different light as she sits in your waiting room?

When you are prepared to broach the topic of nutrition or food with your patients, be yourself. Have a strategy, but be conversational and try to avoid overly technical language or medical jargon. Talk in frank terms about evidence-based strategies for improving health with nutrition. And above all, always keep in mind that you cannot judge a book by the cover: you must take the time to read the whole story.

Theoretical Approaches to Nutrition Counseling

There are a number of theoretical approaches to nutrition counseling that can be enacted to affect behavior change. In the one-on-one or group counseling environment, it may be helpful to think of yourself more of as a coach than as a teacher. If you keep goal-setting a person-centered and patient-directed activity, you can help guide your clients to set, plan for, work toward, and achieve their own goals. Ultimately, however, *they* need to be in the driver's seat if the changes are truly going to "stick."

■ The Health Belief Model

The Health Belief Model (HBM) was developed in the 1950s to help social psychologists in the US Public Health Service more clearly understand why people did not participate in programs designed to prevent and detect disease.[72,73] HBM is constructed on the assumptions that a negative health condition or disease state is avoidable, that taking a particular action can lead to avoidance of such a condition or disease state, and that the individual maintains the power to exert control over the behavior that can lead to positive changes or outcomes.

For example, an individual with chronic kidney disease can choose to acknowledge that chronic kidney disease is not inevitable, that limiting phosphorus intake can mitigate kidney damage, and that with the right amount of knowledge and education, the person can control his phosphorus intake in order to improve kidney function. Table 2–28 outlines the basic constructs of the HBM.

■ The Transtheoretical Model and Stages of Change

The Transtheoretical Model, also called the Stages of Change Model, is applicable in many counseling environments, and can also be helpful to identify where a client is with regards to his or her readiness to change nutrition behaviors. The model has been designed to help explain behavior changes related to smoking cessation, stress management, and diet improvements, and it consists of six stages: precontemplation, contemplation, preparation, action, maintenance, and termination. In some models, relapse is added as a seventh stage. The practitioner can use the Stages of Change to determine what stage a particular learner or patient may be at. Table 2–29 defines the individual stages and provides an application statement for each stage based on an individual who has received a recommendation to begin walking 30 minutes per day in

Table 2-28. Health belief model constructs and nutrition application.

Health Belief Model Construct	Definition	Nutrition Application Perception Statement
Perceived susceptibility	Belief about the likelihood of contracting a disease or getting a particular medical condition	"I believe that because my family has a strong history of colon cancer that I also am at risk for colon cancer."
Perceived severity	Belief about how serious a disease or medical condition is	"My uncle had diabetes and lost his left foot. I know it is a serious condition with life-changing consequences."
Perceived benefits	Belief in the effectiveness of recommended actions to reduce risk or severity of disease or medical condition	"If I work on decreasing my saturated fat and increasing my dietary fiber, maybe I can avoid having to take a statin drug for my cholesterol."
Perceived barriers	Belief about impediments to success in preventing or treating the disease or medical condition	"Only rich people can afford all the fruits and vegetables I should probably be eating to help me lose weight."
Cues to action	Strategies intended to promote readiness	"When I learned that I had prediabetes and that it meant I might get diabetes, I got scared and decided to do something about my eating habits."
Self-efficacy	Belief or confidence in one's own ability to take positive action	"I know it's going to be hard to maintain a gluten-free diet to help my celiac disease, but I saw my neighbor do it, and I think I can do it too."

order to control high blood pressure as an alternative to beginning on a blood pressure lowering medication (Figure 2–10).[13,74]

■ Cognitive Behavioral Therapy

Cognitive behavioral therapy (CBT) represents the blending of two therapies, cognitive therapy (CT) and behavioral therapy.[75] CBT assumes that behaviors are learned and that these behaviors are linked to both internal and external triggers that lead to problem behavior. CBT encourages the person to examine his or her thoughts and beliefs, to analyze how they affect moods and actions, and to direct changes in

Table 2-29. Stages of change and nutrition application.

Stage	Definition	Sample Statement at Stage	Techniques for Counselor
Precontemplation	No intention to take any action within the next 6 months	"I'm really busy at work right now and probably will be through the holidays and then into tax season. Starting a walking program right now just isn't going to work with my schedule."	• Validate lack of readiness • Help clients to clarify that the decision belongs to them • Encourage re-evaluation of current behaviors • Encourage self-exploration (not action)
Contemplation	Intends to take action within the next 6 months	"OK, I am too young to be so out of breath just walking up these stairs! I think by my birthday I need to get into a routine where I walk every day to get in shape."	• Validate lack of readiness • Help clients to clarify that the decision belongs to them • Encourage evaluation of pros and cons of behavior change • Identify and promote new, positive outcome expectations
Preparation	Intends to take action within the next 30 days and has taken some behavioral steps in this direction	"Those new walking shoes I just bought were sure expensive. But it is an investment in my health, and I am going to use them soon, no matter what!"	• Identify and assist in problem solving • Assist client to identify social supports • Verify that client has the underlying skills for behavior change • Encourage initial small steps

Stage	Description	Actions
Action	Changed overt behavior for less than 6 months	"I've been walking on my lunch break every day for a few weeks now, and I'm surprised it wasn't as bad as I thought it would be."	• Continue reinforcing the decision to act • Focus on restructuring cues and social support • Promote self-efficacy for handling obstacles • Combat feelings of loss by echoing long-term benefits that the client has identified
Maintenance	Changed overt behavior for more than 6 months	"I've been walking either on my lunch break or before or after work for 30 minutes every weekday, for the last 9 months."	• Plan for follow-up support • Reinforce internal rewards and health benefits • Discuss coping with relapse
Termination, or in alternate case, Relapse	**Termination:** No temptation to relapse and 100% confidence **Relapse:** Resumption of previous behavior	"Doing my daily walk is now just part of my routine. I don't even think twice about it. I know that it helps keep my weight at a good spot and my blood pressure down, and most importantly, I don't have to take any medications." Relapse statement (patient reverts to Preparation phase): "I have stopped walking and am back to my old sedentary ways. But I'm bringing my shoes with me to work tomorrow, so I can exercise on my lunch break."	• For relapse: evaluate triggers for relapse—what caused the relapse? • Reassess motivation and barriers.

Data from Glanz et al., 2008; Academy of Nutrition and Dietetics, 2012.

Stages of change

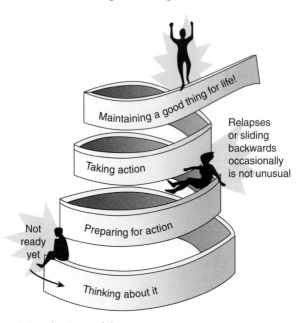

Maintaining a good thing for life!

Relapses
or sliding
backwards
occasionally
is not unusual

Taking action

Not
ready
yet

Preparing for action

Thinking about it

Figure 2–10. The stages of change.

behavior that reflect a more positive health outlook. With CBT, the intervention targets identification of erroneous thoughts and beliefs, such as, "I can't lose weight" or "Carbohydrates are fattening", and modifies those thoughts and beliefs. With behavioral therapy, individuals are encouraged to experience a heightened awareness about environmental triggers to eating (smells, emotions, social situations, etc) and to modify those stimuli and responses.[13] Practitioners of CBT may encourage participants to keep records and journals of eating events, associated feelings and emotions, surroundings, and other thoughts and beliefs in order to identify triggers of problematic behavior. Other cognitive behavior strategies include goal setting, action planning, management of barriers, and self-monitoring.[76]

Cognitive Behavior Therapy: What Does the Evidence Say?
There is strong evidence to support the claim that cognitive-behavioral therapy (CBT), of short, intermediate, or long duration targeted to reduce cardiovascular disease and diabetes risk factors, diabetes management, and/or weight loss, results in health/food behavior change in adults counseled in an outpatient/clinic setting.[39]

- ■ Motivational Interviewing

Although motivational interviewing (MI) was originally developed to address addictive behavior, it is also adaptable for use in nutrition counseling. MI assumes that people digress from their path to goal achievement due to a lack of motivation. Motivational interviewing has been described as "an empathetic person-centered counseling approach that prepares people for change by helping them resolve ambivalence, enhance intrinsic motivation, and build confidence to change."[77] One way in which the motivational interview can promulgate change is by practicing OARS: asking **O**pen-ended questions, providing **A**ffirmation statements, practicing **R**eflective listening and **S**ummarizing (Table 2–30).[78] The motivational interviewer works to promote a focus on strategies that will help motivate the client to build the commitment required to make a behavior change.[79] The basic principles of MI are outlined in Table 2–31, and specific strategies involved in MI are covered in Table 2–32.[78,80]

Other Behavior Change Strategies: What Does the Evidence Say?

There are strong data suggesting that when combined as part of a behavioral program, the use of self-monitoring (such as keeping a food diary), meal replacements or structured meal plans, and reward and reinforcement results in health or food behavior change in adults who are counseled in an outpatient or clinic setting.

There are fair data suggesting that the behavioral strategies of problem-solving, social support, and goal-setting result in health or food behavior change in adults who are counseled in an outpatient or clinic setting.

There are limited data suggesting that the behavioral strategies of cognitive restructuring and the use of MI alone result in health/food behavior changes in adults who are counseled in an outpatient or clinic setting.

When used as an adjunct to cognitive-behavioral program, there is strong evidence suggesting that MI results in health/food behavior changes in adults who are counseled in an outpatient or clinic setting.[39]

Table 2–30. The OARS of motivational interviewing.

Open-ended questioning
Affirmations
Reflective listening
Summaries

Data from Miller et al., 2002.

Table 2–31. Basic principles of motivational interviewing.

Express empathy
Put yourself in the other person's shoes in order to understand that person's perspective
Develop discrepancy
Highlight and intensify obvious discrepancies between current behavior and stated goals to the point where changing from current behavior becomes the recognizable course of action
Avoid escalating resistance
Monitor for and avoid approaching signs of resistance, such as discussions that become argumentative, reluctant or full of denial; change course if resistance escalates
Roll with resistance
When resistance does occur: go with it; create a supportive environment where the client can contemplate expressing fears about change without feeling judged
Support self-efficacy
Promote the client's belief and confidence that he or she can achieve the stated goal

Data from Bauer and Sokolik, 2002.

Table 2–32. Strategies for motivational interviewing.

Allow clients to come to their own conclusions about pros and cons of proposed change
Assist with, but do not push clients into decision making
Give examples of how others in similar situations have acted or decided
Reinforce the idea that ultimately, the client is the best judge of what will work
Do not project your ideas about how the client should feel regarding his or her condition
Present an array of options and choices
Clarify goals when necessary
Acknowledge that failing to reach a decision to change does not constitute a failed session
Anticipate fluctuating levels of commitment
Express empathy with the client's situation

Data from Rollnick et al., 1992.

Nutrition Counseling Tips

Your individual nutrition counseling style is more likely to be a compilation of bits and pieces of the aforementioned models and constructs than to fit nicely into one of its defined boxes. Just as there is no one diet or weight loss plan that works for all people, there is no one approach to nutrition counseling that is appropriate for all patient types. The following recommendations are provided for you to consider as you work toward becoming more comfortable broaching sensitive food and diet topics with your patients and to help you develop your own nutrition counseling style.

■ Use Evidence Based Medicine

Take a look around our food environment and you will see that opinions are everywhere. *This* is the new super food…*that* is the new dream diet. It seems that everywhere we turn, we are being pushed in different directions with regards to food and nutrition. One day butter is better for you, the next day margarine is. Egg yolks are in; egg yolks are out. Eat small frequent meals; never eat between meals. How can a busy practitioner possibly process and stay on top of all of this information, not to mention put it into usable pieces of data for our patients and clients?

If you start to feel overwhelmed about your ability to stay on top of the latest food and nutrition information, save your sanity by turning to evidence-based medicine. The term evidence-based medicine (EBM) is thought to have first been used by investigators from McMaster's University during the 1990s. EBM has been defined as "a systemic approach to analyze published research as the basis of clinical decision making", and then more formally defined by Sacket et al., who stated that EBM was "the conscientious and judicious use of current best evidence from clinical care research in the management of individual patients."[81] In our lightning fast era of web searches, quasi-professionals, and self-diagnoses, the validity of EBM far surpasses any other sources of information. On the other hand, not using EBM may challenge your professional liability (Table 2–33).[82]

Table 2–33. The five steps of evidence-based public health.

1. Identify the problem
2. Assess the extent of the problem
3. Propose a solution
4. Implement program
5. Assess compliance and impact

Data from King, 2007.

What is the USDA's Nutrition Evidence Library?

The USDA's Nutrition Evidence Library (NEL) specializes in conducting systematic reviews to inform federal nutrition policy and programs. The NEL evaluates, synthesizes, and grades the strength of the evidence that supports recommendation statements. The NEL employs an objective and transparent methodology to define the state of food and nutrition-related science, and the library is a readily available resource for food and nutrition research that is accessible to the public. You can access the NEL at: http://www.nutritionevidencelibrary.gov/.

In 2005, the Dietary Guidelines Advisory Committee (DGAC), the group who is responsible for setting forth the revised *Dietary Guidelines for Americans* (DGAs) every 5 years, was advised to focus their analysis on scientific evidence that links diet and health.[82] The 2005 DGAC used a modified systematic review process to address its research questions. For the 2010 revision of the *Dietary Guidelines for Americans*, the DGAC used a new method that drew from the newly established USDA Nutrition Evidence Library. The 2010 process involved conducting evidence-based, systematic reviews of the research related to the major questions addressed by the guidelines. Of the 180 questions posed, 130 were addressed using this method.[37]

Websites such as the USDA's Nutrition Evidence Library (http://www.nutritionevidencelibrary.gov/), the National Guideline Clearinghouse (http://guideline.gov/), and the Academy of Nutrition and Dietetics Evidence Analysis Library (http://andevidencelibrary.com) are useful starting points for obtaining the most current and up-to-date nutrition and food-related recommendations.

■ Stay Current

In our rapidly evolving healthcare and food environments, we are constantly inundated with information. Patients and clients turn to practitioners to help them decipher confusing and conflicting messages. It is certainly a challenge to stay current, but there are an ever-increasing number of resources to help you do so. While you can never read all of the most recent published scientific literature, there are credible newsletters that will summarize it for you! Consider subscribing to mailed, hard copy summary health letters such as University of California, Berkeley's Wellness Letter, The Center for Science in the Public Interest's (CSPI) Nutrition Action Health Letter, and Tufts Health & Nutrition Letter. Get electronic news and updates from reputable nutrition sources such as the Harvard School of Public Health's The Nutrition Source page, Nutrition.gov, or the Mayo Clinic, and sign up for your professional association's weekly email newsletters.

Another way to stay current is to be aware of what is obsolete. In nutrition, diet therapies that have shown to be ineffective through scientific research have a habit of sticking around in day-to-day practice long after they have been disproven. For example, in the past geriatric patients would be placed on overly restricted diets (eg, low-cholesterol, low-fat, sodium-restricted, and calorie-controlled diabetic diets) while in hospitals or long-term care facilities; however, authoritative nutrition bodies now assert that these overly restrictive diet orders should be avoided because they promote inadequate nutrient intake in these individuals.[13] The overarching goal of nutrition therapy for those who are ill is to promote the least-restrictive diet. Promoting liberalized diets may involve a certain level of "unlearning" on the part of the practitioner, who hears, sees, and reads about specific dietary recommendations for disease states, but does not understand that ordering such a restrictive diet may actually promote undernutrition in sick patients. Table 2–34 contains a list of previously used therapeutic diets and nutrition approaches that are now considered to be obsolete. Look around your place of work and note how many of them you still see regularly implemented in practice.[13]

■ Establish Rapport

As with any new relationship, establishing good rapport is an essential first step in the nutrition counseling process. Rapport can be defined as a harmonious relation.[83] Without this good foundation of rapport, your counseling session can quickly go awry. Human beings are naturally reticent to talk about highly personal and sensitive topics such as weight, exercise, diet, and disease. If you make your patients feel comfortable with you and create a judgment-free zone and environment, they are going to be more likely to divulge information that will be essential for patient-driven problem solving. Table 2–35 contains some tips for establishing rapport in a counseling session.

■ Know Your ABC's

Behavior modification theories are based on the notion that our behaviors involve three factors: antecedents or signals that lead to a behavior, the actual behavior, and the consequences of that behavior. Behavior modification approaches can be summarized as identifying the ABCs of your actions: identify the **a**ntecedent, acknowledge the **b**ehavior, and examine the **c**onsequence.

Take the case of Sylvia, a working mother who is trying to lose weight. Sylvia was busy this morning, and she skipped lunch during her workday. She tells herself she wants to exercise and go for a walk when she arrives home. She walks in the house, through the kitchen, and passes an open bag of potato chips on the counter. Famished from not having eaten all day, she devours the bag of chips. Sylvia then starts to feel bad about having consumed the chips, and instead of going for her walk, she decides to start cooking dinner so she can at least get one productive thing done that day. Sylvia makes a healthy dinner for her

Table 2–34. Examples of obsolete therapeutic diets.

Kidney Disease

- Renal diet: a single diet for all renal diseases
- Low-protein diet
- 60 gram protein, 2 gram sodium, and 2 gram potassium diet

Pressure Ulcers

- High-protein, high-kilocalorie diets without consideration of individual protein and energy needs, increased fluid requirements, obesity, and changes in GI tolerance that are associated with malnutrition

Diabetes

- The ADA (American Diabetes Association) diet that has never been clearly defined
- Diets for diabetes that prescribe one set calorie level or one set of percentages of macronutrient distribution
- No concentrated sweets, no sugar added, low sugar, liberal diabetic diets may all unnecessarily restrict sucrose, fructose (eg, fruits), or lactose (eg, milk or yogurt)

GI Diets

- Clear liquid diets traditionally used for diarrhea are high in sugar, promote hyperosmolality, and may exacerbate diarrhea
- Diets for diverticular disease have historically recommended avoidance of nuts, seeds, and hulls despite a lack of supporting literature
- The use of very low fat or fat-free diets is no longer required for the treatment of gallbladder disease
- Recommending a bland diet or utilizing milk or to treat heartburn or bland and "sippy" diets for peptic ulcers are obsolete practices
- With pancreatitis, use of the traditional progression from clear liquid diet to a full liquid diet that is high in fat and lactose-containing foods may exacerbate symptoms and those who have been NPO for long periods of time have lowered levels of lactase; rather, progression should be to a solid, low-lactose, low-fat, high-protein diet that promotes tolerance during the recovery phase
- Historically, patients with pancreatitis were routinely placed on TPN in order to provide nutrition; however, research has now shown that early initiation of enteral feeds promotes GI function and assists with faster recovery and shorter hospital length-of-stay

Cirrhosis and Hepatitis

- Diet was historically protein-restricted; understanding now is that protein restriction leads to inadequate intake and related malnutrition—very few patients are protein sensitive or intolerance, and most do not need a protein restriction
- Fat and caffeine restriction in hepatitis is now only indicated if symptoms of the liver disease dictate

Urolithiasis/Urinary Stones

- The use of a low-calcium diet for stone prevention is outdated and no longer recommended

Data from Academy of Nutrition and Dietetics, 2012.

Table 2–35. Tips for establishing rapport in a counseling session.

Do your background research before the client arrives, and greet the client by name
Use a firm but not overpowering handshake and make eye contact when greeting the client
Introduce yourself briefly and then ask open-ended questions of the client for his or her introduction
Avoid the urge to interrupt unnecessarily, to pass judgment, or to convey bias in your communications
Offering the client a glass of water, coffee, or tea may help set the stage for a conversational rather than confrontational session

family but doesn't eat much of it, since she is full from eating the chips and feeling badly about skipping her exercise.

As a counselor, you can help Sylvia identify the ABCs of her behavior and suggest changes that can redirect these ABCs in a more positive direction. In the scenario just presented, the antecedents were skipping lunch and the presence of the potato chips on the table. The behaviors were eating all of the chips and then not walking. The consequences were her feelings of guilt from overeating and not participating in the healthy meal she made for her family.

How can Sylvia redirect her ABCs into a more healthful direction? Imagine now a different scenario whereby Sylvia makes herself a healthy lunch in the morning before leaving for work. She eats her lunch at work, and when she arrives home after her workday, she is hungry, but not famished. Sylvia enters her house where she encounters her workout clothes and an orange she left for a snack on a chair next to the door in the morning when she left for work. She eats her healthy snack, puts on her walking clothes, and takes a brisk walk. When she returns, she feels rejuvenated and is energized to cook a healthy meal for her family. Sylvia eats the healthy meal and feels satisfied. In this version, the antecedents (having had a healthy lunch and placed her orange and working clothes in an easily accessible place) drove the behaviors (the walk and subsequent healthy meal cooking) that led to the positive consequence (emotions of contentment or satisfaction).

■ Acknowledge Different Learning Styles

An effective counselor acknowledges that there are many different types of learners. When it comes to food and nutrition, your experience with learning styles is likely to run the gamut. You will encounter the "Just tell me what to eat and I'll do it!" type, while your next patient may say, "If you teach me about carbohydrates, I can work them into my meal planning for diabetes management." Some people are more number-oriented and want percentages and numbers of calories, while others are word-oriented and respond well to "eat more" and "eat less" messages. You have visual learners who will easily conceptualize portion size comparisons when given standard household measurements, but you will also have kinesthetic learners who will conceptualize portion sizes by touching and feeling food models. Be prepared to counsel using various techniques because not everyone learns in the same manner. A few simple questions directed at the outset of your session or appointment regarding the patient's preferred learning style can set you, as the educator, on the right path.

■ Individualize Your Approach

Just as a prescribed calorie level for all people with diabetes has fallen out of favor, so has the "one-size-fits-all" approach to nutrition counseling. The conventional wisdom now maintains that any nutrition information you disseminate should be individualized and tailored to fit the patient or client. Whereas *you* may eat three meals per day, your client might work a swing shift schedule that impedes his or her ability to do so. A plan that works for one person might not be appropriate for another. Ask clients to tell you about their usual day, their typical eating patterns, personal diet and weight history, and perceived barriers to success in order to provide you with data needed to create an individualized meal plan. Chapter 1 contains more information on healthy meal planning.

■ Avoid Bias

The term social distance refers to the variations in characteristics that may exist in the clinician-patient relationship.[74] Age, race, gender, and lifestyle have the potential to either strengthen or lessen the patient-provider bond. In a judgment-free environment, practitioners are encouraged to express empathy, share understanding, show attentiveness, and ask questions about the patients' beliefs and value system in order to elicit communication, respect, and information from the client that can help improve his or her nutritional status.

■ Practice Reflective Listening

Reflective listening is an essential skill for an effective listener to have. It helps fill in gaps in communication and to avoid misunderstanding. There are three primary levels of reflective listening:

- Repeating or rephrasing: listener uses synonyms or substitutes phrases, staying close to what the speaker has said
- Paraphrasing: listener provides a restatement that reaffirms the tone and intent of what the speaker has said

- Reflection of feeling: listener highlights the emotional content of speakers' statements—this is considered to be the deepest form of listening.[84]

Examples of reflective listening statements include, "So you feel like cutting back on your number of fast food meals is going to be a challenge?," "It sounds like you have identified a number of higher fiber fruit options that you can take to work for between meal snacks," and "You are wondering if reducing the amount of wine you drink is going to affect your ability to have a good time in social situations." While restating the patient's words may seem repetitive, it ensures that you understand what they are saying, and it gives them the opportunity to clarify information that may have previously been misinterpreted.

■ Ask Open-Ended Questions

Open-ended questions allow respondents to tell their own story without feeling that they have to take the answer in a prescribed direction. One way to think about asking more open-ended questions is to focus on asking *less* closed questions. A closed question is one that leads the respondent in a particular direction, more simply put: a yes/no question. "Did you have breakfast this morning?" implies that I, as the counselor expect that you, as the respondent, eat breakfast. Even if you didn't eat breakfast, you might *say* you did because the question indicates that the questioner places some value on this thing called "breakfast." Additionally, including "this morning" as part of the question implies that I think you woke up in the morning, which, depending upon your schedule or personal preference, could be entirely untrue. A better way to reframe that question as an open-ended question would be to ask, "Tell me about the first thing or things you ate or drank after getting up today." More examples of open question lead-ins include:

- How can I help you with ____?
- Help me understand ____?
- When are you most likely to ____?
- When have you tried before to make a change?
- When might you be most ready to ____?
- How would you like things to be different?
- What are the good things about ____ and what are the less-than-good things about ____?[84]

When asking open-ended questions, start with words like who, what, when, where, how, and why as opposed to words like did, could, and would.

■ Set SMART Goals

The Academy of Nutrition and Dietetics recommends the following sequence of steps for helping clients set goals related to diet. The practitioner serves to:

Table 2-36. Writing SMART goals and objectives.

Specific	• Limit to one action verb • Avoid vague terms • The more specific, the more measurable the outcome is
Measurable	• Focus on "how much" change is desired • Objective should provide a reference point from which deviation and change can be measured
Achievable	• Attainable within time frame • Attainable with given resources
Realistic	• Accurately address the scope of the problem • If objective does not directly relate to the goal, it is not helpful
Time-phased	• Time frame indicating when objective will be accomplished • Time-phased goals set the stage for planning and evaluation of the intervention

Data from CDC, 2009.

- Facilitate client identification of nutrition-related goals
- Evaluate the pros and cons of goal(s) and ask the client to prioritize one goal
- Ask the client to describe how he or she plans to accomplish the goal and ask questions to help the client clarify important details of the plan
- Determine when, where, and how frequently they will do this
- Identify a way to measure if the goal was attained
- Identify nutrition subgoals (eg, a subgoal for a long-term goal of eliminating less than healthful snacks would be to eliminate the morning doughnut snack and determine a realistic alternative.)
- Establish client commitment, including the identification of obstacles that might prevent goal attainment and providing resources that may be helpful in goal achievement

When working with clients to craft goals and objectives, aim for outcomes that adhere to the SMART criteria. A SMART objective is one that is: specific, measurable, achievable, realistic, and time-phased or timely. Table 2–36 contains more detail on writing SMART objectives.[85]

■ Assign Homework

Although you may think of homework in the context of younger patients and clients, you may be surprised to learn that many adults actually *like* homework! As part of your goal setting in nutrition counseling, consider assigning homework for your client to complete between sessions. As part of your summary statements at the end of a session, you might work with the client to identify, for example, two food-related and one exercise-related homework assignments. Keep these assignments client-directed; remembering that you "telling" someone what to do in the next day/week/month is less effective than that person telling you what he or is she is likely to do. Examples of food-related homework may include:

- I will take two pieces of fruit with me to work for my between-meal snacks; I will place them on my desk and not let myself leave work until I have eaten those two pieces of fruit.
- I will go through my pantry and remove all of the processed and package high-salt and high-fat junk foods and either throw them out or donate them.
- I will measure out the amount of fluid allowed by my fluid restriction at the beginning of each day for the next week to help me stay within my fluid limits.
- I will try one new vegetable before our next session.

Examples of exercise-related homework assignments:

- I will go for a 20-minute walk on my lunch break at least one day during this upcoming work week.
- I will reactivate my gym membership this week.
- I will establish an exercise partner who I can work out with at least two times per week before our next session.

When working with clients on identifying useful homework assignments, start small and think baby steps. As a provider, your goal in this role might be as simple to help your clients stay reasonable. If Barbara hasn't been off the couch in months, it is unlikely that she will immediately start going to the gym 6 days per week. Even if she does, the change is too dramatic, making it unlikely to result in sustainable behavior change. A more realistic homework assignment might be for Barbara to walk around the block five separate times before your next session.

■ Track Outcomes Besides Weight

Too often in nutrition counseling, the focus is on weight. "I lost five pounds, and I feel great" can easily turn into, "I didn't lose as much weight as I intended, and now I feel discouraged." Encourage your clients to focus on positive outcomes that *don't* come from the scale. It is inspiring for patients to be able to tighten their belts one more notch, to watch their pant size go down and for them to see muscles develop where fat once existed. Celebrate nonweight-related victories such as improvements in lab values, reductions in blood pressure, increasing exercise capacity, and improved sleep patterns. For weight loss, while it is important to track weight regularly, highlight other areas of progress to discourage an overemphasis on weight. Many clients are inclined to weigh themselves every morning in order to track their weight loss, but this may set them up for disappointment. It may be prudent to have them only weigh themselves one time per week, or once every 2 weeks, in order to focus on the behaviors they are changing, as opposed to a number on the scale.

▪ Plan for Pitfalls

Thomas Edison once said, "I have not failed. I've just found 10,000 ways that won't work." Your journey with patients to their food and nutrition goals will no doubt encounter obstacles, roadblocks, and failures. Relationships do not disintegrate because of setbacks, but rather because of an inability to deal with setbacks. As a practitioner, you are the coach that helps your clients and patients deal with setbacks. In anticipation of potential hiccups, be proactive and brainstorm with your clients what might go wrong with the set plan. In diet therapy, it may help to think of an informal approach called "cruise management." If a client is getting ready to go on a cruise, he or she is going to encounter a pretty predictable food situation: trapped on a boat in the middle of the ocean with innumerable opportunities to eat coupled with an inherent pressure to eat like you're getting your money's worth! Visualize scenarios that may arise, talk about how the scenario might be handled, and offer suggestions for mitigating damage. Holidays, social gatherings, and family reunions present challenging environments for keeping to a set plan. Setbacks are inevitable, but being prepared for those inevitable setbacks promotes success. Remind your clients, "If you fail to plan, you plan to fail."

▪ Know Your Limits (Otherwise Known as: Refer to the Dietitian)

In many areas of the healthcare arena there is an increasing awareness about the relationship between diet and disease. No matter what your specialty area is, as healthcare practitioners, we all have a role to play in the dissemination of food and nutrition information: dentists caution about refined sugar intake, therapists work on food relationships, exercise physiologists promote physical activity, kidney specialists caution about sodium...the list goes on. While a rising tide does truly lift all boats, it is important to know your limits. A heightened awareness regarding evidence-based nutrition practice is a useful tool for the practitioner, but that same practitioner should know when to refer his or her patient to a specialist or an RD for further expert instruction. Research the options in your current setting. Is there a diabetes clinic for low-income patients where they can meet with a certified diabetes educator (CDE)? Who is the registered dietitian at your patient's dialysis center, and can he or she create a more tailored meal plan for the patient? Where is the nearest WIC office where your client can sign up for benefits and take a breastfeeding class taught by a lactation educator? It is not expected that you know the answer to every question your patient will present, but you certainly should know where to get the information from, or know who does know the answer, and know how to connect the dots in your role as a nutrition advocate for your patients.

Group Counseling

The group approach to nutrition counseling is not designed to be a form of therapy, but rather to create an environment that seeks to find solutions to common nutrition problems.[86] In some cases, group counseling may provide advantages that are not attainable in the "one-on-one setting," such as emotional support and group problem solving. In groups, participants have the opportunity to learn from each other through what is known as the "modeling effect." Additionally, group participants encourage each other to reevaluate their own belief systems through the interactions and experiences with others in the group. Potential drawbacks to group counseling include individuals who are reticent to share in a group setting may not have their opinions or voices heard, personality differences may lead to one or a few members dominating the discussion, poor role modeling may occur, and it may be challenging for the facilitator to meet the needs of all group members.[79] Table 2–37 contains a list of some helpful tips for successfully facilitating a group counseling session.

Group Counseling: What Does the Evidence Say?

Three positive-rated random controlled trials that evaluated individual versus group counseling targeted to weight or diabetes management in middle-aged subjects. These short-duration studies found group counseling to be significantly more effective than individual counseling (Evidence Grade II – fair).[39]

Table 2–37. Tips for leading successful group counseling sessions.

Set the stage: select an appropriate room and environment with a seating arrangement that is conducive to sharing ideas; closing the door may promote a feeling of security

Limit the size: an ideal group size is 6 to 12 people

Build a better group: interview prospective members; group people together with common interests or health conditions; some mix may be good, but too much disparity may confuse participants

Encourage buy-in: collecting a fee can encourage attendance as participants have a sense of ownership; conduct financial business at the beginning of the meeting

Be consistent: the same person should lead the group each session

Run a tight ship: arrive early, start and conclude at scheduled times, provide session overview, follow a lesson plan, and redirect inappropriate conversation

Be proactive about attendance: call those who missed the meeting, inquire about reasons for not attending, and express concern for well-being to help retention

References

1. Danaei G, Ding E, Mozaffarian D, Taylor B, Rehm J, Murray CJ. The preventable causes of death in the United States: comparative risk assessment of dietary, lifestyle, and metabolic risk factors. PLoS Med 2009;6(4):e1000058.

2. Adams KM, Kohlmeier M, Zeisel SH. Nutrition education in U.S. medical schools: latest update of a national survey. Acad Med 2010;85(9):1537–1542.

3. McAlpine D, Wilson A. Trends in obesity-related counseling in primary care: 1995-2004. Med Care 2007;45(4):322–329.

4. ABC Good Morning America. Doctor Reprimanded for Calling Patient Fat. New York: August 24, 2005.

5. Post R, Mainous A III, Gregorie S, Knoll M, Diaz V, Saxena S. The influence of physician acknowledgment of patients' weight status on patient perceptions of overweight and obesity in the United States. Arch Intern Med 2011;171(4):316–321.

6. Castaldo J, Nester J, Wasser T, Masiado T, Rossi M, Young M, et al. Physician attitudes regarding cardiovascular risk reduction: the gaps between clinical importance, knowledge, and effectiveness. Dis Manag 2005;8(2):93–105.

7. Wynn K, Trudeau J, Taunton K, Gowans M, Scott I. Nutrition in primary care: current practices, attitudes, and barriers. Can Fam Physician 2010; 56(3):E109–E116.

8. Ray S, Udumyan R, Rajput-Ray M, Thompson B, Lodge K, Douglas P, et al. Evaluation of a novel nutrition education intervention for medical students from across England. BMJ Open 2012;2(1):e000417.

9. Kafatos A. Is clinical nutrition teaching needed in medical schools. Ann Nutr Metab 2009;54(2):129–130.

10. Nightingale J, Reeves J. Knowledge about the assessment and management of undernutrition: a pilot questionnaire in a UK teaching hospital. Clin Nutr 1999;18(1):23–27.

11. US News & World Report. Nurse Practitioner: Adult. Education: Graduate Schools; 2011.

12. Kemper K, Amata-Kynvi A, Dvorkin L, Whelan J, Woolf A, Samuels R, et al. Herbs and other dietary supplements: healthcare professionals' knowledge, attitudes, and practices. Altern Ther Health Med 2003;9(3):42–49.

13. Academy of Nutrition and Dietetics. Normal nutrition. 2012. Retrieved from: Nutrition Care Manual August 2, 2012. http://www.nutritioncaremanual.org; Academy of Nutrition and Dietetics. Nutritional indicators. 2012. Retrieved from: Nutrition Care Manual August 2, 2012. http://www.nutritioncaremanual.org

   Academy of Nutrition and Dietetics. The nutrition care process. 2012. Retrieved from: Nutrition Care Manual August 2, 2012. http://www.nutritioncaremanual.org

   Academy of Nutrition and Dietetics. Weight management. 2012. Retrieved from: Nutrition Care Manual August 2, 2012. http://www.nutritioncaremanual.org

Academy of Nutrition and Dietetics. What is the evidence regarding the difference in effectiveness for individual- vs. group-based nutrition counseling? June 2007. Retrieved from: Evidence Analysis Library September 26, 2012. http://andevidencelibrary.com

Academy of Nutrition and Dietetics. What is the validity and reliability of the Malnutrition Universal Screening Tool (MUST) in identifying nutrition problems in adult patients in acute care and hospital-based ambulatory care settings? December 2007. Retrieved from: Evidence Analysis Library August 4, 2012. http://andevidencelibrary.com

Academy of Nutrition and Dietetics/American Society for Parenteral and Enteral Nutrition. Consensus statement of the Academy of Nutrition and Dietetics/American Society for Parenteral and Enteral Nutrition: characteristics recommended for the identification and documentation of adult malnutrition (undernutrition). J Acad Nutr Diet 2012;112: 730–738; Academy of Nutrition and Dietetics. Nutrition counseling. 2012. Retrieved from: Nutrition Care Manual September 22, 2012. http://www.nutritioncaremanual.org

14. Charney P, Malone AM. ADA pocket guide to nutrition assessment. 2nd ed. Chicago, IL: American Dietetic Association; 2009.

15. American Society for Parenteral and Enteral Nutrition (A.S.P.E.N.) Board of Directors and Clinical Practice Committee. Definition of terms, style, and conventions used in A.S.P.E.N. Board of Directors–approved documents. ASPEN; July 2010.

16. Naber TS, de Bree A, Nusteling K, Eggink L, Kruimel J, Bakkeren J, et al. Prevalence of malnutrition in nonsurgical hospitalized patients and its association with disease complications. Am J Clin Nutr 1997;66: 1232–1239.

17. Keller H. Malnutrition in institutionalized elderly: How and why? J Am Geriatr Soc 1993;41:1212–1218.

18. McWhirter J, Pennington CR. Incidence and recognition of malnutrition in hospital. BMJ 1994;308:945–948.

19. Kruizenga H, Van Tulder M, Seidell J, Thijs A, Ader H, van Bokhorst-de van der Schueren M. Effectiveness and cost-effectiveness of early screening and treatment of malnourished patients. Am J Clin Nutr 2005;82(5): 1082–1089.

20. Mowe M, Bohmer T. The prevalence of undiagnosed protein-calorie undernutrition in a population of hospitalized elderly patients. J Am Geriatr Soc 1991;39:1089–1092.

21. Kelly I, Tessier S, Cahill A, Morris S, Crumley A, McLaughlin D, et al. Still hungry in hospital: identifying malnutrition in acute hospital admissions. Q J Med 2000;93:93–98.

22. Stratton R, King C, Stroud M, Jackson A, Elia M. 'Malnutrition Universal Screening Tool' predicts mortality and length of hospital stay in acutely ill elderly. Br J Nutr 2006;95:325–330.

23. Ukleja A, Freeman K, Gilbert K, Kochevar M, Kraft M, Russell M, et al. Standards for nutrition support – adult hospitalized patients. Nutr Clin Pract 2010;25(4):403–414.

24. Ferguson M, Capra S, Bauer J, Banks M. Development of a valid and reliable malnutrition screening tool for adult acute hospital patients. Nutrition 1999;15:458–464.

25. Heimburger D. Malnutrition and nutritional assessment. In: Longo D, Fauci A, Kasper D, Hauser S, Jameson J, Loscalzo J, eds. Harrison's Principles of Internal Medicine. New York, NY: McGraw Hill; 2012 [chapter 75].

26. Joint Commission on Accreditation of Healthcare Organizations. Comprehensive Accreditation Manual for Hospitals. Chicago, IL: Joint Commission on Accreditation of Healthcare Organizations; 2007.

27. Arizona WIC Program. WIC Anthropometrics Model. Women, Infants, and Children (WIC) Competent Professional Authority (CPA) Training Program. Phoenix, AZ; 2007.

28. Lee RD, Nieman DC. Nutritional Assessment. New York, NY: McGraw Hill; 2007.

29. Kuczmarski MF, Kuczmarski RJ, Najjar M. Descriptive anthropometric reference data for older Americans. J Am Diet Assoc 2000;100(1):59–66.

30. National Heart Lung and Blood Institute. Aim for a healthy weight. 2012. Retrieved from: Assessing Your Weight and Health Risk September 1, 2012. http://www.nhlbi.nih.gov/health/public/heart/obesity/lose_wt/risk.htm#limitations

31. Heimburger DC. Nutritional assessment. In: Heimburger DC, Arg JD, eds. Handbook of Clinical Nutrition. Philadelphia, PA: MOSBY Elsevier; 2006:254–256.

32. Chumlea W, Guo S, Roche A, Steinbaugh M. Prediction of body weight for the nonambulatory elderly from anthropometry. J Am Diet Assoc 1988;88(5):564–568.

33. Flegal K, Kit B, Orpana H, Graubard B. Association of all-cause mortality with overweight and obesity using standard body mass index categories: a systematic review and meta-analysis. JAMA 2013;309(1):71–82.

34. Jeffreys M, McCarron P, Gunnell D, McEwen J, Smith G. Body mass index in early and mid-adulthood, and subsequent mortality: a historical cohort study. Int J Obes Relat Metab Disord 2003;27(11):1391–1397.

35. Zheng W, et al. Association between body-mass index and risk of death in more than 1 million asians. N Engl J Med 2011;364(8):719–729.

36. Pronsky Z, Crowe S J, Elbe D, Young V, Epstein S, Roberts W, et al. Ideal body weight calculations. In: Pronsky Z, Crowe S J, Elbe D, Young V, Epstein S, Roberts W, et al., eds. Food Medication Interactions; 2010:357.

37. US Department of Agriculture. USDA's nutrition evidence library (NEL).2010. Retrieved from: http://www.nutritionevidencelibrary.gov/. September 22, 2012; US Department of Agriculture, Agricultural Research Service. USDA automated multiple-pass method. September 29, 2012 Retrieved from: Products & Services September 9, 2012. http://www.ars.usda.gov/Services/docs.htm?docid=7710

38. US Department of Agriculture. Researchers Produce Innovation in Dietary Recall. Agriculture Research; June 2004.

39. Academy of Nutrition and Dietetics. Based on the available evidence, which nutrition screening tools have been found to be valid and reliable

for identifying nutrition problems in adult patients in acute care and hospital-based ambulatory care settings? December 2007. Retrieved from: Evidence Analysis Library September 26, 2012. http://andevidenceli brary.com; Academy of Nutrition and Dietetics. Nutrition care process. December 2007. Retrieved from: Evidence Analysis Library September 26, 2012. http://andevidencelibrary.com

40. Kruizenga H, Seidell J, de Vet H, Wierdsma N, van Bokhorst-de van der Schueren M. Development and validation of a hospital screening tool for malnutrition: the short nutritional assessment questionnaire (SNAQ). Clin Nutr 2005;24(1):75–82.

41. Nestle Nutrition Institute. (n.d.). Overview: what is the MNA(R)? Retrieved from: MNA(R) Mini Nutritional Assessment August 26, 2012. http://www.mna-elderly.com/default.html

42. MNA-International Group. Validation of the mini nutritional assessment short-form (MNA-SF): a practical tool for identification of nutritional status. J Nutr Health Aging 2009;13(9):782–788.

43. Anthony P. Nutrition screening tools for hospitalized patients. Nutr Clin Pract 2008;23 (4):373–382.

44. Detsky A, McLaughlin J, Baker J, Johnston N, Whittaker S, Mendelson R, et al. What is subjective global assessment of nutritional status? JPEN J Parenter Enteral Nutr 1987;11(1):8–13.

45. Center for Substance Abuse Treatment. Screening and assessment. Chapter 4 In: C. f. Treatment, Substance Abuse Treatment: Addressing the Specific Needs of Women. Rockville MD: Substance Abuse and Mental Health Services 2009.

46. Mueller C, Compher C, Druyan ME. The American Society for Parenteral and Enteral Nutrition (A.S.P.E.N.) Board of Directors. A.S.P.E.N. Clinical Guidelines. Nutrition screening, assessment, and intervention. J Parenter Enteral Nutr 2011;35(1):16–24.

47. Jensen G, Bistrian B, Roubenoff R, Heimburger D. Malnutrition syndromes: a conundrum vs continuum. JPEN J Parenter Enteral Nutr 2009;33(6):710–716.

48. Soeters P, Schols A. Advances in understanding and assessing malnutrition. Curr Opin Clin Nutr Metab Care 2009;12(5):487–494.

49. World Health Organization. International Classification of Diseases, 9th Revision Clinical Modification. Geneva; 1975.

50. National Alliance for Infusion Therapy and the American Society for Parenteral and Enteral Nutrition Public Policy Committee and Board of Directors. Disease-related malnutrition and enteral nutrition therapy: a significant problem with a cost-effective solution. Nutr Clin Pract 2010;25(5):548–554.

51. Jensen G, Mirtallo J, Compher C. Adult starvation and disease-related malnutrition: a rational approach for etiology-based diagnosis in the clinical practice setting from the International Consensus Guideline Committee. JPEN J Parenter Enteral Nutr 2010;34(2):156–159.

52. Academy of Nutrition and Dietetics. ADA conclusion statements and accuracy of resting metabolic rate measurement vs. estimations. 2009. Retrieved from: Evidence Analysis Library September 26, 2012. http://

andevidencelibrary.com; Academy of Nutrition and Dietetics. Does serum albumin correlate with weight loss in four models of prolonged protein-energy restriction: anorexia nervosa, non-malabsorptive gastric partioning bariatric surgery, calorie-restricted diets or starvation. August 2009. Retrieved from: Evidence Analysis Library September 2, 2012. http://andevidencelibrary.com

53. Bernstein L, Bachman T, Meguid M, Ament M, Baumgartner T, Kinosian B, et al. Measurement of visceral protein status in assessing protein and energy malnutrition: standard of care. Prealbumin in Nutritional Care Consensus Group. Nutrition 1995;11(2):169–171.

54. World Health Organization. Nutrition. 2012. Retrieved from: Micronutrient deficiencies September 1, 2012. http://www.who.int/nutrition/topics/ida/en/index.html

55. Ravel R. Clinical Laboratory Medicine: Clinical Application Of Laboratory Data. 5th ed. St. Louis: Mosby; 1989.

56. National Research Council. Dietary Reference Intakes for Energy, Carbohydrate, Fiber, Fat, Fatty Acids, Cholesterol, Protein, and Amino Acids (Macronutrients). Washington, DC: The National Academies Press; 2005.

57. American Dietetic Association. International Dietetics & Nutrition Terminology (IDNT) Reference Manual. Chicago, IL: American Dietetic Association; 2011.

58. Litchford MD. Nutrition Focused Physical Assessment: Making Clinical Connections. Greensboro, NC: Case Software; 2012.

59. Hammond K. Nutrition focused physical assessment. Support Line 1996;18(4):4.

60. Centers for Disease Control and Prevention. Target heart rate and estimated maximum heart rate. March 30, 2011. Retrieved from: Physical Activity January 31, 2013. http://www.cdc.gov/physicalactivity/everyone/measuring/heartrate.html

61. Bohannon R. Grip strength impairments among older adults receiving physical therapy in a home-care setting. Percept Mot Skills 2010;111(3):761–764.

62. Kaburagi T, Hirasawa R, Yoshino H, Odaka Y, Satomi M, Nakano M, et al. Nutritional status is strongly correlated with grip strength and depression in community-living elderly Japanese. Public Health Nutr 2011;14(11):1839–1899.

63. Otto D, Wang X, Tijerina S, Reyna M, Farooqi M, Shelton M. A comparison of blood pressure, body mass index, and acanthosis nigricans in school-age children. J Sch Nurs 2010;26(3):223–229.

64. European Pressure Ulcer Advisory Panel and National Pressure Ulcer Advisory Panel. Prevention and treatment of pressure ulcers: quick reference guide. Washington, DC: National Pressure Ulcer Advisory Panel; 2009.

65. Bergstrom N, Horn S, Smout R, Bender S, Ferguson M, Taler G, et al. The National Pressure Ulcer Long-Term Care Study: outcomes of pressure ulcer treatments in long-term care. J Am Geriatr Soc 2005;53(10):1721–1729.

66. Cashman M, Sloan S. Nutrition and nail disease. Clin Dermatol 2010;28(4):420–425.
67. Williams ME. Examining the Fingernails. 2008. Retrieved from: MedScape Education September 9, 2012. http://www.medscape.org/view article/571916_2
68. US National Library of Medicine. PubMedHealth. 2012 Retrieved from: Dehydration September 9, 2012. http://www.ncbi.nlm.nih.gov/pubmed health/PMH0001977/
69. National Institutes of Health Office of Dietary Supplements. Dietary supplement fact sheets. October 11, 2011 Retrieved from: Vitamin A, Vitamin D, Vitamin E, Vitamin K September 9, 2012. http://www.ods.od.nih.gov/factsheets/list-all/
70. Pope V, Kline W. The personal characteristics of effective counselors: what 10 experts think. Psychol Rep 1999;84(3 Pt 2):1339–1344.
71. Murphy B, Dillon C. Interviewing in Action: Process and Practice. Pacific Grove, CA: Brooks/Cole; 1998.
72. Hochbaum G. Public Participation in Medical Screening Programs: A Socio-Psychological Study. Washington, DC: US Department. of Health, Education, and Welfare; 1958.
73. Rosenstock I. What research in motivation suggests for public health. Am J Public Health 1960;(50):295–302.
74. Glanz K, Rimer B, Viswanath K. Health Behavior and Health Education: Theory, Research, and Practice. 4th ed. San Francisco, CA: Jossey-Bass; 2008.
75. National Institute of Mental Health. Health topics. September 21, 2012. Retrieved from Psychotherapies September 21, 2012. http://www.nimh.nih.gov/health/topics/psychotherapies/index.shtml
76. Gohner W, Schlatterer M, Seelig H, Frey I, Berg A, Fuchs R. Two-year follow-up of an interdisciplinary cognitive-behavioral intervention program for obese adults. J Psychol 2012;146(4):371–391.
77. Kraybill K, Morrison S. Assessing Health, Promoting Wellness: A Guide for Non-Medical Providers of Care for People Experiencing Homelessness. Rockville, MD: Center for Mental Health Services, Substance Abuse and Mental Health Services Administration; 2007.
78. Miller W, Rollnick S. Motivational Interviewing Second Edition, Preparing People for Change. New York, NY: The Guilford Press; 2002.
79. Bauer K, Sokolik C. Basic Nutrition Counseling Skill Development. Belmont, CA: Wadsworth/Thomson Learning; 2002.
80. Rollnick S, Heather N, Bell A. Negotiating behavior change in medical settings: the development of brief motivational interviewing. J Mental Health 1992;1:25–37.
81. Claridge J, Fabian T. History and development of evidence-based medicine. World J Surg 2005;5:547–553.
82. King JC. An evidence-based approach for establishing dietary guidelines. J. Nutr 2007;137:480–483.
83. CDC. Establishing rapport. December 16, 2008 Retrieved from: Behavioral Risk Factor Surveillance System September 22, 2012. http://www.cdc.gov/brfss/training/interviewer/04_section/11_rapport.htm

84. Substance Abuse and Mental Health Services Administration's (SAMHSA) Homelessness Resource Center (HRC). Homelessness resource center library. 2007. Retrieved from: Motivational Interviewing: Open Questions, Affirmation, Reflective Listening, and Summary Reflections (OARS) September 23, 2012. http://www.homeless.samhsa.gov/Resource/View .aspx?id=32840&AspxAutoDetectCookieSupport=1

85. CDC. Program evaluation: healthy youth. 2009. Retrieved from: Writing SMART Objectives September 23, 2012. http://www.cdc.gov/healthyyouth/ evaluation/pdf/brief3b.pdfHelm K. Group process. In: 86. Helm K, Klawitter B. Nutrition Therapy Advanced Counseling Skills. Lake Dallas, TX: Helm Seminars 1995:207–213.

3

Finding Your Weigh: Mastering Weight Management

- Energy Balance

The First Law of Thermodynamics

The regulation of body weight is dependent on the maintenance of energy balance, a concept that is described by the first law of thermodynamics. According to this law, energy can neither be created nor destroyed, but can be exchanged in different forms. The human body (a chemical device) takes in chemical energy (calories from food and beverages) and converts it into other forms of energy such as mechanical work and heat.[1] The thermodynamics law states that:

$$Energy\ intake\ (food) = Energy\ expended\ (heat, work, biosynthesis) + Energy\ stored$$

Imbalance in this equation results in a change in body weight. If the energy intake is greater than the energy expended, the excess energy must be stored (positive energy balance); and, if energy expenditure exceeds that of energy intake, a decrease in body weight occurs (negative energy balance). Because of the law of thermodynamics, this occurs with absolute certainty. With less certainty, however, is that of the regulation of body weight, which involves complex signaling systems and compensatory changes in appetite and metabolic efficiency.[2]

Metabolic Efficiency

The amount of energy an individual must exert to perform a given amount of work is termed *metabolic efficiency*, and metabolic efficiency varies among different individuals. When compared to a person with low metabolic efficiency, a person who has a high metabolic efficiency will expend less energy to perform a certain task. A person with a high metabolic efficiency is better able to preserve body weight when expenditure exceeds intake (negative energy balance), but will be more inclined to gain weight when intake exceeds expenditure (positive energy balance). Although current research points toward the existence of a *set point* that makes weight loss or weight gain progressively difficult, the first law of thermodynamics does not explain the genetics of body weight regulation and metabolic efficiency.[2]

Energy Storage

Evolutionary adaptations have resulted in a human body that is very good at acquiring and storing energy; furthermore, we have a large capacity to store this energy in the form of adipose tissue (fat). Each kilogram of fat yields 7700 kcal when metabolized (approximately three to four times the average daily adult energy requirements).[3] The first law of thermodynamics dictates that if energy intake is greater than energy expenditure, the excess energy must be stored. However, what cannot be explained by the first law of thermodynamics is the reason why men and women distribute fat in different parts of their bodies, or how fat distribution changes with age, or why some medications can produce weight gain, while others produce weight loss.[4]

Appetite

Sensations that promote food ingestion or rejection (appetite) are central to the maintenance of energy balance, although the mechanisms are unclear. Appetite can be divided into three components[5]:

- Hunger: the sensations that promote food consumption, including metabolic, sensory, and cognitive aspects
- Satiation: the sensations that regulate meal size and duration
- Satiety: the sensations that determine the inter-meal period of fasting

Normally, the sensations of hunger subside once eating begins and as it proceeds, then eventually satiation becomes the more dominant sensation, causing the cessation of eating. With satiation, a period of abstinence from eating occurs, and satiety begins. Although the mechanisms that regulate appetite (hunger, satiation, and satiety) and food intake have a physiologic basis, they are also likely to be strongly influenced by environmental factors (eg, the availability of food, sensory stimulation, etc), and/or cognitive factors (eg, habitual meal times, health beliefs).[5] Hunger is on the opposite end of the scale from satiation and satiety, but one is not merely the absence of the other. Satiation and hunger can be present at the same time, and the relationship between appetite and food intake can be disrupted by numerous factors. These potentially disrupting factors include a lack of availability of food, or social constraints that cause one to refrain from eating when hungry. Other factors include boredom, availability of palatable food, or emotional stress that may cause one to eat in the absence of hunger.[5] Therefore, the relationship between appetite and food intake is weak, and because appetite is a subjective construct, it makes direct measurement challenging in scientific studies. Researchers are left to rely largely on the indirect measurements of appetite, including questionnaires, biomarkers (eg, leptin, ghrelin, cholecystokinin, glucagon-like peptide, and peptide YY), and eating patterns (eg, meal frequencies and meal timing). But, despite a long history of research, the mechanisms to control appetite remain poorly characterized and cannot be explained adequately or simply by the first law of thermodynamics.[5]

- ■ Factors Affecting Energy Intake

As obesity research evolves, it becomes more obvious that body weight regulation cannot be explained entirely by just the laws of thermodynamics. What researchers do know, however, is that eating is a behavior that links the individual's *external* physical environment with the individual's two distinct *internal* physiological systems that govern food intake: the homeostatic system and the hedonic system. Both of these systems are regulated centrally, but they do not appear to be integrated. Disturbance in the homeostatic pathways or inappropriate sensitization of the hedonic system may lead to reduced appetite control. Table 3–1 more thoroughly describes how these systems work.[6]

- ■ Factors Affecting Energy Expenditure

Energy expenditure is a fundamental property of life. In research settings, total energy expenditure (TEE) represents a measurement obtained over a 24-hour period. TEE is usually measured after an overnight fast, conducted in a thermoneutral room, and while the individual rests quietly in a reclined position.[7] TEE is defined as the sum of the five metabolic components, which are listed in Table 3–2, along with their role in metabolism.[3,7,8-12]

Other factors affecting energy expenditure are gender, weight, height, age, body surface area, fat mass (or lean body mass), and ethnicity. Fat-free mass is well known for its metabolic activity and influence on resting metabolic rate (RMR). In general, the greater the percentage of fat-free mass, the greater the RMR. The RMR can also be impacted by age, declining approximately 2–3% with each decade of life.[12]

Quantifying Body Weight

- ■ Realistic Weight Goal Setting

In order to guide weight management goals and successfully document outcomes, baseline weight and health indexes are required. These indexes should be capable of reflecting short- and long-term changes in body fat and should strongly correlate with health risk. In addition, measurements of body weight status must be clinically useful, noninvasive, inexpensive, easy to obtain, and reliable.[6] Tables 3–3 and 3–4 list useful weight calculations and weight standards that are used to determine ideal body weight and fat status, respectively (in adults).[13-18] However, the advantages and disadvantages of using these must be carefully weighed by the practitioner before determining the most appropriate standard for use.

- ■ Accommodations for Amputation

Evaluation of a patient's present body weight relative to ideal body weight is a key factor in assessing nutritional status, but this becomes

Table 3–1. Two internal physiological systems that govern food intake.

Homeostatic System		Hedonic System	
Main functions	Key hormone drivers for initiating food intake	Main functions	Key hormone drivers for initiating food intake
• Comprises long-term signaling from adipose tissue • Episodic signaling from the gut generated in response to an eating episode (rise and fall with eating patterns)	• Leptin • Insulin • Ghrelin • Cholecystokinin • Glucagon-like peptide • Peptide YY • Others	• Deals with the cognitive, motivational, and emotional aspects of food intake (perceived pleasantness, liking, and wanting)	• Endocannabinoids • Serotonin • Dopamine
• Interaction between these two sets of the signals reflects the brain's recognition of the current dynamic state of energy stores and the changing nutrient flow derived from eating • Central regulation of energy balance tunes hunger and fullness sensation that accompany eating behaviors		• Represents the main interface with the external environment • Initiation of an eating episode often starts as a cognitive decision, in the absence of a depletion signal • Inappropriate sensitization of this network likely leads to weight gain, since palatability, via this system, is a very powerful determinant of food intake	

Data from American Dietetic Association, 2009.

Table 3–2. Components of total energy expenditure (TEE) and their role in metabolism.

Components of TEE	% of TEE	Role in Metabolism
Resting energy expenditure (REE) or resting metabolic rate (RMR) • Further broken down into basal metabolic rate (BMR) that accounts for rate of energy expenditure fasted, rested, and in supine conditions in a thermoneutral environment 12–18 hours after a meal (more difficult to monitor; therefore, RMR is more widely used)	~65–75	• Largest component of TEE • Rate of energy expenditure when at rest (but not basal) • Consists of involuntary activities that are necessary to sustain life, eg, circulation, respiration, nerve activity, hormone secretion, and blinking and sleeping, basal and arousal metabolism • Usually not susceptible to change, but may decrease in response to an energy deficit, weight loss, and a smaller body size
Activity energy expenditure (AEE)	~15–30	• Takes many forms: minimal muscular movement required for tasks of daily living (grooming, dressing, feeding, basic household chores); earning a living; or other routine requirements of life: recreation, sports, leisure-time, etc • Can be significantly increased when one increases their activity and may decrease in response to an energy deficit, weight loss, and a smaller body size • Energy expended during weight-bearing activities increases proportional to body mass • Energy expended during nonweight-bearing activities has little relationship to body mass • Any strategy to improve weight management must include substantial emphasis on increasing this component

(*Continued*)

Table 3-2. Components of total energy expenditure (TEE) and their role in metabolism. (*Continued*)

Components of TEE	% of TEE	Role in Metabolism
Thermal effect of food (TEF)	~10	• Energy required for digesting, absorbing and assimilating, and storing nutrients; energy expenditure increases for 4-8 hours after a meal is ingested • Impacted by caloric content, composition of the macronutrients and the individual's diet, and decreases with age • TEF of the Macronutrients: 20-30% for protein, 5-15% for carbohydrates, and 0-3% for fat • With a decreased energy intake, will decrease by ~10% of the decrease in energy intake
Facultative (adaptive) thermogenesis	Varies depending on the individual	• The regulated production of heat in response to environmental changes in temperature and diet • Can be rapidly switched on and rapidly suppressed by the nervous system
Anabolism/growth	Varies depending on the life stage	• At certain life stages extra energy expenditure for growth, pregnancy, or lactation are needed

Data from Wang et al., 2001; Foster and Nonas, 2004; McArdle et al., 2000; Joosen and Westerterp, 2006; Himms-Hagen, 1989; Schoeller and Buchholz, 2005; Shils et al., 1999.

Table 3–3. Selected weight calculations.

Weight Calculation	Description/ Interpretation	Advantages	Disadvantages
% Ideal body weight (IBW)	$= \dfrac{\text{actual wt (ABW)}}{\text{IBW}} \times 100$ • Assesses degree of under/over nutrition ≥200% morbidly obese ≥150% obese ≥120% overweight 80–90% mild malnutrition 70–79% moderate malnutrition <69% severe malnutrition	• Appropriate parameter for a healthy adult population	• Limited use when assessing the degree of malnutrition in an ill population • Requires accurate measurement of frame size
% Usual body weight (UBW)	$= \dfrac{\text{ABW}}{\text{UBW}} \times 100$ • Assesses degree of malnutrition 85–95% mild malnutrition 75–84% moderate malnutrition <74% severe malnutrition	• More useful parameter to use with an ill population • Useful when assessing changes in weight status	• Requires accurate measurement of body weight • Interpretation is affected by fluid status • May be dependent on patient memory
% Weight loss	$= \dfrac{\text{UBW} - \text{ABW}}{\text{UBW}} \times 100$ • Assesses severity/ significance of the weight loss Significant weight loss: • 5% over 1 month • 7.5% over 3 months • 10% over 6 months Severe weight loss: • >5% over 1 month • >7.5% over 3 months • >10% over 6 months		

Data from Shronts, 1989.

Table 3-4. Selected weight standards available to determine ideal body weight and fat for healthy adults.

Weight Standard	Description	Advantages	Disadvantages
Metropolitan life insurance tables (MLIT), 1983	• Values are based on weights associated with the lowest mortality rates	• Frame size was determined by elbow breadth • 90% of the weights were obtained by direct measurement	• No data available on the height measurements • Individuals were measured wearing clothes and the weight of clothes was estimated • Findings on an insured population may not represent the entire population • Cannot be used with an elderly population
Hamwi method	Males: 106 pounds for the first 5 feet; 6 pounds for each inch over 5 feet Females: 100 pounds for the first 5 feet; 5 pounds for each inch over 5 feet Generally add +/− 10% to create a range that accommodates for differences in frame size	• Easy to use	• Fairly low and restrictive range of IBW, especially for women, that may establish unrealistic weight goals

Body mass index (BMI)	$= \dfrac{\text{Weight (pounds)}}{\text{height squared (inches}^2)} \times 703$ <18.5 underweight 18.5-24.9 normal 25-29.9 overweight 30-34.9 obese 35-39.9 severely obese >40 extremely obese	• A practical approach to measuring body fat in the clinical setting • More accurate measure of total body fat than body weight alone • A direct calculation based on height and weight, regardless of gender	• Overestimates body fat in persons who are very muscular and males of large stature • Can underestimate body fat in persons who have lost muscle mass
Waist circumference (WC)	High risk circumference Men: >40 inches (102 cm) Women: >35 inches (88 cm)	• Most practical tool to evaluate abdominal fat before and during weight loss treatment • Provides an independent prediction of risk over and above that of BMI	• For those with BMI ≥35, WC adds little to the predictive power of the disease risk classification of BMI

Data from Shronts, 1989; Dalton, 1998; National Heart, Lung, and Blood Institute (NHLBI), 1998; US Department of Agriculture and US Department of Health and Human Services, 2011.

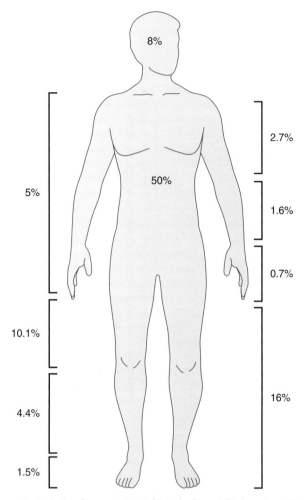

Figure 3-1. Ratio of segment weight to body weight for amputations. (From Osterkamp LK. Current perspective on assessment of human body proportions of relevance to amputees. J Am Diet Assoc 1995;95(2):215–218.)

even more complex if the patient has an amputation. Most of the body's metabolic activity occurs in the trunk and head. When evaluating the nutritional status of an amputee, the ratio of segment weight to body weight must be considered.[19] Figure 3–1 shows the most current evidence-based data on the ratio of segment weight to body weight. When calculating an individual's ideal body weight, the practitioner must deduct the missing body part ratio from the weight standard that is used. See Chapter 2 and Table 3–4 for information on calculating ideal body weight.

■ Determining Energy Needs

The balance between energy intake and energy expenditure has important health implications. Determining energy needs is a basic component of nutritional assessment.[20] The restoration of energy balance is the focus for the medical management of weight loss or weight gain, and subsequently, it affects morbidity and mortality. Achieving energy balance is often a difficult task due to the complex interaction of the components of energy expenditure (resting metabolic rate [RMR], activity energy expenditure, and TEF) and energy intake (calorie availability and consumption).[21]

The RMR, the largest single component of total caloric expenditure, can be measured directly, indirectly, or estimated by equations. As discussed in Chapter 2, although indirect calorimetry is the most accurate method for determining RMR in various stages of health and disease states, it is used primarily as a research tool and is impractical in clinical use due to a number of factors. Indirect calorimetry measurement (obtained with the bedside metabolic cart with face mask or canopy) offers good accuracy, but is also often impractical and expensive for clinical practice. Hand-held indirect calorimeters have been found to have comparable reliability and validity as to traditional calorimeter measurement[22] and are becoming more widely used as tool in clinical practice; however, estimation using mathematical calculations developed by direct and indirect calorimetry measures is by far the most common method of determining energy needs.[21]

Determining RMR via Hand-Held Indirect Calorimetry

In more recent years, the ability to indirectly measure the RMR has become available to clinical practice with portable tools, including the MedGem®, Korr™, and New Leaf™. Actual measurement of the RMR, if conducted properly, should be more accurate than predictive equations.[21] The clinician must understand the conditions that need to be controlled for, in order to ensure a resting state, and thus an accurate reading. Table 3–5 lists these conditions and how they can be controlled.[20]

In order to assess the validity of some indirect calorimetry measurements of RMR, the respiratory quotient (RQ), or the ratio of V_{CO_2} to V_{O_2} can be applied to the interpretation of the RMR measurement. RQ measures of <0.70 or >1.00 suggest protocol violations or inaccurate gas measurement.[20]

Determining RMR via Predictive Equations

Five of the most commonly used RMR prediction equations are listed in Table 3–6 (and are also discussed in Chapter 10).[21,23,24] Of these five equations, the Mifflin-St Jeor predicted RMR within 10% of measured RMR in more nonobese and obese individuals than any other equation, having the most narrow error range, and thus, has been found to be the most reliable and accurate for estimating RMR using actual body

Table 3–5. Conditions required of an indirect calorimetry measurement to achieve a resting state and an accurate test of RMR.

Conditions Affecting RMR	Control of Condition
Meals (thermic effect of food [TEF])	Minimum fast of 5 hours
Snacks (thermic effect of food [TEF])	Minimum fast of 4 hours
Alcohol	Minimum abstention of 2 hours
Nicotine	Minimum abstention of 2 hours and 2 ½ hours after removal of nicotine patch
Caffeine	Minimum abstention of 4 hours
Activities of daily living	Minimum rest period of 10–20 minutes
Moderate aerobic or anaerobic exercise	Minimum abstention of 2 hours
Vigorous exercise	Minimum abstention of 14 hours
Physical comfort	Assure comfort level with measurement position and repeat measures should be in the same position
Room temperature	Assure a room temperature of 20°C–25°C (68°F–77°F)
Testing environment	Assure a room that is quiet with mild lighting
Gas collection device	Vigorous adherence to prevent air leaks with proper placement of face mask and nose clip
Steady-state interval and measurement duration	10-minute test duration with the first 5 minutes discarded, and remaining 5 minutes having a coefficient of variation of <10% for V_{o_2} and V_{co_2}

Data from Compher et al., 2006.

weight. Limitations do exist, however, when applied to certain age, stress levels, and ethnic groups.[6,21]

Determining Total Energy Requirements

Once the RMR of the individual is determined, the practitioner must use clinical judgment to assess the individual's activity factors, and desired weight loss or weight gain, in order to determine the total daily

Table 3–6. Resting metabolic rate (kcal per day) prediction equations for adults.

Name of Equation	Formula
Mifflin-St Jeor	Men: RMR = 9.99 × weight (kg) + 6.25 × height (cm) − 4.92 × age +5 Women: RMR = 9.99 × weight (kg) + 6.25 × height (cm) − 4.92 × age −161 Not recommended as a predictive equation in the critically ill
Penn State equation (PSU2010)	Also referred to as modified Penn State equation RMR = Mifflin(0.71) + V_E(64) + T_{max}(85)-3085 Use for patients with BMI >30 and aged >60 where V_E = Minute ventilation
Harris-Benedict	Men: RMR = 66.47 + 13.75 × weight (kg) + 5.0 × height (cm) − 6.75 × age Women: RMR = 665.09 + 9.56 × weight (kg) + 1.84 × height (cm) − 4.67 × age Not recommended as a predictive equation in the critically ill
Owen	Men: RMR = 879 + 10.2 × weight (kg) Women: RMR = 795 + 7.18 × weight (kg)

Ireton-Jones	Legend:
	• B = Diagnosis of burn (present = 1, absent = 0)
	• O = Obesity, body mass index (BMI) >27 kg/m^2 (present = 1, absent = 0)
	• S = Sex (male = 1, female = 0)
	• T = Diagnosis of trauma (present = 1, absent = 0)
	• Spontaneously breathing: 629−11(A) + 25(W)−609(O)
	  Ventilator dependent (original):
	  1925−10(A) + 5(W) + 281(S) + 292(T) + 851(B)
	• Ventilator-dependent (revised):
	  1784−11(A) + 5(W) + 244(S) + 239(T) + 804(B)
	Although indirect calorimetry is the best method for determining RMR in the critically ill, if it is necessary to use predictive equations, the Ireton-Jones has the best predictive accuracy

(Continued)

Table 3-6. Resting metabolic rate (kcal per day) prediction equations for adults. (*Continued*)

Name of Equation	Formula
WHO/FAO/UNU	**Men:** 18-30 years: 15.4 × weight − 27 × height (m) + 717 31-60 years: 11.3 × weight + 16 × height (m) + 901 >60 years: 8.8 × weight + 1128 × height (m) − 1071 **Women:** 18-30 years: 13.3 × weight + 334 × height (m) + 35 31-60 years: 8.7 × weight − 25 × height (m) + 865 >60 years: 9.2 × weight + 637 × height (m) − 302

WHO/FAO/UNU, World Health Organization/Food and Agricultural Organization/United Nations University; kg, kilograms (actual weight); cm, centimeters; and m, meters.

Data from Frankenfield et al., 2005; Ireton-Jones et al., 1992; Ireton-Jones and Jones, 2002.

energy needs. If the individual is ill, then additional calculations will be required to determine energy needs taking into consideration an injury factor. Table 3–7 lists the appropriate formula to be used for calculating TEE in either an ill or healthy individual.

Activity factors

The activity factor used is determined by how active the individual is on a daily basis and the type of activity. Table 3–8 defines "activity levels," according to the *Dietary Guidelines for Americans, 2010*.[18]

Clinical judgment should be used to determine the most appropriate activity factor. Just as there are various formulas available to determine RMR, there are also various activity factors that can be used.

Table 3-7. Determining the total energy expenditure (TEE).

Healthy Individual	Ill Individual
TEE = RMR × Activity Factor ± 500 calories[a] (for desired weight loss or weight gain, if applicable)	TEE = RMR × Activity Factor × Injury Factor ± 500 calories[a] (for desired weight loss or weight gain, if applicable) + fever factor

[a]Based on 500 calories × 7 days per week = 3500 (1 pound = 3500 calories).

Table 3–8. Activity levels defined.

Activity Level	Activity Level Definition
Sedentary	A lifestyle that includes only the light physical activity associated with typical day-to-day life
Moderately active	A lifestyle that includes physical activity equivalent to walking about 1.5-3 miles per day at 3-4 miles per hour, in addition to the light physical activity associated with typical day-to-day life
Active	A lifestyle that includes physical activity equivalent to walking more than 3 miles per day at 3-4 miles per hour, in addition to the light physical activity associated with typical day-to-day life

Data from US Department of Agriculture and US Department of Health and Human Services, 2011.

Tables 3–9 and 3–10 list the activity factors for the healthy and ill individual, respectively.[25]

For the sick individual, an injury and fever factor must be considered when determining TEE. Table 3–11 describes the injury and fever factor used for the appropriate condition.[26]

Table 3–9. Three sources for determining activity factors for the healthy individual.

Activity Level	Activity Factor	
	Female	Male
Very light (driving, typing, sewing, ironing, and cooking)	1.3	1.3
Light (walking 3 mph, house cleaning, golf, and child care)	1.5	1.6
Moderate (walking 4 mph, dancing, tennis, and cycling)	1.6	1.7
Heavy (running, soccer, basketball, and football)	1.9	2.1
Sedentary	1.0	1.0
Low activity	1.12	1.11
Active	1.27	1.25
Very active	1.45	1.48
Light	1.56	1.55
Moderate	1.64	1.78
Heavy	1.82	2.1

Data from Kushner and Blatner, 2005.

Table 3–10. Determining activity factors for the Ill individual.

Activity Level	Activity Factor
Comatose	1.1
Confined to bed	1.2
Confined to chair	1.25
Out of bed	1.3
Normal activities of daily living (ADLs)	1.5

Data from Kushner and Blatner, 2005.

Table 3–11. Injury and fever factor.

Injury or Fever	Factor
Surgery	
Minor	1.0–1.2
Major	1.1–1.3
Skeletal trauma	1.1–1.6
Head trauma	1.6–1.8
Pressure ulcers	
Stage I	1.0–1.1
Stage II	1.2
Stage III	1.3–1.4
Stage IV	1.5–1.6
Infection	
Mild	1.0–1.2
Moderate	1.2–1.4
Severe	1.4–1.8
Burns (% body surface area [BSA])	
<20% BSA	1.2–1.5
20–40% BSA	1.5–1.8
>40% SA	1.8–2.0
Fever (for every 1 degree over normal)	
Fahrenheit scale	add 7% of RMR
Centigrade scale	add 13% of RMR

Data from Campbell et al., 2005.

Simplifying Estimation of Energy Needs

Determining calorie needs can be a complicated process, but it is an important step in the medical management of weight control. For a healthy individual, the practitioner can refer to the *Dietary Guidelines for Americans, 2010* for estimated calorie needs per day by age, gender, and physical activity level. These are based on estimated energy requirements (EER) equations, using reference heights (average) and healthy reference weights. To learn more, visit: http://www.health.gov/dietaryguidelines/. Appendix B contains the USDA recommended meal patterns for different calorie levels.

Calories per kilogram method (cal/kg)

In certain conditions, estimating total energy needs may be calculated using the simplified approach of kcal/kg/day (also covered in Chapter 2). When using this method of estimation, the practitioner must use clinical judgment and take into account the patient's weight status and goals, age, sex, level of physical activity, and metabolic stressors—all of which may impact estimated energy needs. Table 3–12 provides the evidence-based kcal/kg/day for the specific overall healthy adult.[27]

- Energy and Protein Accommodations for Amputation

In amputees, energy and protein needs vary depending upon the location of amputation. In the immediate postoperative phase, patients who have undergone surgery for the amputation of a limb are moderately

Table 3–12. Kcal/kg/day needed for the overall healthy adult.

Health Condition	Kcal/Kg/Day
Sedentary or very obese individual	22 kcal/kg/day (based on desirable body weight)
Low activity level, or for age >55	28 kcal/kg/day (based on desirable body weight)
Consistent moderate activity	33 kcal/kg/day (based on desirable body weight)
Consistent strenuous activity	40 kcal/kg/day (based on desirable body weight)
Weight maintenance for a healthy older adult	Women: 25–35 kcal/kg/day Men: 30–40 kcal/kg/day
Weight maintenance for an underweight, or chronically or acutely ill older adult	25–30 kcal/kg/day Higher for weight gain

Data from Academy of Nutrition and Dietetics, 2012.

Table 3-13. Level of amputation and how it increases metabolic energy consumption.

Level of Amputation	Metabolic Energy Increase
Transmetatarsal (partial foot)	10-20%
Symes (ankle joint)	0-30%
Transtibial (below the knee)	40-50%
Transfemoral (above the knee)	90-100%
Bilateral transtibial	60-100%
Hip disarticulation	>100%

Data from Office of the Surgeon General, Department of the Army, 1998.

to severely stressed, requiring protein in the range of 1.2–2.0 g/kg body weight/day. In the long-term phase, protein requirements return to normal.[27] Table 3–13 contains information about average energy consumption increase at different levels of lower limb amputation.[28]

Medical Nutrition Therapy for Overweight and Obesity

The global pandemic of overweight and obesity is a major public health concern that shows no signs of abating. In the United States, there is a minority (35%) of individuals at a healthy BMI, with 65% being either overweight or obese.[29] There is no question that obesity results from energy imbalance; however, the energy balance concept does not take into account the many other factors that contribute to the regulation of food intake and the variety of genetic, social, cultural, environmental, and behavioral factors that appear to be contributing to the problem. Obesity does increase health risk and the cost of health care ($147 billion healthcare dollars were spent on obesity-related costs in 2008 alone), with the stigma of obesity leading to traumatization of both children and adults, and causing people to experience prejudice in social and economic situations.[4,30] Therefore, the need for the adoption of effective strategies that will prevent and treat overweight and obesity is crucial.

■ Goals of Weight Management Therapy

While the goal for most individuals should be to achieve an ideal body weight to reduce the risk of developing chronic diseases, this is easier said than done. The following section provides a number of suggestions for promoting realistic weight loss and helping to maintain a healthy weight:

Slow or Stop Weight Gain

The first public health goal for overweight and obese people in the United States, as well as an individual's weight management goal, is to stop the gradual weight gain that occurs each year.[29] Obesity will continue to increase if the average adult weight gain in the United States of 1–2 pounds per year is not stopped. Prevention of further weight gain requires the least modification of energy balance, because it has been estimated that modifying energy balance by only 100 kcal/day would be sufficient for most of the population.[29]

Reduce Body Weight

A 10% reduction in body weight from baseline should be the initial goal of weight loss therapy, with 6 months being a reasonable time frame for meeting this goal. When this goal is achieved, additional weight loss can then be attempted, if indicated through further assessment. Weight loss should occur at a rate of 1–2 pounds per week, usually promoted by a calorie deficit of 500–1000 kcal/day. A more restrictive regimen may be needed once weight loss begins to plateau after 6 months, which is expected due to a lesser energy expenditure at the lower weight. These have been shown to be realistic, achievable, and sustainable goals by a number of authoritative nutrition bodies.[15,31]

Maintain the Weight Loss

Unless a weight maintenance program that consists of dietary therapy, physical activity, and behavior therapy is continued indefinitely, experience has shown that lost weight usually will be regained. If patients are unable to achieve a significant weight reduction, an important goal is to prevent further weight gain; thus, participation in a weight maintenance program is also warranted.[15,31]

▪ Effectiveness of Weight Management Therapy

A comprehensive weight management program that includes diet, physical activity, and behavior modification is necessary to promote weight loss and weight maintenance. A combination of the therapies has been shown to be more successful than using any one intervention alone. Greater weight loss, decreases in abdominal fat, and increases in cardiorespiratory fitness are produced with the combination of a reduced calorie diet and increased physical activity, than with diet alone or physical activity alone. When weight loss occurs, approximately 75% is from fat and 25% from lean tissue.[15,31]

Reduction in energy intake of 500–1000 kcal/day to achieve a 1- to 2-pound weight loss per week is the first recommendation in obesity treatment; however, the desired rate of weight loss and ultimate weight loss goal should be realistic and achievable for that individual (eg, a person with a strong family and personal history of obesity should not immediately strive for a weight in the normal range).[15,31] Failure usually results when attempts to achieve goals defined by external criteria are made, which can lead to a lowered self-esteem, weight regain, and impediments to future weight loss success. Overall, caloric requirements for each individual should be based on daily energy intake, daily energy expenditure, and an average weight loss goal of 1 pound per week beginning after the first month of the program.[32]

Diet Therapy for weight loss should last at least 6 months, or until weight loss goals are achieved. After this initial 6 months, a priority should be the implementation of a weight maintenance program, with dietary therapy optimally lasting at least another 6 months. It has been found that a greater frequency of contacts and the amount of time spent with the individual and the practitioner will lead to better outcomes.[15,31]

The National Weight Control Registry (NWCR, introduced in Chapter 2), established by Rena Wing, PhD, and James O. Hill, PhD, is the largest prospective investigation of long-term successful weight loss maintenance. Through the initial research of the NWCR, the investigators concluded that losing weight and keeping the weight off are two totally different processes, and therefore require different behaviors.[29] Both diet and physical activity were the only common denominators in how over 5000 individuals studied by the NWCR lost their weight. The purpose of the NWCR was to identify the common characteristics of these 5000 individuals who maintained a mean weight loss of approximately 30 pounds and kept it off for at least a year (a group that is often referred to as "successful losers").[33] There were few similarities in the type of diet that was used for weight loss. Researchers have found that the people in the registry participate in levels of physical activity that burn an average of 400–500 calories per day, equivalent to 60–75 minutes of brisk walking or 35–40 minutes of jogging.[3,34,35] The people in the registry eat, on an average, about 1400 calories per day, limit fast foods, sugars, and sweets, consume multiple servings of fruits and vegetables, and watch less television than do the nonlosers.[36-38] Some of the common characteristics of successful losers are also listed in Table 3–14.[29]

Table 3–14. Common characteristics of "successful losers."

Eat a low-fat diet but are aware of total calories consumed
Eat breakfast almost every day
Use self-monitoring in that they weigh themselves frequently and often record their food intake and physical activity
Engage in very high levels of physical activity

Data from Hill et al., 2005.

■ Assessment & Monitoring Parameters

Before managing an individual's condition of overweight and obesity, several parameters must first be assessed. Assessment involves classifying the individual's degree of overweight and obesity and determining their overall risk status (relative to risk at normal body weight). Assessment can also include determining the individual's motivational, nutritional, and medical factors that will allow successful participation in weight loss and/or weight management. These same assessment parameters are used to monitor one's progress once the program has begun.

Classifying Degree of Overweight and Obesity

Determining the degree of overweight and overall risk status (relative to risk at normal body weight) is the first step in the assessment process. BMI and waist circumference (WC) are used to classify overweight and obesity, estimate the risk for disease, identify treatment options, and determine the effectiveness of therapy during reassessment. BMI and WC are correlated to obesity or fat mass and risk of other diseases.[15,31] Table 3–15 describes this classification and correlation.[15]

Table 3–15. Classification of overweight and obesity by BMI, waist circumference, and associated disease risk.

	BMI (kg/m^2)	Obesity Class	Disease Risk[a] WC: men ≤40 inches women ≤35 inches	Disease Risk[a] WC: men >40 inches women >35 inches
Underweight	<18.5			
Normal[b]	18.5–24.9			
Overweight	25.0–29.9		Increased	High
Obesity	30.0–34.9	I	High	Very high
	35.0–39.9	II	Very high	Very high
Extreme obesity	≥40	III	Extremely high	Extremely high

WC, waist circumference.

[a]Relative disease risk for type 2 diabetes, hypertension, and CVD (not absolute risk—a summation of risk factors).

[b]Increased WC can also be a marker for increased risk, even in persons with normal weight.

Data from National Heart, Lung, and Blood Institute (NHLBI), 1998.

Indicators for Weight Management

Obesity increases morbidity and mortality, and assessment of an individual's absolute risk factors is necessary in order to provide adequate and comprehensive care. The relationship between weight and health is a two-way street, and reversing weight gain can impart meaningful health outcomes. There is strong evidence that weight loss and adult weight management reverse the risk factors associated with many health conditions and in many population groups. The disease risk factors affected by weight loss and maintenance of a healthy weight include coronary heart disease, type 2 diabetes, gallstones, gynecological abnormalities, hypertension, metabolic syndrome, osteoarthritis, sleep apnea, and stress incontinence.[15,31,39] Successful weight loss and management has been shown to reduce the risk factors associated with diabetes and cardiovascular disease, high blood pressure, serum triglycerides, total serum cholesterol, LDL cholesterol, and the risk for certain types of cancer such as endometrial, breast, prostate, and colon cancer.[15,31]

Other risk factors that heighten the need for weight reduction in obese individuals include cigarette smoking and physical inactivity. For overweight individuals with two or more risk factors associated with their weight status, the NHLBI recommends weight loss intervention, while the *Dietary Guidelines for Americans, 2010* recommend working toward achieving an ideal body weight, even if individuals are only mildly overweight.[15,18]

Motivation

The importance of one's own motivation to participate in weight loss or weight management therapy cannot be underestimated. Successful weight loss and management is dependent on the involvement and investment of the individual; it also requires a major investment of time and effort by the healthcare team. Table 3–16 contains a list of factors

Table 3–16. Factors to consider when determining readiness to change.

Reasons or specific motivators
Previous history of successful and unsuccessful attempts at weight loss
Family, friends, and work-related support
Understanding of causes and risks of obesity
Attitude toward exercise and physical activity
Ability to participate in exercise and physical activity
Time available for weight loss interventions
Financial considerations and limitations

Data from National Heart, Lung, and Blood Institute (NHLBI), 1998.

that should be evaluated and considered during the assessment phase to determine the readiness of the individual to implement the plan.[15]

Medical Considerations

Physiological causes of increased body weight (eg, endocrine abnormalities, neurological disturbances, medication use, or underlying disease state) should be ruled out with a thorough medical examination. Before making physical activity recommendations, practitioners should screen for musculoskeletal problems and cardiorespiratory fitness. A psychological evaluation may also be indicated, and barriers to successful weight loss should be considered. Possible psychological barriers include depression, anxiety, post-traumatic stress disorder, addictions, bipolar disorder, use of psychotropic medications, eating disorders, and disordered eating, as studies have shown excessive weight problems to occur in high frequency alongside these conditions.[6] There are several classes of drugs that can increase body weight, including psychotropic medications, antidepressants, epileptic agents, insulin, glucocorticoids, and sulfonylureas.[32] Ideally, before beginning nutritional intervention for overweight and obesity, appropriate treatment for any medical concerns should be addressed.

■ Dietary Interventions

Despite the complex and multifactorial nature of obesity, the simple action of food restriction is an important component of weight loss, particularly for those prone to overeating. Research from the NWCR showed that there were few similarities in the type of diet that was used to achieve weight loss among the successful 5000 individuals who maintained a weight loss of approximately 30 pounds for a mean of greater than 6 years. These participants showed that there are many effective diets to lose weight, as long as energy intake is less than energy expenditure.[29] Ideally, documentation of food intake should be managed by the individual to ensure that the appropriate average weight loss goal is achieved. Chapter 2 provides more information about self-documentation of dietary and exercise patterns.

Reduced Calorie Diets

Reduced calorie diets have been found to reduce total body weight by an average of 8% over 3–12 months.[15,31] Depending on the individual's health risk, caloric restriction may be moderate to severe. For most people, a moderate calorie deficit or low-calorie diet (LCD) is indicated, and a more severe caloric restriction or very low calorie diet (VLCD) should be reserved for those individuals facing more serious health risks and who do not show improvements with an LCD.

Low-calorie diet (LCD)

Traditionally, an LCD is defined as a diet that provides a caloric intake of 1200 kcal/day for a woman and 1500 kcal/day for a man. On an average, an LCD has been shown to produce weight loss of 13–17 pounds within 20–24 weeks.[32] However, as both anecdotal and published material suggest, a more individualized approach is more likely to bring success than a prescribed calorie number. It is also prudent to remember that as individuals lose weight, their energy requirements decline; thus, a lower-calorie diet may be indicated. Should calories need to be adjusted to less than 1200 calories per day, a daily vitamin and mineral supplementation is advised.

Very low calorie diet (VLCD)

For those patients who need to lose more weight at a faster pace than what can be achieved with an LCD, a VLCD may be indicated. VLCDs are those (usually commercially prepared formulas) with 800 calories or less that stand to replace all other usual food eaten. VLCDs produce weight loss of 3.3 pounds per week in women and 4.4 pounds per week in men, with a total loss averaging 44 pounds after 12–16 weeks. Within 3 weeks, VLCDs have demonstrated improvements in glycemic control, systolic and diastolic blood pressure, and decreases in serum concentrations of triglycerides, LDL-C, and total cholesterol. It is believed that the short-term success of VLCDs compared to LCDs is more due to the structure of the diet versus the calorie difference, because when obese patients follow a conventional diet, caloric intake has been found to be underestimated by as much as 40%. Thus, adherence may be improved with portion- and calorie-controlled servings and liquid diets.[32] However, long-term (>1 year) weight loss from the VLCD is not different from that of the LCD.[15]

Initiating LCDs

A moderate caloric deficit or LCD should be used as the initial approach for obese individuals attempting weight loss for the first time. For those individuals, with a BMI of 25–34, who may have failed previously at weight loss but are motivated to lose weight, this regimen is also indicated.[32] A practical way to create a caloric deficit of 500–1000 kcal below estimated energy needs is by reducing dietary fat and/or carbohydrates. The most frequently recommended diet by governing health authorities is a low-fat, reduced-energy diet, because it is the most well-studied weight-loss dietary strategy.[6] Low-fat diets without targeted caloric reductions have been found to help promote weight loss by producing a reduced caloric intake, but when coupled with a total caloric reduction, produce greater weight loss than low-fat diets alone.[31] Although fat is the most energy-dense macronutrient, its effect on satiety is weak.[6]

The *Dietary Guidelines for Americans, 2010* are a useful tool to serve as the meal planning guide for otherwise healthy individuals, and for determining the basic nutritional proportions of the LCD. In addition, the LCD should be realistic for the individual's current eating habits, lifestyle, other coexisting medical conditions, and potential nutrient-drug interactions. Unless there is a diagnosis of congestive heart failure, edema, or renal insufficiency, the individual should aim to drink at least 1.5–2 quarts per day of water. Protein requirements may need to be adjusted for individuals with renal disease, diabetes, or other metabolic disorders, and changes in scheduling or medication dosages may be required due to the energy restriction and weight loss.[32]

LCDs are certainly not for the faint of heart or casual dieter, as they require discipline and attention to detail, not to mention significantly reduced food intake. LCDs should be approached only under a qualified and trained healthcare professional's guidance. Potential complications of an LCD include ketosis (especially with very low carbohydrate intake), excessive loss of lean body mass, arrhythmias, dehydration, and tendency for recidivism to the higher calorie intake levels.[32]

A severe caloric deficit or VLCD (250–799 calories daily) is usually a liquid formulation of food and, as with LCDs, should be individualized. Indications for a VLCD may include: (1) high or very high health risk due to BMI alone (BMI ≥35); (2) BMI ≥30 with serious comorbid conditions; and (3) failed prior weight-loss attempts. Unless the healthcare provider deems that the patient faces a major health risk and can safely use this diet, VLCDs are not recommended due to insufficient evidence showing long-term weight loss with usually more weight regained long term. Thus, indiscriminate use of VLCDs is a medical liability. Table 3–17 lists the requirements for and contraindications of VLCDs.[32]

Due to the reduction in anabolic hormones—such as insulin, insulin-like growth factors, and growth hormone—that occurs with aging and due to the associated nitrogen loss with low caloric intake, VLCDs are not recommended in the elderly. Potential complications and side effects associated with VLCDs and patient counseling recommendations are presented in Table 3–18.[32]

Eating Frequency and Patterns

Regular meal pattern

Reduced obesity risk has been associated with the consumption of four to five meals/snacks per day (including breakfast). In contrast, greater obesity risk has been associated with the consumption of three or fewer meals, and with the consumption of six or more meals per day.[40] In men, lower total daily energy intake and body weights have been correlated with higher eating frequency, with less conclusive data being available for women. Additionally, it is believed that consumption of greater calories during the day or the morning contributes to less risk of obesity, compared to greater evening consumption of calories.[6,31]

Eating breakfast

Despite lowering daily energy intakes, skipping breakfast leads to an increased risk of high BMI and obesity. Impulsive snacking appears

Table 3–17. Requirements for VLCDs and contraindications of VLCDs.

Requirements for VLCDs	Contraindications of VLCD Use
Demonstration of motivation to adherence	BMI ≤30 due to increased risk of negative nitrogen balance
Commitment to participate in a weight loss maintenance program	Recent myocardial infarction
≤65 years of age	Cardiac conduction disorder
The VLCD should provide: • Daily protein of at least 1 g/kg desirable body weight • High biological protein (from lean meat, fish, or fowl if solid meal, or if liquid, from dairy sources, eg, soy, or albumin) • Minimum of essential fatty acids • Recommend allowances of vitamins, minerals, and electrolytes • Up to 100 grams of carbohydrate	History of cerebrovascular, renal, or hepatic disease
	Type 1 diabetes mellitus
	Major psychiatric disorders
	Gallbladder disease
	Alcoholism
	Cancer
	Infection
Close supervision with weekly healthcare provider consultations during rapid weight-loss period and every 2–4 weeks thereafter	Acute substance abuse
	Anorexia or history of other eating disorder
Basic serum chemistry, to include electrolytes and liver function tests, at each visit	Human immunodeficiency virus
Duration of use should not exceed 12–16 weeks to avoid excessive nitrogen loss, gallstone accretion, and relapse or recidivism	

Data from American Association of Clinical Endocrinologists/American College of Endocrinology (AACE/ACE) Obesity Task Force, 1998.

to be reduced in people who eat breakfast, with less calories also being consumed at later meals. Studies have shown that normal-weight individuals and people who maintain weight loss tend to eat breakfast regularly. Their breakfasts generally consist of high-fiber cereal that constitutes about 20% of their daily caloric needs. Higher BMIs, however, have been associated with breakfasts that are calorically dense.[6,31]

Portion Control

A comprehensive weight management program should include portion control at meals and snacks because it has been shown to result in reduced energy intake and weight loss. As portion size increases at a meal, caloric intake also increases; however, despite the increase in energy intake, the increased food consumption is not associated with

Table 3–18. Complications and side effects of very low calorie diets.

Complication	General Information
Cholelithiasis	• Most common complication of VLCD therapy, occurring in approximately 25% of patients • Earlier realimentation may minimize cholelithiasis • About 1/3 of gallstones formed during a VLCD disappear in the first 6 months after dieting • Not associated with more conservative weight-loss approaches that rely primarily on behavior modification
Loss of lean body mass	• Prescribe daily, moderate exercise as preventive measure • Do not prescribe VLCD for longer than 16 weeks
Sudden death	• Can occur rarely in medically vulnerable patients with comorbidities, especially if caloric intake is <600 kcal/day • Ensure completion of informed consent form
Ketosis, lipolysis	• May produce increase in serum uric acid; uric acid levels peak in 1-2 weeks, then usually return to normal • Ketosis may alter taste sensation, diminish appetite, and provide a sense of well-being
Side effects	
Cold intolerance, dry skin, and brittle nails	• Caused by VLCD-induced reduction in resting metabolic rate of 15-30% • Important to counsel patient, especially during winter months • Counsel patient to use moisturizing lotion, avoid deodorant soap, and keep nails well trimmed
Hair loss	• Tends to occur when diet lasts >14 weeks; due to diminished metabolic rate • Usually alleviated by gradual realimentation
Dry mouth	• Counsel patient to increase water intake and prevent dehydration
Fatigue	• Probably due to reduced energy intake • Counsel patient to get plenty of rest, eat all prescribed items in food plan, participate in only moderate activities, and drink plenty of fluids
Dizziness	• May be due to postural hypotension or diuresis, which can result in decreased blood volume and lead to orthostatic hypotension • In the second week of the diet, the physician may add 3 grams of sodium chloride (bouillon) daily to prevent postural hypotension, as VLCDs provide only about 1 g/day • Counsel patient to increase water intake by 1 quart daily and to rise slowly to allow blood pressure to adjust

(Continued)

Table 3–18. Complications and side effects of very low calorie diets. (*Continued*)

Complication	General Information
Headache	• Counsel patient to maintain food plan, without skipping meals • Provide patient with list of acceptable headache medications; avoid aspirin and nonsteroidal anti-inflammatory drugs, in order to reduce risk of gastrointestinal bleeding
Muscle cramps	• May be caused by changes in electrolyte balance or physical activity • Counsel patient to increase water intake and perform stretching exercises frequently
Diarrhea	• Provide patient with list of medications • Counsel patient about increased water intake to prevent dehydration
Halitosis	• Counsel patient to pay more attention to dental hygiene, use mouthwash, chew sugarless gum, and drink water after taking a supplement
Abdominal cramps	• Due to prolonged reduced caloric intake • Provide patient with list of medications, if needed

Data from American Association of Clinical Endocrinologists/American College of Endocrinology (AACE/ACE) Obesity Task Force, 1998.

feelings of fullness. As such, the increased energy intake does not lead to less caloric intake at subsequent meals, and consequently, increased daily energy intake results. In order to reduce the energy load of consumed foods, practitioners should encourage portion control to their patients, with the goal of decreasing the energy load of consumed foods. Studies have shown that portion control at meals and snacks does result in reduced energy intake and weight loss. Strategies for implementing portion control include:

- Advising on the energy content of regularly consumed food (eg, energy intake of two cups of sweetened ice tea per day vs one cup per day)
- Using premeasured foods with known calorie amounts
- Replacing higher-energy-density foods with lower-energy-density foods (eg, substituting a cookie for fruit)
- Reducing the energy density of foods (eg, by increasing the vegetable content of a casserole)
- Advising on being aware of "portion distortion" of food, drink, and dinnerware in the marketplace that gives the perception of appropriate amounts to consume at a single occasion (see Chapter 2 for more information on portions for meal planning)

Meal Replacements

Meal replacements include liquid meals, meal bars, and calorie-controlled packaged meals that contain a known energy and macronutrient content. Consuming up to one or two meal replacements daily has been found to be a beneficial component of comprehensive weight management programs. This is especially true for people who have difficulty with portion control and self-selection and for those who are easily overwhelmed by an environment that provides a surplus of palatable, energy-dense, and nutrient-poor food choices. Compared to reduced calorie diets, studies have shown an equivalent or greater weight loss with isocaloric structured meal replacement plans.[6,31]

Nutrition Education

In order to properly adjust to an LCD, nutrition education should be individualized and included as part of a comprehensive weight management program. Studies have shown that nutrition education may lead to improved food choices and increased knowledge. Cooking classes that include recipe modification have been shown to promote behavior change and result in improved dietary habits. Table 3–19 contains a list of topics that should be included in nutrition education.

Table 3–19. Topics to include in nutrition education.

Reading nutrition labels
Recipe modification
Food composition: fats, carbohydrates (including fiber), and protein
Food preparation aimed at avoiding high-calorie ingredients (eg, limiting added fats and oils during cooking)
New habits of purchasing food (eg, having a snack before grocery shopping so as to avoid impulse buys, making a grocery list, and sticking to it)
Avoiding overconsumption of high-calorie foods (such as those high in fat and carbohydrate content)
Maintaining adequate water intake and good hydration
Reducing portion sizes
Limiting alcohol consumption
Avoiding sugar-sweetened beverages
Including regular physical activity in addition to dietary changes

Low-Glycemic Index Diet

The glycemic index (GI) is a value that is expressed relative to the blood glucose response observed after ingestion of 50 grams of a carbohydrate-containing test food, usually glucose or white bread. In theory, after the consumption of a high-glycemic index food, an early and sharp increase in blood glucose occurs, which subsequently causes a strong insulin response. The insulin response then promotes rebound hypoglycemia as a result of the clearance of glucose from the blood. Theoretically, this response is believed to stimulate the appetite, leading to increased energy intake, positive energy balance, and subsequent weight gain.[5] Despite the basic understanding of the GI of various foods, research on low-GI foods, and thus, low-GI diets have failed to show effectiveness as a weight loss or weight management strategy, and are therefore not recommended. Even less conclusive than the effects of consumption of low-GI foods on energy intake and weight loss is the effect on body fat mass. Further research is needed to determine the effect of low-GI foods on body fat composition.[6,31] Chapter 6 contains more information on the glycemic index and glycemic load.

High-Calcium Diet

The DRIs for calcium were last revised in 2010. For males, the RDA for calcium is 1000 mg for men aged 19–70. For females, the RDA is 1000 mg for women aged 19–50 and 1200 mg for 51- to 70-year-olds. Several studies in white and black adults have shown that calcium intake below these levels is associated with increased body weight, body fat, BMI, waist circumference, hypertension risk, and relative risk of obesity. It is not clear, however, if this is a result of an overall poor diet—as milk-drinkers tend to exhibit healthier overall habits than nonmilk drinkers. Additional studies establishing a causal relationship between total daily calcium intake, calcium supplementation or dairy intake, and weight management are needed before definitive statements about these relationships can be made.[6,31]

At this time, current nutrition recommendations maintain that as a component of a comprehensive weight management program, individuals should be encouraged to incorporate three to four servings of low-fat dairy per day. It is not clear, however, what the effect of dairy and/or calcium at or above the recommended levels on weight management is.[6,31] What we do know, however, is that most American adults average only half of their recommended intakes of calcium. Thus, the inclusion of the recommended dosage not only has beneficial effects on the overall health (eg, bone health, blood pressure control), but it may also be beneficial for weight management.

Low-Carbohydrate Diet

The rationale for carbohydrate restriction is that with the resulting lower glucose availability, the body is directed away from fat storage and toward fat oxidation, due to changes in insulin and glucagon concentrations.[41] A low-carbohydrate diet causes the depletion of glycogen stores, and the resultant diuresis produces an initial dramatic weight loss. With a very low-carbohydrate diet (eg, 20 g/day), it is the production of ketones that may be responsible for sustaining fuel utilization in the brain, and this may be responsible for decreasing hunger, and therefore improved diet adherence.[6,31] Although the definition of a low-carbohydrate diet is a nutritional intake of less than 200 grams of carbohydrate per day, it is more likely that a carbohydrate intake in the range of 50–150 g/day leads to metabolic changes associated with the production of ketones.[41] (The DRI recommendations state that the minimum number of grams of carbohydrates to be consumed by an adult are 130 grams per day, although to achieve the Acceptable Macronutrient Distribution Range for carbohydrates—which is 45–65% of total energy—most adults need significantly more than 130 grams of carbohydrate.)

The focus on a reduction in carbohydrate, rather than reducing calories and/or fat may be a short-term strategy or approach for weight loss. Although research indicates that reducing carbohydrate intake to <35% of calories does result in reduced energy intake, in comparison studies of diets designed to be isocaloric, no significant differences in body weight or fat loss during the first 6 months were found between those consuming low-carbohydrate diets compared to other diets. In studies that have shown a greater body weight and fat loss with the consumption of low-carbohydrate diets, as compared with reduced calorie diets (both resulting in reduced calorie intake) the differences were only significant for the first 6 months, and after 1 year, there were no differences found.[40]

The safety of long-term, extreme restrictions of carbohydrates (<35% of calories) has not been evaluated, and because of the limited research, caution should be used in suggesting a low-carbohydrate diet for even short-term use, especially in patients with osteoporosis, kidney disease, and elevated low-density lipoprotein (LDL) concentrations. Because the low-carbohydrate diet tends to be high in protein, and protein-dense foods are usually high in fat and saturated fat, there is concern for an increased cardiovascular disease risk with these diets. Despite the likelihood of increased risk from such a nutrient profile, at this time there is inconclusive evidence to validate these concerns.[6,15,31]

When considering the effect of a low-carbohydrate diet, it is wise to remember that weight control is not the only factor that determines health. The habitual reduction in the carbohydrate composition of a diet may limit fruits, vegetables, and whole grain intakes, and causes a greater challenge in meeting the vitamin, trace element, fiber, and phytochemical recommendations suggested for total health and well-being.[11] In addition, it is impossible to reduce the carbohydrate content of the diet without affecting the proportion of at least one other macronutrient, protein, and/or fat; thus, this also has implications for total health. Currently, the scientific evidence suggests that in order to meet all nutrient recommendations, a weight-loss diet should be moderate in carbohydrate, moderate in fat, and one-fourth to one-third of energy requirements should be contributed by protein.[11] Surely, much of the population consumes excessive amounts of carbohydrate, often in the form of nutritionally void refined carbohydrates, but eliminating carbohydrate altogether is not a viable solution to this problem.

Vegetarian Diet

Therapeutic use of a vegetarian diet has been found to be an effective approach to weight loss, both in the short-term and long-term. Simply following a well-balanced vegetarian diet alone, without regard to calorie level, can result in initial weight loss for some individuals.[42] Studies have shown that those following a vegetarian diet tend to be leaner than those who include meat in their diets. In addition, a vegetarian diet that is rich in fruits, vegetables, whole grains, and legumes is high in fiber. Dietary fiber not only leads to a reduction in calories, but also increases satiety and reduces hunger. Research has also demonstrated that vegetarians have a higher RMR (contributed by higher levels of norepinephrine), likely resulting from their higher carbohydrate and lower fat intakes. Avoiding meat and focusing on a low-energy, high nutrient-dense vegetarian diet pattern, rich in whole grains, vegetables, legumes, and dietary fiber, while reducing total caloric content, leads to greater weight loss when compared to those who include meat in their diets.[42]

In addition to the beneficial effects of the fiber of a vegetarian diet, omega-3 fatty acids from food sources, such as fish, are believed to influence satiety and consequently affect energy restriction and weight management. Similar benefits have also been observed with omega-3-rich supplements. There is also observational data available suggesting that leptin (a hormone that promotes satiety and controls energy intake and expenditure) is lowered in obese individuals who consume omega-3-rich foods, thereby resulting in weight loss.[42]

Not all vegetarian diets are created alike, and it is possible to assemble a vegetarian meal plan that is not well balanced. Adherents to a vegetarian diet, no matter what type of vegetarianism they ascribe to, are advised to limit excessive consumption of full-fat dairy foods and refined carbohydrates and to assure adequate protein intake from plant-based sources, fish, and seafood (if applicable). While it is certainly possible to follow a well-balanced vegetarian meal plan, there is particular interest in assuring that vegetarians achieve adequate protein, omega-3 fatty acids, iron, zinc, iodine, calcium, and vitamins D and B12 from foods or dietary supplements in levels that prevent deficiency.[6]

■ Physical Activity Interventions

Physical activity should be included as part of a comprehensive weight management program. Unless medically contraindicated, the accumulation of at least 30 minutes (and if possible, 60 minutes) or more of moderate intensity physical activity on most, and preferably all days of week, should be the long-term goals established for promoting weight loss in overweight and obese adults.[3,15] The participants in the NWCR, on an average, expended nearly 3000 kcal per week in moderate to vigorous physical activity, which would require somewhere between 60 and 90 minutes of brisk walking per day.[3,35]

Effects of Physical Activity

Physical activity has a number of beneficial effects as part of a weight-loss regimen, beyond just promoting weight loss. Other benefits include[3,15]:

- Mobilization of fat from visceral adipose tissue
- Moderate reduction in abdominal fat
- Preservation of lean body mass
- Modest weight loss, independent of the effect of caloric reduction through diet
- Maintenance of weight loss
- Increases in cardiorespiratory fitness, independent of weight loss
- Improved fitness, health, and overall well-being

Physical Activity Precautions

For some individuals, starting a physical activity regimen may require supervision in order to avoid injury. It is important that individuals be assessed for physical activity readiness by a qualified healthcare professional before undertaking a new routine. Some precautions for physical activity for weight loss include[3,15]:

- Start with simple, less strenuous exercises that can be gradually intensified, especially in the extremely obese individual (Table 3–20 lists types of physical activities)
- Consider exercise testing for cardiopulmonary disease, based on the individual's age, symptoms, and concomitant risk factors
- Administer the Physical Activity Readiness Questionnaire (PAR-Q) to assess the medical readiness of beginning an exercise program (to learn more and to download the PAR-Q form, visit: http://www.csep.ca/english/view.asp?x=698)
- Determine if adjustment in medications are needed
- Assess orthopedic or balance problems and consider nonweight-bearing activities

Setting Realistic Physical Activity Expectations

Although the effects of physical activity on weight loss and management mentioned above are significant, the resulting increase of the REE from physical activity is not consistent in all individuals. This is due mainly to the fact that in order to offset reductions in REE that result secondary to energy restrictions, only moderate- to high-intensity activities (50–75% VO_2 max) are vigorous enough to do this; thus, lower-intensity activities (<50% VO_2 max) have no effect on the REE.[3]

Table 3-20. Types of physical activities.

Purposeful		Lifestyle
Less Strenuous	**More Strenuous**	
• Walking • Swimming • Water aerobics • Chair aerobics • Recumbent stationary cycling • Chair dancing	• Fitness walking • Cycling • Rowing • Cross-country skiing • Aerobic dancing • Rope jumping • Jogging[a] • Competitive sports[a]	• Walking up stairs instead of using the escalator or elevator • Exiting public transportation prior to the actual destination and walking the difference • Parking further away from an entrance • Gardening • Walking a dog • Walking while talking on the phone or in the airport waiting on a flight

[a]Be careful to avoid injury; can lead to orthopedic injury; create a safe environment.

In the short term, increasing activity energy expenditure (AEE) may not be as significantly effective as caloric restriction is, because many overweight or obese individuals are quite sedentary and unfit. The *metabolic engine* of the overweight, obese, and sedentary individuals is not large enough to burn a sizeable number of calories. In addition, these individuals usually cannot exercise for more than a few minutes past 40–50% of their maximal capacity.[3] On an average, 1 kcal/kg of body weight per hour is expended; therefore, if an individual weighs 100 kilograms (220 lbs) only ~200 kcal per hour is burned while walking at 2 mph and ~250 kcal when walking at 2.5 mph. For individuals in this category, walking at a faster pace may not be feasible. Unfortunately, this individual would have to walk ~35 hours in order to metabolize 1 kg (2.2 lbs) of body fat. However, in these cases, it is important to note that sitting expends only 100 kcal per hour, so walking at 2 mph is better than sitting.[3] Table 3–20 compares a number of purposeful versus lifestyle physical activities.

■ Behavioral Interventions

In order to achieve weight loss, behavioral modification should focus on increasing energy expenditure and reducing energy intake, primarily by concentrating on the individual's current behavior while also recognizing the role of genetics and cultural influences on weight. Treatment involves the restructuring of the individual's environment in order to reduce the behaviors that are thought to impede weight loss, along with close monitoring of those behaviors. Key features of a behavioral modification program include: self-monitoring, goal-setting, stimulus control, problem-solving, cognitive restructuring, relapse prevention, and nutrition and exercise. Successful behavior therapy is the key to long-term maintenance of a healthy body weight,[43] and a number of behavior modification concepts are covered in Chapter 2.

Self-monitoring, which involves keeping specific detailed records of the behaviors that support or sabotage weight-loss efforts, is often considered one of the most important components of behavioral therapy. This type of information can lead to self-discovery of eating in response to stress, depression, or boredom. Self-monitoring may also lead the individual to recognizing that being in the company of certain people leads to overeating or inactivity.[43] Goal-setting is another important component of behavioral therapy, and this strategy includes setting goals related to weight, calories, fat content, or other components of the diet, as well as to establishing physical activity goals.

In order to reduce an individual's engagement in behaviors that are known to sabotage weight loss efforts, modifying the physical environment through stimulus control is another recommended behavioral intervention. Stimulus control includes techniques such as carrying healthy snacks to work to reduce trips to the vending machine, or eating breakfast at home to avoid eating the donuts available in the break room.[43] Problem-solving is another behavioral intervention that assists individuals to identify potential barriers to carrying out their program. Possible solutions to these barriers are identified, time for implementation of the solution is given, then the effectiveness of the solution is evaluated.[43]

Many overweight individuals are unaware that they have poor self-esteem that interferes with their weight loss efforts. Recognition and modification of their thoughts and beliefs related to weight are taught through cognitive restructuring, by helping the individuals replace negative and punitive statements with those that are empowering, encouraging, and affirming.[43]

Because lapses are inevitable in weight loss efforts, relapse prevention is key component of behavioral interventions. Practitioners can help patients and clients prepare for lapses (and in turn avoid full relapses) by envisioning potential barriers to success and brainstorming to overcome these barriers as part of the ongoing nutrition counseling process.

■ FDA-Approved Medication Interventions

In the absence of the recommended one-pound per week weight loss after at least 6 months on a weight loss regimen that includes an LCD, increased physical activity, and behavioral therapy, it is then that careful consideration to the use of pharmacological therapy may be given.[15,6] At the time of this writing there are now three long-term-use FDA-approved drugs available for weight loss in the United States, two of which were only recently approved after greater than a decade of very limited FDA-approved weight loss medications. Short-term use of weight loss drugs is not helpful, since obesity is a chronic disease, and therefore the practitioner should include drugs only in the context of a long-term treatment strategy.

Medications for weight loss should only be used as part of a comprehensive program that includes diet, physical activity, and behavioral therapy, and potential drug side effects must be continually monitored for.[15] The FDA-approved weight loss medications, lorcaserin and controlled-release combination of phentermine/topiramate, are both indicated in combination with diet and exercise for obese adults, and for overweight adults with at least one weight-related condition, such as hypertension, type 2 diabetes, or dyslipidemia. Lorcaserin is flagged as a potential drug of abuse and DEA scheduling is still being evaluated. All of these medications listed in Table 3–21 are not without safety concerns and warrant cautious use.

The major role for these medications is to assist the individual in complying with diet and/or physical activity weight loss plans. Studies have shown that not all individuals will respond to pharmacological therapy; thus, there are responders and nonresponders to drug therapy. A good guideline to assess if drug therapy should be continued is to assess if the individual has lost at least 2 kilograms (4.4 lbs) in the first 4 weeks after initiating therapy. If not, long-term response is unlikely and, therefore, the drug should be discontinued.[15] For the weight loss medication, Qsymia, research has found that patients who did not lose at least 3% of their body weight after 12 weeks of treatment were unlikely to lose weight and maintain weight loss. Therefore, this medication (as well as Belviq) is recommended to be discontinued if after 12 weeks the patient has not lost at least 5% of their body weight.[17]

■ Surgical Interventions

The demand for weight loss surgery (WLS) has been fueled by the increase in obesity and lack of effective dietary and pharmacological treatment. In the morbidly obese, the most effective therapy available for weight management that can also result in improved quality of life and resolution of obesity-related comorbidities is bariatric surgery.[31] Bariatric surgery procedures are categorized as being either restrictive or malabsorptive and restrictive. Table 3–22 compares the basic types of bariatric surgery and Figures 3–2, 3–3, 3–4 and 3–5 show the difference between a normal stomach and one that has undergone, Roux-en-Y gastric bypass, a gastric sleeve, and adjustable gastric banding (ie, lap band).[44]

The effectiveness of WLS is increased when it is accompanied by both pre- and postoperative comprehensive therapy, as well as appropriate treatment during hospitalization. Table 3–23 describes the nutrition intervention during these three phases.[31] At this time, there is no evidence to support any specific protocol of post-WLS diet stages; therefore, facilities can develop their own protocols, or adapt protocols from other more experienced WLS facilities. Except for frequency of meals,

Table 3–21. FDA approved weight loss medications.

Medication	Orlistat (Xenical)	Lorcaserin Hydrochloride (Belviq)	Phentermine and Topiramate Extended-Release (Qsymia)
Approved by FDA	1999	June 2012	July 2012
Dosing	• 120 mg by mouth three times per day before meals • Available over the counter as 60 mg reduced dosage	• 10 mg twice per day	Starting dose: • 3.75 mg/23 mg of phentermine/topiramate daily for 2 weeks Usual dose: • 7.5 mg phentermine/46 mg extended-release topiramate Select dose: • 15 mg/92 mg topiramate for select patients who do not reach their weight loss goal
Mechanism of action	Inhibits pancreatic lipase and inhibits absorption of up to 30% dietary fat (only effective if fat is included in the diet)	Activates the serotonin 2C receptor in the brain, which may lead to fullness with less food intake	Phentermine acts as a sympathomimetic amine anorectic, and topiramate is an antiepileptic and also prevents migraine headaches
Adverse effects	Serious: • Anaphylaxis • Angioedema • Fat-soluble vitamin deficiencies • Hepatotoxicity Common: • Bloating • Steatorrhea • Distention • Fecal urgency	Serious: • Serotonin syndrome • Heart attack • Stroke • Confusion • Disturbances in memory • Sleepiness • Hallucinations • Euphoria • Disassociation • Priapism	Serious: • Increased heart rate • Heart attack • Stroke Common: • Parenthesis • Dizziness • Altered taste sensation • Insomnia • Constipation • Dry mouth

(Continued)

Table 3–21. FDA approved weight loss medications. (*Continued*)

Medication	Orlistat (Xenical)	Lorcaserin Hydrochloride (Belviq)	Phentermine and Topiramate Extended-Release (Qsymia)
		Common: • Headache • Dizziness • Fatigue • Nausea • Dry mouth • Constipation • Hypoglycemia (with diabetes) • Back pain (increased with diabetes) • Cough (increased with diabetes)	
Contraindications	• Chronic malabsorption syndrome • Cholestasis	• Recent or unstable CVD, CHF, or CVA since can increase heart size and heart rate • Pregnancy or considering	• Glaucoma • Hyperthyroidism • Pregnancy or considering (can cause birth defects); negative pregnancy test needed • Recent or unstable CVD or CVA
Precautions	• History of hyperoxaluria • History of calcium oxalate nephrolithiasis • History of anorexia nervosa or bulimia nervosa • History of organ transplant	• Heart valve dysfunction	• Regular heart monitoring for all patients • Females must use effective contraception and have monthly negative pregnancy test during treatment
Expected weight loss	Average of 2.89 kg per year (average of 5%)	Average of 3–4% per year	Average of 6.7% per year for the smaller dose and 8.9% per year for the larger dose

Data from National Heart, Lung, and Blood Institute (NHLBI), 1998; Clinical Endocrinology News, 2012; Endocrine Today, 2012.

Table 3-22. Basic types of bariatric surgery.

Types of Bariatric Surgery	Specific Procedures
Restrictive only *(least risk for long-term diet-related complications)*	• Laparoscopic adjustable gastric band (LAGB): adjustable band placed around upper portion of the stomach to restrict portion size; the smaller portion of stomach where food enters is 1 ounce in size • Gastric sleeve: stomach is surgically reduced in size to 1 ounce; long and narrow "sleeve" is about the width of a pen; sphincter is maintained at the bottom of the sleeve to allow for slower emptying; remainder of the stomach is removed from body during surgery, causing decrease in hormones and appetite
Malabsorptive & Restrictive *(highest risk for long-term diet-related complications)*	• Roux-en-Y gastric bypass (RYGBP): stomach is surgically reduced to 1 ounce size using upper portion just below the esophagus; remainder of stomach left inside the abdomen for gastric juices to drain to "y" portion of surgery where lower part of intestine is reconnected to the new stomach pouch • Biliopancreatic diversion, with or without duodenal switch: similar, but more extensive than the Roux-en-Y; less often used than the RYGBP

Data from Cummings et al., 2008.

the nutritional therapy is the same for all surgical procedures. In order to avoid potential complications, including postsurgical issues, all WLS require lifelong medical monitoring and follow-up.[31]

■ Specific Populations and Circumstances

Pediatrics

Overall, the evaluation process for assessing the pediatric population (children and adolescents) at risk of overweight or obesity is similar to the process for evaluating adults; however, the method for quantifying weight status must be modified due to the growth changes with age and sex for children and adolescents. According to the Centers for Disease Control and Prevention guidelines, all children aged 2 years and older should be screened for overweight and obesity. The CDC has developed BMI tools that track the BMI-for-age and BMI-for-sex.[45] The CDC BMI-for-age and BMI-for-sex growth charts are included as Appendix C.

For the pediatric population, underweight is defined as less than the 5th percentile of BMI-for-age, overweight is defined as a BMI

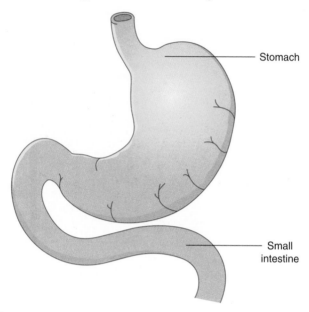

Figure 3–2. Normal stomach.

≥85th percentile and <95th percentile, and obesity is defined as a BMI ≥95th percentile for children of the same age and sex.[46] A healthy weighted child or adolescent is one who's BMI-for-age is 5th percentile to less than the 85th percentile (Table 3–24). A simplified online tool for calculating the BMI percentile for children and adolescents has also been designed and is available at: http://apps.nccd.cdc.gov/dnpabmi/. Because underestimation or overestimation of the BMI-for age and –sex, can occur for early- and late-maturing children, caution should be used for pubertal status influences (Kushner & Blatner, 2005).[25]

Assessment in the pediatric population, in addition to BMI, should include a physical examination and the evaluation of the child's medical history, and psychological and environmental factors for both the child and their family. Assessment and treatment include understanding how the below factors have led to the child's unhealthy weight and working on lifestyle goals that result in improved behaviors and ultimately a healthy weight[25]:

- What foods and beverages are stocked by the parents in the home, and what type of access does the child have to snacks and beverages?
- What are the families' rules concerning television, video games, dining out, and snacking?

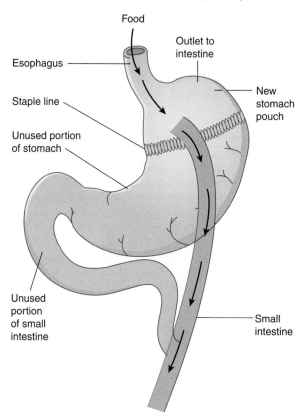

Figure 3–3. Roux-en-Y gastric bypass.

- What are the families' attitude concerning physical activity and exercise, and how much time is spent together as a family being active?
- What is the child's access to money for the purchase of food eaten away from home and at school and what type of food is eaten when away from home?
- How often does the family dine out together in a usual week and how often do they share meals together?
- What type of food is served at home and is it served family style (left on the table) or is it distributed from the kitchen and second servings limited?

Placing children on "diets" should be avoided if at all possible, and rather, the focus should be on optimizing healthy lifestyle choices. In addition, improvements in lifestyle behaviors should be emphasized

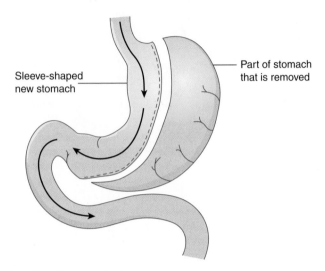

Figure 3–4. Sleeve gastrectomy.

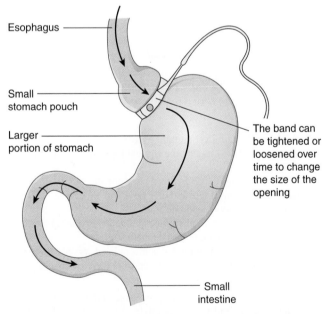

Figure 3–5. Adjustable gastric banding.

Table 3–23. Preoperative to postoperative nutrition interventions for bariatric surgery.

Preoperative Intervention	Hospitalization Intervention	Post-Surgical Intervention
First visit: provide information on what to expect concerning food and fluids during the hospital stay and following discharge, such as: Instruct patient on bariatric surgery protein supplements (low-sugar and low-fat) that all patients require	• Educate on postoperative bariatric surgery nutrition therapy and discharge nutrition therapy for the specific bariatric surgery procedure	• First 2 weeks limit volume to ¼ cup (4 tablespoons) each meal, for a total of three cups high-protein, low-fat, low-sugar bariatric liquid protein supplement, with 1 ounce sipped every 15 minutes between meals and two cups other liquids sipped, eg sugar-free noncarbonated beverages, broth or sugar-free popsicles, and ½ cup yogurt or sugar-free pudding throughout the day
• Advise patient to test various high-protein liquid supplements to find one they like	• Monitor for nausea and vomiting	• Advance eating plan to "pureed" bariatric surgery nutrition therapy, 2 weeks after surgery, until 4 weeks postsurgery; blend all foods to consistency of applesauce; wait 30 minutes to start consuming fluids
• Advise patient to purchase and try other items they will need, including pureed meats, canned tuna, cream soups, cream of wheat, etc.	• Nursing staff dispenses the 1 ounce fluid per hour on postoperative day one and 2 ounces fluid per hour on postoperative day 2	• Progress to "soft" bariatric nutrition therapy, 4 weeks postsurgery
• Discuss importance of vitamin and mineral supplementation for after the procedure; have the patient start taking a liquid or chewable multivitamin and mineral supplement (eg, Flintstones Complete or Centrum Junior), chewable calcium tablets (calcium citrate with vitamin D), and emphasize need to take these for life, no matter how good they feel	• Reinforce the importance of sipping the fluid between meals so as not to become dehydrated; no straws	• Eat foods in this order: (1) protein, (2) vegetables and fruit, and (3) starchy mashed potatoes and strained cooked cereal
• Discuss the importance of physical activity	• Reinforce no fluids with meals or for 30 minutes after meals	• Assess nutritional adequacy of patient's nutritional intake for protein (60–80 grams per day) and adequate fluids (since high protein can lead to dehydration), and at least 30 grams of carbohydrate per meal (minimum 130 grams per day)
	• Monitor for dumping syndrome (RYGBP), and avoid sugar and sweets; high fat, starchy foods may also contribute to dumping syndrome	

(Continued)

Table 3–23. Preoperative to postoperative nutrition interventions for bariatric surgery. *(Continued)*

Preoperative Intervention	Hospitalization Intervention	Post-Surgical Intervention
• *Second visit:* discuss potential failure of the surgery, along with further education, including: • Potential reasons for failure: -Not making lifestyle behavior changes -Drinking liquids with meals (stretches stomach pouch) -Not stopping eating when they feel full (stretches stomach pouch) -Emotional issues associated with eating • Discuss behavior strategies for avoiding overeating • Reinforce the recommendations about volume of foods and fluids		• Three small feedings per day (1/2 cup) plus high-protein liquids for banded gastroplasty and five to six mini-feedings per day (1/4 to ½ cup per meal) for RYGBP, followed forever • Assess weight loss regularly • Have patient always return to clinic with a 3-day food record • Conduct a 24-hour recall when the patient is in the clinic • No alcohol or chewing gum • Reinforce patients regular use for vitamin and mineral supplements • Reinforce cessation of eating when full, and making lifestyle changes • Reinforce patient's need for regular physical activity to aid in maximum weight loss and maintenance of lower weight • Concentrate on behavioral changes

Data from Academy of Nutrition and Dietetics, 2009.[9]

Table 3-24. Children and teens weight status category based on BMI-for-age percentile.

Weight Status Category	Percentile Range
Underweight	Less than the 5th percentile
Healthy weight	5th percentile to less than the 85th percentile
Overweight	85th to less than the 95th percentile
Obese	Equal to or greater than the 95th percentile

instead of specific number of pounds to lose, because setting unrealistic weight expectations can lead to discouragement by both the child and their parents. Childhood overweight and obesity is a family condition, and as such, the family needs to make many, if not all, of the changes that ultimately lead to healthy changes for the child.[47]

Older Adults

The risk of coronary artery disease, dyslipidemia, and insulin resistance increases with age, partially due to an increase in abdominal obesity. With increasing age, especially among individuals 75 years and older, several epidemiological studies suggest that the relationship between BMI and mortality weakens. The lowest morality is believed to result in the BMI range of 25–30 for adults age 55–74, a BMI range that would be considered overweight in younger adults. At the other extreme, an association has been found with increased body weight and lower levels of functioning in the elderly, with disability predicted at a higher BMI.[25]

Although BMI is the most commonly used measurement for classifying obesity, the BMI may actually underestimate adiposity in the elderly, since aging is associated with a decrease in muscle mass, or sarcopenia. Frailty, disability, and loss of independence result from sarcopenia. When determining the type and intensity of potential weight-management programs for the elderly, a comprehensive evaluation should consider BMI, the presence of comorbid conditions, and the ability to perform normal daily activities of living, such as bathing, dressing, getting in and out of bed and chairs, doing housework, and ambulating.[25] See Chapter 4 for additional information on weight management in the older adult.

Pregnancy

At the first prenatal visit, the healthcare practitioner should determine the overweight and obese pregnant woman's pre- or early-pregnancy BMI. Based on this BMI, the practitioner should then utilize the Institute of Medicine (IOM) guidelines to determine how much weight the woman should gain throughout her pregnancy (see Chapter 4), and this information should be shared with the patient. Epidemiological evidence suggests that when the healthcare professional emphasizes the appropriate recommendation for weight gain within the IOM guidelines, success in reaching these goals is more likely. Additionally, the healthcare practitioner should not advise the overweight and obese pregnant woman to lose weight during pregnancy, but instead should emphasize the important of eating healthful foods as outlined in the *Dietary Guidelines for Americans*.[48] Being physically active should be encouraged for the overweight or obese pregnant female, and the American Congress of Obstetricians and Gynecologists (ACOG) guidelines for exercising during pregnancy, should also be emphasized (see Chapter 4). At the first prenatal visit, all obese pregnant women should be screened for gestational diabetes, and even if results are initially negative, repeat screenings should occur throughout the pregnancy.[48]

Promoting Weight Gain

Just as is the case with obesity, being underweight can also have significant health risks. Those who are underweight are prone to infections due to a weakened and compromised immune system. Underweight individuals tend to have lower muscle mass and may have disrupted hormone regulation. The intake and absorption of vital nutrients may be compromised in the underweight, which can lead to an increased risk of anemia and osteoporosis. It can also lead to amenorrhea and potential pregnancy complications in women of child-bearing age.

There may be several reasons why a healthcare provider may promote a high-calorie diet and weight gain. A person may require increased nutrient density because they are unable to consume adequate amounts of foods due to weakness resulting from illness, dementia, problems with chewing or swallowing, or mouth pain. Other reasons for increased nutrient needs may include cancer, HIV/AIDS, burns, trauma, fractures, or increased physical activity. In addition, the individual's living environment, use of prescription drugs, eating habits, presence of depression, or the inability to shop or prepare food may also cause him to be underweight. Table 3–25 contains more information about possible reasons for underweight and the contributing reasons for underweight.[27]

■ Goals of Promoting Weight Gain

The most important factor for promoting weight gain is to design a meal plan that allows the individual to take in more calories than burned. This is accomplished by having the individual consume a high-calorie nutrition plan with multiple feedings throughout the day. Providing adequate calories is very important in order to spare protein for repair and building of lean body tissue, and to avoid protein breakdown.[27]

■ Effectiveness of Promoting Weight Gain

Studies have shown that supplementation with calorie-containing products and foods produce a small but consistent weight gain that leads to shorter length of hospital stays and a protective effect against mortality. An extra 500–1000 calories per day, depending on an individual's needs and goals, is a healthy target to promote a 1–2 pound per week weight gain. Protein needs to promote increased muscle mass range from 1–2 g/kg body weight/day.[27]

■ Assessment and Monitoring Parameters

Assessment begins with determining the individual's degree of underweight status then exploring the cause(s) (eg, medical, environmental, psychological, and cognitive) (such as those listed in Table 3–25). Just as with any individual, a comprehensive assessment of their nutritional

Table 3–25. Possible reasons for underweight.

Reason for Underweight (BMI <18.5 kg/m²)	Contributions to Reasons for Underweight
Inadequate food intake	Poor dentition, poorly fitting dentures, mouth soreness, inability to swallow or difficulty swallowing (dysphagia), lack of appetite, nausea, vomiting, inability to purchase or prepare food due to economic conditions, living arrangements, lack of transportation, and mental or physical illness
Overexercise or high activity levels	Elite athletes engaged in highly active sports, wandering behavior associated with dementia, eating disorder such as anorexia nervosa or exercise bulimia
Past medical history that includes undernutrition	Poor fetal growth or fetal malnutrition, stunting during periods of growth, weight loss induced by illness or disease, failure to thrive
Poor absorption and/or poor utilization of food and nutrients	Digestive disorder such as celiac disease, Crohn's disease and ulcerative colitis (UC), cystic fibrosis, surgery, or radiation therapy to GI tract; other chronic inflammatory or infectious diseases
Disruptions in normal metabolism	Malignant neoplasms, hyperthyroidism, diabetes
Mental illness, psychological, or emotional stress	Major depression, psychoses, and stress

Data from Academy of Nutrition and Dietetics, 2012; Robertson and Jameson, 2012.

status should be completed (see Chapter 2 for more information). Generally, recent significant weight loss and/or BMI <18.5 should trigger the practitioner to consider the need for promoting weight gain. Another widely accepted justification for weight gain is in those who are at less than 85% of their ideal body weight (see Chapter 2 for determining ideal body weight). An REE measurement should also be conducted as part of the assessment for managing underweight.[27] The same assessment parameters are used to monitor progress.

- ## Dietary Interventions for Weight Gain

Make Calories Count

In order to tip the scales to positive energy balance, incorporating foods that are calorie-dense, but still nutritionally healthful, is key. The practitioner should avoid recommending added calories from foods such as soft drinks, chips, fast foods, processed sugars and desserts, and fast foods, as these types of foods are filled with empty and unhealthy calories. Instead, weight gain diets should include nutritionally dense, calorie-rich foods that provide healthy protein, vitamins, minerals, and antioxidants, with guidance from the *Dietary Guidelines for Americans*.[18] Foods low in calories that promote satiety such as tea, coffee, diet sodas, light, or diet foods should be avoided.[27]

Incorporating extra calories into routine meals and snacks can easily be accomplished without increasing food volume. For example, double-strength milk can be made with whole milk and dry-powdered milk for double the calories, calcium, and protein. This high-calorie milk can then be consumed as is, or included in other foods, such as mashed potatoes, puddings, smoothies, or shakes. The water used to make foods such as oatmeal, pancake mixes, puddings, soups, etc, can be replaced with milk or double-strength milk in order to boost caloric intake. Other dairy products, such as cheese, cream cheese, cottage cheese, yogurt, sour cream, ice cream, and evaporated milks, are also calorie- and nutrient-dense and can be incorporated into meals and snacks. Sweets can also be incorporated in routine meals and snacks with the use of honey on toast, muffins, or cereals. Sugar, jam, jelly, or chocolate syrup can also be used wisely in a healthy meal plan to promote weight gain.[27]

Healthy fats from foods such as with olive oils, flaxseed oil, fish oil, or almond, walnuts, cashews, or peanuts (and/or the nut butters), and avocados can make a significant contribution to total caloric and nutrient intake.[27] In addition, fish oils, which are high in omega-3 fatty acids, have also been shown to stimulate lean muscle and tissue growth.

Make Protein Count

Healthy proteins, such as cooked dried beans, hummus, or edamame (boiled green soy beans), can easily be incorporated into spreads, dips, or salads, or they can also be eaten as is. Eggs or egg substitutes are also nutrient-dense and can be incorporated into meals. Tuna, salmon, and chicken can be used in salads or patties, along with eggs for nutrient-dense meals. Protein powders such as whey protein can also be mixed in with foods, such as smoothies, yogurt, puddings, cereals, or casseroles.[27] As previously mentioned, the addition of large amounts of protein should be done with caution in individuals with renal insufficiency. For healthy individuals who are increasing protein intake, be sure to recommend an increase in fluids and water to avoid dehydration and constipation.

Eating Frequency

Frequent snacking or grazing between meals is an acceptable practice for promoting ideal weight gain. An energy-dense snack of nutritious foods that are found desirable by the individual is recommended every 2–3 hours. Meal replacements, such as nutritious energy bars or drinks, are also acceptable. It is not unusual to have the greatest appetite in the morning due to fasting all night; therefore, this time period should be taken advantage of, and additional calories consumed, at the breakfast meal. Also, this is the time when the individual may have more energy to invest in food preparation for the rest of the day.

Most fluids and beverages should be consumed between meals because they usually have fewer calories and tend to make one feel full. Sipping fluids to help swallow food at meal-time is acceptable; however, the majority of fluids should be encouraged between meals to allow room for solid foods in the stomach at meal-time.[27]

▪ Physical Activity Interventions

Just as with promoting weight loss, the key to successful weight gain is balance. Not only is a balanced diet necessary, but a balanced exercise regimen is also crucial. Physical activity that includes weight training promotes increased lean body mass (muscles), which is very important for promoting an ideal body weight and preventing further deterioration in muscle tissue. Physical activity can also lead to an increase in appetite, which can ultimately lead to a desired additional caloric intake. When starting a resistance-training program to promote weight gain, an individual should start with light weights and gradually increase the weight. For patients who may be bedridden, in a wheelchair, or suffering from severe fatigue, the use of isometrics and resistance training with bands is an acceptable alternative to weights. While other conventional exercises may not be an option for those who are physically weak, emphasizing walking or other usual normal daily activities is important.

▪ Medication Interventions

Pharmacological intervention is often needed to help with weight gain in addition to activity and a healthy diet. Although appetite stimulant such as Megace (megestrol acetate) or Marinol (dronabinol) may help improve the appetite and lead to weight gain, the resulting weight may result in fat weight, not muscle weight. In addition, like all drugs, undesirable side effects may ensue.

Eating Disorders and Disordered Eating

Eating disorders (EDs) and disordered eating (DE) are complex psychiatric conditions with diagnostic criteria based on psychological, behavior, and physiologic characteristics and require a collaborative approach by an interdisciplinary team of mental health, nutrition, and medical specialists. Although diet therapy is integral in the treatment of EDs and DE, not just any registered dietitian or advanced practice nurse is qualified to treat this population of patients. The healthcare professional treating EDs and DE must understand the psychological and neurobiological aspects of EDs, and have advanced training to effectively work with this population. In addition, this specialized professional must understand that with dietary changes and weight management, risks for eating pathology further increases.[49] Therefore, it is beyond the scope of this book to significantly elaborate on diet therapy for EDs and DE, other than to describe the diagnostic criteria noted below.

- Diagnostic Criteria

The severity and type of EDs vary considerably. Table 3–26 compares the diagnostic criteria from the fourth edition of the *Diagnostic and Statistical Manual of Mental Disorders* (DSM) to the proposed revision for the newest DSM (5th edition), reflecting current research.[49]

Additional Resources

There are numerous reputable scientific resources available on the subject of managing weight. In addition, the internet offers countless information on diets and weight loss, most of which is not scientifically based, may be misleading, and perhaps even contributes to the worsening of the obesity crisis. The practitioner must be aware of reputable web-based resources available to clients, and the practitioner must also use said resources for their own professional knowledge. The National Agricultural Library's Food and Nutrition Information Center offers a lengthy list of reputable resources on weight management and obesity at: http://www.nal.usda.gov/fnic/pubs/bibs/topics/weight/consumer. pdf. One of the resources that can be accessed via this link is the NHLBI Obesity Education Initiative, Practical Guide Identification, Evaluation and Treatment of Overweight, and Obesity in Adults. The appendices of this government publication contain basic information and meal and physical activity tools that promote a healthy weight.

Table 3–26. Comparison of proposed revisions in diagnostic criteria for eating disorders.

Disorder	DSM IV	Proposed DSM V
Anorexia nervosa Types: restricting or binge-eating/purging	• Exaggerated drive for thinness • Refusal to maintain a body weight above the standard minimum (eg, <85% of expected weight) • Intense fear of becoming fat with self-worth based on weight or shape • Evidence of an endocrine disorder	• Restricted energy intake relative to requirements leading to a markedly low body weight • Intense fear of gaining weight or becoming fat or persistent behavior to avoid weight gain, even though at a markedly low weight • Disturbance in the way in which one's body weight or shape is experienced
Bulimia nervosa	• Overwhelming urges to overeat and inappropriate compensatory behaviors or purging that follow the binge episodes (eg, vomiting, excessive exercise, alternating periods of starvation, and abuse of laxatives or drugs) • Similar to anorexia nervosa, individuals with bulimia nervosa also display psychopathology, including a fear of being overweight	• Recurrent episodes of binge eating with a sense of lack of control with inappropriate compensatory behavior • Self-evaluation is unduly influenced by body shape and weight • The disturbance does not occur exclusively during episodes of anorexia nervosa
Binge eating disorder	• Classified under eating disorders not otherwise specified	• Repeated episodes of overconsumption of food with a sense of a lack of control with a list of possible descriptors such as how much is eaten and distress about the episode • Frequency described as at least once a week for 3 months
Eating disorders not otherwise specified	• Considered to be partial syndromes with frequency of symptoms that vary from above diagnostic criteria • Distinguishing feature of binge eating disorder is binge eating, with a lack of self-control, without inappropriate compensatory behaviors	• Diagnostic criteria to be established for binge eating disorder • Possible descriptions of eating problems such as purging disorder and night eating syndrome

Data from American Dietetic Association, 2011.

For assistance with locating qualified professionals who work with individuals with EDs and/or DO, please visit the Anorexia Nervosa and Associated Disorders website at www.anad.org. The Eating Disorder Referral and Information Center at www.edreferral.com is also an excellent resource.

References

1. Frayn K. Metabolic Regulation: a Human Perspective. 3rd ed. West Sussex, United Kingdom: Wiley-Blackwell; 2010.

2. Dokken B, Tsau T. The physiology of body weight regulation: are we too efficient for our own good? Diabetes Spectrum 2007;20(3):166–170.

3. Foster G, Nonas C. Managing Obesity: a Clinical Guide. Chicago, IL: J Am Diet Assoc; 2004.

4. Bray G, Champagne C. Beyond energy balance: there is more to obesity than kilocalories. J Am Diet Assoc 2005;105(suppl 5):S17–S23.

5. Mattes R, Hollis J, Hayes D, Stunkard A. Appetite: measurement and manipulation misgivings. J Am Diet Assoc 2005;105(suppl 5):S87–S97.

6. American Dietetic Association. Position of the American Dietetic Association: vegetarian diets. J Am Diet Assoc 2009;109(7):1266–1282. American Dietetic Association. Position of the American Dietetic Association: weight management. J Am Diet Assoc 2009;109(2):330–346.

7. Wang Z, Heshka S, Boozer C, Heymsfield S. Resting energy expenditure: systematic organization and critique of prediction methods. Obes Res 2001;9(5):331–336.

8. McArdle W, Katch F, Katch V. Essentials of Exercise Physiology. 2nd ed. Lippincott Williams and Wilkins; 2000.

9. Joosen A, Westerterp K. Energy expenditure during overfeeding. Nutr Metab (Lond) 2006;12(3):25.

10. Himms-Hagen J. Role of thermogenesis in the regulation of energy balance in relation to obesity. Can J Physiol Pharmacol 1989;67(4):394–401.

11. Schoeller D, Buchholz A. Energetics of obesity and weight control: does diet composition matter? J Am Diet Assoc 2005;105(5 suppl 1):S24–S28.

12. Shils M, Olson J, Shike M, Ross A. Modern Nutrition in Health and Disease. New York, NY: Lippincott Williams and Wilkins; 1999.

13. Shronts E. Nutrition Support Dietetics, Core Curriculum. Silver Spring, MD: American Society for Parenteral and Enteral Nutrition; 1989.

14. Dalton S. The dietitians' philosophy and practice in multidisciplinary weight management. J Am Diet Assoc 1998;98(10 suppl 2):S49–S54.

15. National Heart, Lung, and Blood Institute (NHLBI). The clinical guidelines on the identification, evaluation, and treatment of overweight and obesity in adults: the evidence report. Bethesda, MD. 1998. Retrieved from: May 2, 2012. http://www.nhlbi.nih.gov/guidelines/obesity/ob_gdlns.pdf.

16. Clinical Endocrinology News (2012). FDA Oks Lorcaserin Despite Cardiac Concerns. Vol. 7, No. 7. Morristown, New Jersey: International Medical News Group, LLC/Elsevier; & http://www.fda.gov/NewsEvents/Newsroom/PressAnnouncements/ucm309993.htm

17. Endocrine Today (2012). Phentermine/Topiramate Combo Wins FDA Approval for Weight Loss. Vol 10, No. 8. Healio.com/Endocrinology, Thorofare, New Jersey: Slack, Inc.; & http://www.fda.gov/NewsEvents/Newsroom/PressAnnouncements/ucm312468.htm

18. US Department of Agriculture and US Department of Health and Human Services. Dietary Guidelines for Americans, 2010, 7th ed. Washington, DC: US Government Printing Office; 2011.

19. Osterkamp L. Current perspective on assessment of human body proportions of relevance to amputees. J Am Diet Assoc 1995;95(2):215–218.

20. Compher C, Frankenfield D, Keim N, Roth-Yousey L, Group EA. Best practice methods to apply to measurement of resting metabolic rate in adults: a systematic review. J Am Diet Assoc 2006;106(6):881–903.

21. Frankenfield D, Roth-Youssey L, Compher C. Comparison of predictive equations for resting metabolic rate in healthy nonobese and obese adults: a systematic review. J Am Diet Assoc 2005;105(5):775–789.

22. Spears K, Kim H, Behall K, Conway J. Hand-held indirect calorimeter offers advantages compared with prediction equations, in a group of overweight women, to determine resting energy expenditures and estimated total energy expenditures during research screening. J Am Diet Assoc 2009;109(5):836–845.

23. Ireton-Jones C, Turner WJ, Liepa G, Baxter C. Equations for the estimation of energy expenditures in patients with burns with special reference to ventilatory status. J Burn Care Rehabil 1992;13(3):330–333.

24. Ireton-Jones C, Jones J. Improved equations for predicting energy expenditure in patients: the Ireton-Jones Equations. Nutr Clin Pract 2002;17(1):29–31.

25. Kushner R, Blatner D. Risk assessment of the overweight and obese patient. J Am Diet Assoc 2005;105(suppl 5):S53–S62.

26. Campbell C, Zander E, Thorland W. Predicted vs measured energy expenditure in critically ill, underweight patients. Nutr Clin Pract 2005; 20(2):276–280.

27. Academy of Nutrition and Dietetics. Underweight. 2012. Retrieved from: Nutrition Care Manual January 11, 2013. http://www.nutritioncaremanual.org Academy of Nutrition and Dietetics. Normal Nutrition. 2012. Retrieved from: Nutrition Care Manual May 2, 2012. http://www.nutritioncaremanual.org Academy of Nutrition and Dietetics. Musculoskeletal Conditions. 2012. Retrieved from: Nutrition Care Manual January 11, 2013. http://www.nutritioncaremanual.org.

28. Office of the Surgeon General, Department of the Army. Rehabilitation of the injured combatant. In: D. o. Office of the Surgeon General, Textbook of Military Medicine, Part IV (p. 92). Washington, DC; 1998.

29. Hill J, Thompson H, Wyatt H. Weight maintenance: what's missing. J Am Diet Assoc 2005;105(5 suppl 1):S63–S66.

30. Finkelstein E, Trogdon J, Cohen J, Dietz W. Annual medical spending attributable to obesity: payer-and service-specific estimates. Health Aff 2009;28(5):w822–w831.

31. Academy of Nutrition and Dietetics. Medical Nutrition Therapy and Adult Weight Management. Feb 2009. Retrieved from: Evidence Analysis Library May 2, 2012. http://andevidencelibrary.com

32. American Association of Clinical Endocrinologists/American College of Endocrinology (AACE/ACE) Obesity Task Force. AACE/ACE position statement on the prevention, diagnosis, and treatment of obesity. Endocr Pract 1998;4(5):297–350.

33. Wing R, Hill J. Successful weight loss maintenance. Annu Rev Nutr 2001;21:323–341.

34. Catenacci V, Ogden L, Stuht J, Phelan S, Wing R, Hill J, et al. Physical activity patterns in the National Weight Control Registry. Obesity 2008; 16(1):153–161.

35. Harvard School of Public Health. (n.d.). How to get to your healthy weight. Retrieved from: The Nutrition Source January 11, 2013. http://www.hsph .harvard.edu/nutritionsource/healthy-weight-full-story/#references.

36. Phelan S, Wyatt H, Hill J, Wing R. Are the eating and exercise habits of successful weight losers changing? Obesity 2006;14:710–716.

37. Raynor D, Phelan S, Hill J, Wing R. Television viewing and long-term weight maintenance: results from the National Weight Control Registry. Obesity 2006;14:1816–1824.

38. Phelan S, Wyatt H, Nassery S, Dibello J, Fava J, Hill J, et al. Three–year weight change in successful weight losers who lost weight on a low–carbohydrate diet. Obesity 2007;15(10):2470–2477.

39. Flegal K, Kit B, Orpana H, Graubard B. Association of all-cause mortality with overweight and obesity using standard body mass index categories: a systematic review and meta-analysis. JAMA 2013;2(309(1):71–82.

40. Academy of Nutrition and Dietetics. In healthy adults, how effective (in terms of client adherence and weight and loss maintenance) is a regular meal and snack pattern? July 2005. Retrieved from: Evidence Analysis Library January 31, 2013. http://andevidencelibrary.com. Academy of Nutrition and Dietetics. In healthy adults, how effective, in terms of weight loss and maintenance, are low carbohydrate diets (defined as <35% kcals from carbohydrate)? November 2005. Retrieved from: Evidence Analysis Library January 31, 2013. http://andevidencelibrary.com.

41. Westman E, Feinman R, Mavropoulos J, Vernon M, Volek J, Wortman J, et al. Low-carbohydrate nutrition and metabolism. Am J Clin Nutr 2007;86(2): 276–284.

42. Thedford K, Raj S. A vegetarian diet for weight management. J Am Diet Assoc 2011;111(6):816–818.

43. Berkel L, Poston W, Reeves R, Foreyt J. Behavioral interventions for obesity. J Am Diet Assoc 2005;105(5 suppl 1):S35–S43.

44. Cummings S, Apovian C, Khaodhiar L. Obesity surgery: evidence for diabetes prevention/management. J Am Diet Assoc 2008;108(4 suppl 1): S40–S44.

45. Centers for Disease Control and Prevention (CDC). Clinical growth charts. August 4, 2009. Retrieved from: Growth Charts May 26, 2012. http:// www.cdc.gov/growthcharts/clinical_charts.htm.

46. Centers for Disease Control and Prevention. About BMI for children and teens. September 13, 2011. Retrieved from: Healthy Weight - It's Not a Diet, It's a Lifestyle! January 11, 2013. http://www.cdc.gov/healthyweight/ assessing/bmi/childrens_bmi/about_childrens_bmi.html.

47. Ponder S, Anderson M. Teaching families to keep their children S.A.F.E. from obesity. Diabetes Spectrum 2008;21(1):50–53.

48. American Dietetic Association and American Society of Nutrition. Position of the American Dietetic Association and American Society for Nutrition: obesity, reproduction, and pregnancy outcomes. J Am Diet Assoc 2009;109(5):918–927.

49. American Dietetic Association. Position of the American Dietetic Association: nutrition intervention in the treatment of eating disorders. J Am Diet Assoc 2011;111(8):1236–1241.

4

From Infants to Ancients: Nutrition Throughout the Lifecycle

Nutrient needs vary greatly throughout the various stages of life. Achieving adequate nutrient status during infancy, promoting healthy eating habits in toddlers, and encouraging balanced food intakes and proper weight management throughout childhood and adolescence all set the stage for the best possible transition into a healthy adulthood. This chapter will cover the unique nutrient needs specific to each stage of life, from preconception to pregnancy, breastfeeding, infant weaning, childhood feeding practices, school-age child, adolescent, and older adult.

Preconception Nutrition

Assessing and addressing a woman's nutritional status *before* she conceives makes it far easier to encourage optimal birth outcomes than trying to intervene *after* she is already pregnant. The preferred place to start when approaching preconception nutrition is weight status. As obesity rates in the general population trend upward, it follows that more women hoping to conceive will also struggle with their weight. Achieving a healthy weight before conception is ideal because both underweight and overweight reduce the likelihood of conception.[1]

Overweight and obese women who become pregnant are at increased risk for having babies with neural tube defects, congenital abnormalities, preterm delivery, and fetal mortality. These women are also more likely to have preeclampsia, postpartum anemia, and cesarean delivery. Overweight and obesity affect the mother and child's health status after birth, as babies born to mothers with high prepregnancy BMIs are more likely to be macrosomic at birth and be obese during childhood, and less likely to successfully initiate successful and adequate breastfeeding.[2-5] Being significantly underweight prior to pregnancy also negatively affects conception rates, as inadequate body weight and low percent body fat decreases the woman's likelihood of ovulation, regular menstruation and, in turn, conception.

Research has established that it takes obese women longer to conceive as compared to normal-weight women, with the problem being even more prevalent amongst obese cigarette smokers.[6-8] The state of obesity is characterized by excessive fat tissue, and this fat tissue is essential for regulating sex hormone availability and for storing lipid steroids such as androgens. The ability to produce and regulate estrogen and sex hormone-binding globulin is associated with weight status.

Obesity is also linked to increased risk of polycystic ovarian syndrome (PCOS), a condition that causes menstrual interruptions and chronic anovulation. Furthermore, the association between obesity and insulin resistance may play a negative role on overall fertility.[9]

While achieving a healthy body weight prior to becoming pregnant is ideal, women should be counseled that pregnancy is NOT the time to lose weight. This is a discussion topic that clinicians may find difficult to broach with overweight and obese women who are eager to become pregnant. The challenge for the practitioner is to tactfully convey the facts: a healthy preconception weight not only maximizes the likelihood of becoming pregnant, but also improves the mother and baby's health during pregnancy and after birth. Patients and clients may be surprised, and perhaps even inspired, to learn that roughly 25% of ovulatory infertility in the United States may be attributed to overweight and obesity in women of reproductive age.[6]

Even modest weight loss can have discernable benefits for fertility. Among women with PCOS, just 5% weight reduction has been linked to improved fertility.[9] Weight loss enhances chances of fertility by improving menstrual function, ovulation, and infertility in obese women.[7] Bariatric surgery also appears to have positive reproductive effects, with documented improvements in fertility occurring in women with weight loss in the arena of 23–97 pounds.[10] Women who have undergone weight loss surgery are advised to maintain a diet of 1000–1200 calories per day before getting pregnant, to supplement with a multivitamin and additional vitamin B_{12}, and to wait until their weight loss stabilizes (somewhere between 12 and 18 months following surgery) before seeking obstetric care from a specialist in high-risk pregnancy.[1] Meal planning for postbariatric surgery patients who are pregnant should be done under the supervision of a trained Registered Dietitian (RD).

The Academy of Nutrition and Dietetics and the American Society for Nutrition recommend that overweight and obese women in the preconception state should be advised about successful, evidence-based weight loss practices and healthful eating, including information about diet and supplementation with folic acid. These women should be counseled on the benefits of exercise in helping to achieve an ideal weight, but also educated about the maternal and fetal complication risk factors that do exist for pregnant women who are overweight or obese.[1] Chapter 3 contains more information about weight loss interventions, which could be implemented during preconception.

Nutrition During Pregnancy

- ### From Merely Surviving to Absolutely Thriving

There is no shortage of nutrition and weight-related concerns that a pregnant woman experiences: "I think I've gained 100 pounds!," "I feel like I'm always hungry!," "This baby is making me nauseous!," "This baby is making me fat!"…these are just a few of the many complaints that practitioners of pregnant women may hear. For many women, pregnancy is the first time that they have seriously ever considered—or perhaps even been interested in—their own nutritional status. And unfortunately, the inadequate state of nutrition that plagues the nonpregnant female population (eg, low iron intake, low calcium intake, excessive caloric intake, and inadequate fiber intake) is just as prevalent among the pregnant female population. But, whereas the nonpregnant adult population can survive with less than optimal nutritional status, such a situation is contraindicated in, and should be discouraged during pregnancy. It is incumbent upon the practitioner to counsel women in a manner that shifts nutritional status from *merely surviving* to *absolutely thriving.* Nutrition interventions in pregnancy should be designed and implemented with two overarching goals in mind: (1) to promote optimal birth weight of the baby, and (2) to support adequate nourishment for the mother.[11] Pregnant women should be screened for nutrition risk and those who are identified as being at high nutrition risk should be referred to a RD. Table 4–1 contains a sample Prenatal Nutritional Risk Screen that can be used to quickly determine risk level.[11]

▪ Weight Gain Guidelines for Pregnancy

Of paramount importance to the mother and the baby's health is the attainment of appropriate weight gain rates during pregnancy. The Institute of Medicine revised their weight gain during pregnancy guidelines in 2009. These revised guidelines are based on prepregnancy BMI and are outlined in Table 4–2.[12] Many pregnant women are surprised to learn that in their first trimester, no additional calories above baseline needs are required. This "no increase in calories" suggestion dovetails nicely with the next piece of advice; weight gain of 0–5 pounds during the first trimester is recommended and should be expected in women with a healthy or high prepregnancy BMI. Beginning at the start of the second trimester, women should expect to gain approximately 1 pound per week for the duration of their pregnancy. This promotes a total weight gain of 25–35 pounds by the end of pregnancy for a woman with a normal prepregnancy BMI (18.5–24.9). Adolescents and teenagers who become pregnant should aim for a 28–40 pound weight gain by the end of pregnancy.[13]

For women carrying multiples (twins or triplets), weight gain recommendations are increased. A healthy prepregnancy weighted woman carrying twins should gain 1.5 pounds per week beginning at the end of the first trimester or beginning of the second trimester. For triplets, 1.5 pound per week weight gain should start shortly after conception, with total weight gain around 50 pounds expected by the end of pregnancy. Table 4–3 outlines guidelines for weight gain with twins based on prepregnancy BMI.[12]

The American Congress of Obstetricians and Gynecologists (ACOG) recommends assessing and documenting BMI at the first prenatal visit

Table 4-1. Prenatal nutrition risk screen form.

Prenatal Nutrition Risk Criterion	Risk Total
Identified inadequate food resources to meet needs during pregnancy	3
Is vegetarian	1
Stated avoidance of certain foods or food groups because of allergy, intolerance, fad diet, or religious or cultural reasons	2
Is on a weight-reduction diet, or has to follow a special diet	2
Is craving or eating unusual foods or nonfood items (eg, ice or laundry starch)	2
Stated lifestyle is unlikely to meet nutrition needs (eg, lives in a women's or homeless shelter, has an overactive lifestyle, lives alone)	3
Is <16 years of age	3
Last pregnancy was <2 years ago or is breastfeeding while pregnant	3
Was underweight before pregnancy	3
Was overweight before pregnancy	1
Has had severe hyperemesis gravidarum that has caused weight loss	3
Multiple gestation	2
Has another diagnosis (eg, history of eating disorder, hypertension, pregnancy-induced hypertension, diabetes, and hyperlipidemia)	3
Key: 0–5 points is low risk, 6-10 is medium risk, and >10 is high risk	

Data from Academy of Nutrition and Dietetics, 2012; Worthington-Roberts, 1997; Williams SR. Nutrition assessment and guidance in prenatal care. In: Worthington-Roberts BS, Williams SR, eds. *Nutrition in Pregnancy and Lactation*. 6th ed. Dubuque, IA: Brown & Benchmark; 1997:220–253.

and discussing the IOM weight gain guidelines there too. Research suggests that women who are introduced to and advised to follow the IOM guidelines by their practitioner are more likely to stay within these guidelines.[14] Currently, 37% of healthy-weight women and 64% of overweight women gain more weight during pregnancy than recommended by the IOM guidelines.[15,16] Tempering weight gain during pregnancy not only helps to maximize birth outcomes, but also assists in mitigating postpartum weight retention. On the other hand, women who experience high gestational weight gain and who are unable to lose the excess weight following pregnancy are at increased risk of becoming and remaining obese later in life. The number one predictor of 1-year weight retention after delivery is the amount of weight gained during pregnancy.[17]

Table 4-2. Institute of Medicine 2009 recommendations for total and rate of weight gain during pregnancy, by prepregnancy BMI.

Prepregnancy Weight Category	BMI	Total Pregnancy Weight Gain (lbs)	Rate of Weight Gain in 2nd and 3rd Trimesters (Mean Range in lbs/wk)
Underweight	<18.5	28-40	1(1-1.3)
Healthy weight	18.5-24.9	25-35	1(0.8-1)
Overweight	25.0-29.9	15-25	0.6(0.5-0.7)
Obese	≥30.0	11-20	0.5(0.4-0.6)

Data from Institute of Medicine and National Research Council (US) Committee to Reexamine IOM Pregnancy Weight Guidelines, 2009.

While limiting weight gain during pregnancy is challenging for many, conceptualizing a 30-pound weight gain during pregnancy proves troublesome for others. This is particularly true for women with a history of or an active eating disorder. Women with eating disorders are advised to seek treatment and not to attempt pregnancy until disordered eating is under control. For those expressing apprehension about gestational weight gain, practitioners can help allay fears and promote adequate caloric intake and weight gain by carefully defining and explaining the components of weight gain during pregnancy. The weight gained during pregnancy is certainly not all fat, as some women mistakenly believe. While some of the weight gained during pregnancy is indeed from increasing maternal fat stores, additional weight is contributed by the growing fetus, amniotic fluid, placenta, uterus, higher maternal blood volume, amassing breast tissue, and extracellular fluids. Figure 4–1 outlines the weight contributions of these changes during pregnancy.[13]

Table 4-3. Institute of medicine recommendations for weight gain for twins.

Prepregnancy Weight Category	BMI	Total Pregnancy Weight Gain with Twins
Underweight	<18.5	Insufficient data
Healthy weight	18.5-24.9	37-54 pounds
Overweight	25.0-29.9	31-50 pounds
Obese	≥30.0	25-42 pounds

Data from Institute of Medicine and National Research Council (US) Committee to Reexamine IOM Pregnancy Weight Guidelines, 2009.

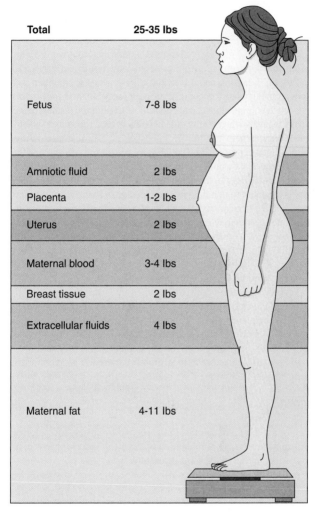

Total	25-35 lbs
Fetus	7-8 lbs
Amniotic fluid	2 lbs
Placenta	1-2 lbs
Uterus	2 lbs
Maternal blood	3-4 lbs
Breast tissue	2 lbs
Extracellular fluids	4 lbs
Maternal fat	4-11 lbs

Figure 4–1. Components of weight gain in pregnancy.

■ Calorie Needs During Pregnancy

Estimated energy requirements for pregnant women are no different than for nonpregnant women until the beginning of the second trimester.[2] Essentially, no increase in calories is needed until the beginning of the second trimester. This is reflected in the pregnancy weight gain recommendations indicating 0- 5-pound weight gain in the first trimester. Theoretically, a woman would not gain weight if she does not increase her caloric intake above baseline levels. In reality, this of course is easier said than done. From the moment they find out they are pregnant, many women adopt an "eating for two" strategy, a practice that leads to excessive caloric intake and early and unnecessary maternal weight gain.

Concentrating on calories can help women curb early gestational weight gain. Learning about baseline calorie needs to maintain weight *before* pregnancy helps encourage proper energy balance *during* the first trimester. Teaching patients and clients how to examine restaurant menus for calorie levels when dining out, and how to read food labels when eating at home can help heighten awareness about caloric intake during the various stages of pregnancy. The DRIs for pregnancy recommend that in the first trimester, a woman consumes only her baseline estimated energy requirement (EER) (ie, the same number of calories she needed before she was pregnant to maintain her body weight). In the second trimester, an additional 340 calories on top of baseline needs are required, and in the third trimester, baseline calories should be increased by 450 calories.[12,18] For example, a woman who could maintain her prepregnancy weight on a 2000-calorie diet per day would eat 2000 calories during the first trimester, 2340 calories during the second trimester, and 2450 calories during the third trimester. Table 4–4 reviews how to calculate EER for nonpregnant adolescents and adult women, and uses the physical activity value coefficients from Table 4–5, and Table 4–6 addresses utilization of EER with pregnancy during each of the three trimesters.[19]

Whereas a primiparous woman with minimal nutrition knowledge might go into pregnancy thinking she has entered a food and fat free-for-all, practitioners can help promote adherence to recommended calorie guidelines by providing real-life examples of sample 340- and 450-calorie snack and meal ideas. These additional calories should come from nutrient-dense, small meals and snacks that stay within the slightly elevated calorie ranges. Table 4–7 provides some sample meal and snack ideas for an extra 340 calories in the second trimester, 450 calories for the third trimester, or a combination of three 150-calorie snacks to reach 450-calorie snacks in the third trimester.

Table 4–4. EER for nonpregnant women.

Estimated Energy Requirement (EER) in Women 14–18 Years of Age
EER: = 135.3 – (30.8 × age in years) + physical activity[a] × [(10.0 × weight in kg) + (934 × height in meters)] + 25

Estimated Energy Requirement (EER) in Women 19 Years and Older
EER: 354 – (6.91 × age in years) + physical activity[a] × [(9.36 × weight in kg) + (726 × height in meters)]

[a]See physical activity coefficients in Table 4–5.
Data from Institute of Medicine, 2006.

Table 4-5. Physical activity coefficients (PA Values) for use in EER equations for adolescents or adult women.

	Sedentary (PAL 1.0-1.39)	Low Active (PAL 1.4-1.59)	Active (PAL 1.6-1.89)	Very Active (PAL 1.9-2.5)
Physical activity level (PAL) description	Typical daily living activities plus: household tasks, walking to the bus	Typical daily living activities plus : 30–60 minutes of daily moderate activity such as walking at 5-7 km/hour	Typical daily living activities plus at least 60 minutes of daily moderate activity	Typical daily living activities plus at least 60 minutes of daily moderate activity plus an additional 60 minutes of vigorous activity or 120 minutes of moderate activity
14–18 years of age	1.0	1.16	1.31	1.56
19 years and older	1.0	1.12	1.27	1.45

Data from Institute of Medicine, 2006.

■ Macronutrient and Micronutrient Needs During Pregnancy

On top of an overall increase in total calories needed during the second and third trimesters, pregnant women also have elevated macronutrient and micronutrient needs throughout the entirety of pregnancy. Many of the increased vitamin and mineral needs are covered with the intake of

Table 4-6. Equations to estimate energy requirement for pregnant women by trimester.

Estimated Energy Requirement (Kcal/Day) = Nonpregnant EER + Pregnancy Calories	
1st trimester	EER = Nonpregnant (adolescent or adult) EER + 0
2nd trimester	EER = Nonpregnant (adolescent or adult) EER + 340
3rd trimester	EER = Nonpregnant (adolescent or adult) EER + 452

Data from Institute of Medicine, 2006.

Table 4-7. Sample 340-, 450-, and 150-mini-meal and snack ideas.

340-Calorie Mini-Meal or Snack Ideas for the 2nd Trimester
- A small peanut butter and jelly sandwich and fruit: 1 piece of whole wheat bread (100 calories) with 1 tablespoon of peanut butter (100 calories), 1 tablespoon of jelly (60 calories), and 1 medium-sized apple (80 calories)
- Or try some cereal: 1½ cups of raisin bran cereal (150 calories), 1 cup nonfat milk (90 calories), and 1 medium-sized banana (100 calories)
- A quesadilla: 1 medium flour tortilla (150 calories), ¼ cup 2% milk shredded cheese (80 calories), and 2 tablespoons guacamole (100 calories)
- Pita, veggies, and hummus: 2 small whole wheat pita breads (75 calories each) plus ½ cup hummus (175 calories) and some cut-up veggie sticks (carrots and celery, 25 calories)

450-Calorie Mini-Meal or Snack Ideas for the 3rd Trimester
Keep in mind 450 is only 90 more calories than 340
- Small pasta meal: 1 cup cooked spaghetti (225 calories), ½ cup marinara sauce (100 calories), and 1 medium-sized meatball (125 calories)
- Yogurt parfait: 1 cup nonfat yogurt (200 calories), 1 cup high fiber cereal (100 calories), 1 cup blueberries (85 calories), and 1 cup raspberries (65 calories)
- Even a hamburger can work: Fully-cooked hamburger made from 4 ounces extra lean ground beef (190 calories), 1 whole wheat hamburger bun (200 calories), lettuce, tomato, pickle, mustard, and 1 slice reduced-fat cheese (70 calories)

150-Calorie Snack Ideas
Combine three of these for the 450 extra calories needed in the 3rd trimester
- 5 cups of air popped popcorn is 150 calories
- 1 cup of edamame in their shells
- 1 packet of hot chocolate prepared with 1 cup of nonfat milk
- 1 piece of whole wheat toast with 1 slice of melted reduced fat cheese
- 6 oz (¾ cup) plain nonfat yogurt with ½ cup blueberries
- 3 cups of watermelon cubes

a daily prenatal vitamin. The nutrients of particular concern, and those that may prove challenging to achieve optimal levels during pregnancy, include carbohydrate, protein, folate, calcium, and iron.

Carbohydrate Needs During Pregnancy

Carbohydrate needs jump from a minimum of 130 grams per day in the nonpregnant state to 175 grams per day during pregnancy.[19] For many women, this may not prove problematic, as a typical 2000-calorie diet with 55–65% of calories coming from carbohydrate would already provide well over the minimum at 275–325 grams of carbohydrate. But for a woman with diabetes, a history of low-carbohydrate dieting, or other "carbo-phobic" behaviors, achieving this minimum level of carbohydrate intake may prove challenging. A simple 24-hour recall or diet interview may reveal substandard carbohydrate intake. It is important to encourage at the very minimum 175 grams of carbohydrate in order to prevent ketosis and to assure adequate blood sugar levels during pregnancy.

Recommended sources of dietary carbohydrate include whole grains, fruits, vegetables, legumes, and low-fat or nonfat dairy foods, if tolerated. Care should be taken to assure that excessive carbohydrate intake from refined and added sugars is avoided. Focusing on the healthier sources of carbohydrate can also help meet increased fiber needs during pregnancy, as whole grains, fruits, vegetables, and legumes are not only good sources of complex carbohydrate, but also generally high in fiber. Pregnant women need 28 grams of fiber per day.

Protein Needs During Pregnancy

The DRIs recommend 46 grams of protein per day for the nonpregnant woman. That increases to 71 grams per day during pregnancy.[19] Considering that most North Americans consume excess calories, and that many of these calories come from protein, there are many people who are already exceeding their protein intake levels due to high consumption of animal foods. Animal protein foods contain complete protein, but may also contribute excessive fat, saturated fat, and calories that contribute to weight gain. A pregnant woman with a well-balanced diet that contains even modest amounts of protein at each meal and snack will likely have no trouble meeting the 71 grams per day pregnancy protein recommendation.

As is also the case with carbohydrate, concern for inadequate protein intake arises for pregnant women who have a history of dieting, restrictive eating patterns, and, in the case of protein, vegetarianism. While it is quite possible to achieve a minimum of 71 grams of protein per day on a well-planned vegetarian diet during pregnancy, certain women are at risk for under-consuming protein, and they should be educated about increasing intake to assure a minimum of 71 grams per day. For each additional fetus, it is recommended to achieve another 25 grams of protein per day.[13] Deficient protein intake often tracks alongside inadequate caloric intake. Women who are suspected to be under eating during pregnancy must also be considered for potentially not eating enough protein.

Lean meats, low-fat and nonfat dairy, nuts, seeds, legumes, and eggs are all good sources of dietary protein for pregnant women. The difference between nonpregnant-protein needs (46 grams per day) and pregnancy needs (71 grams per day) is 25 grams of protein per day. While 25 grams of protein might sound like a lot, it can easily be achieved by adding just the equivalent of an additional 3 ounces of chicken breast or 3 cups of milk per day. Educating women about various ways to incorporate an additional 25 grams of protein per day into their meal plan can help promote adequate fetal growth and development. Table 4–8 contains some examples of high-protein foods that can be incorporated easily into the diet of a pregnant woman.[20]

Table 4–8. Protein content of selected foods.

Food	Serving	Protein (g)
Chopped, cooked chicken breast	½ cup	21 g protein
Cooked salmon	4 oz	23 g protein
Tofu	8 oz	23 g protein
Peanuts, roasted	¼ cup	9 g protein
Nonfat milk, soymilk, or yogurt	8 oz	8 g protein
Black beans, canned	½ cup	8 g protein
Reduced-fat cheese	1 oz (1 slice)	8 g protein
Peanut butter	2 tablespoons	8 g protein
Soymilk	8 oz	6- to 7-g protein
Egg	1 large	6 g protein

Data from US Department of Agriculture, Research Service, 2012.

Folate Needs During Pregnancy

Folate comes from the Latin word "folium," meaning "leaf"; therefore, not surprisingly, folate is a water-soluble B vitamin found in large amounts in dark, green leafy vegetables. Folic acid is the synthetic form of folate, and it is most often consumed in supplements and fortified and enriched foods. During pregnancy, folate is involved in fetal and placental growth, and in the prevention of neural tube defects (NTDs).

In 1996, in an effort to reduce NTDs, the FDA authorized the inclusion of folic acid in enriched grain products. Folate enrichment compliance was made mandatory in 1998. The goal of this enrichment program was to prevent NTDs, acknowledging in part that neural tubes form at the earliest stages of pregnancy, often before a woman knows she is pregnant. Establishing adequate baseline folic acid levels in women of childbearing age is integral to preventing NTDs such as spina bifida and anencephaly. Mandatory folate enrichment in grain products in the United States resulted in a 19% reduction in NTD birth prevalence as compared to the pre-enrichment program, dropping the birth prevalence of NTDs from 37.8 per 100,000 live births (1995–1996) to 30.5 per 100,000 live births (1998–1999).[21]

The folic acid DRI increases from 400 micrograms in nonpregnancy to 600 micrograms in pregnancy.[19] Prior to conception, women who are trying to get pregnant are encouraged to get at least 400 micrograms of folic acid every day from folic acid-fortified foods or supplements. To help achieve this goal, a good rule of thumb for women on birth control is to start taking prenatal vitamins as soon as they stop using contraception.

Table 4–9. Folate content of selected foods.

Food	Serving	Folate (mcg)
Total™ Raisin Bran	1 cup	400 mcg folate
Spinach, boiled, and drained	1 cup	263 mcg folate
Lentils, cooked	½ cup	179 mcg folate
Asparagus, boiled, and drained	½ cup spears	134 mcg folate
Spaghetti, cooked	1 cup	102 mcg folate
Sunflower seeds, dry roasted	¼ cup	76 mcg folate

Data from US Department of Agriculture, Agricultural Research Service, 2012.

The folic acid percent daily value on the Supplement Facts Panel for dietary supplements is based on 400 micrograms per day. Most prenatal vitamins on the market contain 800 micrograms folic acid. There is a tolerable upper intake level (UL) set for folate at 1000 micrograms per day. Women with very high fortified-food or supplement intakes may unknowingly approach or surpass this upper level. Over-supplementation of folic acid is of concern as it may mask vitamin B_{12} deficiency symptoms. Table 4–9 contains the folic acid content of select foods.[20]

Calcium Needs During Pregnancy

During pregnancy, calcium absorption takes a turn in the right direction and absorption improves as compared to nonpregnancy. The presence of placenta-derived estrogen inhibits bone resorption, promoting the release of parathyroid hormone. This helps maintain the mother's serum calcium levels while at the same time promoting her absorption of calcium in the gut. In this way, calcium absorption improves during pregnancy to help meet fetal bone mineralization needs. This is reflected in the DRI value for calcium, which is 1000 mg per day for both pregnant and nonpregnant women.[22] It is important to note that while the actual DRI values do not increase during pregnancy—because of its enhanced absorption in the pregnant state—most women, pregnant or not, are not meeting the 1000 mg recommendation per day. Brief questioning about milk, yogurt, soymilk, cheese, and other dairy food intake levels can quickly reveal which clients may be achieving substandard calcium intake levels. On average, one cup of milk, soymilk, or yogurt and one ounce of cheese each contain 300 mg of calcium. The calcium content of prenatal vitamins can range anywhere from 200 to 600 mg per capsule, with most national and generic brands being in the 200–300 mg range. Higher levels are not usually included in prenatal vitamins because of the bulky nature of calcium carbonate and because calcium offsets the absorption of other vital nutrients for pregnancy, namely iron. Because of lactose intolerance, dislike of or allergy to dairy foods, some women are unable to meet their calcium needs from a prenatal vitamin plus dietary intake; these individuals should consider taking an additional calcium supplement at a time separate from their prenatal vitamin. All pregnant adult women should be aiming for 1000 mg of calcium per day, from food or supplements. Supplemental intake of calcium should not exceed 500 mg at a time. The UL for calcium is 2500 mg per day. This is rarely achieved from food alone, but can occur with very high calcium supplement intake or high levels of antacids used for intake. Excessive intake is associated with heartburn or gastroesophageal reflux disease.

Iron Needs During Pregnancy

Blood volume during pregnancy may increase by as much as 50%, which in turn increases the maternal need for iron.[23] This is reflected in the DRIs for iron that also increase by 50% for pregnant versus nonpregnancy needs. The DRI for iron for a nonpregnant woman is 18 mg of iron per day. That increases to 27 mg of iron per day during pregnancy.[19] Most prenatal vitamins contain 18–28 mg of iron, which equates to roughly 100–150% DV on the Supplement Facts Panel, considering that the %DV is established for nonpregnant individuals.

Maternal anemia is defined as a hematocrit below 32% and a hemoglobin value below 11 g/dL. The risk for maternal anemia is especially high in women with substandard iron levels prior to pregnancy. Iron deficiency anemia that occurs during pregnancy increases the risk for small-for-gestational-age and preterm babies.[24] Fetal iron stores rise during the second and third trimesters. The transfer of fetal iron from the mother to the baby takes place toward the end of pregnancy, putting prematurely born infants at an increased risk for iron-deficiency anemia.

The UL for iron is 45 mg/day of elemental iron. Excessive iron intake has been identified as being involved in the development of preeclampsia and gestational diabetes.[13] Supplements and prenatal vitamins with high iron content may promote nausea or exacerbate morning sickness. Smaller-sized iron tablets or those that contain less iron may promote prenatal vitamin compliance among pregnant women.[25,26] Table 4–10 summarizes the DRI nutrient intake recommendation difference for nonpregnant versus pregnant women.[19,22]

■ Meal Planning During Pregnancy

Meal planning during pregnancy should ideally mirror healthy meal planning habits during other stages of life. Small, frequent meals are encouraged with a focus on achieving adequate fiber, carbohydrate, protein, calcium, iron, and folic acid intake, all while staying within the elevated calorie guidelines during the second and third trimesters. The USDA has a helpful web-based meal planning tool for expectant mothers on their *ChooseMyPlate.gov* website called the "*Daily Food Plan for Moms.*" Pregnant or breastfeeding women input their height,

Table 4-10. DRI nutrient need comparisons in pregnancy versus nonpregnancy.

Nutrient	Prepregnancy Needs	Pregnancy Needs
Protein	46 g/day	71 g/day
Carbohydrate	130 g/day	175 g/day
Folate	400 mcg/day	600 mcg/day
Calcium	1000 mg/day	1000 mg/day
Iron	18 mg/day	27 mg/day

Data from Institute of Medicine, 2006; Institute of Medicine, 2010.

weight, due date (if pregnant), age, and activity level to generate one of a number of calorie-based meal plans. The meal plans make recommendations on the amount of grains, vegetables, fruit, milk and meat, and bean servings to eat daily. While one size does not necessarily fit all pregnant or breastfeeding women, the simplicity of the tool and its straightforward approach to healthy meal planning serve as an excellent starting point for women looking to achieve the healthiest diet possible during pregnancy and breastfeeding. Table 4–11 outlines meal patterns for pregnancy and breastfeeding based on the USDA's *Daily Food Plan for Moms*.[27]

While many pregnant women may become preoccupied with all of the foods they *cannot* eat during pregnancy, it may be ideal, as a practitioner, to shift the focus to foods that they *can* (and should be)

Table 4-11. USDA meal plan recommendations for various calorie levels.

Calorie Level	Grains	Vegetables	Fruit	Milk	Meat and Beans
1800	6 oz	2½ cups	1½ cups	3 cups	5 oz
2000	6 oz	2½ cups	2 cups	3 cups	5½ oz
2200	7 oz	3 cups	2 cups	3 cups	6 oz
2400	8 oz	3 cups	2 cups	3 cups	6½ oz
2600	9 oz	3½ cups	2 cups	3 cups	6½ oz
2800	10 oz	3½ cups	2½ cups	3 cups	7 oz

Data from US Department of Agriculture, 2012.

eating. Practitioners are wise to use pregnancy as a time to promote the inclusion of new, healthy foods: high-fiber items such as legumes and dried peas and beans, lean sources of protein, whole grains such as whole grain breads, pastas, brown rice, and other grains, snacks consisting of fresh fruits and vegetables and adequate dietary calcium if dairy foods can be tolerated.

■ Foods to Avoid During Pregnancy

Pregnant women often lament about the vast number of foods to be avoided during pregnancy. Even further frustrating is the lack of scientific data backing up many of these claims. "Who says I can't have a few sips of wine?" "Just how bad could unpasteurized cheese really be?" "If I don't eat sushi soon, I'm going to lose it!" It is of course unethical to design studies whereby pregnant participants would be subjected to unhealthy levels of certain agents and then have the potential effects tested on their unborn babies. Armed with a lack of definable safety threshold levels for many food-based substances, but with a desire to prevent transmission of any potentially harmful agents across the placenta, women are left to handle food intake during pregnancy with the time-tested mantra, "When in doubt, leave it out."

Despite variations in some recommendations, there are a few general substances that the majority of health-disseminating groups agree should be avoided during pregnancy. The most important are alcohol, excessive caffeine, illicit drugs, and tobacco. From a food standpoint, pregnant women are advised to avoid raw or uncooked meats, fish, poultry, and eggs. Fish that are high in mercury, such as shark, swordfish, king mackerel, and tilefish, should be avoided, with all other fish (including tuna) limited to no more than 12 ounces per week or less.[28] In addition, hot dogs, luncheon meats, bologna, or other deli meats (unless they are heated until steaming hot) should also be avoided. Raw or unpasteurized milk, and cheese and dairy products made with raw or unpasteurized milk are not compatible with healthy pregnancy guidelines. Furthermore, herbal remedies and supplements as well as vitamin or mineral supplements not recommended or prescribed by a primary care practitioner should be avoided.[11] Table 4–12 summarizes these recommendations.[11,29]

When it comes to artificial sweeteners, erring on the side of caution is again desirable here. Saccharin, while not established as a teratogen, does cross the placenta and also appears in breast milk. While this has not demonstrated any adverse effects on a developing infant or fetus, limiting intake of these agents, by limiting diet sodas and reduced-calorie sweetened foods, is advisable. A sensible recommendation followed by many pregnant women is to limit diet sodas to no more than one per day, and to make that beverage caffeine-free if possible. Limiting caffeine during pregnancy, usually to the equivalent of one cup of coffee or less per day, also makes good nutrition sense. Caffeine does appear to increase the risk of spontaneous abortion in the first

Table 4-12. Foods and substances to avoid during pregnancy.

Beverages	• Alcohol • Excessive caffeine • Some types of herbal tea • Unpasteurized juices • Raw and unpasteurized milk
Meat and poultry	• Raw or uncooked meat, fish, poultry, or eggs • Hot dogs, luncheon meats, bologna, or other deli meats, unless they are heated until steaming hot
Fish	• Raw shellfish such as oysters and clams • Avoid fish high in mercury: shark, swordfish, king mackerel, and tilefish • Limit all other fish to 12 oz or less per week
Dairy products	• Raw and unpasteurized milk and dairy products and cheese made with raw or unpasteurized milk • Soft cheeses made from unpasteurized milk, including brie, feta, camembert, roquefort, queso blanco, and queso fresco
Miscellaneous	• Tobacco • Illicit drugs • Herbal remedies and supplements • Vitamin or mineral supplements not recommended by a PCP • Raw sprouts • Raw-cookie dough or cookie batter • Deli or in-store salads made with mayonnaise such as ham salad, chicken salad, and seafood salad

Data from Academy of Nutrition and Dietetics, 2012; http://www.foodsafety.gov/poisoning/risk/pregnant/chklist_pregnancy.htm.

trimester, although it may not contribute to intrauterine growth restriction (IUGR).[13] Risk factors that do contribute to IUGR include alcohol abuse, clotting disorders, illicit drug addiction, elevated blood pressure or heart disease, kidney disease, poor nutrition, and smoking.[30]

Practitioners counseling pregnant women on foods and substances to avoid during pregnancy sometimes find themselves in undesirable conversational situations, particularly with regards to interfamily dynamics. It is not uncommon to hear, "My mom drank when she was pregnant, and I certainly turned out fine!" or "My friends think I am being overly sensitive in trying to avoid unpasteurized cheeses, lunch meats, and sushi." When faced with these challenges, it is always safer to err on the side of caution. Some practitioners find it helpful for clients if they explain how certain agents cross the placenta, or to stress the magnification effect of these compounds on a fetus versus a grown adult. Regardless of your approach, striking a balance between emphasizing the consequences and severity of effects from not adhering to these guidelines, as well as accentuating the positives of adding more healthful foods during pregnancy, should be attempted in all nutrition for pregnancy recommendations.

■ Food Safety During Pregnancy

While foodborne illness is a concern at any stage of life, pregnant women are particularly susceptible to foodborne illness and infection. Foodborne illness may induce miscarriage or may cause serious health problems for both the mother and the baby. Pregnant women should be advised to follow the four basic tenets of food safety: clean, separate, cook, and chill.

- Clean: Wash hands and surfaces often
- Separate: Do not cross-contaminate
- Cook: Cook foods to proper temperature
- Chill: Refrigerate properly

The USDA recommends internal cooking temperatures of 145°F for whole cuts of beef, lamb, veal and pork, 160°F for ground meat (excluding poultry), and 165°F for all poultry, including whole cuts and ground poultry (Table 4–13).[31]

Listeriosis

Listeria monocytogenes is a bacterium found in water, soil, and plants. Listeriosis occurs after eating a contaminated food source and can cause fetal illness, premature delivery, or spontaneous abortion. Symptoms are similar to that of the flu: fever, chills, muscle aches, upset stomach, or diarrhea. *Listeria monocytogenes* infects 2500 Americans each year, and one in five will die from the illness.[32] The USDA's Food Safety and Inspection Service has provided the following tips to help prevent listeriosis in pregnant women and their babies:

- Do not eat hot dogs, luncheon meats, bologna, or other deli meats unless they are reheated until steaming hot
- Do not eat refrigerated pâté, meat spreads from a meat counter, or smoked seafood found in the refrigerated section of the store; foods that do not need refrigeration, such as canned tuna and canned salmon, are ok to eat, but refrigerate after opening
- Do not drink raw (unpasteurized) milk and do not eat foods that have unpasteurized milk in them
- Do not eat salads made in the store, such as ham salad, chicken salad, egg salad, tuna salad, or seafood salad
- Do not eat soft cheese such as feta, queso blanco, queso fresco, brie, camembert, blue-veined cheese, and Panela unless it is labeled as made with pasteurized milk; make sure the label says, "made with pasteurized milk"; be aware that some Caesar dressings are unpasteurized.

Table 4-13. USDA recommended internal temperature and rest times.

Product	Minimum Internal Temperature and Rest Time
Beef, pork, veal, and lamb Steaks, chops, and roasts	145°F (62.8°C) and allow to rest for at least 3 minutes
Ground meats	160°F (71.1°C)
Ham, fresh, or smoked (uncooked)	145°F (60°C) and allow to rest for at least 3 minutes
Fully cooked ham (to reheat)	Reheat cooked hams, packaged in USDA-inspected plants to 140°F (60°C) and all others to 165°F (73.9°C)
All poultry (breasts, whole bird, legs, thighs, and wings, ground poultry, and stuffing)	165°F (73.9°C)
Eggs	160°F (71.1°C)
Fish and shellfish	145°F (62.8°C)
Leftovers	165°F (73.9°C)
Casseroles	165°F (73.9°C)

Data from US Department of Agriculture, Food Safety and Inspection Service, 2012.

Toxoplasmosis

Toxoplasmosis is caused by *Toxoplasma gondii*, a protozoan parasite. In the United States, 22.5% or approximately 60 million individuals are infected with *Toxoplasma*, but most remain asymptomatic due to robust immunity. *Toxoplasma* infection during pregnancy is highly dangerous and can be transmitted to, and cause congenital infections and retardation, brain or eye damage in the unborn fetus. Transmission can occur to humans in undercooked and contaminated food, especially pork, lamb, and venison, or by contaminated utensils. Cats also spread toxoplasmosis, and as such, women are advised to avoid changing litter boxes during pregnancy. Pregnant women should also avoid adopting or handling stray cats and kittens and should wear gloves when gardening or when coming into contact with soil or sand that may harbor cat feces containing *Toxoplasma*.[33]

Methylmercury

The majority of fish and shellfish in our food supply contain some trace of mercury. Concentrations are higher in fish sourced from waters near areas with industrial mercury pollution. For the general, nonpregnant population, the health benefits of increasing fish and shellfish intake, particularly when it replaces other higher-fat animal protein, outweigh the potential harmful effects of methylmercury toxicity. While pregnant women and young children are also encouraged to include fish and shellfish for their health benefits, limited intake recommendations have been established due to the harmful effects of mercury exposure in these at risk populations. Exposure to mercury *in vitro* or in small children can cause irreversible damage to their developing kidneys and neurological systems.

The EPA and FDA recommend that all women who are pregnant or may become pregnant, nursing mothers, and young children avoid high-mercury content fish, including shark, swordfish, king mackerel, and tilefish. Women and young children may eat up to 12 ounces (two average serving sizes) of fish per week from other lower-mercury varieties. Canned albacore tuna should be limited to no more than six ounces (one can's worth of tuna) per week. Canned light tuna (the pink variety) is lower in mercury than is canned albacore (the chunky white kind). Consumers are cautioned to check advisories about fish caught in local lakes, rivers, and coastal areas and to limit intake of locally caught fish to no more than six ounces per week.

More information about food safety can be found at www.food-safety.gov. Table 4–14 contains more information about potentially hazardous foods during pregnancy and which foodborne illness or infection the food increases risk for.

■ Exercise During Pregnancy

Moderate physical activity during pregnancy does not impart negative effects on the developing fetus.[34] Exercise in pregnancy helps reduce gestational diabetes risk and improves labor outcomes and stress levels. Prenatal exercise reduces subcutaneous fat deposition during midpregnancy and subcutaneous fat retention in late pregnancy.[13] For women in good health standing, American College of Obstetricians and Gynecologists (ACOG), along with the CDC and American College of Sports Medicine (ACSM) all recommend at least 30 minutes of moderate-intensity physical activity on most days of the week.[35] Regular exercise during pregnancy helps reduce backaches, constipation, bloating, and swelling. It is helpful in the treatment and management of gestational diabetes; it also improves energy, mood, posture and muscle tone, strength, endurance, and sleep patterns. Recommended activities during pregnancy include walking, swimming, cycling, and aerobics. Running is safe during pregnancy, although modifications to prepregnancy routines may be needed. Pregnant women should avoid activities that increase the risk of falling, such as gymnastics, horseback riding, water and downhill snow skiing, and contact sports such as hockey, basketball, and soccer. Scuba diving increases the risk of fetal decompression sickness and should also be avoided. (Tables 4–15 to 4–17.)[36]

Table 4–14. Potentially hazardous foods and their contaminants to avoid during pregnancy.

Potentially Hazardous Food During Pregnancy	Escherichia Coli	Listeria	Salmonella	Vibrio	Parasites and Bacteria	Mercury	Campylobacter
Shark, swordfish, king mackerel, and tilefish						✓	
Raw cookie dough, batter			✓				
Soft cheeses: brie, feta, camembert, roquefort, queso blanco, and queso fresco	✓	✓					
Raw or undercooked fish: sushi					✓		
Unpasteurized juice or cider	✓						
Unpasteurized milk	✓	✓	✓				
Deli salads: ham salad, chicken salad, and seafood salad		✓					✓
Raw shellfish: oysters, clams				✓			
Sprouts: alfalfa, clover, mung bean, and radish	✓		✓				
Hot dogs, luncheon meats, cold cuts, and deli-style meat		✓					
Eggnog or undercooked eggs		✓					
Undercooked meat	✓						
Undercooked poultry and stuffing			✓				✓

Table 4–15. Exercise during pregnancy: do's and don'ts.

Exercise During Pregnancy "Do's"
Wear comfortable clothing and a protective sports bra
Drink adequate fluid to prevent dehydration
Engage in activity provided that it feels comfortable: walking, swimming, biking,
  low-impact aerobics, or light jogging
Exercise During Pregnancy "Don'ts"
Don't exercise on your back after the 1st trimester
Don't exercise in hot, humid weather, or with a fever
Don't exercise, or stop exercising if experiencing: vaginal bleeding or leaking,
  dizziness, increased shortness of breath, chest pain, headache, muscle weakness,
  calf pain or swelling, uterine contractions, or decreased fetal movement
Don't engage in activities that increase fall risk: skiing, gymnastics, and
  horseback riding
Don't engage in contact sports: hockey, basketball, soccer, and softball
Don't scuba dive

- ■ Nutrition-Related Complications During Pregnancy

Pregnancy can be a physically uncomfortable and nutritionally disruptive period. Nausea, constipation, heartburn, fatigue, cravings and aversions, cramps, and edema may all impair optimal food intake. Minor adjustments in diet and exercise patterns can help alleviate, or at a

Table 4–16. Absolute contraindications to aerobic exercise during pregnancy.

Uncontrolled type 1 diabetes, thyroid disease, or other serious cardiovascular, respiratory, or systemic disorder
Restrictive lung disease
Incompetent cervix/cerclage
Multiple gestation at risk for premature labor
Persistent 2nd- or 3rd-trimester bleeding
Placenta previa after 28 weeks of gestation
Premature labor during the current pregnancy
Ruptured membranes
Preeclampsia/pregnancy-induced hypertension

Data from American College of Obstetricians and Gynecologists, Committee on Obstetric Practice, 2002; Ferraro ZM, Gaudet L, Adamo KB. The potential impact of physical activity during pregnancy on maternal and neonatal outcomes. Obstet Gynecol Surv 2012 Feb;67(2):99–110.

Table 4-17. Relative contraindications to aerobic exercise during pregnancy.

Severe anemia
Unevaluated maternal cardiac arrhythmia
Chronic bronchitis
Twin pregnancy after 28th week
Extreme morbid obesity
Extreme underweight (BMI <12), malnutrition, or eating disorder
History of extremely sedentary lifestyle
Intrauterine growth restriction in current pregnancy
Previous preterm birth
Orthopedic limitations
Poorly controlled type 1 diabetes, hypertension, seizure disorder, or thyroid disease
Heavy smoker

Data from American College of Obstetricians and Gynecologists, Committee on Obstetric Practice, 2002; Ferraro ZM, Gaudet L, Adamo KB. The potential impact of physical activity during pregnancy on maternal and neonatal outcomes. Obstet Gynecol Surv 2012 Feb;67(2):99–110.

minimum, increase tolerability of these occurrences. The more serious conditions of gestational diabetes and pregnancy-induced hypertension do demand alterations in nutrition and exercise patterns.

Nausea and Vomiting

Nausea and vomiting in pregnancy (NVP) occurs in 70–80% of all pregnancies. NVP is generally limited to the first trimester and tends to resolve by the 14th–16th week of gestation.[37] Hyperemesis gravidarum is a more serious condition characterized by excessive vomiting and weight loss and is encountered in 2–5% of pregnancies.[38] Dietary treatment of hyperemesis involves avoiding offensive foods and agents. Sensitivity to odors is heightened with nausea and vomiting in pregnancy. Cold foods are usually more well tolerated than are hot foods, and foods with little or no odor are also preferred. A food that smells good to the individual will likely also taste good, whereas a strong or foul-smelling food will translate as a poorly tolerated food when ingested. Table 4–18 contains a list of recommended foods that may be tolerated by women experiencing morning sickness or hyperemesis gravidarum.[11] Keep in mind that tolerance during this time is highly individualized: what may sound good to one morning sick mother may not to another.

Table 4–18. Recommended foods for hyperemesis gravidarum or morning sickness.

Cold foods	Ice cream, popsicles, and frozen fruit
Warm foods	Mashed or baked potato, soup, and toast
Spicy foods	Salsa, gingersnaps, gingerbread, and curry
Tart or sour foods	Tomato or vegetable juice, dill pickles, lemons and lemonade, limes and limeade, and citrus juice or soda
Creamy foods	Whole milk, custards, puddings, and yogurt
Crunchy foods	Raw vegetables, chips, fruits, nuts, crackers, or dry cereal
Soft foods	Cake, cottage cheese, cooked carrots, and green beans
Beverages and liquid foods	Fruit juice, ginger ale, soft drinks, water, gelatin, and broth
Salty foods	Chips, salted crackers, dips, pizza, and tomato or vegetable juice
Chocolate foods	Chocolate milk, pudding, ice cream, and fudge sauce

Data from Academy of Nutrition and Dietetics, 2012; http://www.nlm.nih.gov/medlineplus/ency/patientinstructions/000604.htm.

Persistent vomiting during pregnancy may require hospitalization, especially when dehydration is present. Suboptimal levels of electrolytes can lead to cardiac irregularities. Care must be taken to slowly reintroduce nutrition to avoid refeeding syndrome in starved women. For women who are unable to tolerate p.o. feedings, enteral nutrition via tube feeding may be initiated. Tube feeding is preferred to total parenteral nutrition (TPN) because of the lower risk of further complications. TPN is a last resort for feeding in persistent, unresolved cases.

Nonpharmacologic treatments for nausea associated with pregnancy include supplementation with vitamin B6 and ginger. ACOG has endorsed the use of ginger and vitamin B6, stating, "treatment of nausea and vomiting of pregnancy with ginger,…vitamin B6 or vitamin B6 plus doxylamine is safe and effective and can be considered as a nonpharmacologic option."[39] While specific doses of ginger are not recommended, the guideline does reference a controlled trial designed to test the efficacy of ginger in cases of pregnancy-related nausea and vomiting that used a 350-mg dose taken three times per day.[40]

Cravings and Aversions

Dietary changes during pregnancy may not always be voluntary. Some women experience alterations in food cravings and aversions that range from mild to powerful. They may be precipitated by cultural or religious beliefs, family, historical or societal influences, recommendations from healthcare professionals, or simply exposure to food and cooking odors. Contrary to some traditional beliefs, cravings are not indicative of nutrient deficiency. The exception to this rule is ice, which may indicate an iron deficiency. Food cravings and aversions are physical manifestations of normal hormonal changes taking place during pregnancy. While the majority of cravings and aversions are harmless and limited to pregnancy or phases of pregnancy, care should be taken to assure that aversions do not impede optimal intake and that cravings are not contributing to excessive weight gain or to the consumption of potentially harmful substances.

Pica

Pica is the craving for and compulsive ingestion of nonfood, nonnutritive substances. The most commonly craved and consumed items in pica of pregnancy are clay (geophagia), starch (amylophagia), and ice (pagophagia).[41] Other items that have been documented as consumed by an individual with pica include burnt matches, hair, stones or gravel, charcoal soot, cigarette ashes, mothballs, antacid tablets, milk of magnesia, baking soda, corn starch, and coffee grounds.[42]

A woman's race and her geographic location appear to have some bearing on pica behavior during pregnancy. African-American women who have a family history of pica behavior or who live in rural areas appear more likely to experience pica,[42] although its incidence is not tied specifically to any one race, geographic location, or culture. There is some evidence, and some speculation, about the relationship between iron deficiency and pica. The craving of ice and in some cases, other nonfood substances is resolved with iron supplementation and when iron levels are restored to normal ranges, although iron deficiency cannot explain all cases of pica. Calcium deficiency as a cause of pica has also been explored.

Due to the unusual nature of the practice, pica is likely under-recognized or at least certainly, under-discussed in a typical prenatal clinic setting. Practitioners should be aware that while chewing on ice is a relatively harmless practice that may be corrected with simple iron supplementation, more serious complications may arise from consumption of other nonfood substances. Complications of pica can include congenital lead poisoning (if wall plaster or lead-based paint chips are consumed), fecal impaction and childbirth difficulties (if clay is consumed), fetal hemolytic anemia (if the mother eats mothballs and toilet air fresheners) and parotid enlargement, and gastric and/or small bowel obstruction (caused by ingestion of excessive laundry starch).[42]

Pregnancy-Induced Hypertension

A blood pressure reading of 140/90 mm Hg in pregnancy (gestational hypertension) is associated with increased perinatal morbidity and mortality and is regarded as abnormally elevated. The diagnosis of gestational hypertension requires two elevated blood pressure measurements obtained at least 6 hours apart. Preeclampsia is the onset of blood pressure greater than 140/90 mm Hg during pregnancy with proteinuria of more than 300 mg per 24-hour period occurring after week 20 of gestation. Severe preeclampsia is a systolic blood pressure reading of 160 or more or a diastolic blood pressure of 110 mm Hg or more and proteinuria of more than 5 grams in a 24-hour period. Management of preeclampsia involves balancing the health of both the mother and the fetus. The ultimate treatment for preeclampsia is delivery of the fetus and the placenta. Magnesium sulfate is used in the prevention and treatment of eclamptic seizures.[43] Sodium restriction and diuretic use are not appropriate therapies for the treatment of pregnancy-induced hypertension, and they do not lower blood pressure, slow weight gain, or resolve proteinuria.[13] The Academy of Nutrition and Dietetics encourages preeclamptic women to add more protein to meals, aiming for two to three servings of protein per day and to have at least three servings of low-fat or fat-free dairy foods, two to three servings of vegetables, at least two servings of fruit, and three servings of whole grains per day. Alcohol, excessive caffeine, and herbal teas should be avoided.

Gestational Diabetes

Gestational diabetes has historically been defined as any degree of glucose intolerance with onset or first recognition occurring during pregnancy. Due to the large number of pregnant women who have undiagnosed diabetes, the American Diabetes Association has revised their recommendations to include finding of diabetes at a first prenatal visit to receive the diagnosis of overt, as opposed to gestational, diabetes.[44] The current recommendations call for testing women not previously known to have diabetes with the 75-gram oral glucose tolerance test (OGTT) between weeks 24 and 28 of gestation. The revised diagnostic cut-points are: ≥92 mg/dL for the fasting test; ≥180 mg/dL 1 hour after drinking; and ≥153 mg/dL 2 hours after drinking the 75-gram glucose solution. Using the previous diagnostic criteria, approximately 7%, or one in 15 pregnant women were diagnosed with gestational diabetes; this is expected to rise to 18% with the revised criteria.[45]

The overarching goal of diabetes management during pregnancy is to achieve and maintain tight glycemic control. Blood glucose monitoring is recommended at least four times per day. Blood sugar checks should be done in the fasting and postprandial state (usually 1–2 hours after each meal). Table 4–19 outlines the American Diabetes Association's revised screening and diagnostic recommendations for gestational diabetes and for fasting and postprandial blood sugar targets.[44] Ketone testing is recommended for women with inadequate calorie or carbohydrate intake and for women experiencing weight loss.

Dietary changes and regular exercise are used to moderate weight gain among women with gestational diabetes. The diet should contain a minimum of 175 grams of carbohydrate per day, with no less than 45% of calories coming from carbohydrate in order to prevent hyperglycemia. Carbohydrate intake should be spaced throughout the day over a number of meals and snacks. Some women find that limiting carbohydrates to no more than 30 grams at breakfast helps minimize postprandial

Table 4-19. GDM screening, diagnosis, and treatment goals.

Screen when?	24-28 weeks gestation
	For women without previous diabetes diagnosis
Screen how?	75-g OGTT with fasting, 1-hour and 2-hour plasma glucose measurements
Diagnose with GDM after 75 g OGTT (in the morning, after overnight fast of at least 8 hours), with plasma glucose measurement fasting, and at 1 and 2 h, if:	Fasting ≥92 mg/day (5.1 mmol/L)
	1 hour ≥180 mg/dL (10.0 mmol/L)
	2 hour ≥153 mg/dL (8.5 mmol/L)
GDM glucose goals	Preprandial ≤95 mg/dL (5.3 mmol/L)
	1-hour postprandial ≤140 mg/dL (7.8 mmol/L) OR
	2-hour postprandial ≤120 mg/dL (6.7 mmol/L)
HbA1c goals	Can be used in 1st trimester to diagnose type 2 diabetes if HbA1c ≥6.5%
Glucose goals for women, with pre-existing type 1 or type 2 diabetes, who become pregnant	Premeal, bedtime, and overnight glucose 60-99 mg/dL (3.3-5.4 mmol/L)
	Peak postprandial glucose 100-129 mg/dL (5.4-7.1 mmol/L)
	A1C <6.0%

Data from American Diabetes Association, 2013.

hyperglycemia; lunch and dinner carbohydrate can usually be higher without adversely affecting glycemic levels. Table 4–20 outlines a sample plan for distributing carbohydrates over three meals and three snacks to meet the 175 grams minimum needed for optimal growth. Chapter 6 contains more information about meal planning for diabetes.

Nutrition for Breastfeeding

There is no lack of consensus regarding the importance of promoting exclusive breastfeeding from the earliest stages of life: the Academy of Nutrition and Dietetics, American Academy of Pediatrics, World Health Organization, United Nations Children's Fund, American Academy of Family Physicians, Academy of Breastfeeding Medicine, and many other organizations around the world advocate exclusive breastfeeding for the

Table 4-20. Sample carbohydrate distribution during pregnancy with GDM.

Breakfast	15- to 30-g carbohydrate
Snack	30 g carbohydrate
Lunch	45- to 60-g carbohydrate
Snack	30 g carbohydrate
Dinner	45- to 60-g carbohydrate
Snack	30 g carbohydrate
Total	**195- to 240-g carbohydrate**

first 6 months of life. Exclusive breastfeeding is defined as the provision of human milk with no additional supplementation (juice, water, cow's milk, foods, etc) with the exception of vitamins, minerals, and medication supplementation. Globally, one in three babies is exclusively breastfed through 6 months. In the United States, however, just over 14% of infants born in 2006 were exclusively breastfed through 6 months. *The Healthy People 2020* target is to increase this to 25.5%.[46,47]

Breast milk has been associated with immediate and long-term health benefits for both the mother and the child. Infants who are breastfed demonstrate lower rates of chronic diseases such as obesity, hypertension, diabetes, and heart disease; they have less GI issues, fewer ear infections, and lower likelihoods of developing food allergies and intolerances. For the mother, breastfeeding reduces the risk of breast and ovarian cancer, type 2 diabetes, and postpartum depression. In addition, breastfeeding moms return to prepregnancy weight faster than moms who do not breastfeed. Table 4-21 summarizes the benefits of breastfeeding for mother and child.[46]

■ Nutrient Composition of Breast Milk

In addition to the health benefits conveyed by breastfeeding, the nutrient composition of breast milk is uniquely suited to meet the rapid growth needs of infants. A newborn should be expected to feed 10-12 times per day to meet nutrient and energy needs. Human milk provides roughly 20 kcal/oz, although the actual energy density ranges from 20.9 to 26.2 calories per ounce, depending on the fat content of the milk. The fat content varies from mother to mother, and even varies within feeding with lower fat foremilk preceding higher fat hind milk toward the end of a feeding session.[48] The nutrients in breast milk are easily digestible and highly bioavailable. Breast milk is high in fat, providing roughly half of its calories. It is also rich in essential fatty acids, which promotes brain development and provides a concentrated source of calories. Lactose is the main carbohydrate in human milk, which also

Table 4-21. Benefits of breastfeeding for infant and mother.

Breastfeeding Reduces the Baby's Risk of	Breastfeeding Reduces the Mother's Risk of
Chronic diseases such as obesity, hypertension, type 1 and type 2 diabetes, heart disease, hypercholesterolemia, and childhood leukemia	Breast and ovarian cancer
Gastroenteritis and necrotizing enterocolitis	Type 2 diabetes
Otitis media, respiratory illness, and asthma	Postpartum depression
Sudden infant death syndrome (SIDS)	Postpartum weight retention
Developing food allergies and intolerances	Hip fracture and increases her bone density
Breastfeeding Increases the Baby's	**Breastfeeding Increases the Mother's**
Bonding with the mother	Bonding with the infant
Access to safe, fresh milk	Faster shrinking of the uterus
Proper development of jaws and teeth	Disposable income with money saved and not spend on formula feeding
Learning potential; and is associated with higher IQ and school performance through adolescence	Birth spacing potential

Data from American Dietetic Association, 2009.

contains over 100 major milk oligosaccharides that are believed to prevent against respiratory and enteric diseases.[46]

Colostrum, the first milk, is the thick yellowish fluid expressed in the first to third day after birth. Colostrum provides 580–700 kcal/L and is lower in carbohydrate and higher in fat than is the mature human milk produced 2 weeks after birth.[49] The protein content of mature milk is rather low, an important consideration for minimizing nitrogen overload on the developing kidneys. Casein is the primary protein in human milk and its digestive byproducts (casein phosphopeptides) help calcium retain its soluble form and promote calcium absorption.[49]

The micronutrient profile of breast milk is nearly ideal for infancy, with only vitamin D and, in some cases, fluoride needing to be supplemented. The American Academy of Pediatrics recommends that all healthy infants and children should receive at least 400 IU of vitamin D daily; this includes breastfeeding infants, and supplementation is recommended to begin within the first few days of life.[50] Breastfed infants

Table 4–22. Fluoride supplementation schedule.

Age	Community Drinking Water Fluoride Concentration in ppm (1 mg/L)		
	<0.3 ppm	0.3–0.6 ppm	>0.6 ppm
0–6 months	None	None	None
6 months to 3 years	0.25 mg/day	None	None
3–6 years	0.5 mg/day	0.25 mg/day	None
6–16 years	1.0 mg/day	0.5 mg/day	None

Data from US Department of Health and Human Services: Centers for Disease Control and Prevention, 2001.

who are 6 months or older may benefit from fluoride supplementation when the local water supply is not fluoridated or if no other fluoride sources are available to the child.[51] Fluoride supplementation is not needed when the municipal water supply contains 0.7–1.0 ppm of fluoride. If the combination of water, food, and toothpaste contributes less than 0.3 ppm fluoride, then 0.25 mg of fluoride via supplementation is recommended. Table 4–22 outlines a proposed fluoride supplement schedule.[52] Another nutritional advantage of breast milk is its changing composition, from colostrum with its antibody and immune-enhancing factors for infants to mature milk for older infants, breast milk meets the evolving nutrient needs of the growing infant.

While modern infant formulas can very closely replicate the nutritional composition of breast milk (and in the case of iron fortification of formulas, even surpass it), two advantages of breastfeeding exist that cannot be achieved with formula feeding: the provision of immune-enhancing factors present in colostrum and the changing composition of breast milk during feeding. The foremilk fed in the early stages of a feeding is thin and low in fat and calories, whereas the hind milk produced later in the feeding is thick and high in fat. The nutritional composition of the hind milk elicits a feeling of satiety that naturally syncs the baby's fullness to the emptying of the mother's current milk supply from that particular breast. Due to the inappropriate nutrient composition for an infant, cow's milk should not be introduced before 1 year of age. Table 4–23 outlines the comparison of breast milk with infant formula and cow's milk.

- Maternal Diet and Exercise During Breastfeeding

The production of breast milk requires an increase in maternal energy (calorie) intake, which is somewhat offset and counter-balanced by the postpartum mother's need/desire to lose weight. The DRIs for lactation are based on presumed weight loss rates of 0.8 kg (1.76 pounds) per

Table 4-23. Nutrient profile comparison of breast milk with infant formula and cow's milk.

	Breast Milk	Infant Formula	Cow's Milk
Antibody Factors	Colostrum and immune-enhancing factors	None	None
Carbohydrate	Lactose	Same as breast milk	Percentage of carbohydrate is too low
Fat	High (about 55%); optimal for brain development	Same as breast milk	Too low in fat for optimal brain development
Protein	Ideal blend of whey and casein; easy for infant digestion	Same as breast milk	Too high in protein for kidneys and digestion; too high in casein
Iron	Content is low, but ok for full-term babies in first 4-6 months, then supplement	Almost always iron fortified	Trace
Vitamin D	Content is low, AAP recommends supplementation	Varies	Fortified
Calcium	2:1 ratio of calcium to phosphorus ideal for absorption of both	Same as breast milk	Too high in calcium for developing kidneys to handle

month. The average daily maternal milk production in the first postpartum month is 600 mL. This increases to 750–800 mL per day by the fourth through sixth month of feeding and then down to 600 mL/day from months 7 through 12. This equates roughly to an output of 500 kcal/day in the first 6 months and 400 kcal/day in the second 6 months of lactation.[18] Some breastfeeding women continue taking a daily prenatal vitamin while breastfeeding, although the Institute of Medicine says that well-nourished, healthy women do not require regular supplementation.[53] Women with limited intake of dairy foods should consider vitamin D and calcium supplements, minimal meat eaters may need supplemental iron, and vegan women require supplemental vitamin B_{12} and possibly additional micronutrients.

Fluid recommendations for lactating women (aged 19–30) are 3.4 L per day. This is based on the 2.7 L for nonpregnant and nonlactating women (aged 19–30) recommendation plus the average milk output during first 6 months of breastfeeding, which is 0.68 L (from 0.78 L milk that is 87% water = 0.68 L).[54] Because other factors influence hydration status, women are encouraged to pay attention to the color of urine and aim for pale yellow urine as an indicator of adequate hydration.

There are no broad micronutrient supplementation recommendations during lactation. Many breastfeeding women choose to continue their prenatal vitamins as a nutritional "insurance policy," although such practices are not required. Recommendations for vitamin and mineral supplementation during lactation should be tailored to the individual. Women with low dairy intake may need supplemental calcium and vitamin D. Vegan women who abstain from all animal products may need to pay particular attention to calorie, protein, calcium, vitamin D, iron, zinc, and vitamin B_{12} intake levels. Table 4–24 contains sample meal plans for

Table 4–24. MyPlate plan for moms for exclusive breastfeeding and breastfeeding + formula feeding.

Food Group	Servings Recommended for the Exclusively Breastfeeding Mother	Servings Recommended for Breast-feeding and Formula Feeding	What is a 1 Cup or 1-ounce Serving?
Fruits	2 cups per day	2 cups per day	1 cup fruit or juice ½ cup dried fruit
Vegetables	3 cups per day	3 cups per day	1 cup raw or cooked vegetables or juice 2 cups raw leafy vegetables
Grains	8 ounces per day	7 ounces per day	1 slice bread 1 ounce ready-to-eat cereal ½ cup cooked pasta, rice, or cereal
Meat and beans	6½ ounces per day	6 ounces per day	1 ounce lean meat, poultry, or fish ¼ cup cooked, dry beans ½ ounce nuts or 1 egg 1 tablespoon peanut butter
Milk	3 cups per day	3 cups per day	1 cup milk 8 ounces yogurt 1½ ounces cheese 2 ounces processed cheese

lactating women from the *USDA MyPlate for Moms* for both exclusively breastfeeding women and combination of breast and bottle-feeders.

While some micronutrient needs increase during lactation (such as vitamin C, vitamin A, and vitamin E), others stay the same as during pregnancy or the nonpregnant, nonbreastfeeding state. Calcium and vitamin D are two examples of this. The DRIs for calcium (1000 mg) and vitamin D (15 mcg/day) are the same for nonpregnant, nonbreast-feeding, pregnant, and breastfeeding women.[22] This seems counterin-tuitive as the developing fetus and breastfeeding baby would seem to need more calcium and vitamin D from the mother to promote opti-mal bone density. The reality is that in the pregnant and breastfeeding state, the body more efficiently absorbs the amount of calcium and vitamin D taken in, utilizing it more readily than would be seen in the nonpregnant, nonbreastfeeding state. Table 4–25 highlights the nutri-ents of concern and recommended amounts needed per day for pregnant and breastfeeding women as compared to nonpregnant, nonlactating women.[19,22]

Certain foods in the mother's diet may influence the breastfeed-ing infant's behavior. Observational studies and anecdotal experiences indicate that foods such as cabbage, broccoli, cow's milk, and chocolate may trigger infant colic symptoms.[55] Another randomized control trial has found that excluding cow's milk, eggs, peanuts, tree nuts, wheat, soy, and fish lowered likelihood of colic symptoms in infants within the first 6 weeks of life.[56] Women are encouraged to avoid and exclude only those foods that seem to be problematic in their particular baby's behav-ioral outcomes. Avoiding whole classifications of foods may result in

Table 4–25. Recommended dietary allowances of fluid, macronutrients, and micronutrients.

	Nonpregnant, Nonlactating Female	Pregnant Female	Lactating Female
Water (L/day)	2.7	3.0	3.8
Carbohydrate (g/day)	130	175	210
Fiber (g/day)	25	28	29
Protein (g/day)	46	71	71
Folate (mcg/day)	400	600	500
Vitamin C (mg/day)	75	85	120
Vitamin D (mcg/day)	15	15	15
Calcium (mg/day)	1000	1000	1000

Data from Institute of Medicine, 2006; Institute of Medicine, 2010.

nutrient deficiency. Caffeine should be consumed in moderation, and alcohol avoidance is recommended during breastfeeding because of its transfer to breast milk, which can disrupt infant sleep patterns, development, and early learning potential.[57]

■ Supplement Use During Pregnancy and Breastfeeding

Pregnant and breastfeeding women are advised to abstain from taking any herbal products or dietary supplements, with the exception of prenatal vitamins or other micronutrients prescribed for diagnosed nutrient deficiencies. Due to the volatile nature of these products, their potential to cross the placenta, and the unregulated environment of supplement manufacturing and distribution, pregnant and breastfeeding women are advised to avoid any unecessary products entirely.

Diet and Breast Milk Supply, What Does the Evidence Say?

The following information is the Academy of Nutrition and Dietetics Evidence Analysis Library (EAL) conclusion statement for dietary factors affecting breast milk production (or breast milk supply, established lactation).

Which dietary factors would affect breast milk production (or breast milk supply, established lactation)?

The Academy of Nutrition and Dietetics Evidence Analysis Library project has produced the following conclusion statement:

Current available evidence shows no significant effects or relationships between any of the following dietary factors and breast milk production in healthy adult lactating women (mean ± SD BMI ranged from 21.4 ± 0.9 to 25.2 ± 4.2): short periods (less than 10 weeks) of reduced calorie intake (25% to 35% energy deficit), increased or decreased fluid intake (±25% to 50%), increased protein intake (1.5 grams per kg per day), three types of nutrition supplement (ie, Coleus amboinicus soup, fenugreek seeds capsules, and sugar-coated Moloco + B_{12} tablets), and calcium intake. (*Evidence Grade II – fair*).[58]

■ Encouraging and Promoting Successful Breastfeeding

If what they say is true, that "the breast is best," then why doesn't every postpartum mother choose breastfeeding? Many factors may contribute to sub-optimal breastfeeding rates. A lack of knowledge, ingrained family and cultural attitudes, an unsupportive environment (in the hospital, home, or workplace), and personal beliefs about breastfeeding may all influence a mother's decision to breastfeed.[59,60] Some women experience pain associated with breastfeeding, while others express frustration with the time and work it takes. Still others are concerned about or

Table 4-26. Contraindications to breastfeeding.

Infants with galactosemia, maple syrup urine disease, and/or phenylketonuria
Mothers with untreated tuberculosis
HIV-positive mothers
Human T-cell lymphotropic virus type I or II positive mothers
Mothers receiving certain radiation therapies or with exposure to radioactive materials
Mothers with herpes simplex lesions on a breast

Data from American Academy of Pediatrics, 2005; Baby-Friendly USA, Inc., 2010.

unsure how to quantify whether or not the baby is eating enough when breastfeeding. All of these concerns are valid; thus, it is important that practitioners have honest and candid conversations with their pregnant patients to assuage these concerns.

In some cases, breastfeeding is not warranted. Mothers who are HIV positive, who have untreated tuberculosis, are receiving certain radiation or chemotherapy treatments, or who are street or IV drug abusers should avoid breastfeeding their infants. Table 4–26 outlines contraindications for breastfeeding for both the mother and the infant.[61,62]

The healthcare practitioner can play a vital role in creating a supportive environment for successful breastfeeding outcomes. Practitioners can promote prenatal breastfeeding classes, provide information on the nutritional and health benefits of breastfeeding, dispel myths about breast versus bottle feeding, and help anticipate common feeding problems. Additional support can be given by providing referrals to lactation specialists, breastfeeding support programs, and pro-breastfeeding groups such as La Leche League.

Hospitals and birthing centers also play a vital role in breastfeeding promotion. The CDC's Maternity Practices in Infant Nutrition and Care Survey found that women who deliver in a hospital that utilizes board-certified lactation consultant have higher breastfeeding success rates. This appears to be particularly true for women who are at presumed high risk of not breastfeeding such as Medicaid recipients, teenage, or adolescent mothers, and those who deliver preterm or low birth weight babies.[63,64] The Baby-Friendly Hospital Initiative (BFHI) is a global program sponsored jointly by the World Health Organization (WHO) and the United Nations Children's Fund (UNICEF). Its purpose is to encourage and recognize those hospitals and birthing centers that provide optimal standards of care for infant feeding. In the United States, the BFHI has established a list of 10 steps for successful breastfeeding. Table 4–27 outlines these steps.[62]

Table 4–27. Baby-friendly hospital initiative guidelines for baby-friendly designation.

Guidelines and Evaluation Criteria for Hospital/Birthing Center Level Implementation of the United States Baby-Friendly Hospital Initiative
Step 1: Have a written breastfeeding policy that is routinely communicated to all health care staff
Step 2: Train all health care staff in the skills necessary to implement this policy
Step 3: Inform all pregnant women about the benefits and management of breastfeeding
Step 4: Help mothers initiate breastfeeding within 1 hour of birth
Step 5: Show mothers how to breastfeed and how to maintain lactation even if they are separated from their infants
Step 6: Give infants no food or drink other than breast milk unless medically indicated
Step 7: Practice rooming-in—allow mothers and infants to remain together 24 hours a day
Step 8: Encourage breastfeeding on demand
Step 9: Give no pacifiers or artificial nipples to breastfeeding infants
Step 10: Foster the establishment of breastfeeding support groups and refer mothers to them on discharge from the hospital or birth center

Reprinted with permission by Baby-Friendly USA, Inc. (Reproduced with permission from Baby-Friendly USA, Inc., 2010. http://www.babyfriendlyusa.org/about-us/baby-friendly-hospital-initiative/the-ten-steps.)

The following information is the Academy of Nutrition and Dietetics Evidence Analysis Library (EAL) conclusion statements for dietary effects on lactation and the effects of artificial nipples on the duration of breastfeeding.[65]

Which dietary factors would affect breast milk production (or breast milk supply, established lactation)?

The Academy of Nutrition and Dietetics Evidence Analysis Library project has produced the following conclusion statement:

Current available evidence shows no significant effects or relationships between any of the following dietary factors and breast milk production in healthy, adult, and lactating women (mean standard deviation body mass index ranged from 21.4_0.9 to 25.2_4.2): short periods (10 weeks) of reduced energy intake (25–35% energy deficit), increased or decreased fluid intake (25–50%), increased protein intake (1.5 g/kg/day), three types of nutrition supplement (ie, *Coleus amboinicus* soup, Fenugreek seed capsules, and sugar-coated Moloco_B-12 tablets), and calcium intake (*Evidence Grade II – fair*).[2]

What are the effects of artificial nipple on the duration of breastfeeding?

The Academy of Nutrition and Dietetics Evidence Analysis Library project has produced the following conclusion statement:

Overall, evidence suggests a negative influence of artificial nipple on the duration of all types of breastfeeding (from partial to exclusive). Observational evidence consistently showed an association between use of pacifier before 3 months of age and shorter breastfeeding duration in healthy term or full-term infants, after controlling for potential confounding. Data are insufficient to determine whether increasing frequencies of pacifier use or introduction of pacifier use beyond 3 months of age has differential influences on breastfeeding duration. Well-designed randomized control tests with blinded assessments of breastfeeding outcomes are needed to further support the validity of the findings from the observational studies concerning negative influence of pacifier use on the duration of breastfeeding. Data are insufficient to make a conclusion regarding the effects of artificial nipple on the duration of breastfeeding among preterm infants (*Evidence Grade II – fair*).

Supplemental Feeding in Term Or Full-Term Infants

Data from both randomized control trials and observational studies also consistently suggested that supplemental feedings to term infants, regardless of method (bottle or cup), had a detrimental effect on breastfeeding duration, compared to no supplemental feeding.

Preterm Infants

Data are insufficient to make a conclusion regarding the effects of artificial nipple on the duration of breastfeeding among preterm infants.

What are the effects of maternal diet or dietary supplements of n-3 fatty acids on the breast milk composition and infant health outcomes?

The Academy of Nutrition and Dietetics Evidence Analysis Library project has produced the following conclusion statement:

Consistent results from randomized control trials have shown that n-3 fatty acid supplementation (fish oil, cod liver oil, or docosahexaenoic acid [DHA]-rich oil) to pregnant women or breastfeeding mothers can increase n-3 FA levels in both breast milk and infant's plasma phospholipids. There is a dose–response relationship between doses of DHA supplementation and breast milk DHA levels, but the saturation dose remains unclear. Currently, there is no study directly examining the dose-response relationship for other types of n-3 fatty acid supplementation. These positive changes in breast milk n-3 fatty acid compositions, however, do not always show a positive effect on children's visual acuity and cognitive development at long-term follow-up. (*Evidence Grade I – good*).

Breastfeeding Multiples

The birthrate of twins rose 76% from 1980–2009. In 1980, one in every 53 babies born was a twin. By 2009, one in every 30 babies born was a twin.[66] Triplets or higher order birth rate births are not 153.5 per 100,000 live births.[67] The following information about breastfeeding multiples is provided by April Rudat, MS Ed, RD, LDN, the author of "*Oh Yes You Can Breastfeed Twins!*" available at www.dietitianapril.com.

1. *What is the best way for an advanced practice nurse to respond to a woman pregnant with twins, who says she has heard she can't breastfeed?*

"It can be done!" Women need support and reassurance, so reinforcing the physiology of breastfeeding is very important. With increased demand—two babies suckling at the breast instead of just one—there will be an increased breast milk supply and enough milk for twins as long as the mom is exclusively nursing. Use of any formula will interfere with breast milk production; therefore, formula supplementation should be avoided if possible. In addition, pumping initially after every feeding will stimulate the production of prolactin, which helps with maintaining or increasing milk supply. One final fact: historically speaking, wet nurses could produce enough milk to adequately nurse six babies, so, "it can be done!"

2. *What do you think is the single most important factor for those interested in breastfeeding twins? Is it time?*

Some say *time* is necessary for breastfeeding twins, but isn't time necessary for breastfeeding or formula-feeding even one baby? The fact is: babies take time! Therefore, the single most important tip in breastfeeding twins to save time is to *tandem breastfeed*, all the time, at every feeding using the football hold or another comfortable position.

3. *How many feedings per day should a mom breastfeeding twins prepare for—and how long will this take?*

Newborn babies need 8–12 feedings per day; therefore, a mom needs to tandem nurse for best success. At 15–60 minutes per feed, nursing twins one at a time could take as much as 24 hours! Moms of twins should learn tandem nursing immediately after delivery, and have the skill established before leaving the hospital. Moms breastfeeding twins benefit from constant support from a qualified lactation consultant (IBCLC). It is also necessary to have help—an extra set of hands—for the first few weeks until a mom figures out how to get both babies latched on together. It is also important to mention switching sides while nursing: Moms can keep one twin on the left breast and the other twin on the right breast for the entire feeding. There is no need to switch sides during a feeding; instead, the mom can switch babies to the alternate sides for the next feeding.

The mom can keep track using a notebook so she knows which baby got which side at each feeding. Provided that the babies have appropriate urination, stooling, and growth, the mom can be reassured that her milk is providing plenty of nutrition for her twins.

4. *Are there any special nutritional considerations that a mother herself needs to take into mind as she prepares to breastfeed twins?*

To successfully breastfeed in general, the mom needs approximately 200–600 kcal/day per baby. She also needs at least 25 grams or more protein per day, which can easily be done by adding extra dairy foods. There are no fluid recommendations available for mothers, breastfeeding twins, except to "drink to thirst." However, realistically speaking, moms should know this may be a few gallons of water per week! Moms who are breastfeeding twins should consume a variety of all foods, using the USDA's *MyPlate* as a guide (www.ChooseMyPlate.gov) and including 8–12 ounces of safe seafood per week. A mom might want to continue taking a prenatal vitamin, and she should limit or avoid caffeine and avoid alcohol. In breastfeeding twins, a mom should avoid dieting; however, the natural weight loss that occurs after delivery and while breastfeeding—1–2 pounds per week—is safe.

5. *Are there any supplements that you endorse as helping to increase milk supply or are they all a waste of time and money?*

As with breastfeeding in general, many women have historically relied on herbal galactogogues to increase breast milk supply despite the lack of research to support their use. Some common herbal galactogogues used among moms of multiples are fenugreek and "Mother's Milk" teas. Even the prescription drug Reglan is sometimes used as a galactogogue. Women need to do what works for them. My endorsement is for breastfeeding on demand, not using formula if able, and pumping after each feeding in the early days of breastfeeding twins to establish a solid milk supply.

6. *Any final tips you have about encouraging primary care providers to encourage women to breastfeed twins?*

Primary care providers should encourage women, especially moms expecting multiples, to breastfeed! Sometimes, women just need to hear they can do it. Women also benefit from early education on successful lactation during pregnancy and soon after birth, including tips on breastfeeding techniques and resolution of problems. Mothers of twins need to know how to tandem breastfeed before leaving the hospital and need to hear that they should rest, relax, and delegate for success. Any introduction of formula will interfere with breast milk supply, so moms need support to keep up on-demand breastfeeding. Finally, PCPs should avoid any negativity if a mom can only part-breastfeed her twins—any breast milk is better than none at all.

(*Continued*)

7. *And—just out of curiosity—can you breastfeed triplets?*

Women can and do breastfeed triplets. However, they may not be able to provide 100% breast milk for all the babies all the time. With triplets or more, two babies can nurse while one baby receives a bottle of breast milk or formula, and tandem nursing always saves time. Of importance, with twins or higher order multiples, if there is greater than a 1 pound weight difference for a baby, he may need additional feedings or supplementation. Also, with triplets or higher order multiples, a mom should not choose some babies that will be "breastfed babies" and others that will be "formula fed." All babies can receive some breast milk either from the breast or the bottle to receive breast milk's benefits.

Nutrition During Infancy

The *Dietary Guidelines for Americans* include recommendations for those aged 2 years and older. The infancy period is from birth to 1 year. With the assumption that a typical child will be breastfed or formula fed exclusively for the first 6 months of life, this section will cover the infant's nutrition needs from 6–12 months of age.

- ■ Calorie Needs During Infancy

As a proportion of their body weight, calorie needs are higher during infancy than they are at any other time in the lifespan. The average caloric needs of an infant in the first 6 months of life is 108 calories per kilogram of body weight, a recommendation that is based on projected growth rates of breastfed infants. The caloric needs drop slightly from 6 to 12 months to an average of 98 calories per kilogram of body weight.[18] These calorie levels are for typical, healthy infants. It is important to note that a number of factors influence caloric needs in infancy, including the baby's weight and the rate of growth, the number of hours spent sleeping versus awake, their level of physical activity, and the temperature and climate where the baby is located. The DRI estimated energy requirement (EER) for daily calorie needs is based on the following formulas during three different stages of infancy[18]:

- • 0–3 months: (89 calories × weight of infant in kg) + 75
- • 4–6 months: (89 calories × weight of infant in kg) + 44
- • 7–12 months: (89 calories × weight of infant in kg) − 78

- ■ Protein Needs During Infancy

As with calories, the amount of protein needed per kilogram of body weight is significantly higher in infants than in adults. During the first year of life, the body of the rapidly growing infant requires protein at rates that surpass those of any other stage of life. Whereas the adult RDA for protein is 0.8 g/kg body weight/day, infants need 2.2 grams of protein per kilogram of body weight per day in the first 6 months of life and 1.6 g/kg/day in months 6–12. An infant who is fed breast milk or formula is likely receiving sufficient amounts of protein.

■ Fat Needs During Infancy

When compared to the average adult diet, the percentage of calories coming from fat in an infant's diet is significantly higher. Infants need a high fat diet to promote optimal brain growth and development. Breast milk derives 55% of its calories from fat. In comparison, a heart-healthy adult diet should have no more than 35% of calories from fat. Infants lack the ability to fast for long periods of time because they are so rapidly using fats more regularly than adults do in order to create energy. Other nutrients and non-nutrients of concern in infancy are listed in Table 4–28.[68]

■ Weaning Foods

The Academy of Nutrition and Dietetics and the American Academy of Pediatrics recommend exclusive breastfeeding for the first 6 months of life with continued breastfeeding into the second 6 months of life with complementary foods.[69] Due to the unique nutritional needs of infants and their immature and developing GI tracts, the introduction of cow's milk is not indicated until after 12 months of age. By 4–6 months of age, most infants have developed the skills needed to begin accepting solid foods. Cues indicating a baby is ready for weaning foods include the ability to move the tongue from side-to-side without moving the head and sitting with little support.[70] First foods should be introduced with a spoon, in portions of one to two tablespoons per meal, offered one or two times per day. Table 4–29 includes general recommendations for solid food feeding by age.

Table 4–28. Other nutrients and nonnutrients of concern in infancy.

Fluoride	0.1 mg/day for 0-6 months and 0.5 mg/day for 7-12 months old
	Source is usually fluoridated water supply; milk is low in fluoride
	Overconsumption leads to dental discoloration
Vitamin D	AAP recommendations are for 400 IU per day for all infants
	Breast milk is low in vitamin D; formulas are generally fortified
	Inadequate vitamin D intake leads to rickets
Fiber	No consensus recommendations for fiber in infancy
	Baby foods are low in fiber
	Weaning foods with fiber (fruits, vegetables, and grains) are appropriate
Lead	Exposure may be environmental and toxicity interferes with brain development
	Screen for lead poisoning beginning at 9-12 months of age[68]

Table 4–29. Introduction of solid foods by age.

Chronological Age	Solid-Food Feeding Recommendation
1–6 months	Breast milk or formula only
6–7 months	Iron-fortified cereal Introduce cup Fruit: strained or mashed
7–8 months	Iron fortified cereal Vegetables: strained or mashed
8–9 months	Finger foods (crackers, bananas) Chopped (junior) baby food
10–11 months	Bite-sized cooked food
12 months	All table food

The first foods that are introduced around 6 months of life should be cereals. Iron-fortified rice cereal is generally offered first: rice because it is unlikely to cause allergies and is easily digested and iron-fortified as it is around 6 months of life when the fetal iron stores the baby received at the end of pregnancy begin to diminish. New foods should be offered one at a time in order to monitor for any potential allergenic reactions to the newly introduced foods. With regards to the introduction of fruits and vegetables, many parents find that introducing new vegetables is preferential before introducing fruits. The notion is that infants are understandably attracted to the inherent sweetness of fruits and may be less inclined to readily accept vegetables after regular exposure to only fruits.[71]

While commercial baby foods are convenient, they are not a necessary part of the infant's diet. Preparing baby food at home by mashing up cooked foods with a fork or using a blender or food processor is perfectly acceptable. The texture of prepared baby food should be on the soupy side and care should be taken to assure appropriate food preparation, handling, and storage techniques in the home kitchen. For parents who do choose to purchase commercial baby foods, they should be advised that baby food dessert products have no place in the diet of a healthy baby. Keep in mind that the portion sizes of commercial baby food products may not reflect the true needs of the infant, who may require more or less than the standard servings. Parents should learn to look for hunger cues and signs of satiety in the infant, keeping in mind that children (in stark contrast to many adults) are acutely aware of when they are hungry and should be eating, and when they are full and should stop. Table 4–30 contains recommendations for infant feeding

Table 4-30. Infant feeding do's and don'ts.

Feeding Practice	Do	Why?	Don't	Why?
Cow's milk	Introduce sometime after 12 months	Gut and kidneys can handle protein load at this time	Don't feed before 1 year	GI tract and kidneys can't handle and increased risk for allergic reactions
Low- or reduced-fat milk products	OK to give after 2 years	Child has other food sources of fat for brain development	Don't give to child under 2 years of age	Child needs fat from full-fat dairy to promote brain development
Honey	OK for kids over 1 year	Immune system is developed enough to handle potential botulism	Don't give to child under 1 year	Risk of botulism in underdeveloped immune system
Cereal	Start feeding iron-fortified rice cereal around 6 months	Rice is least allergenic of cereals	Feed nonrice cereal first	Other grains introduced first may increase allergy risk
Baby food and weaning foods	Give iron-fortified weaning foods and cereals	Maternal iron stores have depleted by end of baby's 6th month	Feed baby food dessert	Increases affinity for sweets and displaces other important nutrients in the diet
Vitamin C	Include in the weaning diet	Helps maximize iron absorption		
Bottle	Put the baby to bed without a bottle in the crib	Eliminates aspiration risk	Put the baby to bed with a bottle containing sugary substance	Increase aspiration risk and risk of dental caries

Table 4–31. Signs when your baby is ready for solid foods.

Your Baby is Ready for Solid Foods When He or She...
Has good head control and can hold head up without wobbling
Can sit well with little support
Has doubled birth weight and weighs at least 13 pounds
Is still hungry after 8 to 10 breast feedings or after drinking 32 ounces of formula per day
Shows interest in foods that others are eating
Leans toward a food or a spoon with food and opens mouth in anticipation
Is able to move foods from front to back of the mouth
Can pick up and hold a small object by hand
Can self-feed with fingers
Can drink from a cup with your help
Turns away to signal "finished" or "enough"

Adapted from Clemson Cooperative Extension, Home & Garden Information Center HGIC 4102 "Introducing Solid Foods to Infants" October 2008.

"Do's and Don'ts." Table 4–31 presents signs when a baby is ready for solid foods.[72]

Nutrition in Early Childhood: Toddlers and Preschoolers

The rate of growth slows after the first year of life, but still remains remarkably higher in toddlers and preschool-aged children than in later stages of life. By the age of three, the human brain is 90% of its adult size,[73] and there is an established link between the quality of a child's diet and his or her cognitive development.[74] One of the topic areas of *Healthy People 2020* is to increase the proportion of children who are ready for school in all five domains of healthy development: physical development, social-emotional development, approaches to learning, language, and cognitive development.[75]

The CDC recommends that healthcare providers use the WHO growth standards to monitor growth for infants and children aged birth to 2 years in the United States. For children aged 2 years and older, the CDC recommends using the CDC growth charts. The CDC clinical growth charts for infants (birth to 36 months) include one growth chart for length-for-age and weight-for-age and a separate growth chart for head circumference-for-age and weight-for-length. The CDC growth charts for children and adolescents (2–20 years) include one growth chart for stature-for-age and weight-for-age and a separate growth chart for BMI-for-age. For preschoolers (2–5 years) there is also a CDC weight-for-stature growth chart. The CDC clinical growth charts can be accessed at: http://www.cdc.gov/growthcharts/clinical_charts.htm and growth charts are also included as Appendix C.

Plotting a child's growth on the gender-specific BMI-for-age growth chart establishes a baseline for assessing underweight, healthy weight, or overweight and obesity. Children in the less than 5th percentile for BMI-for-age are considered to be underweight. Healthy weight is 5th to less than 85th percentile. Overweight are 85th to less than the 95th percentile, and obese is equal to or greater than the 95th percentile. An online child and teen BMI calculator is available at: http://apps.nccd.cdc.gov/dnpabmi/, and more information about childhood and teen BMI calculations is available in Chapter 3.

▪ Toddler Feeding Practices

Although infant and childhood feeding skills evolve at different rates, most children have completed the weaning process by 12–14 months. The variety of textures and types of foods that are introduced correlate with the child's developmental progress. Toddlers who can wag, wave, or move their tongue from side to side develop the ability to chew with rotary movements. This usually occurs between 12 and 18 months and indicates that the toddler is ready for the introduction of chopped and soft table foods.[70] Between 18 and 24 months, toddlers develop the ability to handle meats, raw fruits, and vegetables. Their dexterity to handle a spoon also improves. As feeding abilities improve, so does the toddler's desire to engage in self-feeding. While parents may perceive this developmental stage as occasionally frustrating (and always messy), it is an important part of developing healthy eating behaviors in children. Toddlers who demonstrate independent self-feeding practices still need to be monitored closely, and parents should avoid giving foods that may increase choking, such as peanut butter, hard candy, popcorn, nuts, whole grapes, raisins, and hot dogs cut in coin shapes.[76] Hot dogs cut in matchstick pieces are safer.

Parents play an important role in developing healthy eating patterns in their children; but the children are still active participants in this equation. Table 4–32 contains a list of recommendations for parents to positively influence child feeding.[27] Table 4–33 lists behavioral milestones in preschoolers that affect eating behaviors.[27] More childhood feeding recommendations for preschoolers can be found at www.ChooseMyPlate.gov/preschoolers.html.

Childhood feeding expert Ellyn Satter recommends a *"Division of Responsibility in Feeding"* approach, stating that parents provide structure, support, and opportunities. Children choose how much

Table 4–32. ChooseMyPlate.gov tips for influencing what and how much your child eats.

Tips for Positively Influencing What and How Much Your Child Eats
Set a good example
Offer a variety of foods
Start small with portions
Follow a meal and snack schedule
Make mealtime a family time
Cope with a picky eater
Help them try new foods
Make food fun

Data from US Department of Agriculture, 2012.

Table 4–33. Preschooler milestones from ChooseMyPlate.gov.

2 Years
    Can use a spoon and drink from a cup
    Can be easily distracted
    Growth slows and appetite drops
    Develops likes and dislikes
    Can be very messy
    May suddenly refuse certain foods
3 Years
    Makes simple either/or food choices, such as choice of apple or orange slices
    Pours liquid with some spills
    Is comfortable using fork and spoon
    Can follow simple requests such as "please use your napkin"
    Starts to request favorite foods
    Likes to imitate cooking
    May suddenly refuse certain foods
4 Years
    Influenced by TV, media, and other children
    May dislike many mixed dishes
    Rarely spills with spoon or cup
    Knows what table manners are expected
    Can be easily sidetracked
    May suddenly refuse certain foods
5 Years
    Has fewer demands
    Usually accepts the food that is available
    Dresses and eats with minor supervision

Data from US Department of Agriculture, 2012.

and whether to eat from what the parents provide. The *Division of Responsibility for Toddlers through Adolescents* states that the parent is responsible for what, when, and where food is eaten while the child is responsible for how much and whether. Satter differentiates between the jobs of parents and children in feeding and eating[77]:

Parents' Feeding Jobs:

- Choose and prepare the food
- Provide regular meals and snacks
- Make eating times pleasant
- Show children what they have to learn about food and mealtime behavior
- Not let children graze for food or beverages between meal and snack times
- Let children grow up to get bodies that are right for them

Fundamental to parents' jobs is trusting children to decide how much and whether to eat. If parents do their jobs with *feeding*, children will do their jobs with *eating*:

- Children will eat
- They will eat the amount they need
- They will learn to eat the food their parents eat
- They will grow predictably
- They will learn to behave well at the table

▪ Calorie Needs in Early Childhood

While growth is still remarkable in the toddler and preschool age groups, the rate of growth and estimated calories per unit of body weight is slower and lower than in infancy. The DRIs include estimated energy requirements (EER) for children aged 0–6 months, 6–12 months, 1–3 years, 4–8 years, and 9–13 years. The EER for children aged 13–36 months is (89 × weight of child in kg – 100) + 20.[18] Starting at 36 months of age, the DRI estimations for calorie needs are based on age, height, weight, gender, and the child's physical activity level. Table 4–34 outlines the calorie needs for standardized boy and girl children based on their PALs, and Table 4–35 shows the same information from *ChooseMyPlate.gov*.[18,27] Table 4–36 demonstrates sample meal and snack pattern and ideas for preschoolers of varying activity levels from *ChooseMyPlate.gov*.[27]

▪ Protein, Carbohydrate, and Fat Needs in Early Childhood

The recommended distribution of macronutrients (protein, carbohydrate, and fat) for children aged 1–3 years is 5–20% of calories from protein, 45–65% of calories from carbohydrate, and 30–40% of calories from fat. For aged 4–18 years, the distribution changes to 10–30% of calories from protein, 25–35% of calories from fat, and continues to be 45–65% of calories from carbohydrate. At all stages of life, carbohydrate should constitute the greatest percentage of calories. Good sources of carbohydrate include whole grains, fruits, vegetables, milk

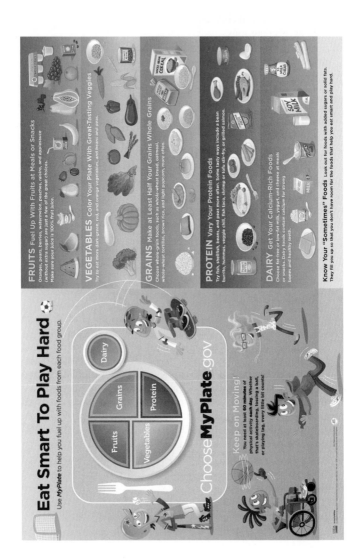

Table 4-34. Estimated calorie needs (EER) for age-specific boys and girls at varying physical activity levels (PALs).

	Reference Height [m (in.)]	Reference Weight [kg (lbs)]	Sedentary PAL (cal/day)	Low Active PAL (cal/day)	Active PAL (cal/day)	Very Active PAL (cal/day)
3-year-old boy	0.95 (37.4)	14.3 (31.5)	1162	1324	1485	1683
3-year-old girl	0.94 (37.0)	13.9 (30.6)	1080	1243	1395	1649
4-year-old boy	1.02 (40.2)	16.2 (35.7)	1215	1390	1566	1783
4-year-old girl	1.01 (39.8)	15.8 (34.8)	1133	1310	1475	1750
5-year-old boy	1.09 (42.9)	18.4 (40.5)	1275	1466	1658	1894
5-year-old girl	1.08 (42.5)	17.9 (39.4)	1189	1379	1557	1854

Data from Food and Nutrition Board, Institute of Medicine, 2005.

Table 4-35. Recommended calorie needs for preschoolers by age and gender from ChooseMyPlate.gov.

	Boys' Daily Calorie Needs			Age	Girls' Daily Calorie Needs		
Age	Less than 30 Minutes/Day Physical Activity	30-60 Minutes/Day Physical Activity	More than 60 Minutes/Day Physical Activity		Less than 30 Minutes/Day Physical Activity	30-60 Minutes/Day Physical Activity	More than 60 Minutes/Day Physical Activity
2	1000	1000	1000	2	1000	1000	1000
3	1200	1400	1400	3	1000	1200	1400
4	1200	1400	1600	4	1200	1400	1400
5	1200	1400	1600	5	1200	1400	1600

Data from US Department of Agriculture, 2012.

Table 4-36. Meal patterning for preschoolers at various calorie levels from ChooseMyPlate.gov.

	Grains	Vegetables	Fruits	Dairy	Protein Foods
1000 calories	3 oz	1 cup	1 cup	2 cups	2 ounces
1200 calories	4 oz	1½ cups	1 cup	2½ cups	3 ounces
1400 calories	5 oz	1½ cups	1½ cups	2½ cups	4 ounces
1600 calories	5 oz	2 cups	1½ cups	2½ cups	5 ounces

Data from US Department of Agriculture, 2012.

and yogurt, and legumes. All individuals aged 1 year and older need a minimum 130 grams of carbohydrate per day.[18]

With regards to protein, the DRIs state that children 1–3 years of age need a minimum of 13 grams of protein per day, whereas children aged 4–8 years require 19 grams of protein per day. Another way to calculate estimated protein requirements is based on kilogram of body weight. Children aged 1–3 years need 1.1 grams of protein per kilogram of body weight, and children aged 4–8 years need 0.95 grams of protein per kilogram of body weight per day.

There are insufficient data to set fat grams per day recommendations for ages 1–3 years and 4–8 years; however, if you use the 35% of calories from fat midpoint for kids aged 1–3 years, this works out to roughly 51 grams of fat per day for a 3-year-old boy with a low-active level calorie requirement of 1324 calories per day and 48 grams of fat per day for a 3-year-old girl with a low-active level calorie requirement of 1243 calories per day. For a low-active 5-year-old boy eating 1466 calories per day with 30% of his calories coming from fat, this would equal 49 grams of fat per day. For a low-active 5-year-old girl eating 1379 calories with 30% of her calories coming from fat, this would equal 46 grams of fat needed per day.

■ Vitamin, Mineral, Fiber, and Fluid Needs in Early Childhood

A child with a well-balanced diet will likely be meeting the majority of his or her daily micronutrient, fiber, and fluid needs. There is not enough data to set a recommended dietary allowance (RDA) for fluid and fiber for kids, but the DRI committee has established recommended adequate intake (AI) levels for fluid and fiber for children. The AI for fluid for children aged 1–3 years is 1.3 liters (1300 mL, 44 fluid ounces, or 5.5 cups) per day. For children aged 4–8 years, the AI is 1.7 liters (1700 mL, 57 fluid ounces, or roughly 7 cups) per day. Children aged 1–3 years should aim to have 19 grams of fiber, and that AI for fiber increases to 25 grams per day for children aged 4–8 years.

Particular nutrients of concern for these age-groups do exist, and they include iron, zinc, calcium, and fluoride. Children who have insufficient iron intakes are at increased risk for iron deficiency and iron deficiency anemia, the most common nutrient deficiency worldwide.[78] Iron is responsible for carrying oxygen in the blood, assisting with energy metabolism, and facilitating adequate nervous system function. Iron deficiency negatively affects cognitive growth. A child's brain is increasingly sensitive to low iron concentrations long before deficits appear in the blood. Symptoms of iron deficiency include a decreased motivation to engage or persist in intellectually challenging tasks, a diminished attention span, and overall decline in intellectual performance.

Iron needs for children aged 1–3 years is 7 mg/day and 10 mg/day for children aged 4–8 years.[18] In order to prevent iron deficiency, children should have a variety of iron-containing foods in their diets. Milk should be consumed, yet limited, after infancy, due to its low iron content. Kids up to 8 years of age should have two cups of milk per day, and children aged 9 years and above should have three cups per day. While milk is low in iron content, meat, fish, poultry, eggs, and legumes are good sources of iron, as are iron-fortified cereals, whole grain breads, and enriched and fortified grain foods. Table 4–37 contains the American Academy of Pediatrics recommendations for iron for infants and toddlers.[79] Table 4–38 contains a list of foods that school-aged children regularly consume that contain approximately 1 mg iron per serving. Note that the percent daily value (%DV) column on the Nutrition Facts panel is based on 18 mg iron/day as 100% DV (for adults). Some children-specific foods may list a %DV column for childhood nutrient needs.

Calcium needs for children also increase with age. Children 1–3 years old need 700 mg calcium per day and those aged 4–8 years need 1000 mg per day.[22] One cup of milk or milk equivalent contains approximately 300 mg calcium. The percent daily value (%DV) on the Nutrition Facts panel is based on 1000 mg per day; therefore, a milk or yogurt product, stating it has "30% DV for calcium," contains 300 mg calcium per serving of that food.

Zinc is an essential mineral required for appropriate growth and development. Zinc needs for children are set at 3 mg per day for 1–3 years and 5 mg per day for 4–8 years. Good sources of zinc include beef, eggs, chicken, lentils, dairy foods, walnuts, and other grain foods. As for fluoride, children obtain this essential mineral primarily from fluoridated municipal water supplies and the use of fluoridated toothpaste. In areas where the water supply is not adequately fluoridated, the American Dental Association, American Academy of Pediatrics, and the American Academy of Pediatric Dentistry recommend following a fluoride supplementation schedule. This schedule is based on the child's age and the fluoride content of the water supply. Children 6–36 months old should have 0.5 mg fluoride/day if water supply is less than 0.3 ppm,

Table 4–37. American Academy of Pediatrics iron recommendations for infants and toddlers.

Term, healthy infants	Sufficient iron for first 4 months of life
	Breastfed: 1 mg/kg/day oral iron beginning at 4 months until iron-rich complementary foods introduced
Formula-fed infants	Adequate iron from formula and complementary foods
	No whole milk before 12 months of age
Infants 6–12 months	11 mg iron/day
	Foods: red meat and vegetables with high iron content
	Liquid iron supplements if food needs are not met
Toddlers aged 1–3	7 mg iron/day
	Foods: red meat, iron-rich vegetables, and fruits with vitamin C
	Can use liquid or chewable supplements
Preterm infants	2 mg/kg iron/day through 12 months
	Iron supplement of 2 mg/kg/day by 1 month of age, continue until weaned to iron fortified formula or complementary foods that give 2 mg/kg/day

Data from Baker, Greer, & Pediatrics, 2010.

Table 4–38. Examples of iron-containing foods for kids, 1 serving = 1 mg iron.

Breads, Cereals, and Grains
   ½ cup spaghetti
   ½ cup noodles, rice, or barley
   1 flour or 2 corn tortillas
Vegetables
   ½ cup green peas
   1 cup vegetable juice
   ½ cup cooked snow peas
Fruits
   4 dried peach halves
   1 tablespoon raisins
Meat and Legumes
   ½ cup meat casserole
   ½ peanut butter and jelly sandwich

and 0.25 mg fluoride per day if local water supply has 0.3–0.6 ppm of fluoride.[80] Care should be taken to avoid excessive fluoride consumption from supplemental sources as this can lead to dental fluorosis, the discoloration or pitting of the dental enamel.

▪ The USDA WIC Program

The USDA's Special Supplemental Nutrition Program for Women, Infants, and Children, more commonly known as the WIC Program, provides nutritious foods, supplements, and nutrition education to improve the health of low-income pregnant, postpartum, and breast-feeding women, infants, and children up to aged 5 years. WIC is a federal grant program administered at the state level, and participation in the program is based on income eligibility standards (≤185% of federal poverty line). WIC services may be provided in county health departments, hospitals, mobile clinics, community centers, military installations, schools, public housing sites, Indian Health Service facilities, or migrant health centers and camps. In addition to income eligibility guidelines, there are two types of nutrition risk that are assessed to help determine WIC eligibility. Medically based risks include anemia, underweight, maternal age, history of pregnancy complications, or previous poor pregnancy outcomes. Diet-based risk is reflected in inadequate dietary patterns, and this risk is identified by a health professional in a screening that is free to program applicants.

WIC participants receive vouchers that can be redeemed when purchasing specific healthy foods and beverages. These products are intended to supplement WIC participants' diets with the nutrients that most benefit this target population. WIC foods include iron-fortified infant and adult cereals, vitamin C-rich fruit or vegetable juice, eggs, milk, cheese, peanut butter, dried and canned beans and peas, and canned fish. New additions to the WIC food package (2007) include soy-based beverages for those who may be lactose intolerant, tofu, fruits and vegetables, baby foods, whole wheat bread, and other whole grains. The WIC Farmers' Market Nutrition Program was established in 1992 and gives additional coupons to WIC participants that they can redeem for fresh produce at participating farmers' markets. WIC promotes breastfeeding as the preferred and optimal nutrition source for infants; however, for women who do not exclusively breastfeed, WIC does provide iron-fortified infant formula. For infants with medical conditions, prescribed infant formulas and medical foods are distributed.

The effectiveness of the WIC program in promoting optimal birth outcomes and childhood and maternal health are well documented. In fiscal year 2010, WIC served 9.17 million women, infants, and children, up from just 88,000 people served in 1974 (its first year of authorization). To truly gauge the reach of WIC, consider this: today, nearly half of all babies born in the United States are to families that receive WIC benefits.[81] Of the 9.17 million individuals who received WIC benefits in 2010, 4.86 million were children, 2.17 million were infants, and

Table 4-39. Summary of health benefits of WIC participation.

WIC reduces fetal deaths and infant mortality
WIC reduces low birth weight rates and increases the duration of pregnancy
WIC improves the growth of nutritionally at-risk infants and children
WIC decreases the incidence of iron deficiency anemia in children
WIC improves the dietary intake of pregnant and postpartum women and improves weight gain in pregnant women
Pregnant women participating in WIC receive prenatal care earlier
Children enrolled in WIC are more likely to have a regular source of medical care and have more up-to-date immunizations
WIC helps get children ready to start school: children who receive WIC benefits demonstrate improved intellectual development
WIC significantly improves children's diets

Data from US Department of Agriculture Food and Nutrition Service, 2012.

2.14 million were women.[82] WIC is an effective nutrition assistance program, and studies conducted by USDA Food and Nutrition Services and other nongovernment entities suggest "that WIC is one of the nation's most successful and cost-effective nutrition intervention programs."[83] WIC works to improve birth outcomes and savings in health care costs, improves diet and diet-related health outcomes, and improves infant feeding practices, immunization rates, cognitive development in children, and preconceptional nutritional status in mothers. Table 4–39 contains a list of the beneficial health outcomes that WIC helps promote.[83] To refer a potential WIC client, encourage the individual to visit the "How to Apply for WIC" page at www.fns.usda.gov/wic/howtoapply/.

Nutrition in Later Childhood: School-Age and Adolescence

■ Energy Needs in Later Childhood

As with other stages of life, the energy needs in school-aged and adolescent children are based on their gender, age, height, weight, and physical activity level. Although the child is still growing, the amount of calories per unit of body weight needed declines in later childhood as compared to infants, toddlers, and preschool-aged children. An online energy-needs, recommended portions-per-day and discretionary calories allotted calculator is available from the Baylor College of

Medicine's Children's Nutrition Research Center at: http://www.bcm.edu/cnrc/healthyeatingcalculator/eatingCal.html. The EER calculations for boys and girls aged 3–8 years and 9–18 years are as follows[18]:

- Boys 3–8 years: EER = 88.5 – (61.9 × age [y]) + PA[a] × {(26.7 × weight [kg]) + (903 × height [m])} + 20
- Boys 9–18 years: EER = 88.5 – (61.9 × age [y]) + PA × {(26.7 × weight [kg]) + (903 × height [m])} + 25
- Girls 3–8 years: EER = 135.3 – (30.8 × age [y]) + PA[b] × {(10.0 × weight [kg]) + (934 × height [m])} + 20
- Girls 9–18 years: EER = 135.3 – (30.8 × age [y]) + PA × {(10.0 × weight [kg]) + (934 × height [m])} + 25

▪ Protein, Carbohydrate, and Fat Needs in Later Childhood

The DRI recommendation for protein for children aged 4–13 years is 0.95 grams of protein per kilogram of body weight per day. As with all other individuals aged 1 year and older, a minimum of 130 grams of carbohydrate per day is required. Carbohydrate should represent 45–65% of total calories, which, for a moderately active 9- to 13-year-old girl consuming 1800 calories, is approximately 200–300 grams of carbohydrate per day and, for a moderately active 9- to 13-year-old boy consuming 2000 calories, approximately 225–325 grams of carbohydrate per day. Fat intake should be 25–35% of total calories, which is roughly 60–67 grams of fat for a 1, 800- to 2000-calorie diet (at 30% of calories coming from fat).

▪ Vitamin, Mineral, Fiber, and Fluid Needs in Later Childhood

It is in the middle school years that children are often allotted their first taste of independence when making food choices. Whether it be money provided to purchase cafeteria lunches, or spare change for vending machine snacks and sodas, children in this developmental period are testing the waters and setting the stage for individual food choices and lifestyles that will impact their health in years to come. Because their bodies are still growing and developing, middle school and adolescent children have nutrient needs that differ from those of fully developed adults. One important micronutrient for this age group is calcium. School-aged children and adolescents are actively laying down bone, and their calcium needs at these ages are higher than at any other time in the lifespan. Males and females aged 4–8 years need 1000 mg calcium per day and 9- to 18-year-olds need 1300 mg calcium per day. Pregnant and lactating 14- to 18-year-olds also need 1300 mg calcium per day.[22] For those in the 1000 mg calcium per day categories, this equates to roughly three servings of dairy or milk equivalents per day. For those in the 1300 mg calcium per day categories, approximately four servings of dairy or milk equivalents per day are required. Middle-school-aged

---

[a]Male PA coefficients 3–18 years: sedentary = 1.00, low active = 1.13, active = 1.26
[b]Female PA coefficients 3–18 years: sedentary = 1.00, low active = 1.16, active = 1.31

children and adolescents should be encouraged to have a variety of non-fat and low-fat (1%) milk and dairy products as part of their regular meal plans. Fluid milk, yogurt, cheese, and calcium-fortified soymilk, almond milk, and rice milk can help meet daily calcium needs. Many children are at risk for not meeting their calcium needs simply because they skip the milk and have soda instead. Children with high intakes of soda and other sugar sweetened beverages traditionally have lower intakes of calcium and vitamin D, phosphorus, potassium, protein, and fiber.[84]

Iron deficiency is not as prevalent in the middle-school and adolescent age groups as it is in earlier childhood, although roughly 4% of 6- to 11-year-old children were discovered to be iron-deficient, according to 1999–2000 NHANES data (compared to 7% of toddlers).[85] Children who adopt vegetarian lifestyles, and particularly female adolescents who have begun menstruating, are at particular risk for developing iron deficiency. Excellent sources of iron include meats, fish, and poultry, but children who do consume these foods should be encouraged to include the lean, nonfried versions of them. In addition, children can also meet their iron requirements through consumption of iron-fortified cereals and enriched and fortified whole grain foods.

Fiber needs are somewhat higher in school age and adolescent males than they are for females. Males aged 9–13 years need approximately 31 grams of dietary fiber compared to 26 grams per day for females aged 9–13 years. Males aged 14 to 18 years need 38 grams of dietary fiber compared to females who need 26 grams per day. Good sources of dietary fiber include whole grains, fruits, vegetables, and legumes. Adequate fluid intake is also important in these stages of the lifecycle, particularly among active children and adolescents. Males aged 9–13 years should aim for 2.4 liters (2400 mL or 81 fluid ounces or 10 cups of water per day) and 3.3 liters (3300 mL or 112 fluid ounces or 14 cups of water per day) for 14- to 18-year-olds. Females aged 9–13 years should be drinking 2.1 liters (2100 mL or 71 fluid ounces or 9 cups of water per day) and 14- to 18-year-olds need 2.3 liters (2300 mL or 78 fluid ounces or 10 cups of water per day). Fluid intake should come primarily from water and milk. Sports drinks are not necessary for these age groups and sodas and other sugar sweetened beverages should be limited or avoided as much as possible.

■ Childhood Obesity

Childhood obesity has more than tripled in the last 30 years. In 1980, 7% of children aged 6–11 years were obese; in 2008, this number rose to 20%. For adolescents, the percentage of obese adolescents increased from 5% in 1980 to 18% in 2008. In 2008, more than one-third of children and adolescents were overweight or obese, putting them well on track to become the two-thirds of the United States' adult population who is also overweight or obese.[65] This rapid increase in childhood obesity is not without its associated health consequences. Obese children and adolescents are at increased risk for cardiovascular disease, prediabetes, and the development of diabetes and bone and joint problems, sleep apnea, and social and psychological disorders related to poor self-esteem. These conditions, which were previously considered to be the disease of adulthood, are now affecting children at young ages.

The root cause of childhood obesity can be attributed to a caloric imbalance: essentially, excessive caloric intake coupled with insufficient energy expenditure.[86,87] The CDC maintains that while caloric imbalance is at the heart of childhood obesity, many institutions, including families, communities, schools, child care settings, medical care providers, faith-based institutions government agencies, the media, and the food and beverage and entertainment industries, all play contributing roles in the ever-expanding waistlines of our youth. The *Healthy People 2020* initiatives include a number of objectives intended to counteract increasing rates of childhood obesity, including[75]:

- Increase the proportion of primary care physicians who regularly assess body mass index (BMI) for age and sex in their child or adolescent patients
- Increase the proportion of physician visits made by all child or adult patients that include counseling about nutrition or diet
- Reduce the proportion of children and adolescents who are considered obese
- Prevent inappropriate weight gain in children and adolescents aged 2–19 years
- Eliminate very low food security among children

Approaches to combating childhood obesity are widespread and focus on improving food environments in schools, households, and communities. Additional strategies include increasing access to fresh fruits and vegetables, encouraging more physical education and activity, decreasing TV, screen-time, and other sedentary behaviors, and reducing intake of sodas, other sweetened beverages, and junk foods that provide empty calories with minimal nutrients. Table 4–40 contains a summary of the CDC recommendations for school-based health programs to promote healthy eating.[88]

▪ Food Allergies

A food allergy is the human immune system's abnormal response to a specific protein found in foods or beverages. Note that it is the *protein* component of the food that will cause the allergic reaction. Food allergies differ significantly from food intolerances (such as lactose intolerance and gluten intolerance) in that food allergies elicit allergic reactions and potentially anaphylactic reactions. Although food intolerances may cause great discomfort, intolerances do not involve the immune system and they are rarely life threatening. It is estimated that 4% of the United States population (12 million Americans) have a food allergy. Food allergy rates are rising among children, and currently, 4% of children under 18 have a food allergy. This prevalence has increased by 18% between 1997 and 2007.[89] While there are over 160 foods that

Table 4-40. CDC guidelines for school health programs to promote lifelong healthy eating.

Policy	Adopt a coordinated school nutrition policy that promotes healthy eating through classroom lessons and a supportive school environment
Curriculum for nutrition education	Implement nutrition education from preschool through secondary school as part of a sequential, comprehensive school health education curriculum designed to help students adopt healthy eating behaviors
Instructions for students	Provide nutrition education through developmentally appropriate, culturally relevant, fun, and participatory activities that involve social learning strategies
Integration of school food service and nutrition education	Coordinate school food service with nutrition education and with other components of the comprehensive school health program to reinforce messages on healthy eating
Training for school staff	Provide staff involved in nutrition education with adequate preservice and ongoing in-service training that focuses on teaching strategies for behavioral change
Family and community involvement	Involve family members and the community in supporting and reinforcing nutrition education
Program evaluation	Regularly evaluate the effectiveness of the school health program in promoting healthy eating, and change the program as appropriate to increase its effectiveness

Data from Centers for Disease Control and Prevention, 1997.

can lead to allergic reactions in humans, eight foods account for 90% of all food allergic reactions.[90] The eight major food allergens are milk, egg, wheat, soy, peanut, tree nut, fish, and crustacean shellfish (Table 4–41). By law, food manufacturers have to list these major food allergens on food packaging if the food contains these allergens or if the food was processed in an area that might have come into contact with these allergens. Currently there is no cure for food allergies; thus, treatment is the total elimination and avoidance of the food.

Did You Know?
The "Big Eight" food allergens include peanuts and tree nuts. Peanuts fall in a separate category because they are not nuts. Peanuts are legumes – related to the dried beans and lentils family.

Symptoms of anaphylactic reactions from food occur within minutes to 2 hours after ingestion and may affect the respiratory and GI

Table 4–41. Eight food allergens account for 90% of food allergies.

The "Big Eight" Food Allergens
Milk
Egg
Wheat
Soy
Peanut
Tree nut
Fish
Crustacean shellfish

systems, skin, and blood. Symptoms include difficulty swallowing, shortness of breath, nausea and vomiting, diarrhea and abdominal cramping, swelling, hives, eczema and rashes, and drops in blood pressure or loss of consciousness. Table 4–42 contains examples of how a child might describe his or her food allergy reaction. Although little is known about preventing food allergies, parents are advised to be aware of the early signs of allergic disease to foods, including eczema, hives, wheezing, repeated diarrhea, and/or vomiting from certain formulas. Rapid administration of epinephrine (adrenaline) is imperative to survival in the event of anaphylaxis, working to reverse symptoms and preventing progression of anaphylaxis. Antihistamines and steroids also aid in recovery, but should be given in addition to, but not in place of, epinephrine.

The first step in establishing a diagnosis of food allergy is usually a skin prick test or blood test (such as Immulite or ImmunoCap) to test for IgE antibodies. Skin prick tests tend to be less expensive than blood tests and can be done in-office. While positive skin prick tests or immunoassays demonstrate if IgE is present in the body, they are not sufficient to predict potential reactions if the patient were to ingest the supposed allergy-causing food.[91] Test results are then compared to results of an in-depth individual history and a possible food allergy to ultimately determine the presence of food allergy. Referral to a specialist and a Registered Dietitian trained in food allergy counseling is recommended for long-term management. It is advisable for individuals with food allergies to maintain a food diary or food-related symptom log for 2–3 weeks at the beginning of treatment. They should record the foods, drinks, condiments, and supplements consumed, along with serving sizes and symptom descriptions. Clinicians who are trained in

Table 4-42. Examples of words a child may use to describe food allergy reaction.

"This food is too spicy"
"My tongue is hot" or "my tongue is burning"
"It feels like something is poking my tongue"
"My tongue (or mouth) is tingling (or burning)"
"My tongue (or mouth) feels like there is hair on it"
"My mouth feels funny"
"There's a frog in my throat"
"There's something stuck in my throat"
"My tongue feels full" or "my tongue feels heavy"
"My lips feel tight"
"It feels like there are bugs in my ears" (to describe itchy ears)
"My throat feels thick"
"It feels like a bump is on the back of my tongue (throat)"

Reproduced from Food Allergy Research and Education, available at: http://www.foodallergy.org/symptoms. With permission.

dealing with food allergies can use these logs to help evaluate nutritional adequacy of the diet and relevant food allergies.

Food Allergy Research and Education (FARE) maintains that, "most children outgrow their food allergies to milk, egg, soy, and wheat by the time they are 10 years old, and often before five years of age." Almost 85% of children with allergies to milk or eggs will outgrow those food allergies, and almost all children with allergies to soy or wheat will outgrow allergies; however, allergies to peanuts, tree nuts, fish, and/or shellfish are generally lifelong allergies. FARE cites statistics showing that approximately 20% of children outgrow peanut allergies and 10% outgrow tree nut allergies.[91]

If food allergy is confirmed, it is important that the child's school be notified. Parents of children with food allergies should be trained to examine all nutrition labels thoroughly. *Food Allergy Research and Education (FARE, formerly the Food Allergy & Anaphylaxis Network)* is a good resource for parents, families, and friends of those with food allergies. The FARE website has a Chef card that individuals with food allergies can download and share with restaurant staff to help them understand the food allergy. The Chef card is available at: http://www.foodallergy.org/managing-food-allergies/dining-out.

■ National School Lunch and Breakfast Programs

While supportive home environments are certainly the foundations upon which healthy childhood eating behaviors are established, some families find that all bets are off when it comes to nutrition and kids leaving the house. Outside of school hours, children of working parents or family members are likely to spend time in center-based care or child-care arrangements with nonparent presence.[92] Inside of school hours, children are no doubt making numerous independent food decisions, some healthier than others. Despite a still-generally negative public outlook, the reality is that in recent years, many school districts have made great strides with nutrition and wellness policies that eliminate the sale of sodas on school grounds, enhance vending and snack cart offerings, and improve the overall nutrition quality and palatability of cafeteria meals. In addition to ancillary food offerings on and near school campuses, much of the food being served during school time comes courtesy of the USDA National School Lunch Program (NSLP).

The NSLP was established under the National School Lunch Act and was signed into law by President Harry Truman in 1946. The program currently operates in over 101,000 public and nonprofit private schools and residential childcare institutions, and in 2010, the program served more than 31 million children, roughly 10% of the entire United States population and 42% of American children under age 18 years.[83,93] Children qualify for the NSLP based on family income eligibility criteria: those at less than 130% of the poverty level are eligible for free meals, those between 130% and 185% of the poverty level are reduced price (for which they can be charged no more than $0.40 per meal), and those from families above 185% of the poverty level pay full price, although full-price meals are generally still somewhat subsidized. The National School Breakfast Program began as a pilot program in 1966 and was made permanent in 1975. In 1998, the National School Lunch Program was expanded to include and cover snacks provided in afterschool educational and enrichment programs for children through 18 years of age.

In its role as a nutrition assistance program for low-income individuals, there are nutritional requirements for meals provided through the National School Lunch and National School Breakfast Programs. School foodservice operations must meet these guidelines in order to receive federal reimbursement for meals provided. It should be noted that these requirements have evolved over the years given the changes in children's nutritional status. In the 1940s and 1950s, the NSLP focused on providing high-caloric foods to children who were at risk for malnutrition and not getting enough calories. Now, with the onset of the childhood obesity epidemic, nutritional requirements focus on lower calorie, nutrient-dense foods.

Schools also have access to and receive USDA entitlement foods of varying nutritive value from agricultural surplus. Compounding the challenges of making nutritious meals that school-aged children will actually eat alongside infusions of not-always-entirely-healthy USDA entitlement foods, school foodservice operations are faced with relatively low reimbursement rates. In 2012, for each free lunch a school provided (provided it served more than 60% free/reduced price lunch in the previous year), the school received $2.94 in reimbursement, $2.54 for reduced-price lunches, and $0.35 for paid lunches. Free breakfasts are reimbursed at $1.55 per meal, reduced-price breakfasts at $1.25, and paid breakfasts at $0.27.[94] Think of your average weekly grocery bill and divide it by the number of healthy meals you prepare each week. Would you have enough resources to make hundreds or thousands of healthy, child-friendly, fresh meals with that per-meal food cost? Despite the inherent challenges facing school foodservice operations, the USDA National School Lunch and Breakfast Programs do provide a valuable source of important nutrients that are vital for optimal growth and performance in children of all socioeconomic backgrounds. In an era of rampant childhood obesity, it is important to remember that for many low-income children, the healthiest, or perhaps the only, foods he or she will have access to in the day, may come from school-based and after-school government-funded foodservice operations and afterschool snack programs.

Nutrition for Adolescents

While developmental rates vary greatly among young individuals, adolescence is generally defined as the time of life between ages 11 years and 21 years. This period of life is characterized by marked physical growth, assertion of independence, consciousness of body image, and changes in activity levels and eating habits. Peer influence drives behavior for many adolescents and can affect decisions made about dieting, alcohol consumption, experimentation with drugs, and other health-related behavioral practices. Nutritional status often declines as adolescents transition from home-based food environments where parents dictate choices to an outside arena filled with independent food choices that often involve foods and beverage selections of minimal nutritional quality.

■ Calorie Needs During Adolescence

The calorie needs for adolescents are based upon individual activity level, basal metabolic rate, and needs required for growth and development. Caloric needs for adolescent males are significantly higher than that of their female counterparts. This discrepancy is due in part to the greater increases in height, weight, and lean body mass that males experience during puberty. The DRIs set energy recommendations for males and females in the 9–13 years of age and 14–18 years age groups and are based on assumptions of a light to moderate level of activity. Males aged 9–13 years need approximately 2279 calories and 14- to 18-year-old males require 3152 calories. Of all of the DRI age and gender groups, the highest calorie needs at any life stage are among the 14- to 18-year-old male population. For females, 9- to 13-year-olds should be consuming 2071 calories and 14- to 18-year-olds need 2368. It is important to note that there is no "one-size-fits-all" calorie number that will meet the needs of all individuals in a given age and gender group. Certain energy estimation calculations are known to overestimate intake needs when compared to actual energy expenditure.[95] Clinicians are advised to estimate energy needs for adolescents on a case-by-case basis, taking into account the individual's height, weight, energy expenditure level, BMI, or weight status (eg, overweight and obesity).

When addressing caloric intake in the adolescent population, practitioners must consider the role that soda and sweetened beverages and snack foods play. According to the *What We Eat in America*, NHANES 2005–2006 data, the percentage of adolescents snacking on any day has increased from 61% in 1977–1978 to 83% in 2005–2006. This represents a mean snacking frequency increase from 1.0 to 1.7 snacks per day in that timeframe; furthermore, adolescents consuming three or more snacks per day went from 9% in 1977–1978 to 23% in 2005–2006.[96] The researchers found that "snacking more times per day was associated with intakes of total calories" and "many of the foods that made the largest contributions to adolescents' intakes at snacks were also high in added sugars, solid fats, or both." By 2005–2006, NHANES data indicates that on average, 526 calories, nearly one-fourth of the day's total intake for adolescents, was coming from snacks. Although snacking is correlated with higher total calorie intake, it was not related to higher BMIs. However, there has been a concomitant increase in adolescent obesity rates over the time period covered in the NHANES evaluation. Today, in the United States, 17% of children and adolescents aged 2–19 years are obese, equating to roughly 12.5 million obese children and teens.[65] Because adolescents do have elevated calorie needs and may be unlikely to meet those needs at three mealtimes, snacking should be an important part of the adolescent's meal plan. It is the *content* of those snacks that nutrition educators, parents, and clinicians should address, rather than the actual snacking behavior itself. Adolescents who are engaged in physical activity and sports should be having healthy snacks before and after practice and athletic events. Healthy snack ideas for adolescents include fresh fruit, nonfat or low-fat yogurt or string cheese, whole grain crackers and pretzels, peanut butter, nuts, trail mix, and popcorn. Adolescents can also be encouraged to approach snacking from a mini-meal standpoint as opposed to an "out-of-the-bag" approach. Having a sandwich or a quesadilla before practice, an extra bowl of cereal, or a smaller portion of leftovers from dinner is a healthier approach than reaching for high-fat and high-salt chips, cookies, and other less nutritive foods.

Data from the NHANES 2005–2008 shows that teenagers and young adults drink more sugary beverages than any other age group.[97] Seventy percent of males and 60% of females aged 2–19 years drink sugary beverages on any given day. Twenty five percent of the population consumes at least 200 calories of sugary beverages per day, equivalent to more than one 12-ounce can of soda. Soda and sweetened beverages provide almost no nutrition other than excessive calories that increase the risk of overweight and obesity. Sodas and sweetened beverages displace other healthy drinks and nutrients from the diet, mainly in the form of milk (including its bygone calcium contributions). Of additional concern is the fact that high intake of carbonated soft drinks has been shown to have an inverse association with bone mineral density in girls.[98] At the very stage in life when calcium intake should be at its highest, sodas and sweetened beverages are robbing the body of important nutrients needed for optimal bone mineral density development. Adolescents should be encouraged to drink water as the primary source of fluid in the diet. Electrolyte replacement sports beverages are indicated only for adolescents exercising vigorously for more than 60 minutes, or in extreme temperature conditions.[99]

■ Protein, Carbohydrate, and Fat Needs During Adolescence

Protein needs during adolescence are based on the DRI recommendations of 0.95 grams of protein per kilogram body weight in 9- to 13-year-old males and females, and 0.85 grams of protein per kilogram body weight in 14- to 18-year-old males and females. Another DRI for protein is presented in terms of grams of protein per day: a 9- to 13-year-old boy or girl needs roughly 34 grams of protein per day, a 14- to 18-year-old male needs 52 grams of protein, and a 14- to 18-year-old female requires 46 grams per day. Adolescents, and in particular, male adolescents, may take an interest in protein needs during their various growth spurts. Protein does play an important role in the development and growth of the human body; however, individuals often overestimate the role of protein, and clinicians are advised to educate adolescents that excessive protein consumption does not lead to increased muscle mass. It is only by repetitive exercise and muscle stimulation that muscle mass can increase. Protein does play a role in muscle recovery, and a snack containing a moderate amount of protein is appropriate following a period of vigorous exercise or weight training.[99] Adolescents should be careful to avoid excessive protein intake as it may contribute unnecessary calories and contribute to unwanted weight gain in some individuals. In general, 10–30% of total calories should come from protein.

Practitioners and parents can encourage adolescents to know their daily protein needs and to read labels to educate themselves about the protein content of various foods. Adolescents, much like adults, are often surprised to see how easy it is to meet daily protein needs with a well-balanced diet. For example, one whole chicken breast contains approximately 50 grams of protein, enough protein for an entire day for a typical adolescent. Care should be taken to promote lean sources of dietary protein, including lean meats, egg whites, nuts, seeds, legumes, and nonfat and low-fat dairy products.

Adolescents, and in particular, female adolescents, may experiment with vegetarianism in their teenage years. The term vegetarian is quite broad and can encompass a variety of eating patterns, although the majority of them are focused on the elimination of at least one type of animal product or animal flesh. While it is certainly possible to have a well-balanced vegetarian diet, care must be taken to assure that the vegetarian lifestyle is not overly restrictive or deficient in important nutrients. If an adolescent has adopted a vegetarian lifestyle for weight-loss purposes, the clinician should carefully assess the individual for a potential underlying eating disorder. Some adolescents will adopt vegetarianism in the earliest stages of eating disorder development as a means to restrict calories and justify the elimination of foods from their diet.

As with other stages of life, the majority of calories in an adolescent's diet should come from carbohydrate. Good sources of carbohydrate include whole grains, fruits, vegetables, milk and yogurt, and legumes. The DRI for carbohydrate is 45–65% of total calories, and the minimum carbohydrate intake for individuals is 130 grams per day. This increases to 175 grams per day for pregnant adolescents and 210 grams for those who may be lactating. Fat intake should be no more than 25–35% of calories and saturated fat should constitute no more than 10% of calories. There are specific recommendations for linoleic and alpha-linolenic acid to support ideal growth and development in adolescents, and those are included in Table 4–43 and the DRI tables are included as Appendix A.

▪ Vitamin, Mineral, Fiber, and Fluid Needs During Adolescence

The particular micronutrients of concern in adolescents are calcium, vitamin D, and iron. Calcium and vitamin D are important for optimal bone development. During adolescence, the human body is actively laying down bone. It is at this life stage that calcium needs are at their highest. All males and females aged 9–18 years should be consuming 1300 mg calcium per day and 15 micrograms (600 IUs) of vitamin D (Institute of Medicine, 2010).[22] Actual vitamin D intake is more difficult to estimate than is calcium because of the role that sunlight exposure plays in vitamin D activation. For calcium, in order to meet the 1300 mg per day recommendation, this equates to roughly four servings of milk or dairy or milk substitutes. Each cup of milk is fortified with 100 IU of vitamin D. If a diet history reveals that the adolescent is not consuming 1300 mg calcium from milk or dairy foods, a simple calcium with vitamin D supplement will help cover nutrient intake gaps. In 2008, the American Academy of Pediatrics revised their vitamin D recommendations, and now say that all infants and children, including adolescents, should have a minimum daily intake of 400 IU of vitamin D beginning soon after birth. This replaces previous recommendations of minimum intake of 200 IU per day beginning in the first 2 months following birth and continuing until adolescence.

Iron needs are increased during adolescence due to the rapid rate of growth, increasing volume of blood that accompanies that growth, and the onset of menarche in female adolescents. Inadequate iron intake

Table 4-43. Dietary reference intakes (DRIs) for adolescents.

	Estimated Energy Requirements (kcal/day)	Carbohydrate (g)	% kcal from Carbohydrate	Fiber (g)	% kcal from Fat	Linoleic Acid (g)	Alpha-linolenic Acid (g)	Protein	% kcal from Protein	Fluid (L)
Males										
9-13 years	2279	130	45-65	31	25-35	21	1.2	34	10-30	2.4
14-18 years	3152	130	45-65	38	25-35	16	1.6	52	10-30	3.3
Females										
9-13 years	2071	130	45-65	26	25-35	10	1.0	34	10-30	2.1
14-18 years	2368	130	45-65	26	25-35	11	1.1	46	10-30	2.3

Data from Institute of Medicine, 2006.

has been linked to poor cognitive development and suboptimal school and work performance. Iron deficiency among adolescents is estimated to be at 9% of 12- to 15-year-old females, 5% of 12- to 16-year-old males, 11% of 15- to 19-year-old females, and 2% of 15- to 19-year-old males.[85] Iron deficiency rates are higher than are iron deficiency anemia rates among adolescents. Less than 1% of males, and less than 2% of females have iron deficiency anemia. The lower rates of iron deficiency among males compared to females can be attributed to their increased likelihood of consuming more iron-rich foods such as meat, fish and poultry, coupled with the onset of menarche that increases iron losses in females.

Iron needs for 9- to 13-year-old males are 8 mg per day and 11 mg per day for 14- to 18-year olds. Females aged 9–13 years need 8 mg of iron and that increases to 15 mg per day for 14- to 18-year-old females. In addition to meat, fish, and poultry, iron-fortified cereals, and enriched and fortified grain supplies are good sources of iron. Dark green leafy vegetables and other vegetables contain lower amounts of iron, in the less absorbable nonheme form. The form of iron found in animal products, called heme iron, is better absorbed. Special attention should be paid to the iron intake levels of vegetarian adolescents, and in particular, female vegetarian adolescents. Vitamin C helps enhance iron absorption; thus, iron deficient adolescents should be encouraged to eat vitamin C-containing foods alongside iron-containing foods, or to take vitamin C supplements in conjunction with iron supplementation.

Adequate dietary fiber intake is important at all stages of life, as it helps to promote regular bowel function, and plays a role in reducing risk for the development of certain types of chronic diseases, such as heart disease, diabetes, and certain types of cancer. Current household level data indicate that adolescent fiber intake in the United States, similar to that of adult fiber intake, falls far short of recommended levels. Currently, adolescent males consume just 14.2 grams of fiber per day, and females eat only 12.3 grams per day.[20] The DRI for fiber for adolescents is 31 grams per day for males aged 9–13 years, and 38 grams per day for 14- to 18-year-old males. All female adolescents aged 9–18 years need a minimum of 26 grams of fiber per day. Snack and junk foods that adolescents gravitate toward are typically low in fiber. These include foods such as potato and tortilla chips, beef jerky, cookies, cakes, and sugary beverages that do not contain the dietary fiber that fruits, vegetables, whole grains, and legumes do. Encouraging more whole grain intake, experimentation with legumes, and utilization of fruits and vegetables both at meals and between meals can help increase an adolescent's daily fiber intake toward the recommended levels.

Fluid intake recommendations for adolescents vary with activity level. While there is no hard-and-fast data about how much fluid an adolescent needs, the AI recommendation states that males aged

9–13 years need 2.4 liters per day, and those aged 14–18 years need 3.3 liters. Females aged 9–13 years should have 2.1 liters per day, and those aged 14–18 years should have 2.3 liters per day. Those with higher rates of physical activity, certain disease states, and medication therapies may have different fluid needs. Adolescents should be encouraged to drink water throughout the day in order to prevent thirst. The feeling of thirst is an indication that the body is already dehydrated. Teaching adolescents to drink water such that they never experience thirst is a useful practice that can be utilized throughout life. Advise adolescents to keep an eye on the color of their urine, which is the best indicator of hydration status. Clear or light, pale yellow urine indicates a well-hydrated state, whereas dark orange or yellow urine indicates dehydration. Teens are often surprised to learn that their urine should not smell. Pungent smelling urine indicates a concentrated waste product and a need for more water to dilute that waste product. Table 4–43 contains a summary of the macronutrient, micronutrient, fiber, and water needs for adolescents.[19]

■ Eating Disorders

Eating disorders and disordered eating behaviors are certainly not limited to the adolescent population; however, it is often in adolescence when individuals, and in particular, females, may first begin experimenting with dieting and food restriction that may lead to an eating disorder. While children of parents with an eating disorder are much more likely to develop eating disorders themselves,[100] even individuals from families with healthy food environments may fall victim to these devastating psychological disorders. There is not one distinct cause of eating disorders, but the focus on thinness from the mass media, peer influences, pressure from coaches and parents, and toxic relationships can all trigger eating disorders. And just as there is not one cause of eating disorders, there is not one discipline that is adequately equipped to treat eating disorders. Successful eating disorder treatment mandates a team-based approach, utilizing highly trained primary care practitioners, registered dietitians, counselors, social workers, and other healthcare practitioners. Advanced practice nurses play a role in screening for disordered eating, but when treatment is indicated, referral to a specialized treatment program is indicated. Chapter 3 contains more information about the diagnostic criteria for various eating disorders.

Just as the treatment of eating disorders involves a multi-disciplinary approach, all avenues of healthcare providers can play a role in helping to prevent eating disorders in adolescents. Avoid being overly critical of weight gain, discourage dangerous and trendy fad diets, promote healthy snack and meal ideas, and encourage physical activity as a means to prevent unnecessary weight gain. Nutrition messaging and programs targeting adolescents should focus on positive body image and the importance of adequate nutrition to achieve maximal potential and optimal growth and development.

Nutrition for Older Adults

"And in the end, it's not the years in your life that count. It's the life in your years." - Abraham Lincoln

How does one age gracefully? This is a question we all ponder as time predictably ticks on. The process of aging is an inevitable part of human life, yet it affects different people in different ways. Some individuals enter the latter years of life full of vim and vigor, while others limp through their final years burdened by chronic disease and pain. Life expectancy in the United States is now at 78.5 years.[67] Nutrition certainly plays a role in the development and prevention of chronic diseases as four of the top 10 leading causes of death for individuals over age 60, cardiovascular disease, cancer, stroke, and diabetes, have nutrition-related risk factors.[101] To state it another way: dietary decisions that one does or does not make over the course of his or her life can significantly impact mortality risk.

- ■ Physiological Changes and Nutrition Impact

The process of aging results in physiological changes that directly impact nutrient and energy needs. Most notable among these changes is the loss of lean body mass, which typically results in a 15% decline in fat-free mass. From ages 30–70 years, lean body mass decreases by 2–3% each decade (Figure 4–2). The aging body also loses muscle, a phenomenon known as sarcopenia, beginning around age 40 years, even in the absence of weight fluctuations.[102,103] As lean body mass and muscle decrease, body fat percentage climbs. By the time males reach their seventies, they have, on average, experienced approximately a 24 pound loss of muscle, going from 53 pounds of muscle to 29 pounds.

20-year-old woman's thigh   64-year-old woman's thigh

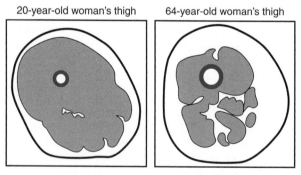

Figure 4–2. Cross section of thighs from a 20-year-old woman and a 64-year-old woman. The younger woman's thigh contains a greater percentage of lean muscle, whereas the older woman's thigh, despite being similar in circumference, contains a greater proportion of fat.

That muscle is gradually replaced by fat. Beyond age 70 years, total weight, including fat mass, starts to drop.[104] The reduction in lean body mass, muscle, and eventually overall weight equates to a decline in energy, fluid, vitamin, and mineral needs.

In addition to declining basal metabolic rates and energy needs, other physiological changes associated with aging impact nutritional status. Immune function declines with age, as does the ability to smell and taste foods. The part of the brain that controls hunger and thirst, the hypothalamus, becomes less active with aging, and leads to an increased risk for dehydration (due to the absence of the thirst mechanism). Changes in the stomach that are associated with aging may lead to delayed gastric emptying. Reduced production of hydrochloric acid leads to lower levels of intrinsic factor, a compound needed for optimal vitamin B_{12} absorption. The pancreas secretes fewer enzymes, which affect digestion and glycemic control. There is an increase in gallstone prevalence, while, at the same time, liver function, liver size, portal blood flow, and vitamin D synthesis in the liver are all on the decline. Reduced mucosal surface area in the small intestine, coupled with reduced digestive enzymatic activity, leads to lowered rates of calcium, zinc, and other micronutrient absorption.

■ Calorie Needs for Older Adults

Adults need fewer calories per day as they age. Of all of the age and gender life stage groups represented in the DRI recommendations, women over age 70 years have the lowest energy needs. The DRIs for "active physical activity level (PAL)" for all adults over age 18 years is 3067 calories per day for males and 2403 calories per day for females.[19] Of course, the needs of an 18-year-old male and a 70-year-old male are dramatically different. The estimated decrease in caloric needs from early to late adulthood is approximately 7–10 calories per year starting at age 19 years, equating to roughly 70–100 calories per decade.[104] Table 4–44 shows how to calculate estimated energy needs using this adjustment factor.

There are a number of other ways to estimate energy needs at the various stages of life. A quick rule of thumb is to apply the kcals/kg approach used in younger adulthood. Give 20–25 kcals/kg/day for weight loss, 25–30 kcals/kg/day for weight maintenance, and 30–35 kcals/kg/day for weight gain. These estimations may need to be adjusted for very overweight or obese, or underweight individuals.

■ Carbohydrate, Protein, and Fat Needs for Older Adults

As with young and middle-aged adults, older adults require at least 130 grams carbohydrates per day, and carbohydrates should still represent 45–65% of their daily energy intake. The protein RDA for older adults is 0.8 g/kg/day, although other research demonstrates a desired protein intake range for elderly of 1.0–1.25 g/kg/day.[105] Protein deficiency is rare in the general American adult population, as well as the

Table 4–44. Estimating adjusted calorie needs for aging past age 19.

Adjusted Male Calorie Needs for Aging	Adjusted Female Calorie Needs for Aging
Sample age: 65 years old	Sample age: 80 years old
19+ male calorie needs: 3067 calories	19+ female calorie needs: 2403
65 years – 19 years = 46 years	80 years – 19 years = 61 years
Subtract 10 cal/day	Subtract 7 cal/day
46 years × 10 cal/day = 460 cal subtracted	61 years × 7 cal/day = 427 cal subtracted
3067 – 460 = 2607 calories per day needed	2403 – 427 = 1976 calories per day needed

older adult groups. Protein needs are higher for individuals with skin breakdown and delayed wound healing, muscle wasting conditions, and compromised immunity. Protein should constitute 10–35% of energy intake for healthy individuals. Fat recommendations in older age are no different than they are in the earlier parts of adulthood. Fat should represent no more than 35% of calories and the focus should be on reducing saturated and *trans* fats in proportion to mono and polyunsaturated fatty acid intake.

- Vitamin, Mineral, Fiber, and Fluid Needs for Older Adults

Although certain elderly populations are at risk for deficiency of a host of micronutrients, the primary vitamins and minerals of concern in the older adult are sodium, calcium, vitamin B_{12}, and vitamin D. The *Dietary Guidelines for Americans, 2010* recommend that all individuals aged 51 years and older, plus African Americans and those with hypertension or any chronic disease, limit their sodium intake to 1500 mg or less per day.[106] This may be a difficult recommendation for an elderly person who relies heavily on packaged, processed, and frozen foods that are laden with salt. Encouraging more fresh fruits and vegetables, whole grains, and minimally processed foods can help meet these rather stringent sodium recommendations.

Calcium and vitamin D intake tend to decline with the reduced food intake that is usually associated with aging. Lower intakes of dairy foods, coupled with reduced effectiveness of converting vitamin D from sunlight, lead to increased needs of calcium and vitamin D in older adulthood. The DRI for calcium for adults all females aged 51 years and above is 1200 mg per day. For males, calcium needs are 1000 mg for 51- to 70-year-olds and 1200 mg for those older than 70 years. Vitamin D DRIs increase to 15 micrograms (600 IU) for males and females age 51–70 years and 20 micrograms (800 IU) for those older than 70 years.[22]

Vitamin B_{12} is also problematic for some older adults due to both declining intakes of animal foods (the only appreciable sources of vitamin B_{12}), and a reduced capacity to absorb vitamin B_{12} because of reduced absorption and lowered intrinsic factor production associated with declining hydrochloric acid production in the stomach. Vitamin B_{12} DRIs are set at 2.4 micrograms per day for all nonpregnant, nonlactating people aged 14 years and older. The DRIs state that, "Because 10 to 30% of older people may malabsorb food-bound B_{12}, it is advisable for those older than 50 years to meet their RDA mainly by consuming foods fortified with B_{12} or a supplement containing B_{12}."[19]

The recommended intake for total water for males and females aged 51 years and older is 3.7 liters (3700 mL or approximately 16 cups) and 2.7 liters (2700 mL or approximately 11 cups), respectively.[19] As previously mentioned, older adults are at increased risk for dehydration due to declining thirst sensations. As they age, individuals should be encouraged to drink water between meals to help conserve stomach space for food at mealtime. For older adults who are concerned with excessive nocturnal urination, encourage them to drink the majority of the water they need each day before lunch, to ensure adequate time for evacuation and reduce anxiety about going to the bathroom at night. Practitioners and family members should be reminded that the signs and symptoms of early dehydration such as confusion and forgetfulness mirror those of dementia and Alzheimer's disease. It may be difficult to assess whether the behavior exhibited is a result of advancing dementia or Alzheimer's disease, or may simply be related to dehydration.

Dietary fiber DRI recommendations are based on grams of fiber per calories consumed. The decline in calorie needs associated with aging also leads to lower fiber intake levels. Males aged 51 years and older should aim for 30 grams of fiber per day and females aged 51 years and older need 21 grams of fiber per day.[19] For older adults in whom inadequate calorie intake is a concern, high-fiber foods are often *not* indicated as they promote satiety and may reduce overall food intake. Spreading fiber intake out over the day, and encouraging fiber from foods such as whole grains, vegetables, fruits, and legumes (instead of fiber supplements), along with adequate water intake can promote regular motility in all adults.

■ Supplementation for Older Adults

When considering the use of vitamin and mineral supplements in older adulthood, practitioners are advised generally to counsel clients and patients to try to get all of the vitamins and minerals they need from foods, not supplements. This recommendation holds true up until a certain age. Many older adults may simply not be consuming enough food to adequately provide 100% of their DRI for all of their micronutrient needs. In many older adults, dietary supplements may be useful tools to help fill these nutrient intake gaps. A simple geriatric (or "Silver") multivitamin with minerals is a cheap and effective way to supplement daily food intake and to assure adequate micronutrient intake. Other individual supplements that may be indicated include calcium and vitamin D, iron, vitamin B_{12}, and additional mineral and vitamin preparations as recommended by the healthcare provider. Care should be taken to inform older adults that "too much of a good thing is not a good thing." Some dietary supplements can build up to toxic levels in the body and many are contraindicated with prescription medications that the individual may be taking. Practitioners are advised to ask all people, regardless of age, to bring in the actual bottles of the supplements they are taking, and to cross-reference with their prescription medication list, searching for possible contraindications. Chapter 12 contains more information about dietary supplements and supplement-drug interactions.

Because the list of potentially used dietary supplements, their indications, recommended dosages, potential usefulness, or ability to cause harm is impossible to remember, practitioners should have access to appropriate references with which to refer their patients and clients. The National Institutes of Health Office of Dietary Supplements website at www.ods.od.nih.gov is a good place to start. Another useful reference is the electronic or print copy of The Academy of Nutrition and Dietetics' publication *The Health Professional's Guide to Popular Dietary Supplements*. While there are no doubt benefits to using dietary supplements for certain documented inadequate intake or deficiencies in certain populations, there are unscrupulous supplement manufacturing companies that market directly to, and prey on, senior citizens. These companies' impressive marketing approaches range from promising to prevent cancer, insomnia, heart disease progression, and even to prolong life. This dishonest approach to selling dietary supplements is particularly harmful for senior citizens on a fixed income. When faced with limited financial resources, older adults are often forced to make decisions on whether or not to purchase healthy foods, or to fulfill medication prescriptions. Those with limited disposable income should not have their financial situation compounded by additional anxiety over whether or not to purchase what are generally worthless *lotions and potions*. Healthcare providers can help by making sound, evidence-based recommendations for the few supplements that may be indicated, and by advising their patients and clients to bypass the rest of the dietary supplement hype.

▪ Exercise and Aging

Exercise is an important component of a healthy lifestyle at all stages of life. Emerging research indicates that exercise and physical activity can be particularly effective in preventing and treating older adults with chronic disease and disabilities. In addition to helping prevent overweight and obesity in the later years of life, regular strength training and balance exercises help reduce the likelihood of falls and associated fractures in the elderly.[107] Many older people may get their recommended exercise in cardiac rehab or other rehab programs or through low-impact activities such as chair-dancing or water aerobics.

ACSM and the American Heart Association (AHA) have developed recommendations for exercise and physical activity for older adults that closely mirror the *2008 Physical Activity Guidelines for Americans*.[102] The ACSM/AHA recommendations are that all adults aim for 150 minutes per week of physical activity for health benefits. For those older adults who cannot achieve 150 minutes of moderate intensity aerobic activity per week due to chronic conditions, they should be as physically active as their abilities and conditions allow. Endurance exercise for older adults is recommended for at least 30 minutes or up to 60 minutes per day. Resistance exercises are advised on at least 2 days per week and frequency exercises also on at least 2 days per week. There are additional guidelines for balance exercises, and free access to the full ACSM/AHA guidelines are available online at: http://journals.lww.com/acsm-msse/Fulltext/2009/07000/Exercise_and_Physical_Activity_for_Older_Adults.20.aspx.

▪ Assessing Nutrition Risk in the Older Adult

In addition to the simple accumulation of years of life, there are other external factors that increase nutrition risk in older adults. The Academy of Nutrition and Dietetics position paper *Nutrition Across the Spectrum of Aging* lists the following risk factors for poor nutrition in older adults: hunger, poverty, inadequate food and nutrient intake, functional disability, social isolation, independent living, depression, dementia, dependency, poor oral health and dentition, chewing and swallowing problems, use of multiple medications, and advanced age.[108] There are a number of validated nutrition risk assessment tools for use in the elderly population that are readily available to practitioners. These include the DETERMINE: Warning signs of poor nutrition health and the Mini Nutritional Assessment (MNA). Chapter 2 contains information on both of these risk assessment tools for malnutrition in the elderly.

In addition to risk assessment tools, there are nutrition education tools that have been developed for the elderly population. Tufts University has developed a "*MyPlate for Older Adults*" that provides food, fluid, and physical activity guidance in conjunction with the *Dietary Guidelines for Americans, 2010*. The University of Florida IFAS Extension has also developed an adaptation of the *MyPlate* nutrition tools that are geared toward older adults (Figure 4–3).

▪ Nutrition Assistance Programs

Due to limited incomes, older adults may qualify for and receive benefits from a variety of nutrition assistance programs. These programs include the USDA's Supplemental Nutrition Assistance Program (SNAP, formerly called Food Stamps), Seniors' Farmers Market

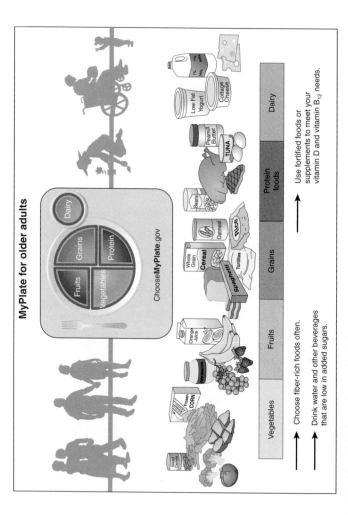

Figure 4–3. MyPlate for Older Adults by Linda B. Bobroff. (Reproduced with permission from MyPlate for Older Americans.) Copyright 2011 Tufts University. For details about the MyPlate for Older Adults, please see http://nutrition.tufts.edu/research/myplate-older-adults

Nutrition Programs, the Commodity Supplemental Foods, the Child and Adult Care Food Program, the Ryan White Comprehensive AIDS Resources Emergency Act, and other programs such as community congregate senior dining programs and Meals on Wheels. The Administration on Aging (AOA) also administers the Elderly Nutrition Program (ENP) that provides grants to support nutrition services to older people throughout the United States. The ENP works to improve the dietary intake of participants and to offer them opportunities to form new friendships and create informal support networks. The ENP provides for congregate and home-delivered meals that can be delivered at senior centers, churches and faith-based settings, schools, or at home. There are nutrition guidelines for the meals that receive federal reimbursement, essentially assuring that each meal provides one-third of the RDA for older Americans for a number of macro- and micronutrients.

References

1. American Dietetic Association; American Society of Nutrition. Position of the American Dietetic Association and American Society for Nutrition: obesity, reproduction, and pregnancy outcomes. J Am Diet Assoc 2009; 109:918–927.
2. American Dietetic Association. Position of the American Dietetic Association: nutrition and lifestyle for a healthy pregnancy outcome. J Am Diet Assoc 2008;108:553–561.
3. The American Congress of Obstetricians and Gynecologists. Nutrition during pregnancy from frequently asked questions: pregnancy. 2011
4. Waller D, Shaw G, Rasmussen S, Hobbs C, Canfield M, Siega-Riz A, et al. Prepregnancy obesity as a risk factor for structural birth defects. Arch Pediatr Adolesc Med 2007;161:745–750.
5. Rasmussen K, Hilson J, Kjolhede C. Obesity may impair lactogenesis II. J Nutr 2001;131:3009S–3011S.
6. Rich-Edwards J, Goldman M, Willett W, Hunter D, Stampfer M, Colitz G, et al. Adolescent body mass index and infertility caused by ovulatory disorder. Am J Obstet Gynecol 1994;171:171–177.
7. Clark A, Thornley B, Tomlinson L, Galletley C, Norman R. Weight loss in obese infertile women results in improvements in reproductive outcome for all forms of fertility treatment. Hum Reprod 1998;13:1502–1505.
8. Bolumar F, Olsen J, Rebagliao M, Saez-Lloret I, Bisanti L. Body mass index and delayed conception: a European multicenter study on infertility and subfecundity. Am J Epidemiol 2000;151:1072–1079.
9. Sarwer D, Allison K, Gibbons L, Markowitz J, Nelson D. Pregnancy and obesity: a review and agenda for future research. J Womens Health 2006;15:720–733.
10. Merhi Z. Weight loss by bariatric surgery and subsequent fertility. Fertility and Sterilization 2007;87:430–432.

11. Academy of Nutrition and Dietetics. Reproduction. October 15, 2012. Retrieved from: Nutrition Care Manual January 31, 2013. http://www.nutritioncaremanual.org

12. Institute of Medicine and National Research Council (US) Committee to Reexamine IOM Pregnancy Weight Guidelines. Weight Gain During Pregnancy: Reexamining the Guidelines. Washington, DC: National Academies Press; 2009.

13. Erick M. Nutrition during pregnancy and lactation. In: Mahan LK, Escott-Stump S. Krause's Food & Nutrition Therapy. St. Louis, MO: Saunders Elsevier; 2008.

14. Olson C. A call for intervention in pregnancy to prevent maternal and child obesity. Am J Prev Med 2007;61:884–891.

15. Keppel K, Taffel S. Pregnancy-related weight gain and retention: implications of the 1990 Institute of Medicine guidelines. Am J Public Health 1993;83:1100–1103.

16. Olson C, Strawderman M, Hinton P, Pearston T. Gestational weight gain and post-partum behaviors associated with weight change from early pregnancy to 1 y postpartum. Int J Obes (Lond) 2003;27:117–127.

17. Phelan S. Pregnancy: a "teachable moment" for weight control and obesity prevention. Am J Obstet Gynecol 2010;202(2):135.

18. Food and Nutrition Board, Institute of Medicine. Dietary Reference Intakes for Energy, Carbohydrate, Fiber, Fat, Fatty Acids, Cholesterol, Protein and Amino Acids (Macronutrients). Washington, DC: National Academy Press; 2005.

19. Institute of Medicine. Dietary Reference Intakes: The Essential Guide to Nutrient Requirement. Washington, DC: The National Academies Press; 2006.

20. US Department of Agriculture, Argicultural Research Service. What We Eat in America. September 29, 2010. Retrieved from: Dietary Intake Data Files March 31, 2012. http://www.ars.usda.gov/Services/docs.htm?docid=13793

21. Honein M, Paulozzi L, Mathews T, Erickson J, Wong L. Impact of folic acid fortification of the US food supply on the occurrence of neural tube defects. JAMA 2001;285(23):2981–2986.

22. Institute of Medicine. Dietary Reference Intakes for Calcium and Vitamin D. Washington, DC: National Academies Press; 2010.

23. Hytten F. Blood volume changes in normal pregnancy. Clin Haematol 1985;14(3):601–612.

24. Scholl T, Hediger M, Fischer R, Shearer J. Anemia vs iron deficiency: increased risk of preterm delivery in a prospective study. Am J Clin Nutr 1992;55(5):985–988.

25. Gill S, Nguyen P, Koren G. Adherence and tolerability of iron-containing prenatal multivitamins in pregnant women with pre-existing gastrointestinal conditions. J Obstet Gynaecol 2009;29(7):594–598.

26. Koren G, Pairaideau N. Compliance with prenatal vitamins. Canadian Family Physician 2006;52(11):1392–1393.

27. US Department of Agriculture. ChooseMyPlate.gov. 2012. Retrieved March 26, 2012, from Health and Nutrition Information for Preschoolers: http://www.choosemyplate.gov/preschoolers

28. US Food and Drug Administration. What You Need to Know About Mercury in Fish and Shellfish. Washington, DC: EPA; 2004.

29. Foodsafety.gov. (n.d.). Foodsafety.gov. Retrieved November 16, 2011, from Checklist of Foods to Avoid During Pregnancy: http://www.foodsafety.gov/poisoning/risk/pregnant/chklist_pregnancy.html

30. US National Library of Medicine. (2010, November 21). PubMed Health. Retrieved November 16, 2011, from Intrauterine growth restriction (IUGR): http://www.ncbi.nlm.nih.gov/pubmedhealth/PMH0002469/

31. US Department of Agriculture, Food Safety and Inspection Service. (2012, October 26). Safe Minimum Internal Temperature Chart. Retrieved January 31, 2013, from Safe Food Handling:http://www.fsis.usda.gov/FACTSheets/Safe_Minimum_Internal_Temperature_Chart/index.asp

32. US Department of Agriculture, Food Safety and Inspection Service. (2011, January 12). Protect Your Baby and Yourself From Listeriosis. Retrieved December 3, 2011, from USDA FSIS Fact Sheets: http://www.fsis.usda.gov/factsheets/Protect_Your_Baby/index.asp

33. Centers for Disease Control and Prevention. (2010, November 2). Toxoplasmosis (Toxoplasma infection). Retrieved December 3, 2011, from Epidemiology and Risk Factors: http://www.cdc.gov/parasites/toxoplasmosis/epi.html

34. Kulpa P, White B, Visscher R. Aerobic exercise in pregnancy. Am J Obstet Gynecol 1989;156:1395–1403.

35. Artal R, Clapp J, Vigil D. (n.d.). ACSM Current Comment: Exercise During Pregnancy. From American College of Sports Medicine: www.acsm.org/docs/current-comments/exerciseduringpregnancy.pdf

36. American College of Obstetricians and Gynecologists, Committee on Obstetric Practice. ACOG commitee opinion. Exercise during pregnancy and the postpartum period. Int J Gynaecol Obstet 2002;77(1):79–81.

37. Jewell D, Young D. Interventions for nausea and vomiting in early pregnancy. Cochrane Database Syst Rev 2003;4:CD000145.

38. Furneaux E, Langey-Evans A, Phil M, Langley-Evans S. Nausea and vomiting of pregnancy: endocrine basis and contribution to pregnancy outcomes. Obstetrical and Gynecological Survey 2001;56:775–782.

39. American College of Obstetricians and Gynecologists. ACOG bulletin: nausea and vomiting of pregnancy. Obstet Gynecol 2004;103:803–814.

40. Fragakis A, Thomson C. The Health Professional's Guide to Popular Dietary Supplements. 3rd ed. Chicago, IL: American Dietetic Association; 2007.

41. Moore D, Sears D. Pica, iron deficiency, and the medical history. Am J Med 1994;97(4):390–393.

42. Worthington-Roberts B. Lifestyle concerns during pregnancy. In: Worthington-Roberts B, Williams S. Nutrition in Pregnancy and Lactation. Dubuque, IA: Brown & Benchmark Publishers; 1997:193–219.

43. Barbieri R, Repke J. Medical disorders during pregnancy. In: Longo D, Fauci A, Kasper D, Hauser S, Jameson J, Loscalzo J. Harrison's Principles of Internal Medicine. 18th ed. 2012. [Chapter 7].

44. American Diabetes Association. Standards of medical care in diabetes - 2013. Diabetes Care 2013;(36 suppl 1):S11–S66.

45. Group HS, Metzger B, Lowe L, Dyer A, Trimble E, Chaovarindr U, et al. Hyperglycemia and adverse pregnancy outcomes. N Engl J Med 2008;358:1991–2002.

46. American Dietetic Association. Position of the American Dietetic Association: promoting and supporting breastfeeding. J Am Diet Assoc 2009;109(11):1926–1942.

47. US Department of Health and Human Services. (2011, November 1). HealthyPeople.gov. Retrieved December 15, 2011, from Healthy People 2020: Maternal, Infant and Child Health Objectives: http://healthypeople.gov/2020/topicsobjectives2020/objectiveslist.aspx?topicid=26

48. Butte N, Garza C, Johnson C, Smith E, Nichols B. Longitudinal changes in milk composition of mothers delivering preterm and term infants. Early Hum Dev 1984;9(2):153–162.

49. Murtaugh MA, Lechtenberg E, Sharbaugh C, Sofka D. Nutrition during lactation. In: Brown J E. Nutrition Throughout the Lifecycle. Cengage Learning; 2011:160–189.

50. American Academy of Pediatrics. Prevention of rickets and vitamin D deficiency in infants, children, and adolescents. Pediatrics 2008;122(5):1142–1152.

51. Kleinman R. Pediatric Nutrition Handbook. 6th ed. Elk Grove Village, IL: American Academy of Pediatrics; 2008.

52. US Department of Health and Human Services: Centers for Disease Control and Prevention. (2001). Recommendations for Using Fluoride to Prevent and Control Dental Caries in the United States. MMWR: Morbidity and Mortality Weekly Report, 50 (RR-14).

53. Institute of Medicine. Nutrition During Lactation. Washington, DC: National Academy Press; 1991.

54. Food and Nutrition Board, Institute of Medicine. Dietary Reference Intakes of Water, Potassium, Sodium, Chloride and Sulfate. Washington, DC: National Academy Press; 2004.

55. Lust K, Brown J, Thomas W. Maternal intake of cruciferous vegetables and other foods and colic symptoms in exclusively breast-fed infant. J Am Diet Assoc 1996;96(1):46–48.

56. Hill D, Hudson I, Sheffield L, Shetlon M, Menahem S, Hosking C. A low-allergen diet is a significant intervention in infantile colic: results of a community-based study. J Allergy Clin Immunol 1995;96(6, Pt. 1):886–892.

57. Mennella J. Alcohol's effect on lactation. Alcohols research and health: The Journal of the National Institute on Alcohol Abuse and Alcoholism 2001;25(3):230–234.

58. Academy of Nutrition and Dietetics. (2008). Dietary factors and milk supply. Retrieved January 12, 2013, from Evidence Analysis Library: http://andevidencelibrary.com

59. Brodribb W, Fallon A, Hegney D, O'Brien M. Identifying predictors of the reasons women give for choosing to breastfeed. J Hum Lact 2007;23(4):338–344.

60. McCann M, Baydar N, Williams R. Breastfeeding attitudes and reported problems in a national sample of WIC participants. J Hum Lact 2007;23(4):314–324.

61. American Academy of Pediatrics. Breastfeeding and the use of human milk. Pediatrics 2005;115(2):496–506.

62. Baby-Friendly USA, Inc. Guidelines and Evaluation Criteria for Facilities Seeking Baby-Friendly Designation. Sandwich, MA: Baby-Friendly USA, Inc.; 2010.

63. Centers for Disease Control and Prevention. (2008). Breastfeeding-related maternity practices at hospitals and birth centers - United States, 2007. MMWR Morbidity and Mortality Weekly Report, 57, pp. 621–625.

64. Castrucci B, Hoover K, Lim S, Maus K. A comparison of breastfeeding rates in an urban birth cohort among women delivering infants at hospitals that employ and do not employ lactation consultants. J Public Health Manag Pract 2006;12:578–585.

65. Academy of Nutrition and Dietetics. (2009). Life Cycle & Nutrition. Retrieved May 25, 2013, from Evidence Analysis Library: http://andevidencelibrary.com

66. Centers for Disease Control and Prevention. (2012, January 4). Three Decades of Twin Births in the United States, 1980-2009. Retrieved from February 20, 2012, CDC NCHS Data Brief: http://www.cdc.gov/nchs/data/databriefs/db80.htm; Centers for Disease Control and Prevention. (2012, October 19). Life Expectancy. Retrieved January 13, 2013, from FastStats: http://www.cdc.gov/nchs/fastats/lifexpec.htm

67. Centers for Disease Control and Prevention. (2011, November 30). Multiple Births. Retrieved February 20, 2012, from CDC FastStats: http://www.cdc.gov/nchs/fastats/multiple.htm; Centers for Disease Control and Prevention. (2011, -September 15). Nutrition, Physical Activity, & Obesity. Retrieved March 26, 2012, from Childhood Obesity Facts: http://www.cdc.gov/healthyyouth/obesity/facts.htm

68. Hagan J, Shaw J, Duncan P. Bright Futures: Guidelines for Health Supervision of Infants, Children and Adolescents. Elk Grove Village, IL: American Academy of Pediatricts; 2008.

69. American Academy of Pediatrics Work Group on Breastfeeding. Breastfeeding and the use of human milk. Pediatrics 2005;115: 496–506.

70. Brown J. Nutrition Through the Life Cycle: Infant Nutrition. Belmont, CA: Wadsworth Cengage; 2011.

71. Academy of Nutrition and Dietetics. (2013). Introducing solid foods. Retrieved January 31, 2013, from Kids eat right: http://www.eatright.org/kids/article.aspx?id=6442459352

72. Satter E. (2012). Child Development - Ages and Stages. Retrieved March 21, 2012, from Ellyn Satter: How to Feed Children: http://www.ellynsatter.com/child-development-ages-and-stages-i-25.html

73. Purves D. Neural Activity and the Growth of the Brain. New York, NY: Cambridge University Press; 2004.

74. Center on Hunger, Poverty and Nutrition Policy. Statement on the Link Between Nutrition and Cognitive Development in Children. Tufts University: School of Nutrition Science and Policy; 1998.

75. Healthy People 2020. (2012, March 1). Early and Middle Childhood Objectives. Retrieved March 21, 2012, from Healthy People 2020 Topics

& Objectives: http://www.healthypeople.gov/2020/topicsobjectives2020/
objectiveslist.aspx?topicId=10

76. Story M. H. Bright Futures in Practice: Nutrition. Arlington, VA: National Center for Education in Maternal and Child Health; 2000.

77. Satter E. (2012). Ellyn Satter's Division of Responsibility in Feeding. Retrieved March 21, 2012, from http://www.ellynsatter.com/ellyn-satters-division-of-responsibility-in-feeding-i-80.html

78. World Health Organization. (2013). Nutrition. Retrieved January 12, 2013, from Micronutrient Deficiencies: http://www.who.int/nutrition/topics/ida/en/index.html

79. Baker RD, Greer FR. Clinical report: diagnosis and prevention of iron deficiency and iron-deficiency anemia in infants and young children (0–3 years of age). Pediatrics 2010;126(5):1040–1050.

80. American Academy of Pediatrics Committee on Nutrition. Pediatric Nutrition Handbook. Elk Grove Village, IL: American Academy of Pediatrics; 2009.

81. US Department of Agriculture, Food and Nutrition Service. (2010, September 21). USDA FNS Newsroom. Retrieved March 30, 2012, from USDA Announces Technology Grants fo rhte Special Supplemental Nutrition Program for Women, Infants and Children: http://www.fns.usda.gov/cga/pressreleases/2010/0477.htm

82. US Department of Agriculture Food and Nutrition Services. (2011, August). Women, Infants, and Children. Retrieved March 30, 2012, from Frequently Asked Questions about WIC: http://www.fns.usda.gov/wic/FAQs/FAQ.HTM

83. US Department of Agriculture Food and Nutrition Service. (2012, February 17). About WIC. Retrieved March 30, 2012, from How WIC Helps: http://www.fns.usda.gov/wic/aboutwic/howwichelps.htm; US Department of Agriculture, Food and Nutrition Service. (2012, February 21). National School Lunch Program. Retrieved March 30, 2012, from Program Fact Sheet: http://www.fns.usda.gov/cnd/lunch/

84. Fiorito L, Marini M, Mitchell D, Smiciklas-Wright H, Birch L. Girls' early sweetened carbonated beverage intake predicts different patterns of beverage and nutrient intake across childhood and adolescence. J Am Diet Assoc 2010;110(4):543–550.

85. Centers for Disease Control and Prevention. Iron Deficiency. United States, 1999–2000. Morbidity and Mortality Weekly Review 2002;51:897–899.

86. Daniels S, Arnett D, Eckel R. Overweight in children and adolescents: pathophysiology, consequences, prevention, and treatment. Circulation 2005;120:S193–S228.

87. Office of the Surgeon General. The Surgeon General's Vision for Healthy and Fit Nation. Rockville, MD: Departmetn of Health and Human Services; 2010.

88. Centers for Disease Control and Prevention. Guidelines for school health programs to promote lifelong healthy eating. J Sch Health 1997;67:9–26.

89. US Department of Health and Human Services and Centers for Disease Control and Prevention National Center for Health Statistics. (2008, October). Food Allergy Among U.S. Children: Trends in Prevalence Hospitalizations. NCHS Data Brief (10).

90. US Food and Drug Administration. (2012, February 2). Food Facts. Retrieved March 30, 2012, from Food Allergies: What You Need to Know: http://www.fda.gov/food/resourcesforyou/consumers/ucm079311.htm

91. The Food Allergy & Anaphylaxis Network. (2011, September 29). Education. Retrieved March 30, 2012, from Outgrowing: http://www.foodallergy.org/page/outgrowing; The Food Allergy & Anaphylaxis Network. (2011, September 29). Education. Retrieved March 30, 2012, from About Food Allergy: http://www.foodallergy.org/section/about-food-allergy

92. Federal Interagency Forum on Child and Family Statistics. (2011). ChildStats.gov. Retrieved March 30, 2012, from America's Children: Key National Indicators of Well-Being, 2011: http://www.childstats.gov/americaschildren/famsoc3.asp

93. US Census Bureau. (2012, January 17). State & County QuickFacts. Retrieved March 30, 2012, from USA: http://quickfacts.census.gov/qfd/states/00000.html

94. US Department of Agriculture, Food and Nutrition Service. Reimbursement rates. http://www.fns.usda.gov/cnd/governance/notices/naps/naps.htm. Accessed July 1, 2013.

95. Gerrior S, WY J, Peter B. An easy approach to calculating estimated energy requirements. Prev Chronic Dis 2006;3(4):A129.

96. Sebastian R, Goldman J, Wilkinson Enns C. (2010, September). What We Eat in America, NHANES 2005–2006 Snacking Patterns of U.S. Adolescents. Food Surveys Research Group Dietary Data Brief.

97. Ogden C, Kit B, Carroll M, Park S. (August, 2011). Consumption of Sugar Drinks in the United States, 2005–2008. NCHS Data Brief, 71.

98. McGartland C, Robson P, Murray L, Cran G, Savage M, Watkins D, et al. Carbonated soft drink consumption and bone mineral density in adolescence: the Northern Ireland Young Hearts project. J Bone Miner Res 2003;18(9):1563–1569.

99. Clark N. Nancy Clark's Sports Nutrition Guidebook. 3rd ed. Champaign, IL: Human Kinetics; 2003.

100. Patel P, Wheatcroft R, Park R, Stein A. The children of mothers with eating disorders. Clin Child Fam Psychol Rev 2002;1:1–19.

101. National Center for Injury Prevention and Control. (2010, June 1). WISQARS Leading Causes of Death Reports, 1999–2007. Retrieved March 31, 2012, from 10 Leading Causes of Death, United States, 2007, All Races, Both Sexes, Age 60 to 85+: 10 Leading Causes of Death, United States, 2007, All Races, Both Sexes, Age 60 to 85+

102. American College of Sports Medicine. Exercise and physical activity for older adults. Med Sci Sports Exerc 2009;41(7):1510–1530.

103. Guo S, Zeller C, Chumlea W, Siervogel R. Aging, body composition, and lifestyle: the Fels Longitudinal Study. Am J Clin Nutr 1999;70(3):405–411.

104. Brown J. Nutrition Through the Life Cycle: Nutrition and Older Adults. Belmont, CA: Wadsworth Cengage; 2011.
105. Campbell W, Crim M, Dallal G, Young V, Evans W. Increased protein requirements in elderly people: new data and retrospective reassessments. Am J Clin Nutr 1994;60(4):501–509.
106. US Department of Agriculture and US Department of Health and Human Services. Dietary Guidelines for Americans, 2010. 7th ed. Washington, DC: US Government Printing Office; 2011.
107. Rizzoli R, Bruyere O, Cannata-Andia J, Devogelaer J, Lyritis G, Ringe J, et al. Management of osteoporosis in the elderly. Curr Med Res Opin 2009;25(10):2373–2387.
108. American Dietetic Association. Position paper of the American Dietetic Association: nutrition across the spectrum of aging. J Am Diet Assoc 2005;105:616–633.
109. US Department of Agriculture. (2011). Nutrient Data Laboratory. The USDA National Nutrient Database for Standard Reference. Washington, DC.

5

Matters of the Heart: Nutrition and Cardiovascular Disease

Heart disease is the number one killer of Americans, accounting for almost 25% of deaths, nearly one in every four people. Heart disease does not discriminate, as it is the leading cause of death for both males and females, as well as for blacks, Hispanics, and whites.[1] In addition to its human toll, heart disease also carries a significant financial impact. In 2010, coronary heart disease cost the United States close to $109 billion in total costs of health care services rendered, medication use, and lost productivity.[2] Despite the bleak mortality statistics and financial impact, the cardiovascular disease (CVD) arena does present many opportunities for Advanced Practice Nurses to effect positive change. Diet and lifestyle play important roles in the prevention and treatment of heart disease, working not only to help reduce the risk of developing heart disease, but also to lower the risk of death from heart disease and the incidence of nonfatal heart attacks, as well as the need to undergo heart bypass surgery or angioplasty.[3]

Preventing Heart Disease

Risk factors for heart disease are classified as being modifiable or nonmodifiable in nature. Age and family history of early heart disease are examples of two nonmodifiable risk factors. Men aged 45 years and older and women aged 55 years and older are at increased risk for developing heart disease. The delayed risk in women is extended until the onset of menopause, which often accompanies elevated low-density lipoprotein (LDL) cholesterol levels. Having a male family member (father or brother) who was diagnosed before age 55, or a female family member (mother or sister) with heart disease onset before age 65 also increases risk.[4] While individuals cannot do anything to alter their advancing age or family history (the nonmodifiable risk factors), the modifiable risk factors can be manipulated with diet, exercise, and lifestyle improvements. For those who are at risk for developing heart disease, the goal of nutrition therapy is to minimize the modifiable risk factors. Modifiable risk factors for heart disease include smoking, high blood pressure, high blood cholesterol, overweight and obesity, a sedentary lifestyle, and poorly controlled diabetes. Table 5–1 outlines the modifiable risk factors and their associated recommendations to lower overall risk of developing heart disease.[4-6]

Table 5-1. Lowering modifiable heart disease risk factors.

Heart Disease Risk Factor	Intervention
Smoking	Smoking cessation
High blood pressure	Increase potassium, lower sodium intake, and increase physical activity to help achieve blood pressure of <120/<80 mm Hg
High blood cholesterol	Increase dietary fiber (particularly soluble fiber) and decrease saturated fat, *trans* fat, and dietary cholesterol to help achieve total cholesterol <200 mg/dL and LDL <160-100 mg/dL
Overweight and obesity	Decrease excessive caloric intake and increase physical activity to lower BMI and waist circumference
Sedentary lifestyle	Engage in regular physical activity to help lower LDL and raise HDL; children and adolescents should do 1 hour or more of physical activity every day, most of which should be moderate- or vigorous-intensity aerobic physical activity
Diabetes	Optimal glycemic control to lower overall CVD risk
Excessive alcohol intake	Avoid overconsumption of alcohol, which elevates blood pressure; limit alcoholic drinks to no more than 1 per day for women and no more than 2 per day for men

Data from US Department of Health and Human Services, 2005; US Department of Health and Human Services, 2008; and US Department of Agriculture and US Department of Health and Human Services, 2011.

Disorders of Lipid Metabolism

- Hypercholesterolemia

High levels of cholesterol and other blood lipids promote the formation of plaque in the arteries. Plaque accumulates and can lead to impaired blood flow, causing ischemia and tissue damage. This is particularly detrimental when the heart and brain vessels are involved.

The causes of high levels of serum cholesterol may be attributable to both genetic and environmental factors. The environmental or lifestyle causes may be related to excessive intake of saturated fat and *trans* fatty acids, lack of dietary fiber (both soluble and insoluble fiber), excess body weight, and a sedentary lifestyle.[7] Cholesterol levels are known to increase with age, particularly for females; as women approach menopause, their declining estrogen levels increase blood levels of cholesterol.[8]

Lipid Goals

The overarching goal of nutrition therapy in hypercholesterolemia (or hyperlipidemia) is to help improve serum lipid levels while managing other risk factors for CVD. The hydrophobic (water-fearing) lipids are transported in the blood packaged with lipoproteins. Very low density lipoproteins (VLDLs) comprise mostly triglyceride and some cholesterol; of the lipoproteins, VLDLs contain the highest amount of triglycerides. They are synthesized in the liver and work to export fat from the liver to the body's cells. Low-density lipoproteins (LDLs) are made up of fat and protein and are responsible for carrying cholesterol, triglycerides, and other lipids in the blood to various parts of the body. High circulating levels of LDL cholesterol can lead to clogged arteries, which is why they are often referred to as the "bad cholesterol." High-density lipoproteins (HDLs) work to remove cholesterol from the cells, returning them to the liver, and are referred to as the "good cholesterol."[9]

The general goals for lipid management in the prevention of heart disease are to achieve total cholesterol under 200 mg/dL, LDL cholesterol below 100 mg/dL (or 130 mg/dL, depending on risk), HDL above 40 mg/dL, and triglycerides below 150 mg/dL. Table 5–2 outlines the National Cholesterol Education Program's (NCEP) lipid

Table 5-2. National Cholesterol Education Program (NCEP) cholesterol classifications.

Total Cholesterol
- Desirable: <200 mg/dL
- Borderline high: 200-239 mg/dL
- High: ≥240 mg/dL

LDL Cholesterol
- Optimal (ideal): <100 mg/dL
- Near optimal/above optimal: 100-129 mg/dL
- Borderline high: 130-159 mg/dL
- High: 160-189 mg/dL
- Very high: ≥190 mg/dL

HDL Cholesterol
- Major heart disease risk factor: <40 mg/dL
- Normal: 40-59 mg/dL
- Gives some protection against heart disease: ≥60

Triglycerides
- Normal: <150 mg/dL
- Borderline high: 150-199 mg/dL
- High: 200-499 mg/dL
- Very high: ≥500 mg/dL

Data from US Department of Health and Human Services, 2005; Grundy et al., 2004; and Expert Panel on Detection, Evaluation, and Treatment of High Blood Cholesterol in Adults, 2001.

Table 5–3. Summary of American Heart Association (AHA) lipid goal guidelines.

Total Cholesterol
- <200 mg/dL

LDL Cholesterol
- <160 mg/dL for those at low risk for heart disease
- <130 mg/dL for those at intermediate risk for heart disease
- <100 mg/dL for those at high risk for heart disease (includes existing heart disease or diabetes)

HDL Cholesterol
- ≥40 for men
- ≥50 for women

Triglycerides
- <150 mg/dL

Data from American Heart Association, 2012.

classification,[4,10,11] and Table 5–3 contains the American Heart Association (AHA) cholesterol guidelines.[12]

■ Interventions to Lower LDL

To lower LDL with dietary interventions, the focus should be on limiting total fat to no more than 25–35% of calories, reducing saturated fat to less than 7% of total calories, limiting or eliminating *trans* fat, and restricting cholesterol to less than 200 mg/day.[13] This eating pattern has the potential to lower LDL cholesterol levels by up to 16%, and reduces the overall risk of developing heart disease.[14] In addition to these nutrition guidelines, the Academy of Nutrition and Dietetics recommends the following nutrition therapy interventions to counteract elevated total and LDL cholesterol:

- Limit intake of saturated fat, *trans* fat, and cholesterol
- Consume adequate calories to maintain or achieve appropriate weight
- Replace saturated fat with monounsaturated or polyunsaturated fat
- Increase intake of omega-3 fatty acids
- Increase intake of fiber—and in particular, soluble fiber[7]

Saturated Fat

Saturated fat in the diet increases LDL cholesterol levels in the blood. A 1% increase in calories from saturated fat can raise LDL cholesterol levels by approximately 2%.[11] Saturated fats are typically solid at room temperature and are found in animal products such as lard, butter, cheese, whole milk, fatty meats, ice cream, and cream. While many vegetable oils are high in the heart-healthy unsaturated fats, the tropical vegetable oils (coconut, palm, and palm kernel oils) are high in saturated fat and should be minimized or avoided.

For individuals with elevated LDL levels, or for those who have, or are at, risk of developing heart disease, saturated fat intake should be kept to less than 7% of the total calories.[15] For an individual on a 1500-calorie diet, this equates to no more than 12 grams of saturated fat; for 2000 calories, no more than 16 grams of saturated fat per day. The daily value (DV) on the Nutrition Facts panel is based on 20 grams of saturated fat per day, a good target to come in under for those that need to lower saturated fat. Cutting back on meat, cheese, and full-fat dairy is a straightforward approach to reducing saturated fat in the diet. Table 5–4 contains information about the top sources of saturated fat among the US population and their saturated fat content.[16]

When providing nutrition counseling for a heart-healthy diet using the food label, teach patients and clients how to identify grams of saturated fat per serving, and how to track their intake against their daily 20 grams of saturated fat budget. Other tips for lowering saturated fat intake include substituting full-fat dairy for nonfat or low-fat (1%) milk and dairy foods, choosing leaner cuts of meat prepared without excessive fat, and selecting olive oil or canola oil in lieu of butter, lard, and higher saturated fat oils when possible. Table 5–5 shows the comparison of higher versus lower saturated fat and calorie food choices. Making these small substitutions can help significantly reduce saturated fat and excess calories.

Saturated Fat and LDL Particle Size

Advances in laboratory technology now allow practitioners to analyze lipoprotein particle size (LDL subfraction); however, no consensus exists on which method or what the standard for measuring particle size should be.[17] There is some evidence to indicate that the size, and not just the sheer number, of LDL particles may play a role in CVD risk. Small, dense LDL particles are thought to elevate heart disease risk by invading artery walls more easily, contributing to atherosclerosis and plaque accumulation more readily, and they may be less easily cleared from the bloodstream than are their larger-sized LDL counterparts. On the other hand, large-sized LDL particles are thought to be more benign than are small-sized LDL particles and less likely to increase CVD risk. Although limited, emerging data indicate that manipulations of sources of dietary fat (eg, replacing saturated with polyunsaturated) and carbohydrate (eg, replacing refined carbohydrates with fiber-containing whole grains) may affect particle size, current dietary education practice for lowering CVD risk should continue to focus on lowering overall dietary saturated fat and minimizing refined sugars.[18] While future findings may dictate changes in saturated fat and carbohydrate dietary recommendations for LDL management, there are currently not enough data to warrant such changes in therapy at this time.[19]

Table 5–4. NHANES top sources of saturated fat in the United States diet.

Ranking	Food Item	Contribution to Saturated Fat Intake (%)	Cumulative Contribution to Saturated Fat Intake (%)	Saturated Fat per Equivalent Serving (g)
1	Regular cheese	8.5	8.5	6 g in 1 oz cheddar cheese
2	Pizza	5.9	14.4	9 g in 8 oz serving
3	Grain-based dessert	5.8	20.2	4 g in 3 oz coffee cake
4	Dairy desserts	5.6	25.8	4 g in ½-cup ice cream
5	Chicken and chicken-mixed dishes	5.5	31.2	7 g in one fried chicken leg
6	Sausage, franks, bacon, and ribs	4.9	36.2	5 g in hot dog
7	Burgers	4.4	40.5	11 g in double-patty hamburger
8	Mexican-mixed dishes	4.1	44.6	7 g in fast food beef, bean, and cheese burrito
9	Beef and beef-mixed dishes	4.1	48.7	12 g in 6 oz slice meatloaf
10	Reduced-fat milk	3.9	52.6	3 g in 8 oz cup

Data from National Cancer Institute, 2010.

Trans Fat

Trans fatty acids raise LDL cholesterol levels and increase heart disease risk. A 2% increase in calories from *trans* fat has been associated with a 23% rise in heart disease risk.[20] Findings from the Nurses' Health Study demonstrated that, after adjusting for age and total caloric intake, relative risk of heart disease was 1.5 times greater for those in the quintile that consumed the most *trans* fat than for those in the lowest quintile.[21]

Table 5-5. Substitution ideas for lowering saturated fat and calories.

Instead Of...			Try...		
	Saturated Fat	Calories		Saturated Fat	Calories
Whole milk (1 cup)	5 g	150	Nonfat milk (1 cup)	0 g	80
Swiss cheese (1 oz)	5 g	100	Low-fat Swiss cheese (1 oz)	1 g	50
70% lean ground beef (3 oz raw)	9 g	280	95% lean ground beef (3 oz raw)	2 g	115
Premium ice cream (1/2 cup)	11 g	270	Sorbet or sherbet (1/2 cup)	0 g	130
Vegetable oil, palm kernel (1 tablespoon)	11 g	115	Canola oil (1 tablespoon)	1 g	115

Trans fat is found in minimal amounts in whole, unprocessed foods. *Trans* fat is much more prevalent in packaged and processed baked goods, fried foods, and snack items that contain stick margarine or vegetable shortening. *Trans* fats are created by hydrogenating or partially hydrogenating liquid vegetable oils. This process not only transforms liquid to solid fats, but also enhances the oxidative stability of the fat. Food manufacturers favor *trans* fats due to their extended shelf life and the favorable texture and mouthfeel that *trans* fat-containing foods impart.[22]

Since 2006, the FDA has required that *trans* fat content of foods be listed on the Nutrition Facts panel. *Trans* fat is listed under the saturated fat on the label and is stated in the nearest 0.5 gram increment when occurring in less than 5 grams per serving, and to the nearest 1 gram increment when above 5 grams. The FDA labeling requirement states that if a food contains 0.5 gram *trans* fat or less per serving (along with total fat less than 0.5 gram per serving, and provided that no other claims about fat, fatty acid, or cholesterol content are made), it may be labeled as 0 gram *trans* fat or bear a footnote saying, "Not a significant source of *trans* fat." This "*trans* fat loophole" leads to confusion among consumers who believe they may be eating *trans* fat-free foods, when they actually do contain *trans* fatty acids.

Because food manufacturers can determine the serving size labeled on their products, many will purposely use a small serving size in order to list the *trans* fat content as 0 gram. This gives the consumer a false sense of security, and when the consumer eats multiple portions, they unknowingly consume a significant amount of *trans* fat. Consumers can work to minimize *trans* fat in the diet by looking for the words "partially hydrogenated" when referring to oils in the ingredients list of food labels and avoid these foods when possible. Cutting back on all high-fat foods also decreases *trans* fat (and saturated fat) intake. The bottom line is: there is no room for *trans* fat in a heart-healthy diet.

The AHA recommends limiting *trans* fat to no more than 1% of calories, while the Academy of Nutrition and Dietetics, the *US Dietary Guidelines for Americans, 2010*, and the NCEP all maintain that dietary *trans* fat should be limited as much as possible.[6,14] Because *trans* fat-containing foods are not consistent with a heart-healthy diet, advise patients to reduce or eliminate packaged and processed baked goods, snack items, and fried foods, and to replace them instead with whole grains, fruits, vegetables, nonfat or low-fat dairy, legumes, and lean protein foods. It is also wise to keep in mind that due to growing public interest in limiting *trans* fats, food manufacturers are routinely removing *trans* fats from foods, but replacing the *trans* fats with equally harmful saturated fats. Patients and clients are advised to pay attention to *both* saturated and *trans* fat content of foods, and to keep in mind that both work to elevate LDL levels and should be minimized in the diet.

Dietary Cholesterol

While reducing saturated and *trans* fat in the diet are effective approaches to lowering overall and LDL cholesterol, patients with elevated LDL should also keep an eye on dietary cholesterol intake. Cholesterol originates from two sources: your body and the foods you eat. About three-quarters of blood cholesterol comes from your liver and other cells, while the remaining quarter comes from the foods you eat.[12] The NCEP recommends limiting dietary cholesterol to no more than 200 mg/day.[11] Dietary cholesterol is only found in foods that come from animals; thus, vegetable-based oils are naturally cholesterol-free. Consumers should not be impressed by French fries fried in "cholesterol-free" vegetable oil, as the saturated fat of that oil is the problem, not the cholesterol. Animal-based foods that are high in cholesterol include egg yolks (but not the whites), shrimp, whole milk, and full-fat dairy foods, such as butter, cream, and cheese. As is the case with saturated and *trans* fat, lowering total fat intake will also serve to lower dietary cholesterol.

Omega-3 Fatty Acids

Omega-3 fatty acids play a role in lowering heart disease risk, not by lowering LDL levels, but, rather, by reducing inflammation and preventing the formation of blood clots. Foods that are rich in omega-3 fatty acids include fatty fish (salmon, mackerel, and tuna, including canned tuna), and fish oil. Omega-3 fatty acids are also found in some plant foods, such as walnuts, flaxseed, canola, and soybean oils. The NCEP recommends eating two fish meals per week.[11] Increasing fish intake not only raises omega-3 fatty acid intake, but if fish is displacing other high-fat protein or meat meals, it is also working to lower total fat and saturated fat intake that would have otherwise been consumed in those foods. For individuals who do not eat fish, they might consider taking 1 gram of EPA plus DHA omega-3 fish oil supplements as a secondary prevention measure.[14]

Dyslipidemia and omega-3 fatty acids from food: what does the evidence say?

The Academy of Nutrition and Dietetics Evidence Analysis Library guidelines recommend consuming dietary sources of omega-3 fatty acids, from 2- to 4-ounce servings of fish per week (preferably fatty fish like mackerel, salmon, herring, trout, sardines, or tuna) and 1.5 grams of plant-based alpha-linolenic acid (from 1 tablespoon canola or walnut oil, 0.5 tablespoon ground flax seed, or <1 tablespoon flaxseed oil) as part of a cardioprotective diet. (Evidence grade: Fair, Conditional).[14]

Dyslipidemia and omega-3 fatty acids from supplements: what does the evidence say?

For individuals who do not eat food sources of omega-3 fatty acids, 1 gram of EPA and DHA omega-3 fatty acid supplements may be recommended as secondary prevention. (Evidence grade: Fair, Conditional).[14]

Dietary Fiber

There are two types of dietary fiber: soluble and insoluble. Many fiber-containing foods have similar amounts of soluble and insoluble fiber, and patients should be cautioned to avoid focusing on the *type* of fiber they are eating, and to instead concentrate on increasing the *total* amount of dietary fiber. With that said, it may be valuable for some populations to know that it is the soluble fiber that conveys heart-healthy benefits, whereas insoluble fiber is more effective for gastrointestinal health. The goal for individuals at risk for or with established heart disease is 25–30 grams of fiber per day. Diets high in fiber and soluble fiber, as components of a cardioprotective diet, have the potential to lower total cholesterol by 2% and LDL cholesterol by 7%.[14]

Soluble fiber, which absorbs water and has a gel-like texture, works to lower CVD risk on two fronts: it increases the excretion of bile acids, while at the same time lowering the hepatic synthesis of cholesterol. In plain English, soluble fiber helps remove LDL from your body, while it also tells your body to make less LDL. For patients with elevated LDL, it may be helpful to liken soluble fiber to a sponge: the fiber soaks up the LDL particles and helps excrete them from the body. Think "S" for soluble and "S" for sponge. Good sources of soluble fiber include fruits,

Table 5–6. Total fiber, soluble fiber, and insoluble content of selected foods.

	Serving Size	Total Fiber (g)	Soluble Fiber (g)	Insoluble Fiber
Whole grain cereals				
Bread: Whole Wheat	1 slice	3	0.7	2.3
Oatmeal: Quaker, quick oats, dry	½ cup	4	2	2
Rice: brown, long grain, and cooked	½ cup	1.8	0.2	1.6
Fruit				
Apple: red delicious, raw, and ripe w/ skin	1 medium (3" diameter)	4.4	1.3	3.1
Avocado: raw, California, and without skin and seed	½ fruit	4.6	1.7	2.9
Mango: fruit without refuse	1	5.4	2.1	3.3
Vegetables				
Potato: sweet, flesh only	½ cup	4.0	1.8	2.2
Broccoli: cooked, boiled, drained, and without salt	1 cup	5.1	2.0	3.1
Carrots: cooked, boiled, drained, and without salt	1 cup	4.7	1.9	2.8
Legumes				
Red kidney beans: can, drained	½ cup	7.2	1.4	5.8
Lentils: dry, cooked, drained	½ cup	7.8	0.6	7.2

Data from US Department of Agriculture Agriculture Research Service; Li, Andrews, & Pehrsson, 2002; and Quaker Oats Company, 2012.

vegetables, legumes, and whole grain cereals. Table 5–6 outlines the soluble fiber and total fiber content of some of these foods.[23-25]

■ Therapeutic Lifestyle Change (TLC) Diet

If LDL is above goal, practitioners are encouraged to recommend initiation of the therapeutic lifestyle changes (TLC) diet. The TLC diet lowers LDL by combining diet, physical activity, and weight management principles. The TLC diet has the following nutrition prescription: less

Table 5–7. Components of the therapeutic lifestyle change (TLC) diet and associated reductions in LDL.

Nutrient	TLC Recommendations	Reductions in LDL
Saturated fat	Decrease to <7% of calories	8–10%
Dietary cholesterol	Decrease to <200 mg/day	3–5%
Soluble fiber	Add 5–10 g/day	3–5%
Plant sterols/stanols	Add 2 g/day	5–15%
Total		20–30%

Data from US Department of Health and Human Services, 2005.

than 7% of calories from saturated fat, no more than 200 mg cholesterol per day, 10–25 grams of soluble fiber per day, and 2 grams of plant stanols/sterols per day. Table 5–7 outlines the nutrient recommendations of the TLC diet and their resulting LDL-lowering potential.[4] The combination of reducing saturated fat and cholesterol intake, while increasing soluble fiber and utilizing plant sterols and stanols, can result in a total reduction of LDL of 20–30%. This is roughly equivalent to the effectiveness of many cholesterol-lowering drugs.[4]

Plant Stanols and Sterols

Plant stanols and sterols are found in small amounts in plant foods. They are extracted from soybean and tall pine-tree oils and are often combined in foods with canola oil. In a fashion similar to that of soluble fiber, plant stanols and sterols impede the absorption of cholesterol from the gut, working to lower LDL, without raising HDL or triglyceride levels. The recommended intake of plant stanols or sterols is 2 grams per day to lower LDL by 5–15% within a few weeks.[4,26] Plant stanols and sterols are found in fortified margarine spreads and salad dressings, milk, yogurt, juices, and snack bars. Advise patients to beware of excess calories from stanol- or sterol-enhanced foods, keeping in mind that their contribution to unwanted weight gain counteracts the potential cholesterol-lowering effects of the plant components.

■ Interventions to Raise HDL

There are a number of dietary interventions for lowering LDL, but not much in the way of food-based ways to elevate HDL. For the treatment of HDL cholesterol below 40 mg/dL, the *Third Report of the Expert Panel on Detection, Evaluation, and Treatment of High Blood Cholesterol in Adults* (ATP III) guidelines recommend first reaching LDL goal and then intensifying weight management and increasing physical activity. If the triglycerides are 200–499 mg/dL, achieve non-HDL goal, and if the triglycerides are <200 mg/dL (isolated low HDL) in coronary heart disease (CHD) or CHD equivalent, consider nicotinic acid or fibrate.[27]

Niacin

It should be mentioned that statins, fibrates, and bile acid sequestrants yield only modest impacts on HDL (5–10%), while omega-3 fatty acids do very little to nudge up HDL. Nicotinic acid is the only drug available that has reliable HDL elevating assets. The HDL response with nicotinic acid is dose-dependent and may raise HDL by as much as 30% above baseline.[28]

The AIM-HIGH trial found that the use of niacin with statin therapy was no more effective at raising LDL in people with established heart disease and low LDL (<70 mg/dL) than was the use of statin therapy alone; however, the use of niacin is still considered to be an effective therapy for lowering triglycerides and raising HDL. In the AIM-HIGH study, use of extended-release niacin at 1500–2000 mg per day (along with statin therapy) increased median HDL cholesterol level from 35 mg/dL to 42 mg/dL, and lowered triglycerides from 164 mg/dL to 122 mg/dL.[29]

Physical Activity

Regular physical activity raises HDL, although the amount of exercise required remains uncertain. Durstine and Thompson have reported that just one intensive exercise session raises HDL.[30] The NCEP's population approach recommends adopting and/or increasing physical activity in addition to weight management and nutrition-related undertakings.[11] The *2008 Physical Activity Guidelines for Americans* recommend 2½ hours of moderate-intensity aerobic activity each week.[5] The evidence-based guidelines of the Academy of Nutrition and Dietetics Evidence Analysis project have found that there is strong/imperative evidence to recommend that "moderate intensity physical activity should be incorporated for at least 30 minutes, most, if not all, days of the week, if not contraindicated…Moderately intense physical activity reduces the risk of CVD events, decreases LDL-C and triglycerides, and increases HDL-C."[14] It should also be noted that CDC recommends 150 minutes of physical activity in addition to 2 days of strength training each week.[31]

Alcohol

Moderate alcohol intake is associated with lower heart disease risk as it has the potential to raise HDL cholesterol concentrations.[32] The exact mechanism by which alcohol raises HDL is unknown. Moderate alcohol intake is defined as no more than one drink per day for women and no more than two drinks per day for men. A serving size of alcohol is defined as a 12-ounce beer, 5-ounce glass of wine, or 1½-ounce serving of 80-proof liquor. For individuals who do not currently drink alcohol, taking up drinking just for the HDL effects is not recommended. Remind patients that excessive alcohol has a deleterious effect on the overall health and increases blood pressure and heart disease risk.

What is moderate alcohol intake?

Moderate alcohol intake is defined as no more than one drink per day for women and no more than two drinks per day for men.

What is a "drink?"

A drink is defined as a 12-ounce beer, 5-ounce glass of wine, 10-ounce wine cooler, or 1½-ounce serving of 80-proof liquor.[33]

Supplements and Disorders of Lipid Metabolism: What Does the Evidence Say?[14]

Vitamin E, vitamin C, and beta-carotene supplements

Dietary sources of vitamin E, vitamin C, and beta-carotene are encouraged. Supplements of these antioxidants have shown no protection for CVD events or mortality; therefore, doses greater than the RDA for these nutrients should not be recommended. *(Evidence Grade: Strong, Imperative).*

Supplemental vitamins, cardiovascular disease, and smoking

Supplemental vitamin E, vitamin C, beta-carotene, and selenium should not be taken with a Simvastatin/niacin drug combination. Supplemental beta-carotene cannot be recommended in individuals who smoke. Research indicates that in these situations, there is an increased risk for CVD. *(Evidence Grade: Fair, Imperative).*

Homocysteine, folate, vitamin B_6, vitamin B_{12}, and cardiovascular disease

Folate, vitamin B_6, and vitamin B_{12} should be planned into the cardioprotective dietary pattern to meet the DRI. If an individual has high serum homocysteine levels (usually greater than 13 μmol/L), these B vitamins may lower serum homocysteine levels by 17–34%. *(Evidence Grade: Fair, Imperative).*

Coenzyme Q10 and disorders of lipid metabolism

If an individual is taking coenzyme Q10 (Co-Q10) supplements, the practitioner may discuss the lack of evidence for the association of Co-Q10 and coronary heart disease events. Research is inconclusive regarding the relationship between Co-Q10 and risk of disease. *(Evidence Grade: Insufficient Evidence, Conditional)*

■ Metabolic Syndrome

The metabolic syndrome (formerly called Syndrome X, and also referred to as the insulin resistance syndrome) is a compilation of metabolic abnormalities that increases the risk of heart disease and diabetes. The metabolic syndrome was first defined by the World Health Organization in 1998, and it has evolved to include the clustering of three

Table 5–8. Clinical identification of the metabolic syndrome.

Metabolic Syndrome is Clinically Identified as Any 3 of the Following:
Abdominal obesity as defined by waist circumference • Men: ≥40 inches (102 cm) • Women: ≥35 inches (88 cm) **Triglycerides** • ≥150 mg/dL **HDL cholesterol** • Men: <40 mg/dL • Women: <50 mg/dL **Blood pressure** • ≥130/≥85 mm Hg **Fasting blood glucose** • ≥110 mg/dL

Data from US Department of Health and Human Services, 2001.

or more risk factors. The five primary risk factors, of which three or more must be present to diagnose, are central obesity, hypertriglyceridemia, low HDL, hyperglycemia, and hypertension. Table 5–8 outlines the inclusion criteria for each risk factor as it pertains to metabolic syndrome.[34]

Excess weight is the primary culprit for metabolic syndrome. Overweight and obesity are related to insulin resistance; however, it is the presence of abdominal obesity (the centralized fat that gathers around the midregion) that increases metabolic risk factors more so than an elevated BMI. Those with abdominal obesity are sometimes referred to as being apple-shaped, and apple-shaped people tend to be those at higher risk for metabolic syndrome. Pear-shaped individuals amass fat in the buttocks and thighs (as compared to the abdominal) regions (see Figure 5–1). The treatment for metabolic syndrome involves weight loss, physical activity, dietary improvements, and smoking cessation. Initial weight loss goals should be in the arena of 7–10% of the total body weight.[14]

With metabolic syndrome, the primary goals of treatment are lowering LDL and cholesterol and managing diabetes if present. The secondary goal is to prevent the onset of diabetes in those who have not already developed it.[35] If the risk factors persist despite these therapeutic lifestyle changes, practitioners are advised to treat hypertension, to use aspirin for CHD patients and reduce prothrombotic state, and to treat the elevated triglycerides and/or low HDL.

■ Hypertriglyceridemia

Elevated triglycerides can occur autonomously or alongside elevated blood cholesterol levels. In spite of the cause or manifestation, hypertriglyceridemia is an independent risk factor for heart disease.[36] The nutritional management of hypertriglyceridemia is very straightforward: eliminate alcohol, cut back on refined carbohydrate and sugars,

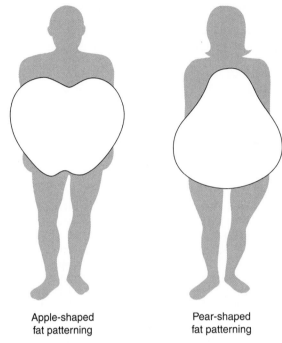

Apple-shaped
fat patterning

Pear-shaped
fat patterning

Figure 5–1. Apple-shaped fat patterning increases risk for metabolic syndrome as compared to pear-shaped fat patterning.

increase whole grains and fiber (especially soluble fiber), and exercise or cut calories to achieve and maintain a healthy weight.

Omega-3 fatty acids may be helpful in lowering triglycerides in some cases, and can be included in the diet from fatty fish and fish oils or as supplements. Supplement with 2–4 grams of docosahexaenoic acid (DHA) and eicosapentaenoic acid (EPA), and when possible, utilize prescription drug omega-3 preparations. Prescription omega-3 preparations contain standardized and known amounts of EPA and DHA, whereas over-the-counter omega-3 supplements may not always.

It may happen that when an individual with elevated LDL adopts dietary changes that lower saturated and *trans* fat intake, serum triglycerides will rise. This occurs when the saturated and/or *trans* fat removed from the diet is replaced with sugars or refined carbohydrate. The key to minimizing elevated triglycerides when reducing saturated and *trans* fat intake is to maintain adequate dietary fiber levels. Encourage individuals to aim for 30 grams of fiber per day, with an emphasis on the heart-healthy effects of soluble fiber.

Almost one-third (31%) of adults in the United States have elevated triglycerides (>150 mg/dL).[37] The primary treatment of elevated triglycerides (those at levels ≥150 mg/dL) is to reach LDL goal.

Table 5-9. ATP III classification for serum triglycerides.

ATP III Serum Triglyceride (mg/dL) Classification	
Normal	<150
Borderline high	150–199
High	200–499
Very high	≥500

Data from National Heart, Lung and Blood Institute, 2001.

Secondary treatment measures include intensifying weight management approaches, increasing physical activity, and, if triglycerides are ≥200 mg/dL after LDL goal is achieved, setting a secondary goal for nonHDL cholesterol at 30 mg/dL higher than the LDL goal.[7] Table 5–9 outlines the ATP III classification for serum triglycerides.[27]

While the goal for triglyceride management remains under 150 mg/dL, the American Heart Association has furthered their recommendations by advocating for a new optimal triglyceride level of 100 mg/dL, although there are currently no data to support the theory that lowering triglycerides to this level is beneficial. Research indicates that replacing saturated fat with unsaturated varieties, engaging in regular physical activity, and losing excess weight can lower triglycerides by 20–50%.[37] Table 5–10

Table 5-10. American Heart Association recommendations for lowering triglycerides.

Sugar	• <5–10% of calories • 100 calories per day for women • 150 calories per day for men • No more than 36 oz sugar-sweetened beverages per week (for a 2000-calorie diet)
Fructose	• <50–100 g/day from both processed and naturally occurring sources
Saturated fat	• <7% of calories
Trans fat	• <1% of calories
Alcohol	• Limit; especially if triglycerides >500 mg/dL
Physical activity	• 150 minutes per week for triglycerides in 150-199 mg/dL range for additional 20-30% triglyceride-lowering effect

A combination of all of the above is the most effective, and may reduce triglycerides by 50% or more

Data from Miller et al., 2011.

contains nutrition recommendations from the American Heart Association for those with triglycerides outside of the normal range.[37]

If triglycerides are greater than 500 mg/dL, the patient is at an increased risk for developing pancreatitis. In this case, the goal is to lower the triglycerides to prevent pancreatitis, adopt a very low fat diet with less than 15% of calories from fat, eliminate alcohol, promote weight management and physical activity, initiate fibrate or nicotinic acid, and, when triglycerides are lowered under 500 mg/dL, turn to LDL-lowering therapies mentioned above.

Hypertension

Hypertension is responsible for more than 7½ million deaths per year worldwide, accounting for 13.5% of total global death, and contributing more than any other individual risk factor.[38] One-third of non-institutionalized adults in the United States aged 20 years and over, and one in three adults worldwide have hypertension.[39,40] In the United States, hypertension has exacted a financial toll of over $73 billion in direct and indirect healthcare costs in 2009.[41] Often referred to as "the silent killer," hypertension has no warning signs or symptoms, and most people with high blood pressure are not aware of their condition. The three food- and weight-related issues that affect hypertension are excess body weight, high sodium intake, and excessive alcohol consumption.[42]

■ Approaches to Lower Blood Pressure

The dietary changes to lower blood pressure include lowering sodium intake, increasing potassium, calcium, and magnesium, and limiting alcohol intake. Lifestyle factors involve increasing physical activity and smoking cessation. *The Dietary Approaches to Stop Hypertension* (DASH) diet principles are covered at the end of this section.

Sodium

There is no question that the majority of people consuming Western diets eat too much sodium. The *Dietary Guidelines for Americans, 2010* recommend limiting dietary sodium to no more than 2300 mg per day. This is restricted even further, to 1500 mg per day, for African Americans, people 51 years or older, and those who have hypertension, diabetes, or chronic kidney disease.[6] The average daily sodium intake for people aged 2 years and older in the United States is 3436 mg, and approximately 87% of adults eat more than the recommended 2.3 grams of sodium per day.[40,41]

Patients and consumers are often unaware of the true sources of sodium in their diet. It is not uncommon to hear, "Oh, I never use salt in my food," or, "We don't even have a salt shaker on the table." Contrary to popular belief, the salt shaker is *not* a primary source of dietary salt in the typical American diet. The majority of salt in the diet comes from packaged, processed, and fast foods. Roughly 77% of sodium is from

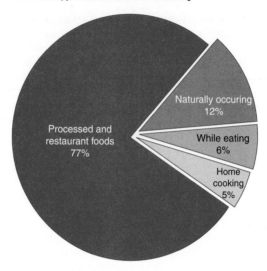

Figure 5–2. Sources of dietary sodium in the typical American diet.

packaged and processed foods purchased at retails stores and restaurants, 5% is added to home cooking, 6% is added from table salt while eating, and 12% comes from naturally occurring sources (Figure 5–2).[43] The impact of sodium from packaged and processed foods is so great and so concentrated that the CDC estimates that 44% of the sodium we eat comes from only 10 different types of foods, listed in Table 5–11.[44] Table 5–12 contains a list of sodium seasoning alternatives for different types of food.[45] Table 5–13 provides some tips to reduce salt and sodium intake from the DASH diet.[46] The DASH diet section of this chapter contains more details about lowering salt intake to reduce blood pressure.

Potassium

Admit it: firing off lists of what *not* to eat is exhausting! Thankfully, when it comes to lowering blood pressure, you can finally tell patients what they *can* eat. Emerging research indicates that increasing dietary potassium may be as important as lowering dietary sodium in controlling blood pressure.[47-49] The easiest part about making potassium recommendations is that foods that are high in potassium, such fruits and vegetables, are also naturally low in sodium. In this case, making *one* recommendation works for you on *two* fronts!

The *Dietary Guidelines for Americans, 2010* recommend at least 4.7 grams of potassium per day.[6] In reality, only about 2% of US adults meet that guideline.[41] The blood-pressure-lowering effects of potassium have largely been established based on studies that analyze food-based

Table 5–11. Top 10 sources of sodium in US diet.

Top 10 Sources of Sodium Account for 44% of Consumption
Breads and rolls
Cold cuts and cured meats
Pizza
Poultry
Soups
Sandwiches
Cheese
Pasta dishes
Meat dishes
Snacks

Data from Centers for Disease Control and Prevention, 2012.

potassium, as opposed to supplements. Encourage patients and clients to obtain their potassium from fresh fruits and vegetables, not from supplements. Salt substitutes often contain potassium chloride in place of sodium chloride. Potassium chloride may prove harmful for individuals with kidney problems or those who are taking medication for heart, kidney, or liver problems. A safer alternative for sodium substitutes is to stick with commercial salt-free seasonings such as Mrs. Dash® or to make your own. Table 5–14 contains a list of herbs and spices, both fresh and dried, to use in lieu of salt when cooking at home.[50] Or make your own salt-free seasoning using the recipe for Spicy Homemade Herb Seasoning listed in Table 5–15.[50,51]

Alcohol

Alcohol intake has a significant effect on blood pressure.[52] Excessive alcohol intake, generally defined as four or more drinks per day for women and five or more for men, increases the risk of stroke. Moderate alcohol intake, defined as no more than one drink per day for females and no more than two drinks per day for males, decreases the risk of ischemic stroke.[53] The Academy of Nutrition and Dietetics Evidence Analysis project has found that current evidence does not justify encouraging those who do not drink alcohol to start doing so for any perceived health benefit related to blood pressure and stroke risk. Furthermore, the Evidence Analysis project supports the Seventh Report of the

Table 5–12. Seasoning foods without salt.

Type of Food	Salt-free Seasoning Ideas
Asparagus	Garlic, lemon juice, onion, and vinegar
Beef	Bay leaf, dry mustard, green pepper, marjoram, fresh mushrooms, nutmeg, onion, pepper, sage, and thyme
Bread	Cinnamon, cloves, dill, and poppy seed
Broccoli	Lemon juice, garlic
Chicken	Green pepper, lemon juice, marjoram, fresh mushrooms, paprika, parsley, poultry seasoning, sage, thyme, and cilantro
Cucumbers	Chives, dill, garlic, onion, and vinegar
Fish	Bay leaf, curry powder, dry mustard, green pepper, lemon juice, paprika, and bell peppers
Green beans	Dill, lemon juice, nutmeg, and marjoram
Greens	Onion, pepper, vinegar, and lemon juice
Lamb	Curry powder, garlic, mint, mint jelly, pineapple, and rosemary
Pasta	Basil, caraway seed, garlic, oregano, poppy seed, and rosemary
Peas	Green pepper, mint, parsley, onion, fresh mushrooms, and garlic
Pork	Apple, applesauce, garlic, onion, and sage
Potatoes	Green pepper, mace, onion, paprika, rosemary, parsley, and oregano
Rice	Chives, green pepper, saffron, and onion
Squash	Cinnamon, nutmeg, mace, and ginger
Tomatoes	Basil, marjoram, onion, and oregano
Veal	Apricot, cinnamon, cloves, and ginger

Data from Gerontological Nutritionists, 2000.

Joint National Committee on Prevention, Detection, Evaluation, and Treatment of High Blood Pressure (JNC7) recommendations recommendations that alcohol consumption should be limited to no more than two drinks (24 oz beer, 10 oz wine, or 3 oz of 80-proof liquor) per day for most men and no more than one drink per day for women and lighter weight people. This has been shown to result in an approximate systolic blood pressure reduction of 2–4 mm Hg.[42,54] Individuals with high blood pressure and greater than moderate alcohol intake are advised to cut back on alcohol or eliminate it entirely from the diet.

Table 5-13. Tips to reduce salt and sodium.

Tips to Reduce Salt and Sodium in Foods	
Condiments	Choose low- or reduced-sodium, or no-salt-added versions of foods and condiments when available
Vegetables	Choose fresh, frozen, or canned (low-sodium or no-salt-added) vegetables
Protein	Use fresh poultry, fish, and lean meat, rather than canned, smoked, or processed types
Cereals	Choose ready-to-eat breakfast cereals that are lower in sodium
Cured foods	Limit cured foods (such as bacon and ham), foods packed in brine (such as pickles, pickled vegetables, olives, and sauerkraut) and condiments (such as mustard, horseradish, ketchup, and BBQ sauce). Limit even lower-sodium versions of soy sauce and teriyaki sauce as these are often still high in sodium
Starches	Cook rice, pasta, and hot cereals without salt. Limit instant or flavored rice, pasta, and cereal mixes, which usually have added salt
Convenience foods	Choose convenience foods that are lower in sodium. Reduce intake of frozen dinners, mixed dishes like pizza, packaged mixes, canned soups or broths, and salad dressing
Canned foods	Rinse canned foods, such as tuna and canned beans; this removes approximately 1/3rd of the sodium content
Spices	Use spices instead of salt; flavor foods with herbs, spices, lemon, lime, vinegar, or salt-free seasoning blends

Data from National Heart, Lung, and Blood Institute, 2006.

Table 5-14. Herbs and spices to use in lieu of salt for home cooking.

Basil	Crushed red pepper	Paprika/smoked paprika
Ground black pepper	Cumin	Parsley
Cayenne pepper	Garlic	Parsley
Chili powder	Ginger	Rosemary
Cilantro	Mint	Salt-free seasoning mix
Cinnamon	Nutmeg	Tarragon
Coriander	Oregano	Thyme

Data from National Institutes of Health, 2010.

Table 5–15. Spicy homemade salt-free herb seasoning.

Ingredients
1 tablespoon cayenne pepper

2 tablespoons garlic powder

2 tablespoons dried basil

2 tablespoons ground savory

2 tablespoons onion powder

2 tablespoons dried sage

1 tablespoon grated lemon zest

2 tablespoons ground mace

2 tablespoons dried thyme

2 tablespoons dried parsley

2 tablespoons dried marjoram

2 tablespoon ground black pepper

Instructions
- Crush or grind all ingredients together
- Let stand at least overnight before using
- Store mixture in an airtight container

Yield
Makes 30 ¾ tablespoon servings

Data from AllRecipes.com.

Magnesium

In its role as a vasodilator, magnesium intake helps regulate blood pressure. A diet rich in green leafy vegetables, nuts, whole grain breads, and cereals helps assure adequate magnesium intake. For individuals whose food patterns result in inadequate magnesium intake, dietary supplements to reach 100% of the DRI may be indicated. Individuals should be encouraged to meet magnesium needs from increasing variety and quality of their diet, as opposed to obtaining magnesium from supplements.[55]

Calcium

Adequate calcium intake has been positively linked to lower blood pressure. *The Dietary Approaches to Stop Hypertension* (DASH) diet (covered in the next section) advocates for the daily inclusion of two to three servings of nonfat or low-fat dairy products. For those who are unable to tolerate dairy, consider obtaining calcium from other sources such as calcium-fortified soy milk or almond milk, tofu made with calcium salts, canned salmon with bones, or frequent consumption of calcium-rich dark green leafy vegetables. Individuals who consume less than the RDA for calcium may consider taking a calcium supplement. Calcium supplements should be limited to no more than 500 mg at one time in order to maximize absorption. The RDA for calcium for males aged 19–70 years and females aged 19–50 years is 1000 mg; the RDA increases to 1200 mg/day for females aged 51 years and older.[56]

Physical Activity

While dietary changes are certainly effective and should be encouraged to lower blood pressure, food is only half the battle. Individuals with hypertension, when not medically contraindicated, should make regular physical activity a part of their efforts to lower blood pressure. Teach patients, and in particular, the "Can't I just take a pill for that?" patients, that exercise can be just as effective at lowering BP as are certain medications. Participating in regular aerobic physical activity, such as jogging or brisk walking, for a period of at least 30 minutes per day, 5 days per week lowers blood pressure on an average by 4–9 mm Hg.[54]

■ The DASH Diet

The *Dietary Approaches to Stop Hypertension* (DASH) is a recommended eating pattern based on findings from two large-scale studies conducted by the National Heart, Lung, and Blood Institute. The DASH study findings confirmed that reducing sodium intake—along with other dietary and lifestyle changes—is an effective therapy for lowering blood pressure. The DASH diet is high in fruits and vegetables and low-fat dairy foods, and low in sodium and saturated fat. It is low in red meat, sweets, and other sugar-sweetened beverages and food. The DASH eating plan includes foods that are good sources of potassium, calcium, magnesium, fiber, and protein. The daily nutrient goals used in the DASH diet (based on a 2000 calorie diet) are outlined in Table 5–16.[46]

The first DASH study involved 459 adults, 50% women, and 60% were African Americans. The participants were randomized to one of three groups: typical American diet, typical American diet plus more fruits and vegetables, or the DASH diet. All of the three groups' sodium levels were about 3000 mg per day. The results were conclusive: those who ate the typical American diet plus more fruits and vegetables and those who ate the DASH diet plan experienced reductions in blood pressure. The DASH or combination diet groups had reductions in systolic BP of 5.5 mm Hg, and diastolic BP was lowered by 3 mm Hg.

In the second DASH study, DASH-sodium, 412 participants were randomized to either a typical American diet group or the DASH diet group and then followed for a month as part of one of three sodium levels: 3000 mg per day, 2300 mg per day, or 1500 mg per day.

Table 5-16. DASH diet nutrient goals.

Nutrient	DASH Diet Daily Goal
Total fat	27% of calories
Saturated fat	6% of calories
Protein	18% of calories
Carbohydrate	55% of calories
Cholesterol	150 mg
Sodium	2300 mg with 1500 mg being most effective for lowering blood pressure
Potassium	4700 mg
Calcium	1250 mg
Magnesium	500 mg
Fiber	30 g

Data from National Heart, Lung, and Blood Institute, 2006.

The most remarkable reductions in blood pressure were seen at the 1500 mg sodium per day level. The *2010 Dietary Guidelines for Americans* recommend sodium intake of no more than 1500 mg sodium per day for African Americans, people aged 51 years and older, and those with hypertension, diabetes, or chronic kidney disease.

The DASH diet eating pattern was designed to be reflective of commonly available foods, in the event that if the study results were positive (which they were), the nutrition recommendations would be easily accessible to the general population. The component of the DASH diet that represents the biggest change for most individuals is the fruits and vegetables aspect. DASH recommends eating four to five servings of fruits and four to five servings of vegetables per day (for a total of 8–10 servings of fruits and vegetables per day). This is a remarkably different approach to fruit and vegetable consumption than most patients, and most healthy individuals, are used to eating. This level of fruit and vegetable intake provides a significant amount of potassium, with minimal salt and calorie contributions. Further dietary recommendations for the DASH diet include eating 2–3 servings of low-fat dairy foods per day, no more than 2300 mg (2.3 grams) sodium per day, weight loss if necessary, and moderate physical activity (at least 3 times per week). This combination of approaches has been shown to lower systolic blood pressure by 4–12 mm Hg.[14] Table 5–17 outlines the food group components of the DASH eating pattern.[46] Table 5–18 offers servings per day on DASH at different calorie levels.[46]

Table 5-17. Sample DASH eating pattern.

Food Group	Servings Per Day	Serving Sizes	Examples & Notes
Grains (with an emphasis on whole grains)	6-8	1 slice bread 1 oz dry cereal 1/2 cup cooked rice, pasta, or cereal	Whole-wheat bread and rolls, whole-wheat pasta, English muffin, pita bread, bagel, cereals, grits, oatmeal, brown rice, unsalted pretzels, and popcorn
Vegetables	4-5	1 cup raw leafy vegetable 1/2 cup cut-up raw or cooked vegetable 1/2 cup vegetable juice	Broccoli, carrots, collards, green beans, green peas, kale, lima beans, potatoes, spinach, squash, sweet potatoes, and tomatoes
Fruits	4-5	1 medium fruit 1/4 cup dried fruit 1/2 cup fresh, frozen, or canned fruit 1/2 cup fruit juice	Apples, apricots, bananas, dates, grapes, oranges, grapefruit, grapefruit juice, mangoes, melons, peaches, pineapples, raisins, strawberries, and tangerines
Fat-free or low-fat dairy	2-3	1 cup milk or yogurt 1 1/2 oz cheese	Fat-free (skim) or low-fat (1%) milk or buttermilk, fat-free, low-fat, or reduced-fat cheese, fat-free or low-fat regular, or frozen yogurt
Lean meat, fish, or poultry	6 or less	1 oz cooked meats, poultry, or fish 1 egg (limit egg yolk intake to no more than 4 per week)	Select only lean; trim away visible fats; broil, roast, or poach; and remove skin from poultry

(continued)

Table 5–17. Sample DASH eating pattern. (*Continued*)

Food Group	Servings Per Day	Serving Sizes	Examples & Notes
Nuts, seeds, or legumes	4-5 per week	1/3 cup or 1 1/2 oz nuts 2 tablespoons peanut butter 2 tablespoons or 1/2 oz seeds 1/2 cup cooked legumes (dry beans and peas)	Almonds, hazelnuts, mixed nuts, peanuts, walnuts, sunflower seeds, peanut butter, kidney beans, lentils, and split peas
Fats and oils	2-3	1 tablespoon soft margarine 1 tablespoon vegetable oil 1 tablespoon mayonnaise 2 tablespoons salad dressing	Soft margarine, vegetable oil (such as canola, corn, olive, or safflower), low-fat mayonnaise, and light salad dressing
Sweets and added sugar	5 or less per week	1 tablespoon sugar 1 tablespoon jelly or jam 1/2 cup sorbet, gelatin 1 cup lemonade	Fruit-flavored gelatin, fruit punch, hard candy, jelly, maple syrup, sorbet and ices, and sugar

Data from National Heart, Lung, and Blood Institute, 2006.

Table 5–18. DASH eating plan for different calorie levels.

Calorie Level	Servings Per Day		
	1600 Per Day	2000 Per Day	3100 Per Day
Grains	6	10-11	12-13
Vegetables	3-4	5-6	6
Fruits	4	5-6	6
Fat-free or low-fat dairy	4	5-6	6
Lean meat, fish, or poultry	2-3	3	3-4
Nuts, seeds, or legumes	3/week	1	1
Fats and oils	2	3	4
Sweets and added sugar	0	≤2	≤2

Data from National Heart, Lung, and Blood Institute, 2006.

- JNC 7 Summary Recommendations

The Seventh Report of the Joint National Committee on Prevention, Detection, Evaluation, and Treatment of High Blood Pressure (JNC 7) provides a guideline for hypertension prevention and management that incorporates many of the recommendations covered in this section on Hypertension.[55] A reference card that summarizes the report findings for primary care practitioners is available at: http://www.nhlbi.nih.gov/guidelines/hypertension/jnc7card.htm. The report supports the approach that a 1600 mg sodium DASH eating plan has effects similar to single-drug therapy for the treatment of hypertension,[58] but that combinations of two (or more) lifestyle modifications can achieve even better results. Table 5–19 contains a list of lifestyle modifications from the JNC 7 and their approximate range of systolic blood pressure reduction.[55,57-63]

Patient Education Tools

There are a host of electronic and print tools available for practitioners to share with patients and clients who are interested in lowering their risk for heart disease and hypertension. Three primary areas for intervention include reading and deciphering of Nutrition Facts panel information, increasing preparation of home-made meals and snacks, and improving quality of choices when eating at restaurants or other establishments outside of home.

Table 5–19. Lifestyle modifications to manage hypertension.

Modification	Recommendation	Approximate Systolic Blood Pressure Reduction
Weight reduction	Maintain a normal body weight BMI: 18.5–24.9 kg/m²	5–20 mm Hg/10 kg weight loss
Follow DASH eating plan	Eat diet rich in fruits, vegetables, and low-fat dairy Reduce content of total fat and saturated fat	8–14 mm Hg
Dietary sodium restriction	Reduce dietary sodium intake to no more than 2.4 g sodium or 6 g salt (sodium chloride)	2–8 mm Hg
Physical activity	Engage in regular aerobic physical activity At least 30 minutes per day, most days of the week	4–9 mm Hg
Moderation of alcohol consumption	Limit consumption to no more than 2 drinks per day for most men and no more than 1 drink per day for women and lighter weight persons 1 drink = 12 oz beer, 5 oz wine, or 1.5 oz 80-proof hard alcohol	2–4 mm Hg

Data from The Trials of Hypertension Prevention Collaborative Research Group, 1997; He, Whelton, Appel, & Klag, 2000; Sacks et al., 2001; Chobanian, AV; Hill, M, 2000; Chobanian et al., 2003; Kelley & Kelley, 2000; Whelton, Chin, Xin, & He, 2002; and Xin, He, Frontini, Ogden, Motsamai, & Whelton, 2001.

■ Label Reading

As covered in Chapter 1, the Nutrition Facts panel contains a host of information, some of it useful, and some of it confusing. Individuals interested in reducing heart disease and hypertension risk are advised to seek information about the recommended serving size, total calories, fat grams, saturated and *trans* fat grams, cholesterol, sodium, and dietary fiber contents of foods. Not all fat and sodium labeling terms are created equal. While a food that claims to be "low-sodium" might sound the same as a "reduced-sodium" food, they are actually distinct claims with specific and separated guidelines mandated by the FDA. Tables 5–20 and 5–21 contain information about what the various sodium- and fat-related claims on food packaging mean. Helping clients and patients understand these claims increases their self-efficacy in selecting heart-healthier food options.[46]

Table 5–20. Sodium labeling language.

Phrase	What it Means
Sodium-free or salt-free	Less than 5 mg of sodium per serving
Very low sodium	35 mg or less of sodium per serving
Low sodium	140 mg or less of sodium per serving
Low-sodium meal	140 mg or less of sodium per 3½ oz (100 g)
Reduced or less sodium	At least 25% less sodium than the regular version
Light in sodium	50% less sodium than the regular version
Unsalted or no salt added	No salt added to the product during processing (this is not a sodium-free food)

Data from National Heart, Lung, and Blood Institute, 2006.

▪ Recipe Resources

Cooking and preparing meals and snacks at home is perhaps the most advisable recommendation for people looking to reduce their CVD risk (and many other chronic and weight-related disease risks for that matter). Cooking at home affords patients the opportunity to control the amount of added fat and sodium in their food, to manage portion sizes, and to improve their overall nutrition profile by increasing the number of servings of fruits and vegetables in their daily diet. Many recipe and cooking websites, magazines, and publications routinely list the nutrition content of their recipes, which is helpful for determining how certain dishes fit into a larger meal plan.

Table 5–21. Fat labeling language.

Phrase	What it Means
Fat-free	Less than 0.5 g fat per serving
Low saturated fat	1 g or less per serving and 15% or less of calories from saturated fat
Low fat	3 g or less per serving
Reduced fat	At least 25% less fat than the regular version
Light in fat	Half the fat compared to the regular version

Data from National Heart, Lung, and Blood Institute, 2006.

The American Heart Association's *"Delicious Decisions"* website is an excellent resource for finding heart-healthy recipes. The site features a Nutrition Center with information about healthy diet goals, as well as a vast repository of heart-healthy recipes. In addition, the AHA has published numerous cookbooks for both general information and special diets that contain nutrition information for the published recipes.

■ Restaurant Resources

While preparing and eating foods at home affords individuals the most control over the content of their diet, the reality is, people eat out. Thankfully, public health organizations and the general public are increasingly pressuring restaurants to post the nutrition information for their menu items. While this information has historically been relegated to hidden parts of difficult-to-navigate restaurant websites, emerging legislation and technology is heightening the visibility of such information. Mobile apps, menu boards, printed menus, and tray cards are now routinely listing calories, fat grams, and sodium, among other dietary components.

When working with clients and patients, ask questions about the restaurants that they frequently visit. What food items do they order? Are they aware of the nutrition content of these items? Do they know where to go to look up the nutrition information of their commonly ordered menu options? In addition to the individual restaurant's website or mobile application, another good resource for finding healthy options at restaurants is the website www.HealthyDiningFinder.com. *Healthy Dining Finder* works directly with restaurants to help identify both healthy dining choices and sodium savvy menu items. Although eating at restaurants on a regular basis can sabotage a well-intended meal plan, there is almost always something that represents a better-for-you option at today's restaurants; the key is putting your patients and clients in touch with the information that they need to make heart-healthier selections.

Coronary Artery Bypass Graft (CABG)

For a patient who has just undergone coronary artery bypass graft (CABG) surgery, the nutrition therapy guidelines are similar to those of other surgical procedures. In the initial stages, the primary goals are to promote wound healing and recovery from surgery with adequate nutrition, and secondarily, to lower LDL cholesterol levels to prevent the restenosis of blood vessels. Other immediate factors that may negatively impact nutrition status include long duration of intubation (which affects swallowing capacity), anorexia associated with polypharmacy, depression or anxiety, and changes in bowel patterns that mandate alterations of fluid regimens.

Nutrition recommendations for the post-CABG patient follow the TLC diet recommendations: less than 7% of daily total energy from saturated fat and *trans* fat, cholesterol less than 200 mg per day, 25–35% total calories from fat including omega-3 fatty acids in place of saturated fat, 50–60% of total calories from carbohydrate, and approximately 15% of total energy from protein. Additionally, fiber should be at 25–30 grams per day with at least half from soluble fiber, plant stanol/sterols (2 grams per day) given as an option, and moderate exercise to expend at least 200 kcal per day. When indicated (in patients with hypertension or to control edema), a sodium restriction of 1500–2300 mg per day may be warranted. Fluid should be given at 35 mL/kg body weight, with adjustments made for edema and increased fluid intake that should accompany increases in dietary fiber consumption.[7]

Practitioners are advised to acknowledge that the inpatient setting is not the most ideal for in-depth nutrition education following a CABG. Individuals who have just undergone a CABG are sick, stressed, may be malnourished, and are preoccupied with many emotions about their own mortality and future quality of life. In the immediate period following the surgery, the medical team should work to maximize nutrition and hydration status and, when appropriate, follow up with an outpatient referral to discuss lifestyle and diet changes that can be made to help prevent further complications of heart disease.

With regards to long-term goals, the guidelines of a standard heart-healthy diet are applicable to the patient who has recently undergone coronary artery bypass graft (CABG) surgery. Diet therapy for the post-CABG patient includes lowering saturated fat, *trans* fat, and dietary cholesterol intake. Therapeutic options such as adding more soluble fiber, or plant stanols and plant sterols, are recommended, as is inclusion of physical activity, when indicated and safe for the patient.[7] As mentioned, all of the principles of the *Therapeutic Lifestyle Changes* (TLC) diet and the nutrition guidelines for lowering LDL and raising HDL are applicable in the long-term for the post-CABG patient.

Heart Failure

Roughly half of heart failure patients are malnourished.[64] Worsening heart failure and shortness of breath cause fatigue that interferes with adequate intake at mealtime. Reduced blood flow to all tissues, including the GI tract, leads to delayed gastric emptying and feelings of fullness, and multiple medications may lead to the loss of certain water-soluble vitamins and minerals, such as riboflavin, vitamin B_6, and thiamin.

The nutrition guidelines of most importance in heart failure include fluid, sodium, alcohol, and total calories. There is an inherent conflict with the implementation of many nutrition guidelines in heart failure:

Table 5–22. Diet therapy for heart failure.

Sodium	<2 g/day for patients with moderate to severe heart failure
Protein	1.37 g/kg in clinically-stable, protein-depleted heart failure patients 1.12 g/kg in adequately nourished
Fluid restriction	<2 L/day for patients with serum sodium <130 mEq/L
Thiamin and potassium	Supplement as needed to compensate for losses in patients on diuretics
Folate, vitamin B-12, and magnesium	Meet DRI for age/gender (see Appendix A)
Alcohol	Limit to 1 drink per day for women and 2 drinks per day for men if alcohol not contraindicated; if alcohol is causative factor of heart failure, abstain

Data from Academy of Nutrition and Dietetics, 2012.

Table 5–23. Nutrition related lab values to monitor in heart failure.

B-type natriuretic peptide (BNP)	Cardiac neurohormone that is the most accurate predictor of heart failure; BNP is high in heart failure BNP is lower in men than in women, inversely related to body weight and increases with age
Serum potassium and sodium	When sodium level drops, initiate fluid restriction
Serum albumin	Easily affected by fluid status, hepatic proteins may be better indicators of protein and nutrition status, as is prealbumin
Serum prealbumin	Use as a marker of visceral protein status; less easily affected by hydration and fluid status than serum albumin

Data from King, Casey, & Rodenberg; Fuhrman, Charney, & Mueller, 2004; and Academy of Nutrition and Dietetics, 2011.

in individuals who are significantly malnourished, overly strict sodium and fluid guidelines can further impede adequate nutrient intake. When not interfering with adequate caloric intake levels, sodium should be limited to less than 2000 mg (2 grams) per day.[14] Fluid restrictions of 2000 mL (2 L) or less are indicated in mild heart failure, with more severe fluid limitations of 1000–1500 mL per day required for diuresis.[65] Protein should be given at a level of 1.37 g/kg in clinically stable, protein-depleted heart failure patients, and 1.12 g/kg in those who are adequately nourished. Because the heart failure patient is in a state of negative nitrogen balance, his or her protein needs will exceed those of the healthy population.[66] Thiamin and potassium should be supplemented, as needed, to compensate for those who are on diuretics. Alcohol should be limited to no more than one drink per day for women and two drinks per day for men, with full elimination recommended in those for whom alcohol has been a contributing factor to the heart failure (Table 5–22).[66]

■ Monitoring Lab Values

Practitioners of patients with heart failure are advised to monitor the laboratory values outlined in Table 5–23.[14,67,68]

References

1. Minino A, Murphy S, Xu J, Kochanek K. Deaths: final data for 2008. Natl Vital Stat Rep 2011;59(10):1–126.

2. Heidenreich P, Trogdon J, Khavjou OA. Forecasting the future of cardio-vascular disease in the United States: a policy statement from the American Heart Association. Circulation 2011;123:933–944.

3. Centers for Disease Control and Prevention. (2012, March 23). Heart Disease. Retrieved April 23, 2012 from Heart Disease Facts: http://www.cdc.gov/heartdisease/facts.htm

4. US Department of Health and Human Services. Your Guide to Lowering Your Cholesterol with TLC. National Institutes of Health, National Heart, Lung, and Blood Institute. Bethesda, MD: NIH; 2005.

5. US Department of Health and Human Services. (2008, October 17). Physical Activity Guidelines for Americans. Retrieved April 23, 2012 from At-A-Glance: A Fact Sheet for Professionals: http://www.health.gov/paguidelines/factsheetprof.aspx; US Department of Health and Human Services. (2008, November 21). Physical Activity Guidelines for Americans. Retrieved April 25, 2012 from Frequently Asked Questions: http://health.gov/paguidelines/faqs.aspx

6. US Department of Agriculture and US Department of Health and Human Services. Dietary Guidelines for Americans, 2010. 7th ed. Washington, DC: US Government Printing Office; 2011.

7. Academy of Nutrition and Dietetics. (2012). Cardiovascular Disease. Retrieved May 6, 2012 from Nutrition Care Manual: http://www.nutrition caremanual.org

8. Grundy S. Nutrition and diet in the management of hyperlipidemia and atherosclerosis. In: Shils M, Olson J, Shike M, Ross A. Modern Nutrition in Health and Disease. Baltimore, MD: Williams & Wilkins; 1999:1199–1216.

9. Rader D. Lipoprotein metabolism. In: Carson J, Burke F, Hark L. Cardiovascular Nutrition: Disease Prevention and Management. Chicago, IL: American Dietetic Association; 2004.

10. Grundy S, Cleeman J, Bairey Merz C, Brewer H, Clark L, Hunninghake D, et al. Implications of Recent Clinical Trials for the National Cholesterol Education Program Adult Treatment Panel III Guidelines. Circulation; 2004.

11. Expert Panel on Detection, Evaluation, and Treatment of High Blood Cholesterol in Adults. Executive summary of the Third Report of the National Cholesterol Education Program (NCEP) Expert Panel on Detection, Evaluation, and Treatment of High Blood Cholesterol in Adults (Adult Treatment Panel III). JAMA 2001;285:2486–2497.

12. American Heart Association. (2012, October 11). About Cholesterol. Retrieved January 13, 2013 from Cholesterol: http://www.heart.org/HEARTORG/ Conditions/Cholesterol/AboutCholesterol/About-Cholesterol_UCM_ 001220_Article.jsp; American Heart Association. (2012, February 22). Lifestyle Changes. Retrieved April 23, 2012 from http://www.heart.org/ HEARTORG/Conditions/HeartAttack/PreventionTreatmentofHeartAttack/ Lifestyle-Changes_UCM_303934_Article.jsp

13. Carson J, Grundy S, Van Horn L, Stone N, Binkoski A, Kris-Etherton P. Medical nutrition therapy for the prevention and management of coronary heart disease. In: Carson J, Burke F, Hark L. Cardiovascular Nutrition: Disease Prevention and Management. Chicago, IL: American Dietetic Association; 2004:109–148.

14. Academy of Nutrition and Dietetics. (2011). Disorders of Lipid Metabolism, Evidence-Based Nutrition Practice Guidelines, Executive Summary of Guidelines. Retrieved May 5, 2012 from Evidence Analysis Library: http://andevidencelibrary.com

15. American Diabetes Association. (n.d.). Fats and Diabetes. Retrieved January 31, 2013, from Food & Fitness: http://www.diabetes.org/food-and-fitness/food/what-can-i-eat/fat-and-diabetes.html

16. National Cancer Institute. (2010, May 24). Risk Factor Monitoring and Methods. Retrieved March 23, 2012 from Top Food Sources of Saturated Fat among US Population, 2005-2006 NHANES: riskfactor.cancer.gov/ diet/foodsources/sat_fat/sf.html

17. Chung M, Lichtenstein A, Ip S, Lau J, Balk E. Comparability of methods for LDL subfraction determination: a systematic review. Atherosclerosis 2009;205(2):342–348.

18. Siri-Tarino P, Sun Q, Hu F, Krauss R. Saturated fat, carbohydrate, and cardiovascular disease. Am J Clin Nutr 2010;91(3):502–509.

19. Ip S, Lichtenstein A, Chung M, Lau J, Balk E. Systematic review: association of low-density lipoprotein subfractions with cardiovascular outcomes. Ann Intern Med 2009; 150(7):474–484.

20. Ascherio A, Hennekens C, Buring J, Master C, Stampfer M, Willett W. Trans-fatty acids intake and risk of myocardial infarction. Circulation 1994; 89:94–101.

21. Willett W, Stampfer M, Manson J, Colditz G, Speizer F, Rosner B, et al. Intake of trans fatty acids and risk of coronary heart disease among women. Lancet 1993;341:581–585.

22. Remig V, Franklin B, Margolis S, Kostas G, Nece T, Street J. Trans fats in America: a review of their use, consumption, health implications, and regulation. J Am Diet Assoc 2010;110(4):585–592.

23. US Department of Agriculture Agriculture Research Service. (n.d.). National Nutrient Database for Standard Reference. Retrieved January 13, 2013 from Nutrient Data Laboratory: http://ndb.nal.usda.gov/ndb/foods/list

24. Li B, Andrews K, Pehrsson P. Individual sugars, soluble, and insoluble dietary fiber contents of 70 high consmption foods. Journal of Food Composition and Analysis 2002;15(6):715–723.

25. Quaker Oats Company. (2012). Quick Oats. Retrieved January 13, 2013 from Quaker Oats: http://www.quakeroats.com/products/hot-cereals/quick-oats.aspx

26. Katan M, Grundy S, Jones P, Law M, Miettinen T, Paoletti R, et al. Efficacy and safety of plant stanols and sterols in the management of blood cholesterol levels. Mayo Clin Proc 2003;78(8):965–978.

27. National Heart, Lung and Blood Institute. Third Report of the Expert Panel on Detection, Evaluation, and Treatment of High Blood Cholesterol in Adults (Adult Treatment Panel III). National Institutes of Health; 2001.

28. Eckel R. The metabolic syndrome. In: Longo D, Fauci A K, Hauser S, Jameson J, Loscalzo J. Harrison's Principles of Internal Medicine. 18th ed. 2012 [chapter 242].

29. AIM-HIGH Investigators: Boden WP, ANderson T, Chaitman B, Desvignes-Nickens P, Koprowicz K, McBride R, et al. Niacin in patients with low hdl cholesterol levels receiving intensive statin therapy. N Engl J Med 2011; 365(24):2255–2267.

30. Durstine J, Thompson P. Exercise in the treatment of lipid disorders. Cardiol Clin 2001;19:471–488.

31. Centers for Disease Control and Prevention. (2011, December 1). How much physical activity do adults need? Retrieved January 31, 2013, from Physical Activity: http://www.cdc.gov/physicalactivity/everyone/guidelines/adults.html

32. De Oliveria E Silva E, Foster D, McGree HM, Seldman C, Smith J, Breslow J, et al. Alcohol consumption raises HDL cholesterol levels by increasing the transport rate of apolipoproteins A-I and A-II. Circulation 2000;102(19):2347–2352.

33. US Department of Health and Human Services. (n.d.). National Institutes of Health, National Institute on Alcohol Abuse and Alcoholism. Retrieved April 25, 2012 from What's a "standard" drink?: http://rethinkingdrinking.niaaa.nih.gov/WhatCountsDrink/WhatsAstandardDrink.asp

34. US Department of Health and Human Services. ATP III At-A-Glance: Quick Desk Reference. National Institutes of Health, National Heart Lung and Blood Institute. NHLBI; 2001.

35. US Department of Health and Human Services. (n.d.). National Institutes of Health, National Heart Lung and Blood Institute. Retrieved April 25, 2012 from Metabolic Syndrome, Treatment: http://www.nhlbi.nih.gov/health//dci/Diseases/ms/ms_treatments.html

36. Austin M, Hokanson J, Edwards K. Hypertriglyceridemia as a cardiovascular risk factor. Am J Cariol 1998;81:7B–12B.

37. Miller M, Stone N, Ballantyne C, Bittner V, Criqui M, Ginsberg HG, et al. Triglycerides and cardiovascular disease: a scientific statement from the American Heart Association. Circulation 2011;123:2292–2333.

38. Arima H, Barzi F, Chalmers J. Mortality patterns in hypertension. J Hypertens 2011;29(suppl 1):S3–S7.

39. World Health Organization. (2012, May 16). World Health Statistics 2012. Retrieved January 13, 2013 from Global Health Observatory (GHO): http://www.who.int/gho/publications/world_health_statistics/2012/en/

40. Centers for Disease Control and Prevention. (2011, February 23). CDC Features, Data & Statistics by Date. Retrieved April 25, 2012 from Americans Consume Too Much Sodium (Salt): http://www.cdc.gov/Features/dsSodium/

41. Institute of Medicine. A Population-Based Policy and Systems Change Approach to Prevent and Control Hypertension. Board on Population Health and Public Health Practice. National Academy of Sciences.

42. Academy of Nutrition and Dietetics. (n.d.). Recommendations Summary Hypertension (HTN) Alcohol Consumption. Retrieved January 13, 2013 from Evidence Analysis Library: http://www.andevidencelibrary.com

43. Mattes R, Donnelly D. Relative contributions of dietary sodium sources. J Am Coll Nutr 1991;10(4):383–393.

44. Centers for Disease Control and Prevention. (2012, February). Where's the sodium? There's too much in many common foods. Vital Signs; Centers for Disease Control and Prevention, National Center for Health Statistics. (2012, January 27). FastStats. Retrieved April 25, 2012 from Hypertension (U.S.): HYPERLINK "http://www.cdc.gov/nchs/fastats/hyprtens.htm" http://www.cdc.gov/nchs/fastats/hyprtens.htm

45. Gerontological Nutritionists. (2000). Gerontological Nutritionists. Retrieved January 13, 2013 from Diet and Disease: http://www2.fiu.edu/~gn/Resources/DietandDisease.htm

46. National Heart, Lung, and Blood Institute. (2006, April). Your Guide to Lowering Your Blood Pressure With DASH. Retrieved January 13, 2013 from DASH Diet: www.nhlbi.nih.gov/health/public/heart/hbp/dash/new_dash.pdf

47. Houston M. The importance of potassium in managing hypertension. Curr Hypertens Rep 2011;13(4):309–317.

48. Karppanen H, Karppanen P, Mervalla E. Why and how to implement sodium, potassium, calcium, and magnesium changes in food items and diets? J Hum Hypertens 2005;19(suppl 3):S10–S19.

49. Suter P, Sierro C, Vetter W. Nutritional factors in the control of blood pressure and hypertension. Nutr Clin Care 2002;5(1):9–19.

50. National Institutes of Health. (2010, Spring/Summer). Tasty Stand-Ins for Salt. NIH Medline Plus, b (2), p. 15.

51. AllRecipes.com. (n.d.). Spicy Herb Seasoning. Retrieved January 13, 2013 from AllRecipes: http://allrecipes.com/recipe/spicy-herb-seasoning/detail.aspx

52. Chen L, Davey Smith G, Harbord R, Lewis S. Alcohol intake and blood pressure: a systematic review implementing a Mendelian randomization approach. PLoS Med 2008;5(3):e52.

53. US Department of Agriculture and U.S. Department of Health and Human Services. (2011). Report of the Dietary Guidelines Advisory Committee on the Dietary Guidelines for Americans, 2010.

54. National Heart, Lung and Blood Institute. JNC 7 Complete Report: The Science Behind the New Guidelines. The Seventh Report of the Joint National Committee on Prevention, Detection, Evaluation, and Treatment of High Blood Pressure - Complete Report. NHLBI; 2004.

55. Chobanian A, Bakris G, Black H, Cushman W, Green L, Izzo JJ, et al. The Seventh Report of the Joint National Committee on Prevention, Detection, Evaluation, and Treatment of High Blood Pressure: the JNC 7 report. JAMA 2003;289(19):2560–2572.

56. Institute of Medicine. Dietary Reference Intakes for Calcium and Vitamin D. Washington, DC: National Academies Press; 2010.

57. Sacks F, Svetkey L, Vollmer W, Appel L, Bra G, Harsha D, et al. Effects on blood pressure of reduced dietary sodium and the Dietary Approaches to Stop Hypertension (DASH) diet. DASH-Sodium Collaborative Research Group. N Engl J Med 2001;344(1):3–10.

58. The Trials of Hypertension Prevention Collaborative Research Group. Effects of weight loss and sodium reduction intervention on blood pressure and hypertension incidence in overweight people with high-normal blood pressure. The Trials of Hypertension Prevention, phase II. The Trials of Hypertension Prevention Collaborative Research Group. Arch Intern Med 1997;157:657–667.

59. He J, Whelton P, Appel LC, Klag M. Long-term effects of weight loss and dietary sodium reduction on incidence of hypertension. Hypertension 2000;35:544–549.

60. Chobanian AV, Hill M. National Heart, Lung, and Blood Institute workshop on sodium and blood pressure: a critical review of current scientific evidence. Hypertension 2000;35(4):858–863.

61. Kelley G, Kelley K. Progressive resistance exercise and resting blood pressure: a meta-analysis of randomized controlled trials. Hypertension 2000;35(3):838–843.

62. Whelton S, Chin A, Xin X, He J. Effect of aerobic exercise on blood pressure: a meta-analysis of randomized, controlled trials. Ann Intern Med 2002;136(7):493–503.

63. Xin X, He J, Frontini M, Ogden L, Motsamai O, Whelton P. Effects of alcohol reduction on blood pressure: a meta-analysis of randomized controlled trials. Hypertension 2001;38(5):1112–1117.

64. Grossniklaus D, O'Brien M, Clark P, Dunbar S. Nutrient intake in heart failure patients. J Cardiovasc Nurs 2008;23(4):357–363.

65. Hunt S, Abraham W, Chin M, Feldman A, Francis G, Ganiats T, et al. ACC/AHA guideline update for the diagnosis and management of chronic

heart failure in the adult: a report of the American College of Cardiology/ American Heart Association Task Force on Practice Guidelines. Circulation 2005;105:e154–e234.

66. Academy of Nutrition and Dietetics. (2012). Heart Failure. Retrieved May 6, 2012 from Nutrition Care Manual: http://www.nutritioncaremanual.org

67. King M, Casey B, Rodenberg R. Heart failure. In: South-Paul J, Matheny S, Lewis E. CURRENT Diagnosis & Treatment in Family Medicine. 3rd ed. Chapter 20. New York, NY: McGraw Hill 2011. Retrieved July 10, 2013 from http://www.accessmedicine.com/content.aspx?aID=8151689

68. Fuhrman M, Charney P, Mueller C. Hepatic proteins and nutrition assessment. J Am Diet Assoc 2004;104:1258–1264.

PWD = people with diabetes

6

A Not-So-Sweet Metabolic Disruption: Diabetes Mellitus

Medical Nutrition Therapy for Diabetes Mellitus: Prediabetes, Type 1, and Type 2

Diet therapy is considered to be the most important component for the treatment of diabetes mellitus.[1] Diet plays a critical role in preventing diabetes, managing existing diabetes, and preventing, or reducing, the potential complications related to poor glycemic, lipid, and blood pressure control. According to the *American Diabetes Association (ADA) Nutrition Recommendations and Interventions for Diabetes Position Statement*, diet therapy is important at all levels of diabetes prevention:

- *Primary prevention*—to prevent diabetes with the use of MNT and public health intervention in those with obesity and prediabetes
- *Secondary prevention*—to prevent complications with the use of MNT for metabolic control of diabetes, type 1, type 2, and gestational
- *Tertiary prevention*—to prevent morbidity and mortality with the use of MNT to delay and manage complications of diabetes, type 1, and type 2

Medical Nutrition Therapy (MNT) provided by a registered dietitian (RD) is recommended by both the ADA and the Academy of Nutrition and Dietetics (AND) for individuals with prediabetes, type 1, and type 2 diabetes, as well as in populations with special circumstances that are affected by metabolic and glycemic disruption.[2,3] It is recommended that an RD, knowledgeable and skilled in MNT, be the team member who plays the leading role in providing nutrition care; however, it is important that all team members be knowledgeable about MNT for diabetes and support its implementation.[4] Table 6–1 lists the recommended series of initial MNT encounters for the person with diabetes (PWD), type 1, or type 2.[3]

After the initial series, and based on the nutrition assessment of learning needs and progress toward desired outcomes, the practitioner can determine if additional diet therapy encounters are needed. Positive outcomes at 1 year and longer (ie, reduction in average glycosylated hemoglobin [HbA1c] levels, improved lipid profiles, improved weight management, adjustments in medications, and reduction in the risk for onset and progression of comorbidities) have been reported with an ongoing series of MNT encounters (Table 6–2). At least annually, a minimum of one follow-up MNT encounter is recommended in order

Table 6-1. Initial series of MNT encounters at diagnosis of diabetes or first referral.

Number of Encounters	Length of Time of MNT Sessions	Time Course to Completion of Series
3-4	45-90 minutes	3-6 months

Data from Academy of Nutrition and Dietetics, 2011.

to reinforce lifestyle changes and to evaluate and monitor outcomes that impact the need for changes in MNT or medication. The practitioner should then determine if additional MNT encounters are necessary.[3]

MNT is also an integral component of diabetes self-management education/training (DSME/T), both in the inpatient and/or in the outpatient settings. MNT is not synonymous with DSME/T; however, DSME/T is an education and training program that helps patients manage their diabetes, whereas MNT consists of more individualized diagnosis, therapy, and counseling related to nutrition.[5] DSME/T programs that are accredited by Medicare consist of 1 hour of individualized assessment and 9 hours of group classes. The "incorporation of nutritional management into lifestyle" is one of the content areas, among others, outlined in the DSME/T curriculum, that are less nutrition-related such as "using medications safely and for maximum therapeutic effectiveness."[5,6]

DSME/T teaches individuals about the interplay among MNT, physical activity, emotional stress, physical stress, and medications, and it is guided by evidence-based standards. In addition, DSME/T helps PWD respond appropriately and consistently to all of these factors, in order to achieve and maintain optimal glycemic control. DSME/T is a critical part of diabetes care, and medical treatment without it is considered inadequate.[7] However, while DSME/T is considered necessary, it is not sufficient for patients to sustain a lifetime of diabetes self-care because initial improvements in metabolic and other outcomes diminish after approximately 6 months. Therefore, most patients will need ongoing diabetes self-management support (DSMS) in order to sustain behavior

Table 6-2. Ongoing series of MNT encounters.

Number of Encounters	Length of Time of MNT Sessions	Time Course to Completion of Series
1-5 individuals or 6-12 group sessions	45-90 minutes	≥1 year and then annually at a minimum or once per month, thereafter for sustained positive outcomes

Data from Academy of Nutrition and Dietetics, 2011.

at the level of self-management needed to effectively manage diabetes.[7] MNT for diabetes patients can be administered only by a licensed/certified registered dietitian or nutritional professional, whereas DSME/T can be administered by a number of qualified healthcare professionals, provided that at least one of the instructors is a registered nurse, dietitian, or pharmacist.[5,6]

■ Effectiveness of Medical Nutrition Therapy for Diabetes Mellitus

The HbA1c is the clinical outcome indicator used to determine the effectiveness of MNT for type 1 and type 2 diabetes. Other outcome indicators include lipid profiles, blood pressure, weight management, adjustment in medications, and reduction in the risk for onset and progression of comorbidities.[4] Studies, both for MNT and for MNT in combination with DMST, have documented decreases in HbA1c ranging from 0.5% to 2.6% (average of ~1% to 2%), which is similar to the effects of many glucose-lowering medications.[4] Although found to be effective at any time in the disease process, MNT appears to have its greatest effect in lowering HbA1c at initial diagnosis.[4,5,7]

Impaired fasting glucose (IFG) and/or impaired glucose tolerance (IGT) are the indicators used for assessing prediabetes.[7,8] In addition, the HbA1c is also now being used as an indicator for prediabetes.[8] Using MNT and lifestyle modification has been shown to reduce the development of diabetes by intervening before its onset.[5,7] In both the Finnish Diabetes Prevention Study (DPS) and the US Diabetes Prevention Program (DPP) lifestyle studies, the development of diabetes was reduced by 58% over 3 years due to intensive lifestyle intervention. Rates remained 39% lower 4 years after completion of the DPS, in association with an increase in physical activity.[5,7]

The body of evidence pointing to the effectiveness of MNT in treating and preventing type 2 diabetes in adults continues to grow. Adapted from the results of the DPS, the Look AHEAD (Action for Health in Diabetes) study is currently underway to test the effects of similar lifestyle interventions in individuals who have already been diagnosed with type 2 diabetes.[9] This trial is planned to extend for 11.5 years; however, in 2009, the researchers published 1-year results in which the intensive lifestyle intervention group lost 8.6% of initial weight compared to 0.7% in the control group.[5,9] Comprehensive diet counseling by an RD was included in the lifestyle intervention, compared to the control group that received basic or "usual" care for diabetes. Significantly greater decreases in HbA1c, systolic and diastolic blood pressure, and triglyceride levels were also observed in the intervention group compared to the control group.[5,9]

By 6 weeks to 3 months, outcomes of MNT interventions are evident and evaluation should be done at these times. If no clinical improvement in glycemic control is evident at 3 months, the practitioner should consider combining MNT with medication therapy, or make an adjustment in medication therapy. Because of the progressive nature of type 2 diabetes, beta-cell function decreases and blood glucose lowering medication(s) may need to be combined with MNT to achieve glycemic goals.[4]

■ Goals of Medical Nutrition Therapy for Diabetes Mellitus

For individuals at risk for diabetes or with prediabetes, MNT goals are to decrease the risk of diabetes and cardiovascular disease (CVD) by promoting healthy food choices and physical activity leading to moderate weight loss that is maintained.[2] Although the etiologies of type 1 and type 2 diabetes differ, MNT goals for both are similar:

- To achieve and maintain blood glucose levels in the normal range or as close to normal as is safely possible, to achieve and maintain a lipid and lipoprotein profile that reduces the risk for vascular disease, and to achieve and maintain blood pressure levels in the normal range or as close to normal as possible
- To prevent or slow the rate of development of the chronic complications of diabetes by modifying nutrient intake and lifestyle
- To address individual nutrition needs, taking into account personal and cultural preferences and willingness to change
- To maintain the pleasure of eating by only limiting food choices when indicated by scientific evidence

Medical Nutrition Therapy for Diabetes Mellitus: Assessment and Monitoring Parameters

The process of MNT for diabetes must first begin with a comprehensive assessment of the individual's nutrition status (see Chapter 2). The individual's diabetes status that is relative to MNT also involves a comprehensive evaluation that begins with investigation of the individual's food intake (initially focusing on carbohydrate intake), their glycemic control, their metabolic control (anthropometric measurements, lipids, and blood pressure), as well as an evaluation of their diabetes medications and physical activity patterns. This information will serve as the basis for implementation of the nutrition prescription, as well as for ongoing monitoring and management of the PWD.[10]

■ Food Intake Assessment and Monitoring

An understanding of the patient's usual personal food habits is required to determine the appropriate approach and individualization for meal planning. Information that is useful includes the following:

- Present and past nutrition interventions
- Present and past meal-planning methods
- Home/family circumstances
- Methods of food preparation
- Food shopping practices

- Dining out approaches
- Use of alcohol
- Use of nutritional supplements
- Issues of disordered eating
- Nutrition history (24-hour recall, usual food intake, food frequency, and/or food records)
- Psychosocial/economic issues (living situation, finances, educational background, and employment)

■ Glycemic Assessment and Monitoring

Glycemic control should be assessed by the practitioner, with the resulting focus of MNT on the achievement of glucose levels in the target range.[3] Current glycemic control standards of three major national diabetes organizations are depicted in Table 6–3.[10-12] Although all three organizations agree on the importance of glycemic control, slight differences are apparent, with the American College of Endocrinology (ACE) being the most aggressive.

Determinants of glycemic control, with the primary determinant being the amount of dietary carbohydrate, include the following[10]:

- Amount of dietary carbohydrate
- Rate of nutrient digestion and absorption
- Insulin resistance and/or secretion
- Type of source of carbohydrate
- Style of food preparation
- Ripeness of food
- Degree of food processing
- Macronutrient distribution

In PWD who have defects in insulin action (insulin resistance), insulin secretion, or both, postprandial glucose response to carbohydrate is impaired.[2] If the PWD has long-term complications from diabetes

Table 6–3. National diabetes' groups glycemic control parameters.

Glycemic Parameter	AAFP	ADbA	ACE
HbA1c	—	7%	6.5%
Fasting glucose	80–120 mg	70–130 mg	≤110 mg
Postprandial glucose	<180 mg	<180 mg	≤140 mg
Bedtime glucose	100–140 mg		
3 am glucose	70–110 mg		

Data from American Academy of Family Physicians, 2010; American Diabetes Association, 2013; American College of Endocrinology, 2002.

(eg, the autonomic neuropathic condition of gastroparesis), delayed digestion and absorption of nutrients will negatively affect glycemic control. The type or source of carbohydrates found in foods also influences postprandial glucose levels (eg, the type of starch [amylose versus amylopectin], style of preparation [cooking method and time, amount of heat or moisture used], ripeness, and degree of processing).[2] The macronutrient distribution of the meal may also influence glucose response.

HbA1c

The HbA1c is the laboratory test used to assess average blood glucose levels over the preceding 2–3 months, and has been shown to be a strong predictive value for diabetes complications.[10] All PWD should receive routine HbA1c testing at initial assessment and as part of continuing care. The frequency of testing the HbA1c should be determined by the clinical situation, the treatment method used, as well as clinical judgment. A twice-a-year testing may only be needed for patients with stable glycemia, whereas an unstable or highly intensely managed PWD may require testing more often than every 3 months. Point-of-care testing (availability of the HbA1c result at the time the patient is seen) has been shown to improve glycemic control due to improved intensification of therapy.[10] Certain conditions can affect the HbA1c results, and these variants (eg, hemolysis or blood loss) must be considered when the HbA1c does not correlate with the patient's clinical situation. In addition, because the HbA1c does not provide a measure of hypoglycemia or glycemic variability, self-monitoring of blood glucose (SMBG) testing should always be used in combination with the HbA1c.[10] The American Diabetes Association is now recommending the use of the term "estimated average glucose (eAG)," which allows the reporting of HbA1c results using the same units (mg/dL or mmol/L) that is routinely available with blood glucose measurements. The relationship between HbA1c and eAG is described by the formula $28.7 \times HbA1c - 46.7 = eAG$.[13] Table 6–4 lists the eAG calculations for a HbA1c value ranging from 6 to 12. A calculator for converting A1C results into estimated average glucose (eAG),[10,13] in either mg/dL or mmol/L, is also available at http://professional.diabetes.org/GlucoseCalculator.aspx.

Self-Monitoring Blood Glucose (SMBG)

Prior to the 1980s, urine was tested to indicate high blood glucose values.[4] Since then, single-point measurement of blood glucose and the laboratory value HbA1c have been used as measures of glycemic control in PWD. SMBG in PWD is an important step in diabetes MNT because the first goal for diabetes MNT is to achieve glycemic control. SMBG is, therefore, required to identify treatment needs, and then evaluate the effectiveness of the treatment plan.

Frequency and Timing of SMBG

For individuals receiving nutrition therapy alone or in combination with glucose-lowering medications, frequency and timing of SMBG

Table 6-4. Correlation of HbA1c with estimated average glucose (eAG).

HbA1c (%)	eAG Mg/dL	eAG Mmol/L
6	126	7.0
6.5	140	7.8
7	154	8.6
7.5	169	9.4
8	183	10.2
8.5	197	10.9
9	212	11.8
9.5	226	12.6
10	240	13.4
10.5	255	14.1
11	269	14.9
11.5	283	15.7
12	298	16.5

Data from Kahn and Fonseca, 2008; American Diabetes Association, 2013.

are dependent on the diabetes management goals and therapies (eg, MNT, diabetes medications, and physical activity). Improved glycemic control has been associated with SMBG when it is incorporated into diabetes education programs. The data collected from SMBG are used to make changes in diabetes management. More frequent SMBG may be indicated in persons experiencing unexplained elevations in HbA1c or unexplained hypoglycemia and hyperglycemia.

SMBG for those with Insulin Dependence

At least three to eight glucose tests per day (more in some insulin regimens) are recommended to determine the adequacy of the insulin dose(s) and to guide adjustments in insulin dose(s), food intake, and physical activity, for persons with type 1, type 2, or gestational diabetes on insulin therapy. Less frequent SMBG may be required once the insulin regimen is established. Improved glycemic control has been reported in intervention studies that included self-management training and adjustment of insulin doses.[4]

Methods of Interpreting SMBG Results

Methods for interpreting SMBG results include a manual review of the logbooks or diaries of the PWD, review of the memory histories, and computations from the individual's glucometer. Note that many glucometers can now be synced with computer software to electronically analyze past meter readings and trends. Whichever method is used, the goals of interpretation of SMBG results are to[14]:

- estimate the degree of blood glucose control and the variation during the day;
- identify the concerns of patient safety in regards to hypoglycemic trends and events;
- understand factors that may influence blood glucose control;
- assess strategies to help achieve improved blood glucose control; and
- reinforce to the PWD how the SMBG data are useful and valuable in their diabetes care.

Ideally, 1–2 weeks of SMBG results should be reviewed. During the review, the practitioner should first identify any episodes of hypoglycemia. The patient should be questioned on whether or not assistance by another individual was required to return to euglycemia, or if management with a fast-acting carbohydrate was adequate. In addition, the cause of the hypoglycemia should be identified, such as if it was the result of a delayed meal or overtreatment of hyperglycemia.[14]

The next step in interpreting SMBG results is to review its consistency and timing. Each time-specific SMBG average should be compared in order to help identify the lowest and highest average, and thus help in determining problem areas. The patient's schedule should be verified as part of the evaluation, because the meter or logbook may not reflect abnormal work schedules (eg, shift workers).[14]

The overall SMBG average and the variability throughout the day should also be assessed. The average should be compared to the HbA1c, as well as to previous results. If using data from an electronic meter download, the goal for an acceptable standard deviation, in the absence of hypoglycemia, is less than half of the average, and times where a higher standard deviation is observed, the data should be evaluated for explanations for the variability.[14]

Both positive and negative trends in basal and prandial control need to be evaluated. The fasting blood glucose is used to evaluate basal trends by comparing bedtime to morning blood glucose values. The prandial trends are evaluated using postmeal blood glucose, while establishing the patient's eating times and routines. For those patients taking insulin, the data should be evaluated for problems of overtreating hypoglycemia, problems with the correction dose, or insulin stacking. For these situations, it may be necessary to adjust the insulin by 10–20%.[14]

Continuous Glucose Monitoring Systems

Continuous glucose monitoring systems (CGMS) are the next generation of glucose monitors that measure glucose in interstitial fluid and provide readings every 5–10 minutes. In addition, they have alarms for high and low glucose readings, and the ability to download data

Table 6–5. Metabolic parameters to assess in diabetes.

Anthropometric	Cardiovascular	Renal
Body weight	High-density lipoprotein (HDL)	Serum creatinine (Cr)
Waist circumference	Low-density lipoprotein (LDL)	Urine albumin
Body mass index (BMI)	Triglycerides (TG)	Glomerular filtration rate (GFR)
	Blood pressure	Blood pressure

and track trends.[4] Persons who may benefit from CGMS include those experiencing unexplained elevations in HbA1c or unexplained hypoglycemia and hyperglycemia. The accuracy of CGMS has been clearly proven, and the trend/data pattern shows less glucose variability and improved glucose control.[4] However, CGMS does not eliminate the need for SMBG because calibration of the CGMS sensors is based on SMBG, and acute treatment decisions should be based on SMBG.

■ Metabolic Assessment and Monitoring

The metabolic parameters to assess in PWD other than blood glucose and HbA1c are listed in Table 6–5.

Anthropometric Parameters

Overweight and obesity are closely linked to type 2 diabetes; therefore, MNT must serve an integral role in its prevention and treatment. As reviewed in Table 6–6, overweight is defined by a BMI ≥25 kg/m² and obesity as BMI ≥30 kg/m², and the risk of comorbidity associated with excess adipose tissue increases with a BMI in these ranges.[2,15] Visceral fat, measured by waist circumference (also listed in Table 6–6), is used in conjunction with BMI to assess risk of type 2 diabetes and CVD.[15] A primary role in the development of type 2 diabetes is believed to be the independent and synergistic relationship between obesity, particularly central obesity (abdominal adiposity), and type 2 diabetes that results in insulin resistance with hyperinsulinemia.[16] A waist circumference ≥35 inches in women and ≥40 inches in men is considered high to extremely high risk.[15] However, in some Asian populations, the risk for type 2 diabetes and CVD appears significant at a BMI of >23 kg/m² and lower waist circumference cut points in Asian populations (≤31 inches in women, and ≤35 inches in men) may be appropriate.[2,17]

The increased risk of type 2 diabetes with increases in body weight has been demonstrated in epidemiological studies. In the Nurses' Health Study, a large prospective cohort study that involved over 121,000 female registered nurses aged 30–55 years, a BMI as low as 22 was found to increase the risk for diabetes. Women with a healthy

Table 6-6. Classification of overweight and obesity by BMI, waist circumference, and associated disease risk.

			Disease Risk[a]	
	BMI (kg/m²)	Obesity Class	WC: Men ≥40 inches Women ≤35 inches	WC: Men ≤40 inches Women ≥35 inches
Underweight	<18.5			
Normal	18.5-24.9			
Overweight	25.0-29.9		Increased	High
Obesity	30.0-34.9	I	High	Very high
	35.0-39.9	II	Very high	Very high
Extreme obesity	≥40	III	Extremely high	Extremely high

WC, waist circumference.

[a]Disease risk for type 2 diabetes, hypertension, and CVD.

Data from National Heart, Lung, and Blood Institute (NHLBI), 1998.

BMI of 24.0–24.9 had up to a five-fold elevated risk when compared with women with a BMI <22. Risk of type 2 diabetes increased by more than 40-fold in those with a BMI >31. Similar results were observed in men from the Professionals' Health Study, which included more than 51,000 U.S. male health professionals, aged 40–75 years. Men with a BMI of 35 were found to have a relative risk of diabetes 42 times higher than that in men with a BMI <23. In addition, when controlling for BMI at 21 years of age, family history, age, and smoking habits, men who gained ≥15 kilograms (33 lb) after age 21 years had 8.9 times higher risk of diabetes than those who were within 2 kilograms (~4.5 lb) of their weight at age 21 years.[16]

There is no question that any intervention that produces weight loss will improve insulin sensitivity because insulin resistance is an adaptation of obesity.[16] Enhancement of glucose metabolism and a reduction of lipid oxidation result from a reduction of fat mass that occurs with weight loss. After weight loss, insulin secretion and plasma insulin concentrations have been shown to decrease substantially.[16] Short-term studies have demonstrated that moderate weight loss (5% of body weight) in subjects with type 2 diabetes is associated with decreased insulin resistance, improved measures of glycemia and lipemia, and reduced blood pressure.[10]

Modest weight loss has been shown to improve glycemic outcomes and contributes to beneficial effects on blood pressure and blood lipids in individuals with type 2 diabetes and insulin resistance; therefore, modest weight loss is recommended for all such individuals who have, or are at, risk for diabetes.[2,4] Unfortunately, weight loss is less likely to be effective in improving glycemic outcomes as the disease progresses and as insulin deficiency, compared to insulin resistance, becomes more prominent.[4] This likely occurs because the central nervous system plays an important role in regulating energy intake and expenditure.[2] Additional antidiabetes medications combined with MNT are necessary, and prevention of weight gain becomes important with insulin deficiency.[4]

A realistic weight loss goal from lifestyle interventions is 5–10% of body weight.[4] A reduced energy intake with reduced total and saturated fats, an increase in dietary fiber and whole grains, and a decrease in sodium are nutritional interventions that are supported by the literature. In addition, physical activity is especially important for its contribution to weight maintenance after weight loss, and thus should be strongly encouraged.[4] However, research on sustained weight loss interventions lasting 1 year or longer resulted in inconsistent effects on the HgbA1c.[10] Although the literature shows inconsistent effects of weight loss on HbA1c, it is important to realize that attrition in lifestyle trials that are 1 year and longer can be a problem, thus making it more difficult to translate research findings to clinical practice.[4] Chapter 3 covers in more detail the various evidence-based dietary interventions for promoting weight loss, which are applicable to most PWD.

■ Cardiovascular Parameters

Patients with type 2 diabetes have an increased prevalence of dyslipidemia, hypertension, atherosclerosis, metabolic syndrome, and polycystic ovary syndrome that are linked to insulin resistance and contribute to their risk of cardiovascular disease (CVD).[10,16] Low levels of HDL cholesterol, often associated with elevated triglyceride levels, are the most prevalent pattern of dyslipidemia in persons with type 2 diabetes.[10] Studies have shown that lifestyle interventions improved several CVD risk factors, including dyslipidemia, hypertension, and inflammatory markers.[2] These same lifestyle interventions have also demonstrated a positive effect on glycemic control.[10] As mentioned in Chapter 5, MNT and lifestyle interventions for improving dyslipidemia involve[10]:

- reductions in saturated fat;
- reduction/elimination of *trans* fat;
- reduction in cholesterol intake;
- increase of omega-3 fatty acids;
- increase in viscous (soluble) fiber (oats, legumes, and citrus);
- increase in plant stanols/sterols;
- weight loss;
- increased physical activity; and
- smoking cessation.

Table 6-7. Blood lipid goals.

LDL Cholesterol	HDL Cholesterol	Triglycerides
Persons WITHOUT overt CVD <100 mg/dL (2.6 mmol/L)	*In men* >40 mg/dL (1.0 mmol/L)	<150 mg/dL (1.7 mmol/L)
Persons WITH overt CVD <70 mg/dL (1.8 mmol/L)	*In women* >50 mg/dL (1.3 mmol/L)	

Data from American Diabetes Association, 2013.

Saturated fat intake should be <7% of total calories, and reducing intake of *trans* fat lowers LDL cholesterol and increases HDL cholesterol.[10] Glycemic control can also beneficially modify plasma lipid levels. Table 6–7 lists the blood lipid goals to reduce the risk of CVD.[10] The first priority of dyslipidemia therapy for most PWD is to lower LDL cholesterol to a target of <100 mg/dL (2.6 mmol/L), unless severe hypertriglyceridemia is the immediate issue. Regardless of baseline lipid levels, statin pharmacological therapy should be added to lifestyle therapy for PWD with overt CVD, and in those without CVD who are greater than 40 years of age and have one or more other CVD risk factors.[10]

Hypertension, which is predictive of the progression of micro- and macrovascular complications of diabetes, can also be prevented and managed through MNT and lifestyle interventions. According to the ADA, MNT and lifestyle interventions for decreasing blood pressure include[10]:

- weight loss;
- moderation of alcohol intake;
- regular aerobic physical activity;
- smoking cessation; and
- *Dietary Approaches to Stop Hypertension* (DASH, see Chapter 5) style dietary pattern that includes less than 1500 milligrams of sodium per day, increased potassium intake through 8–10 servings of fruits and vegetables per day, and low-fat dairy products (2–3 servings per day).

If the PWD is overweight, although there is a great variability in response to weight loss, a modest amount of weight loss has been shown to reduce blood pressure in PWD. Regular aerobic physical activity, such as brisk walking, has an antihypertensive effect. Although chronic excessive alcohol intake is associated with an increased risk of hypertension, a reduction in blood pressure is seen with a light-to-moderate alcohol intake.[2] The DASH-style dietary pattern and smoking cessation are also well-known methods for reducing hypertension. These nonpharmachological strategies may also positively affect glycemia and lipid control.[10]

The ADA Standards of Medical Care in Diabetes state that people with diabetes and hypertension should be treated to a systolic blood pressure goal of <140 mm Hg, noting that lower systolic targets (eg, <130 mm Hg) may be appropriate for certain individuals, such as younger patients, if they can be achieved without imparting undue treatment burden. Patients with diabetes should be treated to a diastolic blood pressure <80 mm Hg. Patients who present with a blood pressure >120/80 mm Hg are recommended to be educated on lifestyle changes to reduce blood pressure. If confirmed blood pressure is ≥140/80 mm Hg, in addition to lifestyle therapy, promptly initiate and titrate pharmacological therapy to achieve blood pressure goals.[10] Chapter 5 contains more information about dietary interventions for cardiovascular disease, including blood pressure management.

■ Renal Parameters

Preventing nephropathy in diabetes, or slowing its progression, is crucial. Compared to the general population, PWD are at an increased risk for renal decompensation and myocardial infarction. To reduce the risk or slow the progression of nephropathy, optimization of blood pressure control and glycemic control are the top priorities. In addition, observation data suggest that dyslipidemia may increase albumin excretion and the rate of progression of diabetic nephropathy. Although observations do not confirm that MNT will affect diabetic nephropathy, in theory, MNT designed to reduce the risk for CVD may also favorably affect microvascular complications such as diabetic nephropathy.[2] Table 6–8 categorizes the renal parameters and their significance that need to be screened annually in PWD.[10]

A random spot collection of albumin-to-creatinine ratio is used for screening microalbuminuria. It is not necessary to conduct the more burdensome 24-hour or timed collection, which often adds little to prediction or accuracy.[10] The earliest stage of diabetic nephropathy in type 1 PWD and a marker of development of nephropathy in type 2 PWD is persistent albuminuria in the range of 30–299 mg/24 hours (microalbuminuria), which is also a well-established marker of increased CVD risk. However, before considering a PWD having crossed the diagnostic threshold, two of three abnormal specimens should be collected within a 3- to 6-month period. Urinary albumin excretion over baseline values may be elevated by infection, fever, CHF, marked hypertension or marked hyperglycemia, or physical activity within 24 hours.[10] The staging of CKD can be done with information on presence of abnormal urine albumin excretion and/or the level of the glomerular filtration rate (GFR). Decreased GFR in the absence of increased urine albumin excretion has been found in a

Table 6–8. Annual screening for nephropathy.

Renal Parameter and Population Measured	Significance	Category/Interpretation
Urine albumin • >5 years in type 1 PWD • In all type 2 PWD	To measure the rate of albumin excretion and gauge the method of treatment	*Spot collection (μg/mg creatinine)* Normal <30 Microalbuminuria 30–299 Macro (clinical)-albuminuria ≥300
Serum creatinine (Cr) • In all adult PWD	To estimate GFR	*Reference range*[a] 0.5–1.0 mg/dL – female 0.7–1.2 – male

eGFR[a]
• In all adult PWD
	Used to stage the level of chronic kidney disease (CKD)	*Stages of CKDGFR*[b]
		1. ≥90
		   Kidney damage[c] *with normal or increased GFR*
		2. 60–89
		   Kidney damage[c] *with mildly decreased GFR*
		3. 30–59
		   Moderately decreased GFR
		4. 15–29
		   Severely decreased GFR
		5. <15 or dialysis
		   Kidney failure

[a]Varies per laboratory.
[b][estimated] Glomerular filtration rate in mL/minute per 1.73 m² body surface area.
[c]Kidney damage defined as abnormalities on pathologic, urine, blood, or imaging tests.

Data from American Diabetes Association, 2013.

substantial percentage of PWD, and serum creatinine should, therefore, be measured at least annually in adult PWD, regardless of the degree of urine albumin excretion, in order to estimate GFR and stage the level of CKD.[10] In PWD who progress to macroalbuminuria (300 mg/ 24 hours), ESRD is likely to ensue.[10]

The practitioner is encouraged to provide continued surveillance to these renal parameters in order to assess both response to therapy and progression of disease. Delay in onset of microalbuminuria and the progression of micro- to macroalbuminuria in patients with type 1 and type 2 diabetes have been shown in large, prospective, randomized studies with intensive diabetes management and the goal of achieving near-euglycemia. In addition, the control of blood pressure was also shown to reduce the development of nephropathy.[10]

■ Pharmacologic Assessment and Monitoring of Antidiabetic Medications

Although MNT, weight management for overweight patients, and physical activity are the cornerstones of therapy for type 2 diabetes, at some point pharmacologic management may become necessary to assist in achieving glycemic and metabolic control.[18] All patients with type 1 diabetes require pharmacologic management of their condition at diagnosis (with insulin), and patients with prediabetes may also benefit from pharmacologic therapy at diagnosis. MNT also assists in the monitoring of pharmacologic therapy so as to avoid potential side effects that often ensue with the use of antidiabetic regimens, the most common side effects being hypoglycemia and weight gain.

There are several different antidiabetic agents, within various drug classes that target different organ systems in order to achieve glycemic control. Table 6–9 categorizes these antidiabetic agents and describes the glycemic parameter most affected, the expected HbA1c reduction, the recommended SMBG that should be tested to assess its effectiveness, the greatest risk for hypoglycemia to occur, and their MNT significance.[18,19] Many of these medications can also be found in combination with other medications, consequently having the properties and side effects of both. Patients with type 2 diabetes may be on one or several different antidiabetic agents, whereas patients with type 1 diabetes, because of their absolute deficiency of insulin, will always require daily injections of insulin, with usually no other antidiabetic agent.

Classes of Antidiabetic Medications
Secretagogues

Secretagogues stimulate the pancreas to secrete insulin, which then reduces hepatic glucose production and improves glucose uptake by muscles. There are two classes of secretagogues: sulfonylureas and nonsulfonylureas.[18]

Sulfonylureas

Sulfonylureas reduce fasting and postprandial glucose levels and have been shown to lower HbA1c levels by 1–2%. Glipizide, glyburide, and glimepiride are drugs in this category.[18] Sulfonylureas are metabolized by the liver and cleared by the kidney, except for glimepiride, which is used cautiously in patients with impaired renal function. In the elderly, sulfonylureas are used at low doses because some patients can have a decreased GFR, even with a normal serum creatinine concentration. Missed meals or snacks could lead to hypoglycemia in patients taking sulfonylureas, which can then cause an increase in appetite and possible weight gain. MNT is important due to its effectiveness for weight management.

Table 6-9. Antidiabetic medications and their MNT significance.

Drugs, Class/Site of Action/System(s) Targeted	Glycemic Elevations Most Affected and Expected HbA1c Reduction	Recommended SMBG Testing for Effectiveness	Greatest Risk for Hypoglycemia	MNT
Secretagogues: Sulfonylureas/Pancreas				
Glipizide Glyburide Glimepiride	Fasting and postprandial and HbA1c 1–2%	2–3 times per day, especially fasting	• 4–6 hours after meals and fasting • With missed meal or snacks	• Emphasize weight management techniques • Appropriate snacks and timing • Take before meal; skip drug if not eating
Secretagogues: NonSulfonylureas/Pancreas				
Repaglinide Nateglinide	Postprandial and HbA1c 0.5–2%	2 hours after meal	• 1 hour after meal • With missed meal or snacks	• Emphasize weight management techniques • Appropriate snacks and timing • Take before meal; skip drug if not eating
Sensitizers: Biguanides/Liver/Muscle/Adipose Tissue				
Metformin	Fasting and postprandial and HbA1c 1–2%	Fasting	• None	• May cause weight loss • Limit foods that can cause GI side effects • Take with food to reduce GI side effects

Sensitizers: Alpha-Glucosidase Inhibitors/Small Intestines			
Acarbose *Miglitol*	Postprandial and HbA1c 0.5–0.8%	2 hours after meal	• None • Treat with glucose tablets (Predigested carbohydrates)	• Must be taken before carbohydrate-containing meals, with first-bite of food • Caution for gastrointestinal side effects and minimize by reducing foods that cause abdominal bloating and flatulence • May cause low serum iron
Sensitizers: Thiazolidinediones/Muscle/Liver/Adipose Tissue			
Rosiglitazone *Pioglitazone*	Fasting and postprandial and HbA1c 1–2%	2–3 times per day, especially fasting	• None	• Reduce caloric consumption to avoid weight gain • Reduce sodium to reduce fluid retention • Can be taken with or without food • Adequate osteoporosis protection
Incretin System: DPP-4 Inhibitors/Small Intestines/Pancreas/Liver/Muscle			
Sitagliptin *Saxagliptin* *Linagliptin* *Alogliptin*	Fasting, postprandial and HbA1c 0.7–1.4%	2–3 times per day	• None	• Weight-neutral • Concentrate on healthy food choices • Can be taken with or without food

(Continued)

Table 6-9. Antidiabetic medications and their MNT significance. (Continued)

Drugs, Class/ Site of Action/ System(s) Targeted	Glycemic Elevations Most Affected and Expected HbA1c Reduction	Recommended SMBG Testing for Effectiveness	Greatest Risk for Hypoglycemia	MNT
Incretin-Mimetic: GLP-1 Receptor Agonists/Small Intestine/Pancreas/Liver/Muscle/Brain/Adipose Tissue				
Exenatide and Exenatide XR *Liraglutide*	Postprandial and HbA1c 0.5–1.5%	2 hours after meal and fasting	• A reactive hypoglycemia if significant hyperglycemia	• Slows gastric emptying and causes feeling of fullness halfway through meals • Can cause some nausea or feelings of satiety early in meals (avoid greasy or acidic foods; and counteract with carbonated beverage or ginger) • Increased water and fiber since potential side effect of constipation • Give 30–60 minutes before eating and do not take after or during eating • Consume at least 30 grams of complex carbohydrate
Amylin Mimetic: Pancreas				
Pramlintide	Postprandial and HbA1c 0.3–0.6%	Before meal and 2 hours after meal	• 2–3 hours after meal	• Slows gastric emptying • Causes feeling of fullness halfway through meals • Can cause some nausea or feelings of satiety early in meals • Consume at least 30 grams of carbohydrate

Dopamine Agonist: Brain					
Bromocriptine mesylate	Postprandial and HbA1c 0.6–0.9%		Postprandial	None	• Take with food within 2 hours of awakening • May cause nausea • Weight-neutral
Sodium Glucose Co-transporter 2 Inhibitors: Kidney					
Canagliflozin	Fasting, Postprandial, & HbA1c 0.91–1.16		Fasting, pre-meals, & postprandial	None	• May increase LDL cholesterol • May increase risk of hypotension
Insulins: Basal Analogs (Long-Acting)					
Glargine Detemir	Fasting and A1c		Fasting and premeals	None	• Timing of meals not an issue if receiving proper dose, but carry snacks in case meal is delayed
Insulins: Mealtime Analogs (Rapid-Acting)					
Lispro Aspart Glulisine	Postprandial and HbA1c		Postprandial	1–1½ hours postinjections	• Insulin to carbohydrate ratio education • Hypoglycemic precautions

(continued)

Table 6-9. Antidiabetic medications and their MNT significance. (*Continued*)

Drugs, Class/ Site of Action/ System(s) Targeted	Glycemic Elevations Most Affected and Expected HbA1c Reduction	Recommended SMBG Testing for Effectiveness	Greatest Risk for Hypoglycemia	MNT
Insulins: Intermediate-Acting (NPH)				
Humulin N *Novolin N*	Fasting and HbA1c	Fasting and premeal and between-meal	• 6-12 hours postinjections	• Eat 3 meals daily with between-meal snacks • Keep carbohydrate content of meals as consistent as possible
Insulins: Short-Acting (Regular)				
Humulin R *Novolin R*	Postprandial and HbA1c	Postprandial and between-meal	• 2-4 hours postinjections	• Insulin to carbohydrate ratio education • Keep snacks available due to unpredictability
Insulins: Premixed Analogs (Combination Basal and Mealtime)				
Lispro protamine/ lispro *Aspart protamine/ aspart*	Fasting, postprandial, and HbA1c	Fasting, premeal, and postprandial	• 1-4 hours postinjections	• Eat 3 meals daily • Keep carbohydrate content of meals as consistent as possible

Data from DeFronzo et al., 2012; Fonseca and Kulkarini, 2008; Chavez and Summers, 2003.

Nonsulfonylureas

Nonsulfonylureas stimulate rapid insulin production by the pancreas and are shown to reduce postprandial blood glucose and to reduce HbA1c by 0.5–2%. Nateglinide and repaglinide are drugs in this category, also known as meglitinides.[18] Nonsulfonylureas have a quicker onset and shorter duration of action (4–6 hours) than sulfonylureas, as well as reduced risk of hypoglycemia and less weight gain. This class is a potential option for patients with erratic meal schedules and those concerned about weight gain. This class should only be taken before meals or large snacks that contain substantial amounts of carbohydrate. Hypoglycemia can occur if taken before low-carbohydrate meals or when a meal is missed. Nonsulfonylureas are cleared hepatically and may be used in patients with renal impairment.

Sensitizers

Sensitizers enhance insulin action and work through a variety of mechanisms. Sensitizers can inhibit gluconeogenesis and glycogenolysis, inhibit hepatic glucose absorption, or increase glucose uptake in fat and muscle. There are three categories of sensitizers: biguanides (metformin), thiazolidinediones, and alpha-glucosidase inhibitors.[18]

Biguanides

Biguanides enhance insulin sensitivity, inhibit hepatic gluconeogenesis, and, to a lesser extent, inhibit glycogenolysis. The only available medication in this class is metformin, which is typically given in two equal doses daily, before breakfast and before supper, but can also be given three times daily with meals, or in a slow-release formulation once daily. Metformin has been shown to lower fasting and postprandial blood glucose levels and to lower HbA1c by 1–2%. Metformin does not cause hypoglycemia when used as a monotherapy and can cause weight loss. Gastrointestinal side effects include abdominal cramping, nausea, diarrhea, and a metallic taste, which can be minimized by starting with a small dose and titrating gradually. Individuals who experience gastrointestinal side effects should limit their intake of gas-producing and high-fiber foods (eg, cauliflower, cabbage, broccoli, lentils, and legumes). A potentially rare fatal adverse effect is lactic acidosis, which can be increased if baseline renal function is abnormal or if there is any other condition affecting the kidneys (eg, dehydration, major surgery, or chronic heart failure).[18] Metformin is typically prescribed as a first line of therapy in individuals with prediabetes, newly diagnosed T2DM, and PCOS.

Thiazolidinediones

Thiazolidinediones (TZDs) enhance insulin sensitivity by increasing the efficiency of the glucose transporter. TZDs are taken once or twice a day and have been shown to lower HbA1C by 1–2% and reduce fasting and postprandial blood glucose levels. TZDs do not cause hypoglycemia when used as a monotherapy, and they have a positive effect on lipids by decreasing triglycerides, increasing high-density lipoprotein cholesterol, and increasing the particle size of low-density lipoprotein cholesterol. The two available TZDs are rosiglitazone and pioglitazone. Rosiglitazone carries a boxed warning for the potential of myocardial infarction and ischemia, and warnings with the use of nitrates, co-administration with insulin, and in patients experiencing an acute coronary event. Pioglitazone does not appear to carry the same cardiovascular risk and may have a protective effect of reducing triglycerides and slightly increasing high-density lipoprotein cholesterol. The most noted side effects of this class are weight gain and mild edema. MNT goals with use are to reduce caloric consumption and reduce sodium to reduce fluid retention.[18] This class should be used cautiously in patients with congestive heart failure.

Alpha-glucosidase inhibitors

Alpha-glucosidase inhibitors (AGI) block the enzyme alpha-glucosidase in the brush borders of the small intestine, which delays absorption of carbohydrates. This class lowers the HbA1c value by 0.5–1%. AGIs are taken before carbohydrate-containing meals, and should not be taken when meals are missed. AGIs should be avoided in people with severe renal or hepatic impairment or any gastrointestinal disease. Side effects include bloating, abdominal cramps, flatulence, and diarrhea. Foods that cause gastrointestinal side effects should be avoided. The two AGIs used in the United States are acarbose and miglitol.[18] Liver function tests should be obtained every 3 months for the first year, then periodically thereafter.

Dipeptidyl Peptidase-IV Inhibitors

Dipeptidyl peptidase-IV inhibitors (DPP4i) are agents that inhibit dipeptidyl peptidase, the enzyme that degrades endogenously secreted incretins, including glucagon-like peptide-1(GLP-1) and glucose-dependent insulinotropic polypeptide. Increased levels of the incretin hormones result in increased insulin secretion and suppression of glucagon secretion. The main effect is the lowering of postprandial blood glucose levels. The HbA1c is lowered by 0.7–1.4%. The most common side effects are headache and nasopharyngitis. The three available DPP4i are sitagliptin, saxagliptin, and linagliptin. Sitagliptin and saxagliptin are metabolized in the liver and excreted mostly in the urine, whereas linagliptin is minimally metabolized and excreted mostly unchanged in the feces. Therefore, in patients with renal insufficiency, the dose of sitagliptin and saxagliptin should be decreased by 50–75%. There is no dose adjustment needed for linagliptin. These drugs are weight-neutral and do not cause hypoglycemia when used with an insulin sensitizer or as a monotherapy.[18]

Glucagon-Like Peptide-1 Receptor Agonists

GLP-1 receptor agonists mimic the action of incretins, such as GLP-1, in the small intestines. This class improves glycemic control through several mechanisms, including increased insulin synthesis and secretion in the presence of elevated glucose concentrations, improvement of first-phase insulin response, slowed gastric emptying, reduced glucagon concentration during glycemic excursions, and reduced food intake. There are currently two noninsulin injectable incretin drugs on the market: exenatide and liraglutide.[18] Exenatide is administered twice daily, or exenatide-extended release is administered once weekly. Liraglutide is injected once daily.

Amylin-Mimetic

An amylin-mimetic is a synthetic version of the naturally occurring hormone, amylin. This class works with type 1 or type 2 diabetes patients who are also using mealtime insulin to reduce postprandial glucose absorption. An amylin-mimetic may allow patients to reduce their insulin requirements by 50%, leads to weight loss, and improves HbA1 levels. The only available amylin-mimetic is pramlintide. A common side effect of this class is nausea, but it is usually transient and can be addressed through slow titration.[18]

Dopamine-Agonist

A dopamine receptor agonist is a relatively new class of an antidiabetic agent that acts on the central nervous system. The precise mechanism of action is unknown, but studies have shown that appropriately timed daily administration (morning) normalizes aberrant hypothalamic neurotransmitter activities that induce, potentiate, and maintain the insulin-resistant, glucose-intolerant state. Morning administration improves glycemic control, particularly postprandial glycemic control in patients with type 2 diabetes without increasing plasma insulin concentrations. This class is weight neutral, and has been shown to decrease the HbA1c by 0.6–0.9% when added to other oral antidiabetic drugs. The most common adverse effect was found to be nausea, but this is transient and can be addressed through slow titration. The only available dopamine-agonist is bromocriptine mesylate.[20]

Sodium–Glucose Cotransporter 2 Inhibitors

The newest class of antidiabetic agents comprises the sodium–glucose cotransporter 2 inhibitor (SGLT-2 inhibitor). At the time of publication, the only SGLT-2 inhibitor approved by the FDA in the United States is canagliflozin. In glucose homeostasis, the role of the kidneys is to reabsorb glucose filtered at the glomerulus via sodium–glucose cotransporters (SGLT-2) that are located in the proximal convoluted tubule. SGLT-2 is a low-affinity, high-capacity glucose transport protein that reabsorbs 80–90% of filtered glucose. This adaptive mechanism helps ensure that the body's energy needs are met during fasting states. Inhibition of SGLT-2 reduces resorption of glucose in the kidney, resulting in increased urinary glucose excretion, with a consequent lowering of plasma glucose levels, as well as weight loss. A1c and both fasting and postprandial glucose levels, are decreased with the use of SGLT-2, independent of insulin secretion or resistance, therefore being effective in both newly diagnosed and long-standing diabetes mellitus. Canagliflozin monotherapy has been found to lower A1c dose-dependently by 0.91–1.16% over 6 months. Since SGLT-2 inhibitors do not directly stimulate insulin secretion, the risk of hypoglycemia is low, and there is no risk of gastrointestinal side effects. Weight loss occurs due to a net loss of calories and there may also be a reduction in blood pressure due to osmotic diuresis.[21] Potential side effects are vaginal yeast infection, urinary tract infection, and postural hypotension. There are potential long-term effects of the dose-dependent increase in LDL cholesterol and impact of treatment on bone density and fractures. This class of medication should be avoided in patients with renal impairment.[22]

Insulin Regimens

Insulin is the most powerful and effective pharmacologic tool available to treat diabetes.[18] The main priority with the use of any type of insulin is to understand the insulin's time to action, peak of action, and duration of action, in order to reduce the very real potential side effect of hypoglycemia; therefore, the insulin therapy needs to be integrated into the person's lifestyle. An appropriate insulin regimen can usually be developed to conform to an individual's preferred meal routine, food choices, and physical activity patterns. Insulin can also be given in combination with oral or other noninsulin injectable diabetes medications.

The practitioner must also understand that the use of insulin therapy will almost always result in weight gain. This weight gain is due to the absolute function of insulin, carrying excess blood glucose into the cells for use as energy (fewer calories are lost from glycosuria), and is also due to the anabolic nature of this hormone. Therefore, the use of MNT and physical activity for weight management should be encouraged in all PWD using insulin. Some types of insulin regimens or inappropriate uses of insulin may cause more weight gain than others, due to the need to eat to counteract hypoglycemia. Patients should be educated on the most appropriate way to correct hypoglycemia to avoid unnecessary weight gain and unnecessary rebound hyperglycemia. Rates of hypoglycemia and degree of weight gain have been found to be greatest with prandial insulin and least with basal insulin. A twice-daily biphasic insulin has been found to be intermediate between these two regimens; thus, the single-best insulin regimen to achieve glycemic control while minimizing hypoglycemia and weight gain is not possible to identify.[18]

Fixed-dose insulin regimens

Fixed-dose insulin regimens are widely used and consist of twice-daily injections of a combination insulin consisting of intermediate- and rapid- or short-acting insulin, administered before breakfast and before dinner. The use of this class requires consistency in timing and in carbohydrate content of meals, but the regimen can be adjusted to accommodate variations in food or physical activity.

Intermediate-acting insulin/rapid- or short-acting insulin regimens

An intermediate-acting insulin dose should be taken at bedtime (instead of predinner) to prevent the blood sugar from peaking while sleeping (between 0100 and 0300) and allow the peak to occur when it is most needed (between 0500 and 0800), when insulin resistance and insulin needs are at their highest due to growth hormone surges that occur during sleep (Dawn phenomenon), or to alleviate the potential for a Somogyi effect. An additional intermediate-acting insulin injection may be required before breakfast because this intermediate-acting insulin's duration of action does not last the entire 24 hours, and the rapid- or short-acting insulin that may be taken before the meal may result in periods of hypoinsulinemia and high glucose levels.

Basal-bolus analog insulin regimen

A basal-bolus analog insulin regimen is a physiological approach to insulin therapy that consists of a long-acting basal insulin given once or twice daily and rapid-acting bolus insulin given before each meal to cover mealtime glucose fluctuations. A basal-bolus analog insulin regimen allows for a more flexible food intake and lifestyle patterning than does a fixed-dose insulin regimen or an intermediate-acting insulin/ rapid- or short-acting insulin regimen, but some patients may initially be intimidated by this type of intensive regimen. The major determinant of bolus insulin doses for individuals on basal-bolus analog insulin therapy is the total carbohydrate content of meals and snacks. To adjust mealtime insulin doses, insulin-to-carbohydrate ratios (ICR) should be determined. The carbohydrate content of meals can be estimated by several different methods of calculation, including carbohydrate counting methods, the exchange system, or experience-based estimation.[2] Improvement in HbA1c without significant increase in severe hypoglycemia was demonstrated in the *Dose Adjustment for Normal Eating* (DAFNE) study group,[23] where participants learned how to use glucose testing to better match insulin to carbohydrate intake. Even though increases in number of insulin injections and blood glucose tests were required, positive effects on quality of life, satisfaction with treatment, and psychological well-being were achieved.[2]

Basal analog insulin regimen

A basal analog insulin regimen consists of one to two injections per day, usually used along with the oral antidiabetic drug, and the dose is titrated to a 3- to 5-day average of the fasting blood sugar. This is often a less intimidating method of initiating insulin for the patient naïve to insulin therapy.

Continuous subcutaneous insulin infusion

Continuous subcutaneous insulin infusion (CSII) or insulin pumps use small amounts of rapid- or short-acting insulin infused through a subcutaneous catheter every few minutes to establish a steady basal insulin, mimicking normal pancreatic function. The patient administers bolus injections prior to the meal through the same catheter. Prior to initiating CSII therapy, most insurance carriers require patients to undergo extensive education and counseling including MNT and carbohydrate counting (Table 6–10).[24]

Table 6–10. Key features of currently available human insulin and analogs.

Insulin Type	Onset (hours)	Peak (hours)	Duration of Action (hours)
Rapid Acting			
Insulin lispro, Insulin aspart, and Insulin glulisine (no clinically significant difference)	5–15 minutes	1–1.5	2–4
Short Acting			
Human regular	0.5	2–4	6–8
Humulin R, Novolin R (no clinically significant difference)			
Intermediate Acting			
NPH insulin	0.5–1.5	6–12	12–18
Human N, Novolin N			
Long Acting			
Insulin glargine	1	None	≥24
Insulin detemir	1	6–12	18–24
Premixed			
Insulin lispro protamine/insulin lispro *Humalog mix 75/25, humalog mix 50/50*	5–15 minutes	1–4	12–18
	5–15 minutes	1–4	12–18
Insulin aspart protamine/insulin aspart *Novolog mix 70/30*	0.5	2–12	12–18
Insulin isophane suspension (NPH)/ regular *Humulin 70/30, Humulin 50/50, Novolin 70/30*			

Data from Cefalu et al., 2004.

■ Physical Activity Assessment and Monitoring

Physical activity is a vital component of diabetes prevention and management, and helps mitigate diabetes complications. At least 2.5 hours of moderate-to-vigorous physical activity each week should be undertaken to prevent type 2 diabetes onset in high-risk adults.[25] In addition, epidemiological studies suggest that higher levels of physical activity may also reduce the risk of developing GDM during pregnancy.[25] Some benefits of physical activity to PWD include[26]:

- reduction of cardiovascular risk factors;
- promotion of a healthy weight;
- reduction in body weight and body fat;
- improvement in blood glucose control and tolerance;
- increase in peripheral insulin sensitivity;
- reduction in insulin requirements;
- improvement in sense of well-being; and
- decrease in stress.

Although physical activity is a crucial component of care, the practitioner is advised to be aware of the individual's potential restrictions for exercise and the metabolic effects and benefits for the PWD, in order to maximize rewards and minimize risks of injury and poor medical outcomes. In general, the PWD who is a casual exerciser may require assistance to maintain euglycemia, by either the adjustment of medications, the amount of food consumed, the timing of meals, and/or the actual physical activity regimen. Management issues for type 1 PWD may be especially challenging due to their complete lack of ability to make metabolic adjustments to manage fuel homeostasis. PWD who are in good metabolic control and without serious complications may be able to freely participate in recreational and competitive exercise, but those with certain diabetes co-morbidities will require further assessment.

Physical Activity with Type 1 Diabetes

Exercise is not reported to improve glycemic control in persons with type 1 diabetes; however, the same benefits from exercise that the non-diabetic population experiences, such as decreased risk of CVD and improved sense of well-being, still apply; thus, regular physical activity should be encouraged in individuals with type 1 diabetes.[4] It is important to note that research regarding the benefits and risks of physical activity on this population is limited. Participation in exercise may pose challenges for a person with type 1 diabetes. If a type 1 PWD has a minimal amount of insulin available due to inadequate insulin therapy, the secretion of catecholamines and glucagon can cause high blood glucose levels during exercise, and if untreated, can lead to the accumulation of ketone bodies and cause diabetic ketoacidosis. It is not necessary to postpone exercise based simply on hyperglycemia, as long as the patient feels well and as long as urine and blood ketones are negative. On the opposite end of the spectrum, if the type 1 PWD has excessive insulin on board, severe hypoglycemia can occur during the activity.[10,25]

For this reason, it is imperative that all type PWD check their blood sugar before activities and always carry some form of rapid-acting glucose (eg, glucose tablets or juice) to treat hypoglycemia.

It has been reported that participation in continuous moderate-intensity exercise (aerobic activity between 40% and 59% of maximum oxygen uptake or 55–69% maximal heart rate) causes an increase in the risk of hypoglycemia, both during and up to 31 hours following the cessation of an activity. Additionally, during sustained high-intensity exercise (approximately 15 minutes at >80% of maximum oxygen uptake), a progressive rise in blood glucose levels can occur.[4] In this case, with high hyperglycemia caused by vigorous activity, additional insulin should only be added after the individual's response to vigorous activity is studied on several occasions.[4] A reduction in insulin dosage is the preferred method to prevent hypoglycemia when exercise is planned. For unplanned exercise, additional carbohydrate is generally required, such that a person of 70 kilograms of weight would need an additional 10–15 grams of carbohydrate per hour of moderate-intensity physical activity, and more if intense activity occurs.[2]

Physical Activity with Type 2 Diabetes

Structured exercise interventions of at least 8 weeks' duration have been shown to lower HbA1c by an average of 0.66% in people with type 2 diabetes, even with no significant change in BMI.[10] Higher levels of exercise intensity are associated with greater improvements in HbA1c and in fitness.[10] For adults over the age of 18 years, the accumulation of 150 minutes of moderate-intensity aerobic physical activity (40–60% of maximal oxygen uptake or 50–70% of maximum heart rate) per week with no more than two consecutive days between bouts of aerobic activity, in addition to resistance/strength training that involve all major muscle groups, three times per week on nonconsecutive days, is recommended.[4,10,25,27] In a meta-analysis of eight randomized, controlled trials and 18 observational studies, people who used pedometers increased their physical activity by 27% over baseline. In this analysis, having a goal (eg, taking 10,000 steps per day) was as an important predictor of increased physical activity.[25]

Independent of weight loss, both aerobic exercise and resistance training have been found to improve glycemic control and reduce CV risk factors. For those individuals already exercising at moderate intensity, to obtain even greater benefits in glycemic control and aerobic fitness, increasing the intensity even more is recommended. For adults over the age of 65 years and for those with disabilities, the adult guidelines should be followed if possible, or if not possible, individuals should be encouraged to be as physically active as they are able.[10] In older men with type 2 diabetes, progressive resistance exercise improves insulin sensitivity to the same or even greater extent as aerobic exercise. Clinical trials have provided strong evidence for the HbA1c-lowering value of resistance training and for an additive benefit of combined aerobic and resistance exercise.[10]

Overall, the improvement in insulin sensitivity and the decrease in the risk for CVD (eg, through reduced LDL levels) and all-cause mortality have been shown with appropriate physical activity.[4] No more than two consecutive days should pass without physical activity, in order to achieve long-term glycemic control.[4,27] Before undertaking exercise that is more intense than brisk walking, sedentary persons with type 2 diabetes should consult a primary care practitioner (PCP). Electrocardiogram (ECG) exercise stress testing for asymptomatic individuals at low risk of CVD is not recommended but may be indicated for those who are at high risk.[25]

Type 2 PWD may have similar hypoglycemic precautions as those persons with type 1 diabetes if they take insulin, sulfonylureas, and/or meglitinides. Because exercise has a potent insulin-like effect on blood sugar levels, hypoglycemia may occur during prolonged exercise when exogenous insulin levels are at their peak.[25] With the exception of β-blockers, some diuretics, and statins, most other medications prescribed for concomitant health problems do not affect exercise. β-blockers are known to blunt heart rate response to exercise and lower maximal exercise capacity, as well as block adrenergic symptoms of hypoglycemia. By reducing coronary ischemia during activity, β-blockers may increase exercise capacity in those with CVD rather than lowering it.[25] Diuretics may lower overall blood and fluid volume, resulting in dehydration and electrolyte imbalances, especially if exercise occurs in the heat. Statin use has been associated with an elevated risk of myopathies, especially when combined with fibrates and niacin.[25]

Physical Activity with Gestational Diabetes

A diagnosis of gestational diabetes (GDM) places the woman at a significantly increased risk for developing type 2 diabetes after pregnancy. Physical activity may be a tool that can prevent both GDM and possibly type 2 diabetes at a later date.[25] Engaging in 30 minutes of moderate-intensity physical activity such as walking, during most days of the week (2.5 hours/week), has been adopted as a recommendation for pregnant women without medical or obstetrical complications.[25] It should be noted that women with GDM who are placed on bed rest can still perform small amounts of exercise. For example, under the guidance of a physical therapist, some women may be able to perform resistance band training in order to keep their muscles toned.

Physical Activity with Long-Term Complications of Diabetes

Before recommending a physical activity program, the practitioner should assess patients for conditions that might contraindicate certain types of exercise, such as those with multiple CV risk factors, or for conditions that predispose to injury, such as uncontrolled hypertension, severe autonomic neuropathy, severe peripheral neuropathy, or history of foot lesions and unstable proliferative retinopathy. The patient's age and previous physical activity level should also be considered, and evaluation for the presence or absence of hyperglycemia or hypoglycemia, prior to any activity, should be taken into account.[10]

Coronary Artery Disease

The area of routine screening for coronary artery diseases (CAD) in asymptomatic PWD remains unclear and practitioners are advised to exercise their own clinical judgment in these circumstances. Those considered to be at high risk should be encouraged to start with short periods of low-intensity exercise and slowly increase the intensity and duration.[10] Known CVD is not an absolute contraindication to exercise. Individuals with angina classified as moderate or high risk should begin exercise in a supervised cardiac rehabilitation program.[25]

Retinopathy

Vigorous aerobic or resistance exercise that greatly increases intraocular pressure and systolic blood pressure is contraindicated in the presence of proliferative diabetic retinopathy (PDR) and severe nonproliferative diabetic retinopathy (NPDR). This is due to the risk of triggering vitreous hemorrhage or retinal detachment. Head-down activities and jumping or jarring activities also increase hemorrhage risk and should be avoided.[10,25]

Peripheral Neuropathy

Decreased pain sensation in the extremities results in increased risk of skin breakdown and neuropathic joint disease (Charcot joint). Prior recommendations have advised nonweight-bearing exercise for patients with severe peripheral neuropathy. More recent studies have shown that moderate-intensity walking may not lead to increased risk of foot ulcers or reulceration in those with peripheral neuropathy. Therefore, individuals with peripheral neuropathy and without acute ulceration may participate in moderate weight-bearing exercise. All individuals with peripheral neuropathy should wear proper footwear and examine their feet daily to detect lesions or abrasions early. Anyone with a foot injury or open sore should be restricted to nonweight-bearing activities. Moderate walking likely does not increase the risk of foot ulcers or reulceration with peripheral neuropathy.[10,25]

CV Autonomic Neuropathy

The risk of exercise-induced injury or adverse event through silent ischemia, heart rate, and blood pressure abnormalities (postural hypotension), impaired thermoregulation, impaired night vision due to impaired papillary reaction, and unpredictable carbohydrate delivery from gastroparesis predisposing to hypoglycemia is greater in those with CV autonomic neuropathy (CAN) than in those without CAN. However, moderate-intensity aerobic training can improve autonomic function in all individuals. Individuals with CAN should be screened and should receive PCP approval and, when possible, an exercise stress test before initiating exercise. Exercise intensity is best prescribed using the heart rate reserve method with direct measurement of maximal heart rate.[10,25]

Nephropathy and Microalbuminuria

Exercise training increases physical function and quality of life in individuals with kidney disease, and may even be undertaken during dialysis sessions. The presence of microalbuminuria does not necessitate exercise restrictions. Persons with overt nephropathy should be screened, have PCP approval, and possibly undergo stress testing to detect CAD and abnormal heart rate and blood pressure responses. Because aerobic capacity and muscle function are substantially reduced in those with CKD, exercise should be begun at a low intensity and volume, while avoiding the Valsalva maneuver and any high-intensity exercises in order to prevent excessive increases in blood pressure.[10,25]

General Guidelines for Physical Activity

In general, appropriate entry-level activities for most people that are unlikely to have adverse consequences beyond sore muscles are walking, yard work, and dancing. Additional time should be devoted to an exercise program as the fitness level improves, but patients should be advised to stop exercising if pain or discomfort is experienced and to seek medical attention if the pain fails to subside. Because elevated blood sugar levels can cause excess water to be lost via the urine, PWD are at increased risk for developing dehydration. In addition, thirst centers in the brain are not activated until a 1% body water loss has occurred. It is, therefore, necessary to assure that exercise be initiated in a hydrated state, and that a fluid consumption schedule be established during exercise.[25] Table 6–11 contains basic fluid guidelines with physical activity.[28]

Fueling the body prior to the activity and replenishing it after the activity are also crucial. Eating a meal or snack within 2 hours prior to

Table 6–11. Fluid consumption schedule for physical activity.

Timing of Activity	Amount of Fluid to Consume	Note
Before activity	16–20 ounces	Consume 2 hours prior
During activity	8 ounces every 15 minutes	For activity lasting >1 hour, replace sodium and carbohydrate
After activity	24 ounces for every pound of body weight lost during the activity	Weigh before and after activity to ensure proper rehydration

Data from Kundrat and Rockwell, 2008.

Table 6–12. Nutrient needs for varying levels of energy source.

Level or Type of Activity	Calories (kcal) (Per Pound of Body Weight)	Carbohydrate (g) (Per kg Body Weight)	Protein (g) (Per kg Body Weight)	Fat (g)
Sedentary	13–15 kcal/lb			
Low activity 30–60 minutes/day	16–18 kcal/lb	2–5 g/kg	0.8 g/kg	20–35% of total kcal
Active 1–1½ hours/day	19–21 kcal/lb	5–7 g/kg	0.8 g/kg	20–35% of total kcal
Endurance exercise			1.2–1.4 g/kg	
Strength training			1.6–1.7 g/kg	

Data from Kundrat and Rockwell, 2008.

exercise increases energy levels and results in an increased number of calories burned. Glycogen stores need to be replenished post exercise, and the muscular microtears that occur with sustained activity need to be repaired within 30 minutes after exercise. During exercise lasting longer than 45–60 minutes, supplemental fluids and calories may be needed, as will more frequent blood sugar testing. When blood glucose remains within 70–150 mg/dL during exercise, muscle efficiency and performance are optimized.[28-31] MNT should be individualized based on the type, amount, and intensity of the exercise performed. Table 6–12 lists nutrient needs for varying levels of activity.[28]

For PWD on antidiabetes medications, in order to minimize risks, self-adjustment of insulin doses and/or intake of carbohydrates must be learned. Unfortunately, there is limited research on the type and amounts of carbohydrate to consume with exercise.[4] For PWD taking insulin or insulin secretagogues, instruction should be provided for safety guidelines to prevent hypoglycemia (eg, frequent blood glucose monitoring, possible adjustments in insulin dose or carbohydrate intake, and the need to carry carbohydrate food/beverages while exercising).[4] The research suggests that the incidence of hypoglycemia may be dependent on baseline glucose levels. Table 6–13 contains information for recommended exercise precautions for PWD taking insulin or insulin secretagogues.[28-32] Overall, developing self-efficacy and fostering social support should be the focus for promoting physical activity among PWD. In order to adopt and encourage maintenance of regular physical activity participation, the encouragement of mild-to-moderate physical activity may be beneficial.[25]

Table 6-13. Exercise precautions with insulin or insulin secretagogue use.

Exercise Situation	Intervention
Pre-exercise glucose levels of <100 mg/dL	Eat 15-30 grams of carbohydrate for every 30-60 minutes of planned activity
Pre-exercise glucose levels >250 mg/dL	Test urine ketones, and if positive, delay exercise and give insulin; supplement with noncaloric fluids to prevent dehydration and clear ketones
Pre-exercise glucose levels >300 mg/dL	Delay exercise regardless of presence of ketones; give insulin; and supplement with noncaloric fluids to prevent dehydration and clear ketones
Mild-to-moderate planned exercise	Reduce premeal insulin by 30-50% based on its intensity and duration; always carry glucose tabs or gels to treat possible hypoglycemia
Unplanned activity with unadjusted insulin	For every 60 minutes of moderate activity, add an extra 15-30 grams of carbohydrate before the activity, plus an additional 15-30 grams following cessation of the activity
For afternoon or evening activity	Aim for a prebedtime glucose of >130 to avoid hypoglycemia during sleep

Data from Rachmiel et al., 2007; Walsh and Roberts, 2000; Hinnen et al., 2001; Dunford, 2006; Kundrat and Rockwell, 2008.

Medical Nutrition Therapy for Diabetes Mellitus: Nutrient Recommendations

- Macronutrients: Carbohydrates, Proteins, and Fats

The optimization of energy intake and the composition of macronutrients are considered the major concentrations for diabetes MNT,[1] which leads us to the question: what is the optimal macronutrient composition of the diet for PWD?

Over the past 100 years, dietary prescriptions for diabetes have varied widely from the very low carbohydrate diets initiated, before insulin was discovered, to the relatively high-carbohydrate, high-fiber diets often endorsed today by some health professionals. One thing has always been consistent, and that is that dietary prescription for diabetes is centered around carbohydrates. The so-called diabetic diets that were used before exogenous insulin became widely available consisted mainly of protein and fats. The optimal diet for a typical PWD (with or without the need for insulin) described by Elliott P. Joslin in 1927 consisted of 100 grams of carbohydrate. In the 1920s and early 1930s, normal or even high-carbohydrate diets were used by many physicians for treating PWD. From the period of 1940 to today, the debate continues with the pendulum swinging back and forth on what is considered to be the best balance of carbohydrate, protein, and fat.[33] Although it is well known that the restriction of calories is essential for the achievement of adequate glycemic and lipid control, mainly through weight loss, the optimal dietary macronutrient composition for PWD remains controversial.[1]

Relative Composition of Dietary Protein

The focus of protein intake for the management of diabetes was originally to preserve lean body mass, although now, dietary protein is believed to play a role in the management of hyperglycemia and body weight.[10] Although glucose produced from ingested protein has been shown in a number of studies to produce increases in serum insulin responses, it has not been shown to have an effect on plasma glucose concentration in type 2 PWD.[2] Insulin deficiency and insulin resistance may be the cause of abnormal protein metabolism, but they are usually corrected with good glycemic control.[2] Diets with protein content of >30% of total energy have been shown in small, short-term studies to reduce glucose and insulin concentrations, to reduce appetite, and to increase satiety; however, the ability of individuals to follow such diets long-term has not been adequately studied.[2] The DRI recommends a macronutrient distribution of protein in the range of 10–35% of energy intake, with 15% being the average adult intake in the United States and Canada.[2] The RDA is 0.8 grams of good-quality protein per kilogram body weight (on an average, equating to approximately 10% of total calories).[2]

Relative Composition of Dietary Carbohydrate

Low-carbohydrate diets have been defined as providing anywhere between 50 and 150 grams of carbohydrate per day.[34] The DRI recommendations state that the minimum amount of carbohydrate that should be consumed by adults is 130 grams per day. Although brain fuel needs can be met on lower-carbohydrate diets, long-term metabolic effects of very low carbohydrate diets are unclear.[2,10] A high-protein diet is not recommended for PWD due to the risk of nephropathy.[1]

Relative Composition of Dietary Fat

Saturated and *trans* fatty acids are the principal dietary determinants of plasma LDL cholesterol; thus, in PWD, the primary goal is to limit saturated fatty acids, *trans* fatty acids, and cholesterol intake so as to reduce the risk for CVD. Because of lack of evidence on the effects of specific fatty acids on PWD, recommendations are consistent with those for individuals with CVD.[10] Restricting fat intake has been shown to decrease overall energy intake and reduce weight, but a low-fat diet that is accompanied by a high-carbohydrate intake (eg, >55% of total energy from carbohydrate) may increase postprandial plasma glucose, insulin, and triglyceride levels, and, in fact, has not been shown to improve fasting plasma glucose or HbA1c compared with a high-monounsaturated fat diet.[2] However, in one meta-analysis, although replacing fat with carbohydrate deteriorated insulin resistance, the adverse effect on triglycerides from the low-fat, high-carbohydrate diet could be avoided by restricting energy intake to a degree sufficient for the attainment of weight reduction.[1]

Even today, it appears that the question above regarding the most optimal macronutrient composition of the diet for PWD still cannot be answered. This is likely due to a lack of consistency in study design and size, and to the fact that the intake of unrefined, carbohydrate-dense foods that are high in fiber is not consistently tested in studies. In addition, cohort sizes are often small, and observation time can be very long (over 5 years in some cases), making it difficult, expensive, and not feasible to follow a controlled diet in a controlled environment for long enough to detect true effects. As a result, the practitioner should encourage consumption of macronutrients based on the DRI for healthy eating, as the research does not support any ideal percentage of energy from macronutrients.[4] The best mix of carbohydrate, protein, and fat appears to vary depending on individual circumstances. Regardless of the macronutrient mix, the total caloric intake must be appropriate to meet weight management goals. In addition, the macronutrient composition will depend on the metabolic status and renal function, as well as individual food preferences.[2,10]

▪ Carbohydrates

Although low-carbohydrate diets may seem to be the logical approach to lowering postprandial glucose, carbohydrate-containing foods are important sources of energy, fiber, vitamins, and minerals. Carbohydrates also contribute to the palatability of the diet, thereby making them important components of the diet for PWD.[2,4,10]

Carbohydrate Intake Consistency

Meal and snack carbohydrate intake for the person with type 1, type 2, and gestational diabetes should be consistently distributed throughout the day. Consistency in carbohydrate intake has been shown to result in improved glycemic control in persons receiving either MNT alone, glucose-lowering medications, or fixed insulin doses.[4] Table 6–14 shows the distribution of 350 grams of carbohydrate over three meals and three snacks.

Carbohydrate and Medication Dose Adjustment

In order to optimize diabetes treatment, it is important to match doses of insulin and insulin secretagogues to the carbohydrate content of the meal. Insulin doses should be adjusted to match carbohydrate intake (insulin-to-carbohydrate ratios) in persons with type 1 or type 2 diabetes who adjust their mealtime insulin doses or who are on insulin pump therapy.[4] This has been shown to improve glycemic control and quality of life without any adverse effects.[4] In addition, insulin secretagogues

Table 6–14. Sample distribution of 350 grams of carbohydrate.

Meal or Snack	Carbohydrate (g)
Breakfast: ½ cup dry oatmeal (27 g), 1 cup nonfat milk (12 g), and ½ cup blueberries (11 g)	50
Snack: whole-wheat pita bread (4″, 15 g), ½ cup hummus (25 g), cucumber, sliced (4 g), and tomato (5 g)	49
Lunch: 3 oz curried chicken kabobs (5 g), 1 cup long grain white rice (45 g), 1 cup boiled greens (4 g), 1 glass Indian lassi made with yogurt, sugar, and water (21 g)	75
Snack: 1 mango (31 g), ¼ cup almonds (4 g), and 1 oz potato chips (15 g)	50
Dinner: ½ cup pinto beans (22 g), 2 corn tortillas (21 g), ¼ cup salsa (4 g), ¼ avocado (3 g), 1 cup squash (10 g), and 1 orange (15 g)	75
Snack: 1 cup ice cream (37 g), ½ banana (13 g), and 1 maraschino cherry (1 g)	51
Total	350

may also cause hypoglycemia if timed incorrectly with the carbohydrate intake. To accomplish appropriate matching of carbohydrate and medication dose, comprehensive nutrition education and counseling on interpretation of blood glucose patterns, and nutrition-related medication management should occur in collaboration with the health care team.[4] Table 6–15 describes the steps to determine an insulin-to-carbohydrate

Table 6–15. Steps in determining and insulin-to-carbohydrate ratio (ICR).

1. Determine the average amount of carbohydrates eaten at each meal and snack through the use of food diaries or establish a carbohydrate budget for the PWD and request that they eat a consistent amount of carbohydrates at meals and snacks from one day to the next.
2. Analyze the SMBG data with the patient and assess if there was an appropriate return of glucose to baseline values following the meal with the amount of mealtime or bolus insulin that was given for the amount of carbohydrate eaten. The ICR is calculated by dividing the number of grams of carbohydrate in the meal or snack by the units of insulin given (Example: 60 grams of carbohydrate were eaten and 6 units of insulin were given; therefore, the ICR is 1 unit of insulin per 10 grams of carbohydrates or ICR = 1:10).

ratio.[35] Note that a person may have a different ICR for different meals or snacks, based on physical activity, insulin needs, and other variables. In addition, ICRs may change with body weight, hormonal changes, and variations in physical activity.

Nutritive Sweeteners: Sucrose, Fructose, and Polyols

It is estimated that 14.6% of energy in the average American adult's diet comes from added sugars. Higher intake of added sugars is linked to higher energy intake and poorer quality of diet, as well as an increased risk for obesity, prediabetes, type 2 diabetes, and cardiovascular disease.[36] The word "nutritive" in the term "nutritive sweetener" implies the understanding that calories (energy) are provided.

Sucrose

As a form of carbohydrate, sucrose and fructose have an energy value of 4 kcal/g. For the individual with type 1 or type 2 diabetes, the total amount of carbohydrate consumed at meals, regardless of whether the source is sucrose or starch, has consistently been reported in the literature as the primary determinant of postprandial glucose levels. As a result, sucrose-containing foods can be substituted for other carbohydrate foods if the individual with type 1 or type 2 diabetes chooses to do so. Research has shown that when sucrose intakes of 10–35% of total energy were substituted for isocaloric amounts of starch, there were no negative effects on glycemic or lipid level responses.[4] However, caution should be advised because intake of other nutrients ingested with sucrose, such as fat, could lead to excess energy intake, and excess sucrose could be substituted for high-quality starches, consequently contributing to inadequate intake of foods with essential nutrients.[2,4]

Fructose

Although fructose has been shown to produce a lower postprandial glucose response in PWD when it replaces sucrose or starch in the diet, there is a concern that fructose may adversely affect plasma lipids (especially triglycerides); therefore, its use as a sweetening agent is not recommended.[2] However, naturally occurring fructose found in nutrient-dense fruits, vegetables, and other foods need not be avoided by PWD, but appropriately incorporated with the total carbohydrate content of the diet.

Polyols

Reduced calorie sweeteners such as sugar alcohols (polyols), like erythritol, isomalt, lactitol, maltitol, mannitol, sorbitol, xylitol, tagatose, and hydrogenated starch hydrolysates, are not fully absorbed from the gut. As such, they provide approximately 2 kcal/g (one-half the calories of other nutritive sweeteners).[2] These nutritive sweeteners are generally recognized as safe (GRAS) by the Food and Drug Administration (FDA). They are found commonly in sugar-free chocolates and sweets, which although labeled as "sugar-free" are not calorie-free, and will elevate blood sugar levels if consumed in excess. In addition to causing glycemic reactions, high intake levels of sugar alcohols have been known to cause gastrointestinal distress, and may carry a label warning about potential laxative effects.

Use of polyols, or sugar alcohols, as sweeteners reduces the risk of dental caries. There is no evidence, however, that sugar alcohols reduce glycemia, energy intake, or weight. Although they appear to be safe, polyols may cause diarrhea in children, or, with excessive amounts in adults, can also cause gastrointestinal side effects.[2] When calculating the carbohydrate content of foods containing polyols, subtracting half of the grams is appropriate.[2]

Nonnutritive Sweeteners

The term "nonnutritive" implies the understanding that "no" calories or energy is provided. Nonnutritive sweeteners (NNS), sometimes called artificial sweeteners, are food additives regulated by the FDA. Currently, there are seven NNS that have been approved by the FDA for use in the United States: acesulfame K, aspartame, Luo Han Guo extract, neotame, saccharin, stevia, and sucralose.[36] The FDA has established an acceptable daily intake (ADI) level for each of these NNS. The ADI assumes a level that is safe to consume per day, but which is not advisable to surpass.[37] Table 6–16 contains a summary of the NNS, their chemical names, sweetness comparison to sucrose, ADI, and common uses in the food supply.[36]

The limited number of studies examining the safety and use of NNS in PWD reports that NNS do not affect changes in glycemic responses. Although research is limited, these products are widely tested and have been proven to be safe in animal studies before being marketed to human populations. In their position paper on the use of nutritive and nonnutritive sweeteners, the Academy of Nutrition and Dietetics states:

> It is the position of the Academy of Nutrition and Dietetics that consumers can safely enjoy a range of nutritive and nonnutritive sweeteners when consumed within an eating plan that is guided by current federal nutrition recommendations, such as the Dietary Guidelines for Americans and the Dietary Reference Intakes, as well as individual health goals and personal preference.[3]

Resistant Starch and High-Amylose Foods

Resistant starch is starch that is physically enclosed within intact cell structures. It is found in some legumes, starch granules (as in raw potato), and retrograde amylose from plants modified by plant breeding to increase amylose content.[2] It has been proposed that foods containing resistant starch or high-amylose foods may modify postprandial glycemic response, prevent hypoglycemia, and reduce hyperglycemia. There are, however, no published long-term studies in PWD to prove these benefits.[2]

Table 6-16. Nonnutritive sweeteners approved for use in the United States by the FDA.

Name	Acceptable Daily Intake (ADI) and Estimated Daily Intake (EDI)	Times Sweeter than Sucrose	Use in Food Supply
Acesulfame K	ADI: 15 mg/kg body weight (BW) EDI: 0.2-1.7 mg/kg BW	200	• Approved for general use, except in meat and poultry • Combines well with other NNS • Stable at baking temperatures
Aspartame	ADI: 50 mg/kg BW EDI: 0.2-4.1 mg/kg BW	160-220	• Approved for general use • Degrades during heating
Luo Han Guo extract	ADI: None determined EDI: 6.8 mg/kg BW	150-300	• Generally recognized as safe (GRAS) • Intended for use as a tabletop sweetener, a food ingredient, and a component of other sweetener blends
Neotame	ADI: 18 mg/kg BW EDI: 0.05-0.17 mg/kg BW	7000-13,000	• Approved for general use, except in meat and poultry • To date, little use in food processing
Saccharin	ADI: prior sanctioned food ingredient, no ADI determined EDI: 0.1-2 mg/kg BW	300	• Limited to <12 mg/fl oz in beverages, 20 mg per serving in individual packages, or 30 mg per serving in processed foods
Stevia	ADI: 4 mg/kg BW EDI: 1.3-3.4 mg/kg BW	250	• GRAS • Intended for use as a sweetener in a variety of food products, including cereals, energy bars, beverages, and as a tabletop sweetener
Sucralose	ADI: 5 mg/kg BW EDI: 0.1-2.0 mg/kg BW	600	• General use • Heat stable for cooking and baking

Data from Academy of Nutrition and Dietetics, 2012.

Glycemic Index and Glycemic Load

Although the primary determinant of postprandial glucose response is the balance between total carbohydrate intake and available insulin, several other factors have been identified that influence the glycemic

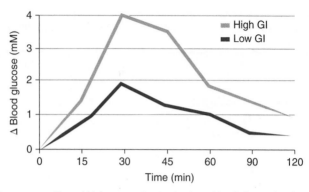

Figure 6–1. Effect of high- versus low-GI foods on blood glucose levels.

response to foods. One of these factors is the glycemic index (GI) of a food, which is the increase above fasting in the blood glucose area over 2 hours after ingestion of a constant amount of that food (usually a 50 grams of digestible carbohydrate portion) divided by the response to a reference food (either glucose or white bread).[2]

In clinical practice, the use of the GI has been questioned due to factors such as the intra- and intervariability of glucose responses, and studies comparing high- versus low-GI diets report mixed effects on HbA1c levels (Figure 6–1). These research studies are complicated by differing definitions of high-GI or low-GI diets or quartiles, as well as possible confounding dietary factors.[4] It is worth noting that when a person consumes a particular food (eg, white bread), the food is rarely consumed on its own. That food is likely to be eaten alongside other foods (eg, turkey, mayonnaise, cheese, lettuce, and tomato). Thus, the blood sugar response to eating is a response to the macronutrient composition of the entire sandwich, not just the white bread.

High-glycemic index foods are those with a GI >70 and include foods such as breads, breakfast cereals, rice, and snack products (including whole grain types), whereas low-GI foods are those with a GI <55 and include legumes, pasta, fruit, vegetables, and dairy.[38] Further limiting the practical use of the GI is the fact that the amount of carbohydrate in a typical serving of food is not taken into account; rather GI values are based on a standard amount of carbohydrate (50 grams). To state this another way, consider the amount of carrots that you would have to eat to consume 50 grams of carbohydrate. It is roughly 1 pound, certainly not a standard serving size of carrots, which actually represents a relatively modest carbohydrate load when considering typical portion sizes of such a food.

To counter the limitations of the GI, scientists sometimes refer to the glycemic load (GL). The GL differs from the GI and takes into consideration the standard serving of a given type of food. To calculate the GL of a food, divide its GI by 100 and then multiply by grams of carbohydrate in one serving. In the example of carrots, with a GI of 39 and approximately 8 grams of carbohydrate per half cup serving,[38,39] the GL is 3.12. Low-GL foods are generally those with a GL of <10, moderate-GL foods have a GL of 11–19, and high-GL foods are those with a GL >20.[40]

If the use of the GI is proposed as a method of meal planning, the practitioner is encouraged to advise the individual with type 1 or type 2 diabetes on the conflicting evidence of effectiveness.[4] It is also important to note that low-glycemic index foods that are rich in fiber and other important nutrients should be encouraged.[2]

Glycemic Index and Weight: What Does the Evidence Say?

The Academy of Nutrition and Dietetics Evidence Analysis project has found that there is good evidence to support the statement that, "Eight randomized controlled trials report no significant differences in energy intake or body weight after the consumption of a low-glycemic index diet" (Evidence Grade I – good).[41]

Fiber

Increased intake of whole grains and dietary fiber has been reported to reduce risk of diabetes, while whole grain-containing foods have been associated with improved insulin sensitivity, independent of body weight. Additionally, increases in dietary fiber intake have been shown to improve insulin sensitivity and result in an improved ability to secrete insulin adequate to overcome insulin resistance.[2] Recommendations for fiber intake for PWD are similar to the recommendations for the general public: follow the DRI of 14 g/1000 kcal,[10] and include a variety of fiber-containing foods, such as legumes, fiber-rich cereals (≥5 grams of fiber per serving), fruits, vegetables, and whole-grain products. These foods provide vitamins, minerals, and other phytochemicals important for good health.[10] Although more usual fiber intakes (up to 24 g/day) have not shown beneficial effects on glycemia, diets containing 44–50 grams of fiber daily are reported to improve glycemia in PWD.

Due to the potential gastrointestinal side effects and undesirable palatability of some high-fiber products, achieving such high-fiber intakes may be difficult. Therefore, it is recommended that PWD include foods containing 25–30 grams of fiber per day, with special emphasis on soluble fiber sources (7–13 grams).[10] As part of a cardioprotective nutrition therapy, studies in participants without diabetes show that diets high in total fiber (17–30 g/day) and soluble fibers (7–13 g/day), as part of a diet low in saturated fat and cholesterol, can further reduce total cholesterol by 2–3% and LDL cholesterol up to 7%.[4]

- ## Protein

High-protein digestibility-corrected amino acid score (PD-CAAS) is the criterion used to categorize protein sources as being of a good or high quality. Sources of high-PD-CAAS proteins include meat, poultry, fish, eggs, cheese, and soy, and the high scores of these items are reflected by the fact that they contain all of the nine essential amino acids. Cereals, grains, nuts, and vegetables are not considered to have a high PD-CAAS because they lack one or more of the essential amino acids. When planning meals, protein intake should be >0.8 g/kg/day to account for the mixed protein quality in foods.[2]

Protein Intake and Normal Renal Function

Research demonstrates that usual protein intake of approximately 15–20% of daily energy intake does not have to be changed for persons with type 1 or type 2 diabetes and who have normal renal function. Usual protein intake in longer-term studies has minimal effects on glucose, lipid level, and insulin concentrations, even though protein intake does cause small amounts of insulin secretion. However, in persons who consume excessive protein choices high in saturated fats, who have a protein intake less than the RDA, or who have diabetic nephropathy, a change in protein intake is warranted.[10]

Protein Intake and Diabetic Nephropathy

Dietary protein restriction has been shown to slow the progression of declining GFR, albuminuria, and occurrence of end-stage renal disease (ESRD) in patients with varying stages of nephropathy.[10] The long-term effect on the development of nephropathy of dietary protein intake of >20% of energy has not been determined; however, a protein intake of <1.0 g/kg/day has been recommended for persons with diabetic nephropathy.[2] Studies have shown that a decrease in protein intake to ~0.7 g/kg/day, but not at a protein intake of ~0.9 g/kg/day, resulted in hypoalbuminemia, or low levels of albumin in the blood.[4] For persons with chronic kidney disease Stages 3 through 5 (late-stage diabetic nephropathy), the potential risk of malnutrition should be monitored via hypoalbuminemia and energy intake. In any case, overall nutritional status should be continually monitored, and changes in protein and energy deficits may occasionally need to be corrected. Chapter 9 contains more information about diet for kidney disease.

- ## Fat

Given that PWD are at a three- to fourfold increased risk for CVD, the amount and type of fat in their diet is an important dietary consideration. This increased risk of CVD is particularly evident in younger age groups and in women. PWD have equivalent CVD risk as persons with pre-existing CVD and no diabetes; therefore, it is imperative that the

MNT for diabetes addresses this risk. Limiting saturated and *trans* fatty acids, as well as reducing dietary cholesterol intake, is the primary goal of MNT for persons with CVD (and thus also for PWD). In addition, other beneficial effects have been reported, including the use of fiber, phytostanols/phytosterols, omega-3 fatty acids, a Mediterranean diet, and other plant-based food approaches.[4] Although fewer studies examining these benefits have been conducted in PWD, because persons with CVD and PWD have equivalent CVD risks, the MNT recommendations are the same for both groups.

Omega-3 Fatty Acids

In individuals with type 2 diabetes who have high triglyceride levels, very long chain omega-3 polyunsaturated fatty acid supplements (primarily consisting of fish oil supplements) have been shown to lower plasma triglyceride levels.[2] Although a small accompanying rise in plasma LDL cholesterol has also been observed, the concomitant rise in the HDL cholesterol (healthy lipoprotein) may counteract this concern.[2] Two or more servings of fish per week (with the exception of commercially fried fish fillets) can routinely and beneficially replace high-saturated fat-containing foods from the diet, in addition to providing valuable omega-3 fatty acids.[2]

Mediterranean Diet

The Mediterranean-style diet incorporates a high-monounsaturated fatty acid (MUFA) dietary pattern. A modified Mediterranean diet, in which polyunsaturated fatty acids were substituted for monounsaturated fatty acids, reduced overall mortality in elderly Europeans by 7%.[2] In a 2-year dietary intervention study, Mediterranean and low-carbohydrate diets were found to be effective and safe alternatives to a low-fat diet for weight reduction in moderately obese participants.[10] A recent randomized trial looking at high-risk individuals in Spain showed that the Mediterranean dietary pattern reduced the incidence of diabetes in the absence of weight loss by 52%, compared to the low-fat control group.[10]

In regards to pancreatic beta-cell health and insulin resistance, fatty acids in monounsaturated oils were found to mitigate the negative effects of saturated palmitic acid on beta-cell death,[42] and unlike circulating saturated fatty acids that have been found to cause pronounced insulin resistance, MUFA did not.[19] It would appear from this research that a Mediterranean diet is beneficial in the role of diabetes management; however, a clearer understanding of the protective mechanisms from differing components of the diet is still warranted.[4]

Trans Fatty Acids

In nondiabetic individuals, reducing *trans* fatty acid intake decreases plasma total and LDL cholesterol. Saturated and *trans* fatty acids are the principal dietary determinants of plasma LDL cholesterol. Thus, minimal intake of *trans* fatty acids is recommended for PWD.[2] This can be obtained primarily through minimizing packaged and processed dessert and snack foods that are the primary sources of *trans* fat in the Western diet.

Dietary Cholesterol

In nondiabetic individuals, reducing dietary intakes of cholesterol decreases plasma total and LDL cholesterol. The recommended daily intake of cholesterol for PWD is <200 mg/day. One egg yolk contains approximately 200 milligrams of cholesterol, so the assumption is that foods such as eggs may be part of a well-balanced diet for PWD, provided that such foods are consumed in moderation.

Saturated Fats

In nondiabetic individuals, reducing saturated fatty acids decreases plasma total and LDL cholesterol. Although reducing saturated fatty acids may also reduce HDL cholesterol, the ratio of LDL cholesterol to HDL cholesterol is not adversely affected.[2] The recommendation for saturated fatty acids for PWD is <7% of total calorie intake per day. As covered previously, circulating saturated fatty acids appear to cause pronounced insulin resistance.[19] Minimizing saturated fatty acid intake is best achieved through a reduction in animal foods such as meats and full-fat dairy, tropical oils, and other added fats.

Plant Sterol and Stanol Esters

The intestinal absorption of dietary and biliary cholesterol can be limited or partially blocked through the routine use of plant sterol and stanol esters. A daily intake of approximately 2 grams of plant sterols and stanols has been shown to lower plasma total and LDL cholesterol in individuals with and without type 2 diabetes. Plant sterols are now being added to a wide range of foods and beverages. Consumers of these products are advised to monitor the excess calories and fat that such products can deliver alongside their potential healthful contributions.[2] Chapter 5 contains more information on the CVD-preventing effects of plant stanols and sterols.

■ Micronutrients and Antioxidants

The vitamin and mineral needs of PWD appear to be no different than for the general population, and there also appears to be no indication for routine supplementation, unless there are underlying deficiencies. Underlying deficiencies are most likely to occur in the high-risk populations of the elderly, women who are pregnant or lactating, strict vegetarians and vegans, those on extreme calorie-restricted diets, those with malabsorption syndromes or cardiovascular disorders, and those with poor overall metabolic and glycemic control.[10] Natural food sources and a balanced diet that meets the RDA and DRI for all micronutrients should be the focus by healthcare providers through nutritional counseling and individualized meal planning, rather than with micro-nutrient supplementation.[10,43]

Historically, there was belief that antioxidant therapy had a beneficial application for PWD because diabetes is considered to exist alongside a state of increased oxidative stress. To date, however, no studies have examined the effects of dietary intervention on circulating antioxidant levels and inflammatory biomarkers. The limited and small clinical studies that have involved functional foods thought to have high antioxidant potential (eg, tea, cocoa, and coffee) in PWD were found to be inconclusive and lack any benefit with respect to glycemic control and progression of complications. In fact, studies have shown a potential harm from high supplemental doses of vitamin E, carotene, and other antioxidants.[10] In PWD and a history of CVD, no beneficial effects on CV outcomes, microvascular complications, or glycemic control were observed.[4] Therefore, due to the lack of evidence of efficacy and concern for long-term safety, routine supplementation with antioxidants is not advised.[10]

Carbohydrate intolerance may be aggravated by a dietary deficiency of chromium, potassium, magnesium, and possibly zinc. The deficiency of potassium or magnesium in serum is readily detectable; however, the detection of zinc or chromium deficiency is more challenging.[10] Beneficial effects on glycemia were achieved with chromium supplementation in the late 1990s in two randomized, placebo-controlled studies in China; but chromium status, either at baseline or following supplementation, was not evaluated. Chromium supplementation was found to have a possible role in the management of glucose intolerance in GDM and in diabetes induced by corticosteroids, according to data from recent small studies. Other well-designed studies in PWD and impaired glucose tolerance, however, have failed to demonstrate any significant benefit for chromium supplementation.[10] In addition, chromium picolinate supplementation has been evaluated in a meta-analysis of randomized, controlled trials, with no benefit demonstrated. Although one small study suggested that chromium picolinate may reduce insulin resistance, the FDA concluded that there was an uncertain relationship between chromium picolinate and either insulin resistance or type 2 diabetes.[10]

Medical Nutrition Therapy for Diabetes Mellitus: Overall Nutrition Recommendations

- ### Primary Prevention: Preventing Diabetes

Because of the strong genetic implications and autoimmune characteristics involved in the development of type 1 diabetes, no diet has been shown to prevent type 1 diabetes. The story, however, is quite different with regards to the prevention of type 2 diabetes. Overweight and obesity, which are both strong risk factors for type 2 diabetes, have been promoted by lifestyle changes characterized by increased energy intake and decreased physical activity.[2] More than 85% of people with type 2 diabetes are overweight or obese.[44] From a practitioner standpoint, this means that when you are talking about type 2 diabetes prevention, you are mostly talking about excess weight gain prevention. The nutrition and diet therapy recommendations for individuals at high risk of developing type 2 diabetes are as follows[2]:

- Lifestyle changes that include moderate weight loss of at least 7% of body weight and regular physical activity of at least 150 minutes/week, with dietary strategies that include reduced calories and reduced intake of dietary fat
- The inclusion of dietary fiber (14 grams of fiber per 1000 kcal) and foods that contain whole grains (at least one-half of total grain intake should be from whole grains)
- Although there is not sufficient, consistent information to conclude that low-glycemic load diets reduce the risk for diabetes, low-glycemic index foods that are rich in fiber and other important nutrients are to be encouraged.

■ Secondary Prevention: Controlling Diabetes

For a person with type 1 or type 2 diabetes, the primary determinants of postprandial glucose levels are carbohydrate intake and available insulin; therefore, managing carbohydrate intake is a primary strategy for achieving glycemic control.[4] It should be mentioned, however, that total energy intake from all the macronutrients (carbohydrate, protein, and fat) cannot be ignored as excessive energy intake may lead to weight gain and consequent insulin resistance.[4] In addition, PWD should be aware of the importance of acquiring appropriate micronutrient intake, including daily vitamin and mineral requirements from natural food sources and a balanced diet.[2] The overall MNT recommendations for controlling diabetes are included in Table 6–17.[10,45]

■ Tertiary Prevention: Controlling Diabetes Complications

Improving glycemic control, lowering blood pressure, and potentially reducing protein intake all work synergistically to modify the progression of diabetes complications, as demonstrated in the Epidemiology of Diabetes Interventions and Complications (EDIC) trial (the follow-up of the Diabetes Control and Complications Trial [DCCT]).[46] In this study, the risk of the combined end point of cardiovascular death, myocardial end point of cardiovascular death, myocardial infarction, and stroke was significantly reduced, and most of the treatment effect was explained by adjustment for HbA1c.[2] The risk reductions achieved exceeded those demonstrated by other interventions such as blood pressure and cholesterol reductions. In *the United Kingdom Prospective Diabetes Study*, CVD risk in type 2 diabetes was also found to be proportionate to the

Table 6–17. Nutrition and diet recommendations for controlling diabetes.

Carbohydrate Recommendations

Carbohydrate intake from fruits, vegetables, whole grains, legumes, and low-fat milk is encouraged in a daily dietary meal plan

A similar amount of carbohydrate should be consumed throughout the day each day, and distributed evenly throughout the day

To achieve glycemic control, the monitoring of carbohydrate intake is a key strategy that can be achieved through carbohydrate counting, exchanges, or experience-based estimation

A modest additional benefit to observing total carbohydrate alone is the use of the glycemic index and glycemic load

Excess energy intake should be avoided; however, foods containing sucrose can be substituted for other carbohydrates in the meal plan; insulin or other glucose-lowering medications should be used if sucrose is added in addition to an established meal plan

A variety of fiber-containing foods are encouraged

When consumed within the daily intake levels established by the FDA, sugar alcohols and NNS are safe

Fat and Cholesterol Recommendations

Saturated fat should comprise no more than 7% of total calories

Limit intake of *trans* fat

Dietary cholesterol limited to no more than 200 mg/day

Omega-3 polyunsaturated fatty acids from 2–3 servings of fish per week

Protein Recommendations

For those with normal renal function and diabetes, modification of protein to 15–20% of energy; or a reduction to protein of 0.8–1.0 g/kg/day

Protein should not be used to treat acute or prevent nighttime hypoglycemia, since ingested protein can increase insulin response without increasing plasma glucose concentrations

Although high-protein diets of >20% of calories from protein may lead to short-term weight loss and improve glycemia, the long-term effects on kidney function are unknown; thus, high-protein diets are not recommended

Micronutrient Recommendations

No clear evidence of benefit for vitamin or mineral supplementation in those who do not have underlying vitamin or mineral deficiencies

Due to lack of evidence of efficacy and long-term safety concerns, routine supplementation with antioxidants, such as vitamin E, vitamin C, and carotene, is not recommended

Supplementation with chromium has not been clearly demonstrated and is therefore not recommended in those without a deficiency

(Continued)

Table 6-17. Nutrition and diet recommendations for controlling diabetes. (*Continued*)

Calorie Recommendations
Adjusting portions to reasonable sizes is essential for optimal glucose and weight control; PWD should be encouraged to consume foods they enjoy, but in smaller portions

Type 1 Diabetes Nutrition Recommendations
Insulin therapy needs to be integrated into the dietary and physical activity patterns
Adjustment of the meal and snack insulin doses based on the carbohydrate content of the meals and snacks needs to be made with the use of rapid-acting insulin by injection or with the use of an insulin pump
Carbohydrate intake on a day-to-day basis should be kept consistent with respect to time and amount when using fixed daily insulin doses
Insulin doses can be adjusted for planned activity, and extra carbohydrate can be given for unplanned activity

Type 2 Diabetes Nutrition Recommendations
In order to improve glycemia, dyslipidemia, and blood pressure, lifestyle modifications that reduce intakes of energy, saturated and *trans* fatty acids, cholesterol, and sodium and that increase physical activity are encouraged
To determine if adjustments in foods and meals are sufficient to achieve blood glucose goals, or if medication(s) will need to be combined with MNT, SMBG should be instituted

Data from American Diabetes Association, 2013; Daly, 2009.

level of HbA1c elevation.[47] The overall MNT recommendations for controlling microvascular and macrovascular complications in diabetes are outlined in Table 6-18.[2,10]

Medical Nutrition Therapy for Diabetes Mellitus: Specific Populations and Circumstances

The goal for MNT for individuals in specific situations is to meet their unique nutritional needs.[2] As with all of the other nutrition-related disease states covered in this book, there is no "one-size-fits-all" approach when it comes to making nutrition recommendations for PWD. For individuals treated with insulin or insulin secretagogues, the goals of MNT are to provide self-management training for safe conduct of exercise,

Table 6-18. Nutrition and diet recommendations for controlling diabetes complications.

Microvascular Complications

In PWD in the earlier stages of CKD, reduce protein intake to 0.8-1.0 g/kg body weight per day

For those in latter stages of CKD, protein reduction to 0.8 g/kg body weight per day should be implemented as this may improve measures of renal function (urine albumin excretion rate, glomerular filtration rate)

Diet therapy that favorably affects CV risk factors (macrovascular) has been found to also favorably affect microvascular complications (eg, retinopathy and nephropathy), and should therefore be implemented

Macrovascular Complications

HbA1c should be kept as close to normal as possible without significant hypoglycemia; the ADA recommends a HbA1c target of <6.5% as long as significant hypoglycemia does not act as a barrier

Diets high in fruits, vegetables, whole grains, and nuts should be part of the daily dietary meal plan

Dietary sodium intake of <2000 mg/day may reduce symptoms of symptomatic heart failure in PWD

A reduced sodium intake of <2300 mg/day and DASH eating plan to lower blood pressure (see Chapter 5), with a diet high in fruits, vegetables, and low-fat dairy products should be implemented

A modest amount of weight loss has beneficial effects on blood pressure and should be encouraged if indicated

Data from American Diabetes Association, 2008; American Diabetes Association, 2013.

prevention and treatment of hypoglycemia, and diabetes treatment during acute illness.[2]

■ Children and Adolescents

Type 1 Diabetes

Developing and implementing an optimal diabetes regimen for children and adolescents requires the consideration of the many unique aspects of care and management of this population, especially those diagnosed with type 1 diabetes. Roughly three-quarters of the cases of type 1 diabetes are diagnosed in those who are less than 18 years of age.[10] Diabetes in children differs in many aspects from diabetes in adults. For children with type 1 diabetes, consider the effects of sexual maturity and physical growth on insulin sensitivity and overall well-being, the ability to provide self-care, whether proper supervision and management during school or day-care activities is being provided, and attention to family dynamics and developmental stages.[10] Children also have unique neurological vulnerability to hypoglycemia and diabetic ketoacidosis (DKA), and as a result, glycemic goals are not the same as they are for adults.[10] Overall, MNT for children and adolescents with type 1 diabetes should be focused on the achievement of optimal blood glucose levels without excessive hypoglycemia, optimal lipid and blood pressure levels, and normal growth and development.[48] The age-specific glycemic and HbA1c goals for children and adolescents are listed in Table 6–19.[10]

Despite the reality that MNT plays a very important role in the treatment of type 1 diabetes in children and adolescents, in practice, it is often the most difficult aspect of treatment. There is no research on the nutrient requirements for children and adolescents with diabetes; therefore, nutrient recommendations are based on requirements for all healthy children and adolescents.[48] Individualized meal planning to accommodate food preferences, cultural influences, and physical activity patterns must be assured, along with the appropriate meal planning approach to assist families in learning the effect of food on blood glucose levels. A child's appetite should also be considered when determining energy requirements and the overall nutrition therapy. Weight gain and growth patterns should be followed on a regular basis to assure adequacy of energy intake. As energy requirements change with age, growth rate, and physical activity, the nutrition prescription will also change. An annual assessment of height, weight, BMI, and the nutrition plan should meet minimal requirements. Such an assessment will also assist in achieving good metabolic control, which is essential for normal growth and development.[48] In an effort to control blood glucose, the withholding of food or requiring a child to eat consistently when without an appetite is to be discouraged.

Table 6–19. Plasma blood glucose and HbA1c goals for children and adolescents with type 1 diabetes.

Age Group	Plasma Blood Glucose Goal Range (mg/dL) Before Meals	Plasma Blood Glucose Goal Range (mg/dL) at Bedtime or Overnight	HbA1c Goal
Toddlers and preschoolers, age 0–6 years	100–180	110–200	<8.5%
School age, age 6–12 years	90–180	100–180	<8%
Adolescents and young adults, age 13–19 years	90–130	90–150	<7.5%

Data from American Diabetes Association, 2013.

If a child becomes overweight, calories should be restricted and/or activity increased, while monitoring the gender-specific BMI-for-age percentile.[48]

Just as in adults, total carbohydrate content of meals and snacks is the most important parameter for determining the premeal insulin dosage and projecting the postprandial response. The same methods of calculation used in adults for determining ICR and estimating the carbohydrate content of meals can be used for children and adolescents.[48] For those who are on fixed insulin regimens and who do not adjust premeal insulin dosages, the carbohydrate intake needs to be consistent.[48]

In many cases, it is common for the newly diagnosed type 1 PWD to be placed on a consistent carbohydrate diet. The person will be prescribed a set amount of carbohydrates to consume at breakfast, lunch, dinner, and snacks. The insulin regimen will then be titrated around this set amount of carbohydrates until optimal glycemic control is achieved. At this point, the person can begin eating more or less carbohydrates with their meals and snacks, then experimenting with ICRs to control the postprandial glucose response.

Type 2 Diabetes

It is only in the last decade that the incidence and prevalence of type 2 diabetes among children and adolescents have been recognized as a critical health concern. Research on the effectiveness of MNT for diabetes in children and adolescents is limited, but, based on the existing evidence pertaining to adults with type 2 diabetes, the ability to prevent and treat type 2 diabetes in children with MNT and lifestyle changes is promising.[2,5] As long as nutritional needs for normal growth and development are maintained, it is reasonable to apply approaches demonstrated to be effective in adults, even though there are insufficient data at present to warrant any specific recommendations for prevention of type 2 diabetes in youth.[2] Although primary prevention efforts most likely focus on weight management in childhood, the potentially important etiology of type 2 diabetes in youth also includes the consideration of early life factors such as general maternal diabetes, glycemic control during pregnancy, and breastfeeding.[49] A cardiovascular disease risk factor profile for youth with diagnosed type 2 diabetes also includes screening for obesity, dyslipidemia, hypertension, or a combination of these factors.[49]

▪ Prepregnancy, Pregnancy, and Lactation

The general diet therapy principles for diabetes in prepregnancy, pregnancy, and lactation are the same as those for nondiabetic women in these life stages (see Chapter 4). The goals for MNT during these special circumstances are to promote the following[50]:

- An adequate nutritional intake that supports a healthy pregnancy
- Optimal glucose control by balancing food/carbohydrate intake with physical activity and insulin treatment

- Adequate but not excessive weight gain
- The learning of appropriate food and exercise behaviors that can contribute to long-term maternal health; this will also result in the promotion of healthy behaviors in the offspring.

■ Prepregnancy

For Type 1 and Type 2 Diabetes

Preconception diabetes care is greatly facilitated when pregnancies are planned; however, in reality, nearly two-thirds of pregnancies in women with diabetes are unplanned. Preconception counseling should be a part of all routine diabetes clinic visits for women of child-bearing age, starting at puberty. Before conception is attempted, HbA1c levels should be as close to normal as possible (<7%), and all MNT goals and interventions should be executed to help achieve this goal. The appropriateness of the use of or ability to continue medications, particularly statins, ACE inhibitors, ARBs, and most noninsulin therapies, should be evaluated prior to conception, as these commonly used drugs to treat diabetes may be contraindicated during pregnancy.[10] Because of the risk for neural tube defects, 400 mcg/day of folate should be consumed in women capable of becoming pregnant. Folate intakes of 600 mcg/day should be consumed in the periconception and prenatal periods through supplementation or consumption of fortified food sources.[50]

For Gestational Diabetes

Obesity, excessive weight gain prior to pregnancy, and increased saturated fat intake are associated with the development of glucose abnormalities in pregnancy and increased risk for developing gestational diabetes (GDM).[10] In order to reduce the risk for the development of GDM in the nondiabetic population, prior to conception, achievement of a normal weight before pregnancy is encouraged.

■ Pregnancy

For Pre-Existing Diabetes

During pregnancy, adequate energy intake facilitates appropriate weight gain rates, and weight loss is generally not recommended (see Chapter 4 for more information on maternal weight gain guidelines during pregnancy). The distribution of energy and carbohydrate intake during pregnancy should be based on the woman's food and eating habits and her plasma glucose responses. Because of a continuous fetal draw of glucose from the mother and the increased risk for hypoglycemia as well as the risk of ketonemia from ketoacidosis or starvation ketosis, maintaining a consistency of times and amounts of food eaten are important considerations. Plasma glucose monitoring and daily food record documentation are important tools that can allow the practitioner to adjust for food and/or insulin intake and monitor for adverse effects.[2] Optimal glycemic and blood

Table 6-20. Optimal glycemic and blood pressure goals during pregnancy with pre-existing diabetes.

Glycemic Parameter	Goal
Premeal, bedtime, and overnight glucose	60-99 mg/dL
Peak postprandial glucose (2 hours after the first bite of food)	100-129 mg/dL
Mean daily glucose	<110 mg/dL
HbA1c	<6.0
Blood pressure	110-129 mm Hg systolic BP 65-79 mm Hg diastolic BP

Data from American Diabetes Association, 2008; American Diabetes Association, 2013.

pressure goals for pregnancy and pre-existing diabetes are listed in Table 6-20.[2,10]

For pregnant women with pre-existing diabetes, a food plan that consists of a daily meal and snack pattern should be developed based on individual preferences. The following list provides suggestions for meal planning for this population[50]:

- Provide adequate calories to meet energy needs and promote appropriate rates of weight gain
- Provide protein at roughly 1.2 g/kg/body weight per day
- Minimum intake of 175 g/day digestible carbohydrate (noting that significantly more carbohydrate will likely be required)
- Distribute carbohydrate throughout the day to promote optimal glycemic control and to avoid hypoglycemia and ketonemia
- Consume a wholesome, balanced diet consistent with ethnic, cultural, and financial considerations, while maintaining the pleasure of eating
- Encourage fiber intake of at least 28 grams per day with use of whole grains, legumes, nuts, seeds, fruits, and vegetables
- Consistently time meals and snacks to minimize hypoglycemia, and in proper relation to insulin doses to prevent hyperglycemia (eat every 2–3 hours and do not fast for more than 10 hours overnight)
- Promote intake of unsaturated fatty acids (omega-6 and omega-3 fatty acids)
- Control fat intake in the interest of long-term maternal health and limit saturated fats and *trans* fats

In order to assess adequacy of nutrient intake and comparison of carbohydrate intake with SMBG records, all food and beverage intake should be recorded continuously or for at least 1 week before each visit.

Folate at 600 mcg/day should be continued during the prenatal period, either with supplementation or with fortified food choices. Supplemental mineral, trace element, and vitamin intake that meets the AI or RDA recommended by the IOM should be continued during all trimesters of pregnancy.[50,51] The supplementation of iron is not necessary unless hemoglobin is <11.0 g/dL in the first and third trimesters, or <10.5 g/dL in the second trimester, and when there is other laboratory evidence of iron deficiency.

In women with type 1 diabetes who may have autoimmune gastritis, folate supplementation may mask signs of vitamin B_{12} deficiency, and obtaining a baseline vitamin B_{12} level may be indicated in these patients.[50] Supplementation of vitamin D and vitamin B_{12} may be needed for vegetarian pregnant women. Evidence to support recommendations for general supplementation of omega-3 fatty acids in a diabetic pregnancy is insufficient. Due to the risk of CVD or hypertriglyceridemia, women with diabetes are encouraged to eat at least two meals of oily ocean fish per week (up to 12 oz/week) to increase omega-3 fatty acids (eicosapentaenoic and docosahexaenoic acids), while avoiding eating fish potentially high in methylmercury (eg, swordfish, king mackerel, shark, or tilefish).[50] Additional nutritional considerations and approaches may be indicated in other medical conditions that are linked to diabetes, including celiac disease, autoimmune atrophic gastritis, nonalcoholic hepatic steatosis, and postgastric bypass surgery.

For Gestational Diabetes

Risk assessment for GDM should be conducted at the first prenatal visit.[52] Clinical characteristics that are consistent with a high risk of GDM are marked obesity, personal history of GDM, glycosuria, or a strong family history of diabetes. Glucose testing as soon as feasible should be undertaken in those at high risk of GDM. If the initial screening is negative, the woman should be retested between 24 and 28 weeks of gestation.[37] MNT should be initiated within 1 week after diagnosis of GDM and include a minimum of three nutrition visits. If a woman is diagnosed with impaired glucose tolerance (IGT) during pregnancy, the same MNT recommendations apply because similar adverse outcomes have been shown to occur with both IGT and GDM.[3] The primary goals of MNT for GDM are promotion of optimal nutrition for maternal and fetal health, with adequate energy for appropriate gestational weight gain, as well as the achievement and maintenance of normoglycemia and the absence of ketosis. This is primarily achieved with a carbohydrate-controlled meal plan. Individual assessment and SMBG are used to determine and modify the specific nutrition and food recommendations, and training patients in carbohydrate counting is imperative. Studies have shown that this approach reduces serious perinatal complications without increasing the rate of cesarean delivery, while also improving the quality of life. Therefore, MNT should be provided to all women with GDM at the time of diagnosis.[2,48]

Table 6-21. Sample distribution of carbohydrates for a GDM meal pattern.

Meal	Number of Servings	Grams of Carbohydrates or Carbohydrate Choices[a]
Breakfast	Limit of 2	30 grams or 2 choices
Noon meal	3-4	45-60 grams or 3-4 choices
Evening meal	3-4	45-60 grams or 3-4 choices
3-4 Snacks	1-2	15-30 grams or 1-2 choices

[a] 1 Choice = 15 grams of carbohydrate.

Clinical outcome measures such as hunger, plasma glucose levels, weight gain, and ketone levels are used to determine the amount and distribution of carbohydrate, as long as a minimum of 175 grams of digestible carbohydrate per day is provided. Three small-to moderate-sized meals, and two to four snacks per day is the generally preferred carbohydrate distribution, with an evening snack to prevent overnight accelerated ketosis. Usually, less carbohydrate is tolerated at breakfast than at other meals, so when planning a meal plan, consider allocating less of the carbohydrate budget to the morning meal and snacks. Maintaining carbohydrate consistency at meals and snacks becomes an even higher priority with the addition of insulin to MNT.[2,48] A sample distribution of carbohydrates for a GDM meal pattern is listed in Table 6–21, with the blood glucose targets for a GDM pregnancy listed in Table 6–22.[10,37,53]

In obese women with GDM (BMI >30 kg/m^2), hypocaloric diets can result in ketonemia and ketonuria. A moderate caloric restriction of 30% of estimated energy needs (to ~25 kcal/kg actual weight per day) may help improve glycemic control without ketonemia, reduce

Table 6-22. Blood glucose targets in GDM pregnancy.

	ADA	ACOG
Fasting	≤95 mg/dL	<95 mg/dL
1 hour postmeals	≤140 mg/dL	<130 mg/dL
2 hours postmeals	≤120 mg/dL	<120 mg/dL

Data from American Diabetes Association, 2013; American Diabetes Association, 2004; American College of Obstetricians and Gynecologists (ACOG) Practice Bulletin, 2001.

maternal weight gain, and reduce plasma triglycerides. How these diets affect perinatal outcomes has not yet been determined; however, fetal macrosomia and unhealthy maternal postpartum weight retention are associated with excess gestational weight gain. Individual energy requirements, and whether a woman is purposefully under-eating to avoid insulin therapy, should be monitored through the use of daily food records, weekly weight checks, and ketone testing. Maternal glucose levels have been shown to decrease, and maternal and fetal outcomes improve, with a restriction of carbohydrates to 35–40% of calories.[2,37,48]

An adjunct to improving maternal glycemia is regular physical activity, which helps to lower fasting and postprandial plasma glucose concentrations. For all individuals capable of participating, planned physical activity of 30 minutes per day is recommended. Brisk walking or arm exercises while seated in a chair for at least 10 minutes after each meal will meet this goal. Regular aerobic exercise with proper warm-up and cool-down should be encouraged. Safety precautions should also be considered,[2,48] and the potential for hypoglycemia in women using pharmacological treatment should be addressed. Contraindications to exercise during pregnancy may include, but are not limited to: pregnancy-induced hypertension, premature rupture of membranes, intrauterine growth retardation, preterm labor or history of incompetent cervix/cervical cerclage, and persistent second or third trimester bleeding. Medical clearance is recommended before initiating an exercise program.[10]

Even though most women with GDM will revert to normal glucose tolerance postpartum, women with GDM are at an increased risk for GDM in subsequent pregnancies, as well as for type 2 diabetes later in life, obesity, and CVD. In order to reduce these subsequent risks, lifestyle modifications after pregnancy that are aimed at reducing weight and increasing physical activity are strongly encouraged.[2] MNT for GDM should emphasize overall healthy food choices, portion control, and cooking practices that can continue postpartum.[2,48,52]

Lactation

Breastfeeding in infants of women with GDM and pre-existing diabetes is strongly recommended, although planning and coordination of care are needed for successful lactation. Because of the calories expended with nursing, in most situations, less insulin is required of breast-feeding mothers. Fluctuations in blood glucose related to nursing sessions have been reported in women who breastfeed, and often a carbohydrate-containing snack is required before or during breast-feeding to prevent hypoglycemia.[2] See Chapter 4 for the recommended energy requirements when breastfeeding. Unless contraindicated, breastfeeding should be encouraged, as the research indicates that even a short duration of breastfeeding results in long-term improvements in glucose metabolism and may also reduce the risk of type 2 diabetes in children.[2]

■ Older Adults

Chapter 4 discusses the age-related changes that can lead to altered nutritional intake. These and other special factors must be considered when managing blood glucose levels, preventing potential acute and chronic complications, and providing self-management education to the older adults with diabetes.

Nutrition

Modest energy restriction (5–10% of body weight) and an increase in physical activity may be of benefit for the obese older adult with diabetes. Energy requirements in this population are generally less than those for a younger individual of a similar weight. In the case of involuntary gain or loss of 10 pounds or 10% of body weight in less than 6 months, a thorough MNT evaluation is indicated in the older adult PWD. A daily multivitamin/mineral supplement is appropriate for those older adults with reduced energy intake.[2] It is important to assess and monitor the older person's fluid intake, due to a decreased thirst mechanism, total body water, renal concentrating ability, and vasopressin effectiveness that can lead to the potential complication of hyperglycemic hyperosmolar nonketotic coma (HHNK) that can occur with acute hyperglycemia and dehydration.[54]

Physical Activity

In order to attenuate the loss of lean body mass that occurs with energy restriction and with advanced age, physical activity is strongly recommended in the geriatric population. Table 6–23 lists the risks and benefits (other than improved glycemic control) of physical activity in the elderly.[25]

Medications

Visual difficulties and decreased fine motor skills may interfere with the ability of the older adult to prepare and self-administer their medications, especially insulin; thus, assistance may be needed. Cognitive

Table 6–23. Risks and benefits of physical activity in the elderly.

Benefits	Risks
Reduces decline in maximal aerobic capacity	Cardiac ischemia
Improves risk factors for atherosclerosis	Musculoskeletal injuries
Slows the age-related decline in lean body mass	Hypoglycemia with use of certain antidiabetic medications
Decreases central adiposity	
Improves insulin sensitivity	

Table 6-24. Medications that can affect glycemic response.

Increase Risk of Hyperglycemia	Increase Risk of Hypoglycemia
Diuretics	Beta blockers
Glucocorticoids	Monoamine oxidase inhibitors
Nicotinic acid	Phenylbutazone
Lithium and other antidepressants	Aspirin in large doses
	Cimetidine

ability and/or confusion from a complicated drug regimen may also be an issue. Response to antidiabetic medications in the elderly may be affected by altered renal function, altered hepatic function, and drugs used to treat coexisting conditions, and all of these can complicate diabetes management. Table 6–24 lists common drugs that can affect glycemia and, in turn, potentially alter MNT.

Hypoglycemia

The risk for hypoglycemia increases in older adulthood as a result of renal changes, slowed counter-regulation, inadequate hydration, use of multiple medications, erratic food intake, and slowed intestinal absorption. Symptoms related to neuroglycopenia include confusion and lack of motor skills, as opposed to the more common epinephrine responses of shakiness, sweating, and weakness that is commonly seen in younger patients. The older person should be educated on how to recognize their own individual signs and symptoms.[24]

Self-Monitoring

Depression and cognitive dysfunction may interfere with self-monitoring and total diabetes care management. Visual acuity and fine motor skills can also interfere with SMBG; therefore, assistance in choosing the appropriate glucometer to meet the individual's needs may be required. In some cases, use of a talking glucometer may be warranted.

Acute Illness

During acute illnesses, increases in counter regulatory hormones occur, and the need for insulin and oral glucose-lowering medications may often be higher than usual. This can lead to the development of hyperglycemia and ketoacidosis. In situations like this, patients should be advised of the following:[2,55]

- Test plasma glucose and ketones more often (at least every 2–4 hours) and report moderate-to-large urine ketones to the healthcare team
- Increase fluid intake and assure adequate hydration

- If plasma glucose is <100, give additional carbohydrate containing liquids or food as tolerated (amount of daily carbohydrate sufficient to prevent starvation ketosis is 150–200 grams or 45–50 grams every 3–4 hours); note that this additional carbohydrate can come from crackers, soup, regular soda or juice, or glucose tablets
- Continue insulin and oral glucose-lowering medications
- Watch for signs of ketoacidosis: nausea, vomiting, abdominal pain, increased drowsiness, fruity odor to breath, and cracked lips, mouth, or tongue

Hypoglycemia

For PWD taking insulin or insulin secretagogues, changes in food intake, physical activity, and medication can contribute to the development of hypoglycemia. Hypoglycemia (plasma glucose <70 mg/dL) requires treatment with the ingestion of glucose or glucose-containing foods. The glucose content, rather than the carbohydrate content of the food, correlates better with the acute glycemic response. Table 6–25 describes the effects of oral glucose supplementation for treatment of hypoglycemia.[2]

Note that response to treatment should be apparent in 10–20 minutes; however, test again in ~60 minutes, as glucose levels begin to fall and an additional treatment may be necessary.

Any form of carbohydrate that contains glucose will raise blood glucose, but pure glucose may be the preferred treatment in hypoglycemia. The glycemic response is not affected by adding protein to the carbohydrate and subsequent hypoglycemia is not prevented by the addition of protein. The acute glycemic response may be retarded and prolonged by the addition of fat. Gastric-emptying rates are twice as fast during hypoglycemia as during euglycemia, with liquid and solid foods having the same response.[2] One helpful way to address hypoglycemia is to recommend and use the "15 and 15" rule: if blood sugar is less

Table 6–25. Effects of oral glucose supplementation for treatment of hypoglycemia.

Amount of Oral Glucose	Resultant Rise on Plasma Glucose Levels	Time to Recovery
10 grams	40 mg/dL	20 minutes
20 grams	60 mg/dL	45 minutes

Data from American Diabetes Association, 2008.
Response to treatment should be apparent in 10–20 minutes; however, test again in ~60 minutes, as glucose levels begin to fall and an additional treatment may be necessary.

than 70 mg/dL, eat or drink something with 15 grams of carbohydrate. Rest for 15 minutes, and then re-check blood sugar. If blood sugar is still below 70, repeat with 15 more grams of carbohydrate, and 15 minutes rest before re-checking.

Acute and Chronic Care Facilities

Acute care facilities

The establishment of an interdisciplinary team that implements MNT and timely diabetes-specific discharge planning is known to improve the care of PWD both during and after hospitalizations. The implementation of a diabetes meal-planning system that provides consistency in the carbohydrate content of meals is an important aspect of care.[2] A hospitalized patient, with or without diabetes, often suffers from hyperglycemia, which is a marker of poor clinical outcomes. In order to optimize glucose control, the interdisciplinary team must integrate MNT into the overall management plan. It is suggested that hospitals implement a consistent carbohydrate diabetes meal-planning system that uses meal plans without a specific calorie level, but has consistency in carbohydrate intake of the meals. The day-to-day carbohydrate content of specific meals and snacks is kept constant, but the individual meal and snack carbohydrate content may vary. The American Diabetes Association no longer endorses a single nutrition prescription or percentages of macronutrients; thus, the term "ADA" diet is no longer used.[2] As with any hospitalized patient, special nutrition issues may arise for the use of liquid diets, pre- and postsurgical diets, and enteral or parenteral nutrition. Table 6–26 provides recommendations for liquid diets and tube feedings. Chapter 10 provides greater detail for these special nutrition issues.[2]

Overfeeding hospitalized patients should be avoided in order to decrease the chance for hyperglycemia. For most patients, calorie requirements range from 25 to 35 kcal/kg/24 hours; however, this will vary based on specific and individualized circumstances. As with all patients, the progression of liquid to solid food consumption should be implemented as rapidly as possible.[2] In the newly diagnosed hospitalized PWD, DSMT/E can be initiated in the hospital, but it is best

Table 6–26. Special nutritional needs of the hospitalized PWD.

Type of Nutrition	Recommendations
Clear or full liquid diets	Nonsugar-free liquids consisting of ~200 grams of carbohydrate per day in equally divided amounts at meal- and snack times
Tube feedings	Either a standard enteral formula (50% of carbohydrate) or a lower-carbohydrate content formula (30–40% of carbohydrate)

Data from American Diabetes Association, 2008.

provided in an outpatient setting when the PWD is better able to focus on the education being provided.

Long-term care facilities

Just as in an acute care facility, an interdisciplinary team approach is necessary to integrate MNT in PWD residing in long-term care facilities, although the imposition of dietary restriction is no longer warranted in the elderly PWD in these settings. There is no evidence to support prescribing diets such as "no concentrated sweets," "no sugar-added," or "liberal diabetic diet" over standardized diets in this population because these obsolete diets unnecessarily restrict sucrose. Instead, PWD in long-term care facilities should be served a regular menu, with consistency in the amount and timing of carbohydrate and special attention paid to individual food preferences. Older patients with diabetes in these facilities may tend to be underweight rather than overweight, which is associated with greater morbidity and mortality, and as such, their nutrition interventions should be tailored accordingly.

Studies have shown that geriatric PWD will eat better when they are given less restrictive diets. To reduce the risk of iatrogenic malnutrition, making medication changes to control glucose, lipids, and blood pressure, rather than implementing food restrictions, may be more appropriate. Specific nutrition interventions will depend on other factors as well, such as age, life expectancy, comorbidities, and patient preferences.[2]

Medical Nutrition Therapy for Diabetes Mellitus: Special Topics

▪ Plant-Based Diets

Plant-based diets (vegan or vegetarian) that are well planned and nutritionally adequate have been shown to improve metabolic control.[3] Among individuals following plant-based and vegetarian diets, diabetes prevalence is relatively low; but it also bears noting that this population is more likely to be engaged in other healthful behaviors that may further contribute to low risk of diabetes. In addition, clinical trials using vegetarian diets have shown improvements in glycemic control and cardiovascular health. Barnard, Scialli, Turner-McGrievy, Lanou and Glass compared the effects of a low-fat vegan diet to those of a diet based on the National Cholesterol Education Program in nondiabetic overweight women, with exercise patterns unchanged.[56] The low-fat vegan diet resulted in significant weight loss, despite the absence of prescribed limits on portion size or energy intake.

Barnard et al. investigated the effects of a low-fat vegan diet consisting of vegetables, fruits, whole grains, and legumes (~10% of energy from fat, 15% from protein, and 75% from carbohydrate) compared to a conventional diabetes diet following ADA guidelines (less than 7% of energy from saturated fat, 15–20% from protein, 60–70% from carbohydrate and monounsaturated fat, and less than 200 mg/day from cholesterol) on glycemic control, weight loss, and plasma lipid levels in type 2 PWD.[57] Portion sizes, energy intake, and carbohydrate intake were unrestricted in the low-fat vegan diet group, while the ADA diet group had nutrient content individualized based on body weight and plasma lipid concentrations. It was found that both diets were associated with modest, sustained weight loss, and yielded comparable reductions in HbA1c, but more individuals in the vegan group were able to reduce medications. Significantly greater reductions were seen in HbA1c and total and LDL cholesterol concentrations in the vegan group, after controlling for these medication changes. There was also a greater reduction of triglycerides in the vegan group compared with the conventional group, and this reduction was attributed to the use of high-fiber and low-glycemic index foods. This is unlike other research studies that have shown elevation in triglycerides with the use of refined carbohydrate diets. However, in this study, weight loss was also likely to have had an effect on lipid levels.

- ▪ Alcohol

With regards to alcohol, the same precautions that apply to the general population also apply to the PWD. If a person chooses to drink alcohol, no more than one alcohol-containing beverage per day is recommended for adult women, and no more than two per day for adult men.[42] This is considered to be light-to-moderate alcohol intake guidelines, whereas three or more drinks per day is considered to be an excessive amount.[2] One alcohol containing beverage is defined as 12 oz beer, 5 oz wine, or 1.5 oz distilled spirits (80 proof), with each serving containing approximately 15 grams of alcohol.[2,42]

Primary Prevention

Observational studies have suggested that light to moderate consumption of alcohol may improve insulin sensitivity and decrease the risk of type 2 diabetes, coronary heart disease, and stroke.[2,42] The associated decreased risk for coronary heart disease does not appear to be due to the concomitant increase in plasma HDL cholesterol.[2] The cardioprotective factors of alcohol cannot be determined by the type of alcohol consumed.[2,42] Although light to moderate alcohol consumption may have some primary prevention benefits, heavy alcohol consumption may be associated with increased incidence of diabetes.[2] Overall, the data do not support recommending alcohol consumption to individuals at risk of diabetes.[2]

Secondary Prevention

For people with a history of alcohol abuse or dependence, pregnant women, and people with medical problems such as liver disease, pancreatitis, advanced neuropathy, or severe hypertriglyceridemia, abstinence from alcohol should be advised.[2] If adults with diabetes choose to consume alcohol, daily intake should be limited to a light to moderate amount.[2]

When ingested with food, moderate amounts of alcohol (served without any mixers) have minimal acute effects on plasma glucose and serum insulin concentrations, but carbohydrate co-ingested with alcohol (as in a mixed drink) may raise blood sugar. For individuals using insulin or insulin secretagogues, alcohol should be consumed with food to avoid hypoglycemia. Evening consumption of alcohol may increase the risk of nocturnal and fasting hypoglycemia. To reduce risk of nocturnal hypoglycemia in individuals using insulin or insulin secretagogues, alcohol should be consumed with food.[2] Excessive amounts of alcohol have been shown to contribute to hyperglycemia.[2]

Tertiary Prevention

Light to moderate alcohol consumption is associated with reductions in blood pressure; however, chronic excessive alcohol intake is associated with an increased risk of hypertension. In patients at high risk for heart failure, alcohol intake is strongly discouraged.[2]

▪ Diet and Genome Interactions

Differences in individual glycemic responses to food are now being explored in some research settings as a function of diet/genome interactions. How individuals react physiologically to their dietary pattern may be influenced by a number of genetic factors. In experiments with mice, overexpression of the Rad gene caused mice eating a high-fat diet to become more insulin resistant and glucose intolerant, compared to mice eating the same diet having normal gene expression. In humans, Rad overexpression has also been identified, thus suggesting that a high-fat diet may have similar impact in some individuals. Eventually, further genetic studies may allow the fine-tuning of individual diets, in order to optimize glycemic control and improve long-term glycemic outcomes.[58]

▪ Wound Healing

As the result of circulation and nerve damage from hyperglycemia, wound healing in PWD is a significant, complex, and multifactorial problem that often leads to amputation in those who develop foot ulcers as a result of recurrent mechanical trauma of daily ambulation. Cellular and inflammatory pathways are involved in wound healing. Hyperglycemia, due to a hyperosmotic effect, leads to loss of water and electrolytes, decreased tissue oxygenation, slowed neutrophil chemotaxis, and impairment of the overall immune response. Diabetes can be viewed as a state of chronic vascular inflammation, as altered glucose and free fatty acid metabolism increase the production of free radicals. This, in turn, increases oxidative stress, endothelial dysfunction, and activation of inflammatory cytokines, leading ultimately to tissue damage and cell death. Increased protein degradation and increased collagen formation as a result of lack of insulin in diabetic wounds impedes the body's ability to heal. Due to this cascade of effects from hyperglycemia on wound healing, prevention is crucial, as is optimum MNT to promote healing.[59] Chapter 10 contains more information for goals of MNT in wound healing.

■ Eating Disorders

The ideal situation and standard of care for both eating disorders and diabetes treatment is most effective when undertaken from a multidisciplinary approach. It is important that the team and the practitioner be knowledgeable in both conditions, and understand the effective treatment strategies for both, which can often appear to have conflicting goals and strategies for treatment. When disordered eating and diabetes occur simultaneously, the initial focus should be on establishing medical stability before addressing specific eating disorder symptoms, with optimal diabetes management to be gradually approached.[60]

One particular form of bulimia can present in eating disordered PWD who are taking insulin. In this form of bulimia, the purging, or getting rid, of calories is achieved by refusing to inject insulin. The PWD may continue to eat normal or even large quantities of food, but because she does not take insulin, the calories are not absorbed and weight loss is achieved. The resulting hyperglycemia from not injecting insulin becomes a major medical concern, because over time, HbA1C values will remain elevated and micro- and macrovascular complications may develop.

MNT goals for PWD and eating disorders should be customized according to the type and the severity of the eating disorder symptoms. For both conditions, the treatment involves using the "total diet" approach, and is aimed at normalizing eating, rather than on specific nutrients or foods, and focusing on "moderation and proportionality in the context of a healthful lifestyle."[60]

Medical Nutrition Therapy for Diabetes Mellitus: Meal Planning Tools and Resources

As part of the ongoing practice of incorporating MNT in the management of your patients' diabetes, you will routinely assess your patients, monitor and evaluate their metabolic parameters, and continue to teach and empower them to take leading roles in the management of their condition. Implementation of the overall MNT nutrient recommendations presented in this chapter requires significant behavioral changes on the part of the patient, and relies on appropriate practitioner meal planning tools and resources.

It may be helpful for the practitioner to prioritize the MNT advice and goals for the patient and have the patient choose one or

Table 6–27. Examples of poorly set goals and S.M.A.R.T. goals.

Poorly Set Goals	S.M.A.R.T. Goals
"I will reduce the amount of fast foods that I eat."	"I will decrease the amount of French fries I eat to less than 1 serving a week for the next 2 months."
"I will increase my physical activity."	"I will walk for 20 minutes, Monday, Tuesday, Wednesday, Friday, and Saturday, for the next month."
"I will eat more vegetables."	"I will replace the chips I eat with a spinach salad at lunch and add a serving of a yellow vegetable dinner at least two times a week for the next month."
"I will decrease the fat content of my diet."	"I will replace the margarine that I use on my food, with a lower calorie olive oil-based spray for the next 3 months."

two primary behavior-change areas he or she is willing to gradually work on. Providing a written copy of the specific goals,[45,61] and helping the patient develop "*S.M.A.R.T.*" goals, is crucial to the process. (See Chapter 2 and Table 2–36 for more information on goal setting). Ideally, both short- and long-term goals should be set. Table 6–27 provides examples of poorly set goals, and an example of a more preferable "*S.M.A.R.T.*" goal.

Opinions about the most effective MNT interventions or strategies are plentiful. There is no single strategy or method that can be recommended for every patient, and the method should be chosen based on the patient's individualized goals and circumstances. Initially, MNT educational tools for the PWD will incorporate the same basic nutrition guidelines that are used for the general population. More simplified resources that illustrate basic nutrition guidelines can be used during initial phases of diabetes MNT to provide "survival skill" education.[45] Even PWD who have more experience with diabetes management find that the day-to-day reality of diabetes management is overwhelming. In addition, they may have suboptimal math skills that limit their ability to correctly calculate carbohydrates and insulin needs. In these situations, finding simplified methods of portion control is necessary.[62] Some of these simplified resources are listed in Table 6–28 along with how they can be used, and where web educational or professional resources can be found.[60-62]

Table 6–29 lists and describes some of these more advanced meal-planning strategies, how they can be used, and where web educational or professional resources can be found.[61,63,64,65]

Table 6–28. Simplified diabetes MNT resource methods or strategies.

Method or Strategy	How It is Used	Web Educational or Professional Resources
ChooseMyPlate	• Mirrors the dietary guidelines and suggests number of servings from each of six food categories • Provides tips for healthy eating	www.choosemyplate.gov
U.S. Dietary Guidelines	• Cornerstone of Federal nutrition policy and nutrition education activities	www.dietaryguidelines.gov
Idaho Plate Method	• A visual method where a dinner plate serves as a pie chart to show proportions of the plate that should be covered by various food groups • Portions of foods and appropriate food choices can be depicted for meals and snacks in assorted forms of the model • Methods of presenting the model range from professional photography to hand-drawn sketches and displays of food models	http://www.diabetes.org/food-and-fitness/food/planning-meals/create-your-plate/ http://www.platemethod.com
Zimbabwe Hand Jive	• Illustrates how to measure the amount of food "imaginatively" in a reasonably accurate manner with one's hands, without scales or other measurement tools	http://medweb.bham.ac.uk/easdec/prevention/portionsize.htm
Guide to Good Eating (National Dairy Council)	• Groups food based on their nutrient content and suggests appropriate number of servings and portions	http://www.eatsmart.org/client_images/gtge-english_1_.pdf
Individualized Menus	• Based on a person's food preferences and treatment goals • Specifies the portions and types of foods to be consumed at meals and snacks	Professionally designed by a nutrition and diabetes specialist
Month of Meals	• 28 days of complete diabetes menus for breakfast, lunch, dinner, and snacks providing 1200, 1500, and 1800 calories per day	http://www.shopdiabetes.org/101-american-diabetes-association-month-of-meals.aspx

(Continued)

Table 6–28. Simplified diabetes MNT resource methods or strategies. (*Continued*)

Method or Strategy	How It is Used	Web Educational or Professional Resources
Meal Replacements	• Involves the use of formulas, shakes or bars, or prepared meals to control portions and simplify food decisions • Formula drinks or bars are used to replace two meals and one snack per day to achieve weight loss and to replace one meal per day for weight maintenance	Examples: Slim-Fast®, Glucerna® Nutrisystem®
Healthy Food Choices	• Simplified exchange list approach • Focuses on the importance of portion control and provides suggestions for making lower-fat and higher-fiber food choices, all of which can lead to weight loss	http://www.shopdiabetes.org/177-healthy-food-choices-25pk.aspx

Data from Brown et al., 2001; Rizor and Richards, 2000; Mian and Brauer, 2009; Delahanty, 2002.

Table 6–29. Advanced diabetes MNT resource methods or strategies.

Method or Strategy	How It is Used	Web Educational or Professional Resources
Exchange lists (Choose Your Foods: Exchange Lists for Diabetes)	• Validated system of meal planning that is designed to provide structure and an understanding of grouping food based on their nutrient content	www.eatright.org www.diabetes.org http://www.shopdiabetes.org/175-choose-your-foods-exchange-lists-for-diabetes-25pk.aspx
Nutrient counting	• A more precise meal-planning method that allows more flexibility with food choices and meal planning than the exchange list method • Can be used for calorie-, and/or fat- and/or carbohydrate counting • Journaling and/or tracking of nutrients are encouraged	http://www.diabetes.org/food-and-fitness/food/my-food-advisor/
Insulin-to-carbohydrate ratios (ICR)	• See section on calculating ICR in this chapter	Professionally assessed and taught by a nutrition and diabetes specialist

Data from Geil, 2008; Wheeler et al., 2008; Delahanty, 2002; King and Klawitter, 2007.

Summary

MNT for diabetes is complex and multi-factorial, and it requires the placement of pre-established systems and a team of health care professionals well-versed in effective diabetes management. In order to assess the need for changes in diabetes MNT, and to ensure successful outcomes, monitoring of HbA1c, lipids, blood pressure, body weight, and renal function is essential. Diabetes MNT is not limited just to the period surrounding to the time of diagnosis; rather it continues throughout life and must continually be re-evaluated based on changes in lifestyle, growth and development, health status, as well as advances in the fields of nutrition and diabetes.

Designing an individualized diabetes self-management nutrition plan takes commitment on the part of both the practitioner and the patient. Successful MNT for diabetes requires a team approach that can effectively empower PWD to take responsibility for their own self-care management through the powerful interplay of food, positive lifestyle decisions, and medication and insulin when necessary.

References

1. Kodama S, Saito K, Tanaka S, Maki M, Yachi Y, Sato M, et al. Influence of fat and carbohydrate proportions on the metabolic profile of people with type 2 diabetes: a meta-analysis. Diabetes Care 2009;32(5):doi: 10.2337/dc08-1716.

2. American Diabetes Association. Nutrition recommendations and interventions for diabetes: a position statement of the American Diabetes Association. Diabetes Care 2008;31(suppl 1):S61–S78.

3. Academy of Nutrition and Dietetics. (2011). ADA diabetes type 1 and 2 evidence-based nutrition practice guidelines for adults. Retrieved May 5, 2012, from Evidence Analysis Library: http://andevidencelibrary.com

4. Franz M, Powers M, Leontos C, Holzmeister L, Kulkarni K, Monk A, et al. The evidence for medical nutrition therapy for type 1 and type 2 diabetes in adults. J Am Diet Assoc 2010;110:1852–1889.

5. Morris S, Wylie-Rosett J. Medical nutrition therapy: a key to diabetes management and prevention. Clinical Diabetes 2010;28(1):12–18.

6. Funnell M, Brown T, Childs B, Haas L, Hosey G, Jensen B, et al. American Diabetes Association: national standards for diabetes self-management education. Diabetes Care 2011;33(suppl 1):S89–S96.

7. Bloomagarden Z. Approaches to treatment of prediabetes and obesity and promising new approaches to type 2 diabetes. Diabetes Care 2008; 33(7):1461–1466.

8. American Diabetes Association. Diagnosis and classification of diabetes mellitus. Diabetes Care 2012;35(suppl 1):S64–S71.

9. Wadden T, West D, Neiberg R, Wing R, Ryan D, Johnson, et al. One year weight losses in the Look AHEAD study: factors associated with success. Obesity 2009;17:713–722.

10. American Diabetes Association. Standards of medical care in diabetes—2013. Diabetes Care 2013;36(suppl 1):S11–S66.

11. American Academy of Family Physicians. (2010, October). Diabetes. Retrieved May 5, 2012, from Monitoring your blood sugar: http://familydoctor.org/online/famdocen/home/common/diabetes/living/779.html

12. American College of Endocrinology. American College of Endocrinology consensus statement on guidelines for glycemic control. Endocr Pract 2002;8:S1.

13. Kahn R, Fonseca V. Editorial: translating the A1c Assay. Diabetes Care 2008;31(8):1–4.

14. Odegard P, Beach J. Blood glucose monitoring: a practical guide for use in the office and clinic setting. Diabetes Spectrum 2008;21(2):100–111.

15. National Heart, Lung, and Blood Institute (NHLBI). Clinical Guidelines on the Identification, Evaluation and Treatment of Overweight, and Obesity in Adults. Bethesda, MD: National Institutes of Health; 1998.

16. Cummings S, Apovian C, Khaodhiar L. Obesity surgery: evidence for diabetes prevention/management. J Am Diet Assoc 2008;108(4 suppl 1):S40–S44.

17. Mian S, Brauer P. Dietary education tools for South Asians with diabetes. Can J Diet Pract Res 2009;70(1):28–35.

18. Fonseca V, Kulkarini K. Management of type 2 diabetes: oral agents, insulin, and injectables. J Am Diet Assoc 2008;108:S29–S33.

19. Chavez J, Summers S. Characterizing the effects of saturated fatty acids on insulin signaling and ceramide and diacylglycerol accumulation in 3T3-L1 adipocytes and C2C12 myotubes. Arch Biochem Biophys 2003;419(2):102–109.

20. Gaziano J, Cincotta A, O'Connor C, Ezrokhi M, Rutty D, Ma Z, et al. Randomized clinical trial of quick-release bromocriptine among patients with type 2 diabetes on overall safety and cardiovascular outcomes. Diabetes Care 2010;33(7):1503–1508.

21. Brown M, Lackey H, Miller T, Priest D. Controlling calories—the simple approach. Diabetes Spectrum 2001;14(2):110–112.

22. DeFronzo RA, Davidson JA, Del Prato S. The role of the kidneys in glucose homeostatis: a new path towards normalizing glycaemia. Diabetes, Obesity and Metabolism 2012;14(1):5–14.

23. Dose Adjustment for Normal Eating (DAFNE) Study Group. Training in flexible, intensive insulin management to enable dietary freedom in people with type 1 diabetes: Dose Adjustment for Normal Eating (DAFNE) randomized controlled trial. BMJ 2002;325(7367):746.

24. Cefalu W, Gerich J, LeRoith D. Council for Advancement of Diabetes Research & Education (CADRE) Handbook of Diabetes Management. New York, NY: Medical Information Press 2; 2004.

25. Colberg S, Sigal R, Fernhall B, Regensteiner J, Blissmer B, Rubin R, et al. Exercise and type 2 diabetes: The American College of Sports Medicine and the American Diabetes Association: joint position statement. Diabetes Care 2010;33(12):e147–e167.

26. Colberg S, Sigal R, Fernhall BR, Blissmer B, Rubin R, Braun B. Exercise and type 2 diabetes: The American College of Sports Medicine and the American Diabetes Association: joint position statement. Diabetes Care 2010;33(12):e147–e167.

27. Sigal R, Kenny G, Wasserman D, Castaneda-Sceppa C. Physical activity/exercise and type 2 diabetes. Diabetes Care 2004;27:2518–2539.

28. Kundrat S, Rockwell M. Sports Dietetics: Practiced, Proven, and Tested Manual. Urbana, IL: Nutrition on the Move, Inc; 2008.

29. Dunford M. Sports Nutrition: A Practice Manual for Professionals. 4th ed. Chicago, IL: American Dietetic Association; 2006.

30. Hinnen D, Guthrie D, Childs B, Guthrie R. Pattern management of blood glucose. In Franz M. A Core Curriculum for Diabetes Education. 4th ed. Chicago, IL: American Association of Diabetes Educators; 2001:173–197.

31. Walsh J, Roberts R. Exercise. In Walsh J, Roberts R. Pumping Insulin. San Diego, CA: Torrey Pines; 2000:157–168.

32. Rachmiel M, Buccino J, Daneman D. Exercise and type 1 diabetes mellitus in youth: review and recommendations. Pediatr Endocrinol Rev 2007;5: 656–665.

33. Wheeler M, Pi-Sunyer F. Carbohydrate issues: type and amount. J Am Diet Assoc 2008;108:S34–S39.

34. Westman E, Feinman R, Mavropoulos J, Vernon M, Volek J, Yancy W, et al. Low-carbohydrate nutrition and metabolism. Am J Clin Nutr 2007; 86(2):276–284.

35. Kulkarni K. Carbohydrate countin: a practical meal-planning option for people with diabetes. Clinical Diabetes 2005;23(3):120–122.

36. Academy of Nutrition and Dietetics. Use of nutritive and nonnutritive sweeteners: position of the Academy of Nutrition and Dietetics. J Acad Nutr Diet 2012;112:739–758.

37. American Diabetes Association. A position statement of the American Diabetes Association: gestational diabetes mellitus. Diabetes Care 2004; 27(1):S88–S90.

38. Atkinson F, Foster-Powell K, Brand-Miller J. International tables of glycemic index and glycemic load values: 2008. Diabetes Care 2008; 31(12):2281–2283.

39. US Department of Agriculture, Agriculture Research Service. (n.d.). National Nutrient Database for Standard Reference. Retrieved January 15, 2013, from National Agriculture Library: http://ndb.nal.usda.gov/ndb/foods/list

40. Foster-Powell K, Holt S, Brand-Miller J. International table of glycemic index and glycemic load values: 2002. J Am Clin Nutr 2002;76(1):5–56.

41. Academy of Nutrition and Dietetics. (2005, November). Low Glycemic Index Diet. Retrieved January 15, 2013, from Evidence Analysis Library: http://andevidencelibrary.com

42. Franz M, Bantle J, Beebe C, Brunzell J, Chiasson J, Garg A. Evidence-based nutrition principles and recommendations for the treatment and prevention of diabetes and related complications. Diabetes Care 2003;26(suppl 1): S51–S61.

43. Welch G, Rose G, Ernst D. Motivational interviewing and diabetes: what is it, how is it used, and does it work? Diabetes Spectrum 2006;19(1):5–11.

44. National Institute of Diabetes and Digestive and Kidney Diseases (NIDDK). (2010, April 7). Do You Know the Health Risks of Being Overweight. Retrieved January 16, 2013, from Weight Control Information Network: http://win.niddk.nih.gov/publications/health_risks.htm

45. Daly A. Healthy lifestyle changes: food and physical activity. In: Childs BP, Cypress M, Spollett G, eds. Complete Nurse's Guide To Diabetes Care. 2nd ed. Alexandria, VA: American Diabetes Association; 2009:24–39.

46. Diabetes Control and Complications Trial (DCCT) Research Group. The effect of intensive treatment of diabetes on the development nad progression of long-term complications in insulin-dependent diabetes mellitus. N Engl J Med 1993;329:977–986.

47. American Diabetes Association. Implications of the United Kingdom Prospective Diabetes Study. Diabetes Care 2002;25(suppl 1):S28–S32.

48. Silverstein J, Klingensmith G, Copeland K, Plotnick L, Kaufman F, Laffel L, et al. Care of children and adolescents with type 1 diabetes: a statement of the American Diabetes Association. Diabetes Care 2005;28(1): 186–212.

49. Mayer-Davis. Type 2 diabetes in youth: epidemiology and current research toward prevention and treatment. J Am Diet Assoc 2008;108: S45–S51.

50. Kitzmiller J, Block J, Brown F, Catalano P, Conway D, Coustan D, et al. Consensus statement of the American Diabetes Association: managing preexisting diabetes for pregnancy: summary of evidence and consensus recommendations for care. Diabetes Care 2008;31(5):1060–1079.

51. Institute of Medicine. Dietary Reference Intakes: Energy, Carbohydrate, Fiber, Fat, Fatty Acids, Cholesterol, Protein and Amino Acids. Washington, DC: National Academies Press; 2002.

52. Metzger B, Buchanan T, Coustan D, de Leiva A, Dunber D, Hadden D, et al. Summary and recommendations of the fifth international work-shop-conference on gestational diabetes mellitus. Diabetes Care 2007; 30(suppl 2):S251–S260.

53. American College of Obstetricians and Gynecologists (ACOG) Practice Bulletin. Clinical management guidelines for obstetrician-gynecologists: gestational diabetes. Obstet Gynecol 2001;98(3):525–538.

54. American Association of Diabetes Educators (AADE). From position statement: special considerations for education and management of older adults with diabetes. 2002.

55. American Diabetes Association. Be prepared: sick day management. Diabetes Spectrum 2002;15(54).

56. Barnard N, Scialli A, Turner-McGrievy G, Lanou A, Glass J. The effects of a low-fat, plant-based dietary intervention on body weight, metabolism, and insulin sensitivity. Am J Med 2005;118:991–997.

57. Barnard N, Cohen J, Jenkins D, Turner-McGrievy G, Gloede L, Jaster B, et al. A low-fat vegan diet improves glycemic control and cardiovascular risk factors in a randomized clinical trial in individuals with type 2 diabetes. Diabetes Care 2006;29(8):1771–1783.

58. Dedoussis G, Kaliora A, Panagiotakos D. Genes, diet and type 2 diabetes mellitus: a review. Rev Diabetic Stud 2007;4(1):13–24.

59. Sheehan P. Foot ulcers, peripheral arterial disease, and risk classification. In: Lebovitz H, ed. Therapy for Diabetes Mellitus and Related Disorders. Alexandria, VA: American Diabetes Association; 2009.

60. Goebel-Fabbri A, Uplinger N, Gerken S, Mangham D, Criego A, Parkin C. Outpatient management of eating disorders in type 1 diabetes. Diabetes Spectrum 2009;22(3):147–152.

61. Delahanty L. Evidence-based trends for achieving weight loss and increased physical activity: applications for diabetes prevention and treatment. Diabetes Spectrum 2002;15(3):183–189.

62. Rizor H, Richards S. All our patients need to know about intensified diabetes management they learned in fourth grade. Diabetes Educ 2000; 26(3):392–404.

63. Geil, P. Choose your foods: exchange lists for diabetes: the 2008 revision of exchange list for meal planning. Diabetes Spectrum 2008;21(4):281–283.

64. Wheeler M, Daly A, Evert A, Franz M, Geil P, Holzmeister L, et al. Choose your foods: exchange list for diabetes. J Am Diet Assoc 2008;108: 883–888.

65. King K, Klawitter B. Nutrition Therapy: Advanced Counseling Skills. 3rd ed. Philadelphia, PA: Lippincott Williams & Wilkins; 2007.

7

A Pain in the Gut: Nutrition in Gastrointestinal Disorders

A healthy digestive system is crucial for optimal nutritional status. Impairments in any segment of the gastrointestinal (GI) tract can quickly undermine adequate nutrient digestion, transport, and absorption. As advanced practice nurses often confront a wide variety of GI complaints, the importance of having a thorough understanding of both the digestive process as well as the relevant diet therapy for gastrointestinal disorders cannot be understated. Every year, digestive diseases affect upward of 70 million people in the United States (approximately 23% of the population).[1] Treating digestive disease accounts for $140 billion in annual medical costs,[2] and 31% of all ambulatory surgical procedures are performed for GI conditions.[3]

The term "digestive disorders" casts a wide net. Because the GI tract stretches from the mouth to the anus, the probability of something going awry in this arrangement of anatomy over the course of a lifetime is highly probable. Underlying disease pathology, medication use, surgical and therapeutic interventions, along with lifestyle choices and exercise patterns, all impact gut health. Regardless of the origination or severity of disruption in the GI tract, dietary manipulation is often an important component of digestive disorder management. By understanding the digestive process, where various nutrients are absorbed in the GI tract, and what dietary practices can be employed to minimize pain and maximize nutritional status, practitioners can help patients use food and nutrition to prevent, manage, and mitigate a variety of GI disorders.

Nutrient Digestion, Absorption, and Transport

The organs that make up the digestive tract consist of the mouth, esophagus, stomach, small intestine, large intestine, rectum, and anus (Figure 7–1). The small intestine includes the duodenum, jejunum, and ileum. The large intestine, also called the colon, houses the ascending, transverse, and descending portions of the colon. The pancreas, liver, and gallbladder, which produce and store digestive juices and enzymes, serve as accessory organs to the GI tract. Select components of the nervous and circulatory systems also play important roles in the digestive process.

In order to obtain the beneficial nutrients from foods you consume, foods must first be broken down, or digested, into their most simple components. The process of digestion allows for the eventual release, transport, and absorption of nutrients that are vital to health.

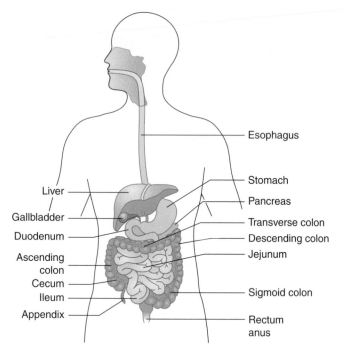

Figure 7–1. The anatomy of the digestive system.

The energy-yielding macronutrients (carbohydrate, proteins, and fats) utilize the digestive process to break their large molecular forms down into smaller, more usable components:

- Carbohydrate digestion involves the breakdown of complex polysaccharides into smaller monosaccharides: glucose, fructose, and galactose.
- Protein digestion requires enzymes to break the large polypeptide proteins down into dipeptides, tripeptides, and individual amino acids.
- Fats are digested down to free fatty acids, monoglycerides, glycerol, phospholipids, and cholesterol.

From a chemical standpoint, digestive juices, or enzymes, are secreted from the salivary glands, stomach, small intestine, liver (via the gallbladder), and pancreas. From a physical standpoint, peristalsis and segmentation mediate digestive travel (Figure 7–2). Peristalsis involves the successive waves of involuntary muscular contraction in the esophagus, stomach, and small intestine that move food through the gut. Segmentation is the periodic squeezing or partitioning of the intestine by its circular muscles, which mixes and then slowly pushes the GI contents along.

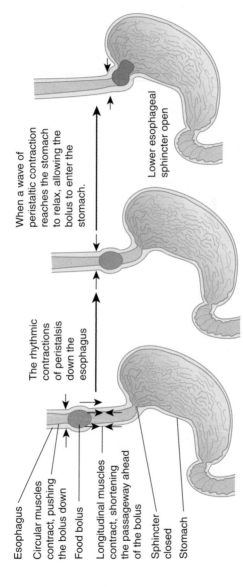

Esophagus

Circular muscles contract, pushing the bolus down

The rhythmic contractions of peristalsis down the esophagus

Food bolus

Longitudinal muscles contract, shortening the passageway ahead of the bolus

Sphincter closed

Stomach

When a wave of peristaltic contraction reaches the stomach to relax, allowing the bolus to enter the stomach.

Lower esophageal sphincter open

Figure 7-2. Peristalsis and segmentation.

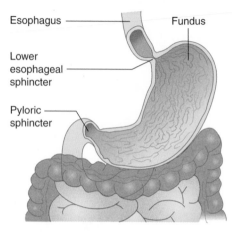

Figure 7–3. The lower esophageal and pyloric sphincters regulate the flow of food in and out of the stomach.

The three primary sphincters that are involved in regulating digestive travel and preventing the backflow of GI tract contents are as follows (Figure 7–3):

- *Lower esophageal sphincter:* located between the bottom of the esophagus and the top of the stomach; prevents acidic contents of the stomach from splashing back up into the esophagus
- *Pyloric sphincter:* located at the bottom of the stomach, between the stomach and the entrance to the small intestine; controls the rate of chyme (combination of stomach secretions and partially digested food) release into the small intestine
- *Ileocecal sphincter:* located at the end of the small intestine and the entrance to the large intestine; prevents contents of the large intestine from re-entering the small intestine

Digestion begins in the mouth, where salivary amylase secreted from the salivary glands begins to act on the starch content of carbohydrate-containing foods. The chewing and swallowing mechanisms progress the bolus of food into the esophagus. Food arriving from the esophagus into the stomach mixes with stomach acid and enzymes that promote protein and lipid digestion. Small amounts of lipid digestion take place in the stomach with the aid of lipolytic enzymes. Here, some proteins are also partially digested with proteolytic enzymatic assistance and are broken down into large peptides. The stomach is responsible for the production of gastric secretions including hydrochloric acid, gastric lipase, mucus, the GI hormone gastrin, and intrinsic factor (a glycoprotein that promotes absorption of vitamin B_{12} in the ileum).

After its journey through the stomach, the resultant chyme then transits to the small intestine. The majority of digestion and absorption of nutrients occurs within the first 100 centimeters of the small intestine.[4] With the exception of fiber and some carbohydrate, digestion and absorption of nutrients is generally completed by the time food remnants transit out of the small intestine. The large intestine is the site of reabsorption of water, electrolytes, and some vitamins.

■ Nutrient Absorption

No nutrient absorption occurs in the mouth or esophagus. There is a small amount of absorption that takes place in the stomach, primarily for alcohol and some medications. The small intestine is where most nutrient absorption occurs, and the anatomy of the small intestine is uniquely constructed to maximize nutrient digestion and absorption. The mucosa of the small intestine is arranged in a pattern of numerous folds that contain fingerlike projections called villi (Figure 7–4). The villi are constantly moving, trapping food and absorbing nutrients. Each fingerlike villus projection contains many additional, smaller hair-like projections called microvilli, which also facilitate absorption. The variety of structural levels of the small intestine increases its capacity for absorption by up to 600 times that of a simple tube.[5]

The small intestine is divided into three sections: the duodenum, the jejunum, and the ileum. The duodenum is approximately 0.5 meter-long, the jejunum is 2–3 meters, and the ileum is 3–4 meters. Most nutrient digestion and absorption occurs in the duodenum and jejunum. Digestive contents move through the small intestine at a rate of 1 centimeter per minute, taking anywhere from 3 to 8 hours to travel the length of the digestive tract.[4] Understanding where nutrients are absorbed along the GI tract can help predict potential nutrient deficiencies when injury or disease afflicts a particular area of the digestive tract. Table 7–1 highlights the location of specific nutrient absorption throughout the GI tract.[6]

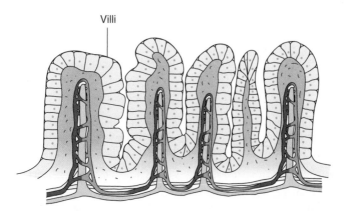

Villi

Figure 7–4. Intestinal villi.

Table 7–1. Primary sites of nutrient absorption.

Organ	Primary Nutrients Absorbed
Stomach	
	Water
	Alcohol
	Minerals: copper, iodide, fluoride, and molybdenum
Small intestine	
Duodenum	Minerals: calcium, phosphorus, magnesium, iron, and copper
	Vitamins: thiamin, riboflavin, niacin, biotin, folate, and vitamins A, D, E, and K
Jejunum	Minerals: calcium, phosphorus, magnesium, iron, zinc, chromium, manganese, and molybdenum
	Vitamins: thiamin, riboflavin, niacin, pantothenate, biotin, folate, vitamin B_6, vitamin C, and vitamins A, D, E, and K
	Lipids
	Carbohydrates: monosaccharides
	Proteins: amino acids and small peptides
Ileum	Minerals: Magnesium
	Vitamins: vitamins C, B_{12}, D, and K, and folate
	Bile salts and acids
Large intestine	
	Minerals: sodium, chloride, and potassium
	Vitamins: vitamin K, biotin
	Short-chain fatty acids
	Water

- ■ Nutrient Transport

When nutrients enter the bloodstream or the lymphatic system, they are transported with the assistance of the circulatory systems. Blood is carried to the digestive system via the arteries, which branch into capillaries to reach every cell in the body. Blood exiting the digestive system travels via the veins, with the hepatic portal vein directing the blood to and from the liver. The liver is the body's major metabolic organ, and it plays a vital role in digestion as it receives and packages absorbed nutrients and filters out harmful agents.

Lipid absorption proves difficult in the watery environment of the GI tract, and fats must utilize protein carriers to facilitate their absorption and transport. The cluster of fat and protein required to transport fats is called a chylomicron, which is a type of lipoprotein. Chylomicrons move throughout the body, with surrounding cells picking off their lipid contents. The shrinking chylomicron eventually travels to the liver, where different lipoproteins are produced. As a result of this lipid transport and absorption process, many diseases of the small intestine can interrupt normal fat digestion and absorption.

The liver produces lipoproteins of varying densities. Very low density lipoproteins (VLDLs) are made up primarily of triglycerides, and they transport lipids to various tissues in the body. Low-density lipoproteins (LDLs) are derived from VLDL, and are composed primarily of cholesterol. They carry cholesterol and triglycerides from the liver to the cells. High circulating levels of LDL are thought to elevate risk of cardiovascular disease. High-density lipoproteins (HDLs) are composed primarily of protein. They are synthesized in the liver and take cholesterol from the cells to the liver in preparation for metabolism and excretion. High circulating levels of HDL are cardioprotective. Table 7–2 summarizes lipoprotein construction, roles, and health implications, and Chapter 5 contains more information on lipoproteins and their role in cardiovascular health.

Table 7-2. Lipoproteins, their content, roles in the body, and health implications.

Lipoprotein	...is Made up of	...and Does:	Health Implications
VLDL: very low density lipoprotein	Mostly triglycerides	• Takes TG from the liver to the body tissues • Made by liver	
LDL: low-density lipoprotein	Mostly cholesterol	• Carries cholesterol and TG from the liver to the body's cells • What is left after the cells remove TG from VLDLs	• Large, light, and lipid-filled • ↑ LDL linked to ↑ heart disease risk • LDL = "Bad" (Less-healthy) cholesterol
HDL: high-density lipoproteins	Mostly protein	• Carries cholesterol back to the liver from the body's cells	• Small, dense, and protein-packed • ↑ HDL thought to be cardioprotective • HDL = "Good" (Healthy) cholesterol

Diet Therapy for Disorders of the Upper GI Tract

- ## Xerostomia

Xerostomia, also called "dry mouth," is a common salivary gland disorder. Healthy salivary glands produce 1–2 liters of saliva per day. Saliva is made up almost entirely of water (99.5%), electrolytes, and protein, and it contains amylase, an enzyme that initiates starch breakdown in the mouth. Saliva is also responsible for the lubrication and moistening of food in preparation for digestion. Saliva is important for dental hygiene because it neutralizes acid, protects teeth from dental caries, washes food away from the oral cavity, and facilitates the bacteriolytic protein lysozyme that further protects dentition from bacteria.

Xerostomia is a common side effect of a number of conditions, including Parkinson's disease, HIV/AIDS, Sjögren's syndrome, diabetes, and other autoimmune diseases.[7] Advancing age, radiation therapy and chemotherapy, nerve damage to the head or neck, and many medications can also result in dry mouth. Prolonged xerostomia can interfere with speech and taste, promote the presence of plaque, cause halitosis, contribute to depression, and negatively affect food intake and nutritional status. Patients often decrease the variety of foods they eat due to discomfort associated with dry mouth.[8]

When xerostomia as a side effect can be predicted, focusing on prevention should be the key, keeping in mind that nutrition, lifestyle, and pharmacologic treatment may also be indicated. Prevention (including products and practices to avoid) and treatment recommendations can be found in Table 7–3.[9]

- ## Dysphagia

Dysphagia is not a specific diagnosis or disease; rather it is the disruption of swallowing, which may be an indicator or symptom of any one of a number of disorders. Dysphagia, or difficulty swallowing, can negatively impact nutritional status if it affects dietary intake. Complications of dysphagia include choking and aspiration. Reduced ability to swallow food safely can result in a variety of nutritional deficiencies. Potential nutritional impacts of untreated dysphagia are outlined in Table 7–4.[10]

National Dysphagia Diets

Determination of safe swallow prognosis in patients with dysphagia involves a team-based clinical approach, with the speech language pathologist ultimately determining the appropriate level of modified diet texture and liquid consistency. In an effort to standardize language for dysphagia, the American Dietetic Association (ADA, now the Academy of Nutrition and Dietetics) published *The National Dysphagia Diet* (NDD) in 2002. The NDD proposes four levels of semisolid and solid foods and outlines inclusion and exclusion of food items for each level. Table 7–5 outlines the specifics of the NDD.[11,12]

Table 7–3. Xerostomia treatment techniques and products to avoid.

Nutrition and Lifestyle	Pharmacologic	Oral Care Practices	Products to Avoid
• Artificial saliva • Gum chewing • Sugarless candy • Increased fluid intake/ frequent sips of water • Sucking on ice cubes • Consumption of foods with high fluid content • Use of humidifier during sleep	• Amifostine • Inorganic thiophosphate, broad-spectrum cytoprotectant • Artificial saliva; available as sprays, lozenges, gels, and swabs	• Mouth rinse: ½ to 1 teaspoon baking soda + 8 ounces water every 2 hours while awake • Biotene products by laclede; include toothpaste, mouth rinse, and chewing gum • Chapstick and moisturizing gels to lips • Pilocarpine	• Sucrose-containing and carbohydrates that stick to teeth and lead to dental caries • Citrus and spicy foods • Dry and hard, nonmoist foods • Caffeine; limit coffee and tea • Tobacco • Alcohol • Alcohol-based mouth washes

Data from Academy of Nutrition and Dietetics, 2012; Radvansky LJ, Pace MB, Siddiqui A. Prevention and management of radiation-induced dermatitis, mucositis, and xerostomia. Am J Health Syst Pharm 2013;70(12):1025–1032.

Table 7–4. Nutritional consequences of untreated dysphagia.

Malnutrition
Aspiration pneumonia
Dehydration
Unintended weight loss
Depression
Mortality
Pneumonia
Decreased rehabilitation potential
Decreased quality of life
Increased length of hospital stay
Increased costs

Data from Academy of Nutrition and Dietetics, 2012.

Table 7–5. The National Dysphagia Diet food considerations.

The National Dysphagia Diet
The National Dysphagia Diet (NDD) is a standardized set of terminology for a progressive diet used nationally in the treatment of dysphagia. The NDD outlines requirements for both food consistency and liquid viscosity.

Dysphagia Pureed (NDD 1)

- Smooth, pureed, homogenous, and cohesive foods of "pudding-like" consistency
- Avoid gelatin, fruited yogurt, unblenderized cottage cheese, peanut butter, and lumpy food including hot cereal and soup
- Avoid scrambled, fried, or hard-boiled eggs; soufflés are allowed
- Mashed potatoes should be served with gravy, butter, margarine, or sour cream
- Pre-gelled slurried breads are allowed

Dysphagia Mechanically Altered (NDD 2)

- Moist, soft-textured foods that easily form a bolus
- Moist, tender ground or finely diced meats
- Soft, tender-cooked vegetables and soft ripe or canned fruit
- Slightly moistened dry cereal with little texture
- No bread, dry cake, rice, cheese cubes, corn, or peas
- Meats should not exceed ¼ inch cube, moistened with gravy or sauce
- Allows canned fruit (except stringy pineapple), cooked fruit, or fresh banana
- Avoids skins, dry fruit, coconut, and seeds
- Allows scrambled, poached, or soft-cooked eggs
- Cooked vegetables should be less than ½ inch and fork-mashable
- Note: Mechanical soft diet includes same foods as above, but allows bread, cakes, and rice

Dysphagia Advanced (NDD 3)

- Food is nearly regular texture with the exception of very hard, sticky, or crunchy foods
- Allows breads, rice, moist cakes, shredded lettuce, and tender, moist whole meats
- Avoids hard fruits and vegetables, corn, skins, nuts, and seeds

Regular

- All foods are allowed

Data from McCallum, 2003; McCullough et al., 2003.

Thickened Liquids

Dysphagia affects not only solid-food swallowing capabilities, but also the ability to safely swallow liquids of varying consistency. The NDD proposed four frequently used terms to label levels of liquid viscosity. Speech language pathologists determine the viscosity of fluid that a patient can tolerate separately from solid-food recommendations. The classification of liquid types is based on measurement using a viscometer. As most commercial establishments do not have a viscometer, commercial

Table 7–6. National Dysphagia Diet liquid consistencies.

NDD Liquid Consistency	Inclusions
Thin liquid	• Regular liquids, no adjustments • Includes anything liquid at room temperature: frozen yogurt, ice cream, and popsicles • Includes clear juices, milk, water, tea, coffee, soda, broth, plain gelatin, high-liquid fruits such as watermelon, grapefruit, and orange sections, or any food that will liquefy in the mouth within a few seconds
Nectar-like	• Falls slowly from a spoon and can be sipped through a straw or cup • Includes nectars, vegetable juices, chocolate milk, buttermilk, thin milkshakes, cream soups, and other properly thickened beverages
Honey-like	• Drops from a spoon, is too thick to be sipped from a straw • Includes tomato sauce
Spoon-thick	• Maintains shape, needs to be taken with a spoon, too thick to drink • Includes pudding, custard, and hot cereal

Data from Academy of Nutrition and Dietetics, 2012.

thickening agents or pre-thickened liquids are generally used to achieve the appropriate level of thickness. The four liquid types in the NDD are outlined in Table 7–6, in the order of least restrictive to most restrictive.[10]

Dehydration risk increases with dysphagia because fluid intake is often limited or suboptimal. While an individual's fluid needs are dictated by disease state, a general rule of thumb is that 30 milliliters of fluid per kilogram of body weight will provide normal daily fluid requirements. Fluid requirements may vary for those with cardiac problems, renal failure, dehydration, obesity, or in those who require fluid restrictions.[13]

Dysphagia: What Does the Evidence Say?

The Academy of Nutrition and Dietetics Evidence Analysis project has found that there is strong, conditional evidence to support the statement that, "Older adults consuming modified texture diets report an increased need for assistance with eating, dissatisfaction with foods, and decreased enjoyment of eating, resulting in reduced food intake and weight loss" (Evidence Grade 1 – good).[14]

■ Gastroesophageal Reflux Disease

Gastroesophageal reflux disease (GERD) occurs when the contents of the stomach splash back up into the esophagus causing irritation

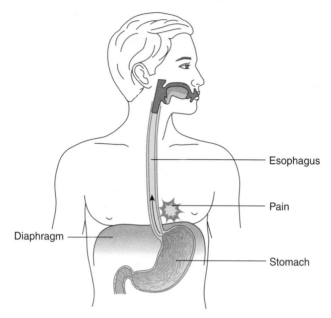

Figure 7-5. GERD.

and a burning sensation (Figure 7–5). Compromised lower esophageal sphincter (LES) pressure can allow the acidic contents of the stomach to re-enter the esophagus, causing dysphagia, heartburn, belching, and increased salivation.[15]

The diet therapy for GERD management includes the following:

1. Avoid foods and agents that reduce LES pressure
2. Restrict foods that increase gastric acidity
3. Improve clearance of contents from the esophagus

Specific recommendations for intervention goals and diet therapy for patients with GERD can be found in Tables 7–7 and 7–8.[16,17]

Citrus Foods and Heartburn: What Does the Evidence Say?

Particular foods are unlikely to damage the gut, although certain classifications of food can increase the production of gastric acid. In some individuals, citrus or tomato-based foods may exacerbate GERD and, in that case, should be eliminated.[14] Practitioners should carefully question about categories of foods that may increase gastric secretion and help design a well-balanced diet that does not include these offending foods. As with many other areas of gastrointestinal nutrition, responses to certain foods are highly individualized and vary from one person to another.

Table 7–7. Nutrition interventions and goals in patients with GERD.

Improve competence of lower esophageal sphincter
Decrease gastric acidity
Improve clearance of esophageal contents
Initiate weight loss if indicated
Identify potential drug–nutrient interactions
Prevent obstruction if esophageal stricture present
Improve overall nutrition intake

Data from Academy of Nutrition and Dietetics, 2012.

■ Hiatal Hernia

A hiatal hernia occurs when the top portion of the stomach and the lower esophageal sphincter protrude through the esophageal hiatus into the thoracic cavity (Figure 7–6). The presence of a hiatal hernia facilitates easy reflux of acid into the esophagus. Hiatal hernia symptoms are similar to those of GERD, and the primary dietary interventions for GERD also apply. Because hiatal hernias and associated GERD are more prevalent in the obese, weight loss efforts should be undertaken if indicated.[18] Those with hiatal hernias should

Table 7–8. Diet therapy for patients with GERD.

Restrict foods that increase gastric acidity, including black pepper, red pepper, coffee (includes decaffeinated), and alcohol
Eliminate foods and agents that reduce lower esophageal sphincter pressure, including chocolate, mint, high-fat foods, and tobacco
Lose weight if indicated
Smoking cessation
Refrain from lying down after eating; remain upright
Restrict eating within 3 hours of bedtime
Avoid tight-fitting clothing
Elevate head of bed while sleeping
Substitute large, high-fat meals with smaller, more frequent lower-fat meals

Data from Academy of Nutrition and Dietetics, 2012; Hasler, 2006.

Normal stomach   **Hiatal hernia**

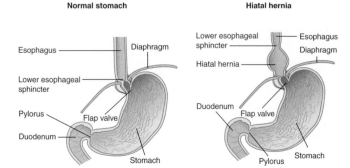

Figure 7–6. Normal stomach and stomach with hiatal hernia.

be advised to avoid high-fat meals and avoid laying down less than 3 hours after eating.

▪ Peptic Ulcer Disease

Peptic ulcer disease (PUD) is characterized by ulceration in the gastric and duodenal mucosa (Figure 7–7). Each year there are 500,000 new cases, and 4 million recurrent ulcers in the United States.[19] Ulcers are five times more likely to occur in the duodenum than in the stomach. Understanding of the etiology of and approach to treating PUD has changed dramatically since *Helicobacter pylori* infection was identified as a primary factor in the development of PUD.[20] It is now believed that 70% of gastric ulcers and 92% of duodenal ulcers are caused by *H. pylori*.[21] The use of NSAIDs, aspirin, and corticosteroids may also contribute to the development of PUD.

Medication use remains the preferred treatment modality for PUD; however, diet and lifestyle choices can alleviate PUD-associated

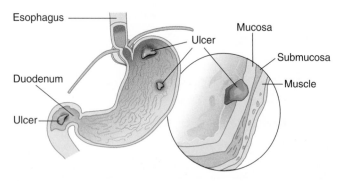

Figure 7–7. Peptic ulcer disease.

pain. The medication treatment regimen for *H. pylori* infection usually involves three or four drugs. Acid suppression is achieved with a proton pump inhibitor (PPI) alongside antibiotic therapy and use of a bismuth-containing agent, such as Pepto-Bismol.[22] In addition to medication, diet and lifestyle choices can ameliorate PUD-associated pain. The approach to nonmedication-related management of PUD focuses on three areas: (1) avoid and/or treat factors that impair mucosal integrity, (2) avoid behaviors that reduce blood flow to the gastric and duodenal mucosa, and (3) avoid factors and foods that stimulate excessive gastric secretions. Table 7–9 outlines the specifics of these three approaches.[23]

Peptic ulcer-associated pain can impede nutritional intake and reduce appetite, resulting in unintended weight loss and potential nutrient deficiencies. Iron deficiency can occur as a result of blood loss. Long-term use of medications that suppress acid secretion can lead to deficits in calcium, iron, and vitamin B_{12} absorption.[24,25]

Abdominal discomfort with PUD generally occurs when the stomach is empty. Common complaints include feelings of an upset stomach, and dull or burning pain either between meals or during the night. In the case of duodenal ulcers, food is likely to help relieve the pain. Antacid use can alleviate pain with both gastric and duodenal

Table 7–9. Factors that exacerbate peptic ulcer disease.

Factors That May Affect Mucosal Integrity
Helicobacter pylori infection Aspirin Nonsteroidal, antiinflammatory drugs (NSAIDs) Alcohol Steroids
Factors That Decrease Blood Supply to Gastric or Duodenal Mucosa
Smoking Stress Injury (eg, Curling's ulcer in a burn injury)
Factors That Increase Acid Secretion
Foods: including pepper, alcohol and caffeine from colas, coffee, including decaffeinated coffee, tea, and chocolate Rapid gastric emptying Stress Other conditions (eg, Zollinger-Ellison syndrome)

Data from Academy of Nutrition and Dietetics, 2012; http://www.nlm.nih.gov/medlineplus/ency/article/000206.htm.

ulcers. Patients should be encouraged to identify and avoid foods that are not well tolerated or that easily irritate the gastric mucosa. In addition to individualized food recommendations, all people with PUD should be advised to avoid foods that may increase gastric acid secretion or that are known to harm the gastric mucosa, including pepper, alcohol, and caffeine from colas, coffee, decaffeinated coffee, tea, and chocolate.

Encouraging small, frequent meals, avoiding fried foods, and smoking cessation are advisable for PUD. Many individuals find that avoiding food for at least 2 hours before bedtime also helps minimize PUD-associated discomfort. Previous diet therapy was based on a notion that milk and milk products could "coat" the stomach and protect against gastric secretions, a therapy formerly called the "sippy diet." It is now known that milk, with its protein content, actually increases gastric secretions. Generally, with active PUD, reduced-fat (2%) milk, whole milk, cream, chocolate milk, and high-fat yogurt are discouraged.[15,23] If tolerated, some patients may wish to include nonfat (skim) milk, low-fat (1%) milk, buttermilk, or low-fat and nonfat yogurt (Table 7–10).[23]

▪ Gastric Surgery

The need for gastric surgery can arise from a multitude of reasons: malignancy, PUD, or surgical weight loss (see Chapter 3). Regardless of the diagnosis or condition necessitating gastric surgery, understanding how such surgeries impact nutrient digestion and absorption can help predict where particular nutrient deficiencies or deficits may arise. Patients undergoing gastric surgery are at increased nutritional risk from potentially poor oral intake, maldigestion, and malabsorption of nutrients. Table 7–11 provides a brief overview of the various surgical procedures.

Normal digestive processes are disrupted with any gastric surgery, either by reducing the capacity of the stomach or by altering the transit time for contents in the gut. Altering the normal digestive process in the stomach may cause a reduction in the production of intrinsic factor. Intrinsic factor is produced by the parietal cells of the stomach and is required for optimal vitamin B_{12} absorption. Gastric surgery often results in sub-optimal vitamin B_{12} status due to reduced intrinsic factor. Hydrochloric acid (HCl) production is also affected by gastric surgery, resulting in further disruption of the normal digestive process. Additionally, bone health suffers as calcium absorption is compromised, resulting in an increased need for calcium and vitamin D supplementation in the postsurgical state.

▪ Dumping Syndrome

Dumping syndrome is a common side effect of gastric surgery. Dumping syndrome can be initiated by alterations in the rate of gastric emptying, innervation to the stomach, and fluctuating stimulation of GI hormones.

Table 7-10. Foods not recommended for people with peptic ulcer disease.

Dairy and Milk Products	Dairy foods can cause more stomach acid, avoid: • Whole milk, chocolate milk • Cream • Dairy products from whole milk or cream
Fats and spices	Fatty foods can exacerbate symptoms, avoid: • High-fat meats and meats that are not tolerated on an individual basis • Fried foods • Chocolate • Butter • Lard • Stick margarine • Hydrogenated oils
Drinks and beverages	• Alcohol • Colas • Coffee (including decaffeinated) • Green or black tea (including decaffeinated) • All caffeinated beverages
Spices	• Pepper • Spicy foods
Miscellaneous	• Avoid eating late at night or right before going to sleep • If you smoke or chew tobacco, stop • Stress can further exacerbate symptoms • Avoid drugs such as aspirin, ibuprofen, or naproxen; instead, take acetaminophen for pain

Data from Academy of Nutrition and Dietetics, 2012; http://www.nlm.nih .gov/medlineplus/ency/patientinstructions/000380.htm.

If normal gastric emptying rates cannot be achieved, a higher osmolar load dumps into the small intestine too quickly, with too much volume to be comfortably accommodated. Approximately half of all Roux-en-Y gastric bypass patients experience dumping syndrome.[26]

Dumping results in abdominal cramping and pain, diarrhea, dizziness, weakness, and tachycardia. These symptoms are present in early dumping syndrome, occurring within the first 10–20 minutes following a meal. Undigested food then transits to the large intestine, where colonic fermentation produces gas, abdominal pain, cramping, and diarrhea. Late dumping syndrome takes place between 1 and 3 hours postmeal, particularly following the consumption of simple carbohydrates. The rapid rate of absorption in the small intestine stimulates insulin

Table 7–11. Gastric surgical procedures.

Gastric Surgery Procedure	Anatomical Effects
Vagotomy	Eliminates innervations from the vagus nerve to parietal cells Results in decreased acid production Results in decreased response to gastrin
Pyloroplasty	Innervations to parietal cells are severed Eliminates part of the vagus nerve that controls gastric emptying Pyloric sphincter is enlarged
Billroth I	Partial gastrectomy or pyloroplasty performed with reconstruction with anastomosis of proximal end of the duodenum to the distal end of the stomach
Bilroth II	Partial gastrectomy with anastomosis of the proximal end of the jejunum to the distal end of the stomach
Roux-en-Y	Partial gastrectomy with creation of a small pouch and anastomosis of jejunum to the upper part of the stomach

release. Insulin, in the presence of hypermotility and decreased transit time, finds no remaining substrate on which to act, causing subsequent hypoglycemia. The symptoms of hypoglycemia, and ultimately, late dumping syndrome, include confusion, weakness, shakiness, and sweating.[27]

Management of dumping syndrome is mediated by dietary modification. Consuming small and frequent meals, avoiding simple carbohydrates (including clear liquids), drinking fluids separate from solid foods, and including supplemental pectin or guar gum to promote increased viscosity of food all can help minimize symptoms. The presence of sugars and sugar alcohols in the GI tract may exacerbate associated GI symptoms. As such, patients are generally advised to avoid sucrose, fructose, and sugar alcohols such as sorbitol, mannitol, and xylitol (commonly found in sugar-free and diet foods, candies, chewing gum, and drinks). Those with dumping syndrome may benefit from laying down following meals.

■ Steatorrhea

Steatorrhea (the presence of fat in the stools) is an indicator of fat malabsorption. Steatorrhea is characterized by the four F's: fatty, frothy, floating, or foul-smelling stools. Those experiencing fat malabsorption for extended periods of time are at risk for developing deficiencies of fat-soluble vitamins. Practitioners should monitor hemoglobin,

Table 7–12. Dietary interventions in a postgastric-surgery patient.

Avoid simple sugars (sucrose, fructose), sugar alcohols (sorbitol, mannitol, and xylitol), and clear liquids (except broth) at the first feeding
First meal postsurgery should contain protein, fat, and complex carbohydrate, and be limited to only 1-2 food items at a time
Patients may experience lactose intolerance
Liquid or puréed foods may be prescribed for 2-3 weeks after surgery, progressing to soft, then regular texture foods
Slowly progress to 5-6 small meals per day
Drink liquids 30 minutes to 1 hour after eating solid food
Lay down after eating
Utilize functional fibers to delay gastric emptying and to mitigate diarrhea
Liquid multivitamin and mineral supplements should be used to meet minimum nutrient needs
Supplements include vitamin B_{12} injections, multivitamin with iron, calcium (1,200 mg/day with no more than 500 m at one time, recommended form is calcium citrate) and vitamin D

Data from Academy of Nutrition and Dietetics, 2012; http://www.nlm.nih.gov/medlineplus/ency/patientinstructions/000173.htm.

hematocrit, ferritin, serum iron, and serum vitamin B_{12} levels to detect deficiencies of iron, vitamin B_{12}, or folate in those with dumping syndrome.[28] Table 7–12 outlines a variety of approaches for dietary management in a post gastric-surgery patient.[27]

Due to alterations in gut transit time, gastric secretion production, and nutrient absorption capacities following gastric surgery, the potential for some nutrient maldigestion and malabsorption does exist. Table 7–13 outlines micronutrients of concern following gastric surgery.[29]

Re-establishing healthy eating patterns within the guidelines and restrictions of postgastric surgery treatment protocols is challenging. Fear of dumping symptoms and fatigue, as well as disinterest in food following surgery, all can impair nutrition status. Table 7–14 outlines foods to include in the recovery phase following gastric surgery,[27] and Table 7–15 lists foods to avoid.[27]

Diet Therapy for Disorders of the Lower GI Tract

The integrity of the lower gastrointestinal system (small intestine, large intestine, rectum, and anus) is of paramount importance to optimal nutrient digestion, absorption, and transport, as more than 98% of all

Table 7–13. Potential micronutrient deficiencies following gastric surgery.

Iron
Folate
Calcium
Vitamin B$_{12}$
Copper
Thiamin
Vitamin A
Vitamin D

Data from O'Donnell, 2008.

Table 7–14. Diet tips and foods to include following gastric surgery.

General Recommendations

After surgery the stomach cannot hold more than 1 cup of chewed food; a normal stomach holds up to 4 cups of chewed food

Take your time at meals: take 20–30 minutes to eat a meal and eat 6 small meals per day instead of 3 big meals

Do not drink anything during a meal and nothing for 30 minutes following a meal

Avoid using a straw, which can introduce unwanted air into your stomach

Milk and Dairy Foods

Recommended foods: buttermilk, evaporated and skim, 1% milk, soy milk without added sugar, yogurt without added sugar, powdered milk, cheese, and low-fat low-sugar ice cream

Select lactose-free foods following surgery

Choose yogurts that contain live, active cultures (but without added sugar)

Drink milk and other liquids between meals, rather than with food

Wait 30–60 minutes after eating solid foods to try beverages

Meat and Protein Foods

Recommended foods: tender, well-cooked meats, poultry, fish, eggs, smooth nut butters, or soy foods made without added fats

Include a protein food at every meal and snack

(Continued)

Table 7–14. Diet tips and foods to include following gastric surgery. (*Continued*)

Grains

Recommended foods: white breads, bagels, rolls, crackers, and cold or hot cereals made from refined wheat or white flour
Look for grains that have less than 2 grams of fiber per serving
Choose cereals with no added sugar

Vegetables

Recommended foods: most well-cooked vegetables without seeds or skins, potatoes without skin, lettuce, or strained vegetable juice

Fruits

Canned, soft fruits without added sugar, bananas, and melons

Fats

Recommended foods: small amounts of oils, butter, margarine, cream, cream cheese, and mayonnaise

Beverages

Recommended foods: decaffeinated coffee, caffeine-free tea, and caffeine-free sugar-free sodas
Sweeten beverages only with artificial sweeteners, not sugar-containing sweeteners

Sweeteners

Recommended foods: artificial sweeteners, and foods or beverages that contain them
Instead of sugar, choose artificial sweeteners such as Sweet 'n Low, Equal, NutraSweet, Splenda, Stevia, Sunnette, or Sweet One

Data from Academy of Nutrition and Dietetics, 2012; http://www.nlm.nih.gov/medlineplus/ency/patientinstructions/000173.htm.

digestion and absorption takes place in the lower half of the GI tract.[30] The lower GI tract essentially finishes what the upper GI tract started: movement of GI contents, secretion of digestive enzymes and juices, and nutrient digestion, absorption, and transport. The small intestine consists of three segments: the duodenum, jejunum, and ileum (Figure 7–8). The arrangement of intestinal tissue folds within the small intestine is uniquely suited to maximizing nutrient absorption.

- ■ Constipation

Constipation can arise from a lack of dietary fiber or as a secondary occurrence related to another condition or disease. Common causes

Table 7–15. Foods to avoid following gastric surgery.

Milk and Dairy Foods

Chocolate milk
Any milk with added sugar
Avoid regular milk if you have lactose intolerance, drink sugar-free soy milk
    products
Do not drink milk or other beverages with food; wait for 30–60 minutes after food
    to drink

Meat and Protein Foods

Fried meat, poultry, or fish
Lunch meats such as bologna or salami
Sausage, hot dogs, or bacon
Tough or chewy meats
Dried peas and beans such as pinto or kidney beans
Chunky nut butters or nuts

Vegetables

Any raw vegetables except for lettuce
Any cooked vegetables served with skins or seeds
Beets
Broccoli, Brussels sprouts, or cabbage
Cauliflower
Collards, mustard, or turnip greens
Corn
Potato skins

Fruits

All raw fruits except for bananas and melons
All dried fruits including prunes and raisins
Fruit juice
Canned fruit packed in sugar or syrup

Beverages

Caffeinated coffee or tea
Alcoholic beverages
Beverages made with sugar, corn syrup, or honey
Fruit juices and fruit drinks
Carbonated beverages
Do not drink beverages with meals and snacks; wait for 30–60 minutes after food
    to drink

(Continued)

Table 7–15. Foods to avoid following gastric surgery. (*Continued*)

Sweeteners
Sugar
Honey, syrup
Sugar alcohols such as sorbitol or xylitol
Foods that list sugar, honey, syrup, xylitol, or sorbitol as one of the first three ingredients

Academy of Nutrition and Dietetics, 2012; http://www.nlm.nih.gov/medlineplus/ency/patientinstructions/000173.htm.

of constipation include obesity, pregnancy, inactivity, irritable bowel syndrome (IBS), or diseases such as diabetes, Parkinson's disease, multiple sclerosis, stroke, spinal cord injuries, and disorders of the thyroid gland, lupus, and scleroderma. Medication may induce constipation, with diuretics, calcium or aluminum antacids, pain medications containing codeine, antidepressants, antihistamines, and iron and calcium supplements being particularly constipating.[31] The use of fiber supplements without adequate fluid intake may also contribute to constipation. Table 7–16 contains potential nutrition diagnoses for constipation.[32]

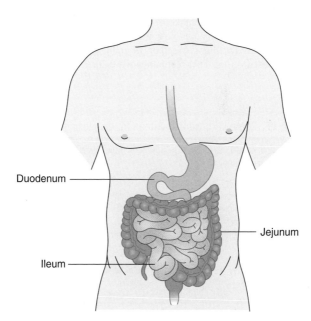

Figure 7-8. The small intestine.

Table 7–16. Possible nutrition diagnoses related to constipation.

Inadequate fluid intake
Inappropriate intake of carbohydrates
Inadequate dietary fiber intake
Undesirable food choices
Food and nutrition-related knowledge deficit

Data from American Dietetic Association, 2010.

Diagnostic Criteria

While general complaints about constipation may vary, the National Digestive Diseases Information Clearinghouse defines constipation as having a bowel movement fewer than three times per week. The Rome III Consensus Criteria more strictly define constipation. Table 7–17 contains the Rome III Consensus Criteria for diagnosing constipation, provided that the criteria are met for the past 3 months, with symptom onset at least 6 months before diagnosis.[33]

Dietary Fiber and Constipation

The most well-known association between constipation and diet is related to the inadequate intake of dietary fiber. While a number of dietary fiber recommendations exist, the Institute of Medicine's Dietary Reference Intake for fiber is based on 14 grams per 1000 calories consumed.[34] Based on the DRI-recommended calorie intake levels, this

Table 7–17. Rome III consensus criteria for diagnosing constipation.

Constipation diagnosis must include two or more of the following (as well as the criteria in the last two rows):
• Straining during at least 25% of defecations • Lumpy or hard stools in at least 25% of defecations • Sensation of incomplete evacuation for at least 25% of defecations • Sensation of anorectal obstruction or blockage for at least 25% of defecations • Manual maneuvers to facilitate at least 25% of defecations (eg, digital evacuation) • Fewer than three defecations per week
Loose stools are rarely present without the use of laxatives
There are insufficient criteria for irritable bowel syndrome

Data from Standards of Practice Task Force of the American Society of Colon and Rectal Surgeons, 2007.

Table 7-18. Dietary Reference Intake adequate intake recommendations for dietary fiber.

Daily Fiber Intake Recommendations for Children
• Babies 0-6 months: no fiber recommendations
• Babies 7-12 months: not enough data to set recommended level
• Kids 1-3 years: 19 grams of fiber per day
• Kids 4-8 years: 25 grams of fiber per day
• Kids 9-13 years: girls need 26 grams, and boys need 31 grams per day
• Adolescents 14-18 years: girls need 26 grams, and boys need 38 grams per day
Daily Fiber Intake Recommendations for Adults
• Female adults aged 50 years and younger: 25 grams of fiber per day
• Female adults aged 51 years and older: 21 grams of fiber per day
• Male adults aged 50 years and younger: 38 grams of fiber per day
• Male adults aged 51 years and older: 30 grams of fiber per day

Data from Institute of Medicine, 2005.

works out to 25 grams per day for adult women and 38 grams per day for men. National household level data indicate that on an average, in the United States, most people consume only 13–15 grams of dietary fiber per day.[35] Table 7–18 contains the DRI for fiber for different age and gender groups.[34]

While it may prove difficult to assess individual fiber intake in a traditional clinical setting, a quick survey of a person's previous 24-hour intake can yield substantial information about the nature (or absence) of dietary fiber in the diet. Diets that are low in fiber also tend to be low in fruits, vegetables, whole grains, and legumes. These same diets tend to be high in dairy, meat, refined carbohydrate foods, and fats. While it is the insoluble fibers that appear to have the greatest effect on constipation, there is no clear evidence in regards to the best type of fiber to alleviate constipation.[36] Insoluble fibers are found in the skins of fruits and vegetables, and in whole grains.

Rather than expend unnecessary energy making specific soluble versus insoluble fiber recommendations, the practitioner is instead advised to encourage an overall, gradual intake of any and all dietary fiber from food sources (as opposed to supplements). A well-balanced diet with fiber-containing foods will naturally have both soluble and insoluble fiber content. Individuals should be cautioned that a sudden spike in dietary fiber intake may lead to undesirable GI side effects. Those with constipation should be counseled to gradually increase their fiber intake, by no more than a few grams per day, and to always assure adequate fluid intake along with increases in fiber. Increasing fiber intake too quickly or without adequate fluid intake can cause gas, bloating, cramping, diarrhea, and general GI

Table 7-19. Quick estimation for determining daily fiber from food records.

To quickly estimate fiber intake from a food record:
1. Multiply the number of fruit and vegetable servings by 1.5 grams
2. Multiply the number of servings of whole grains by 2.5 grams
3. Multiply the number of servings of refined grains by 1.0 grams
4. Add specific fiber amounts for nuts, legumes, seeds, and high-fiber cereals
5. Total to estimate fiber intake per day

Data from Marlett and Cheung, 1997.

discomfort. Table 7–19 offers a quick way to estimate fiber intake from a person's food record.[37]

Functional Fibers

Counseling individuals to increase dietary fiber intake can be challenging in today's food environment. As consumers' interest in fiber grows, so do food manufacturers' offerings of fiber-containing packaged and processed foods. Many packaged and processed foods are increasingly adding isolated or functional fibers to foods that traditionally are low in fiber. These contain ingredients such as maltodextrin, polydextrose, and inulin (from chicory root), among others. In high concentrations, these additives may cause gastrointestinal distress in some individuals,[38,39] although they may be tolerated at more moderate levels by others.[40] Table 7–20 contains some commonly used isolated fibers.

In today's grocery stores, you can purchase yogurt with added fiber, white bread made *with* whole grains (although not always with *much* whole grain), and even low-fat ice cream sandwiches with 3 grams of dietary fiber per serving. While the addition of isolated fibers does increase the dietary fiber count on a food's Nutrition Facts panel, it is important to educate patients and clients that the health benefits of such added fibers are not yet known. According to a position paper on the topic by the Academy of Nutrition and Dietetics, "(w)hether isolated, functional fibers provide protection against cardiovascular disease remains controversial." The paper goes on to say, "longer-term studies of fiber intake which examine the effects of both intrinsic [intact] and functional [isolated] fibers…are required."[41]

Individuals should be encouraged to increase dietary fiber intake from naturally occurring sources of dietary fiber as opposed to isolated or functional fibers added to processed foods. Naturally occurring sources of fiber include fresh and frozen fruits and vegetables, whole grains, dried peas and beans, and lentils, and, to a lesser degree, nuts and seeds. When choosing bread products made with flour, look for the

Table 7–20. List of commonly used isolated (functional) fibers.

Maltodextrin
Inulin (chicory root)
Polydextrose
Oat fiber
Resistant starch
Pectin
Gum

word "whole" as the first ingredient in the ingredient list. Avoid bread products with "enriched wheat flour" as the first ingredient, as these are made with refined, low-fiber wheat flour. Table 7–21 includes tips for increasing dietary fiber.

Fluid Intake

In addition to inadequate dietary fiber intake, insufficient fluid can exacerbate underlying constipation. While there are no consensus guidelines for fluid intake recommendations, some groups recommend increasing fluid intake to at least 64 ounces (eight cups) per day.[42] The best

Table 7–21. Tips for increasing dietary fiber intake.

Leave skins and peels on fruits and vegetables
Use 100% whole-wheat bread instead of wheat or white bread
Try 100% whole-wheat pasta or brown rice
Replace half of white flour in baking with a whole-grain flour
Look for breads and cereals that have the word "whole" as their first ingredient
Steam vegetables quickly to retain color and crunch
Utilize low-sodium canned beans in casseroles, salads, and soups
Explore whole grains: try barley, quinoa, wheat berries, or whole-wheat couscous
Add ½ cup cut fruit to your cereal, oatmeal, or yogurt
Use fruit as a between-meal snack: aim for three servings of fresh or frozen fruit per day

indicator of hydration status is urine color: light yellow or clear urine that is not pungent indicates adequate hydration in most cases. Urine that is dark yellow or orange and urine that has a pungent odor indicate the presence of concentrated waste product and insufficient hydration status.

Three other ways of estimating fluid needs are based on calorie intake, body weight, or calorie intake plus nitrogen consumed. Providing 1 milliliter of fluid per calorie consumed per day is estimated to meet hydration needs in otherwise healthy people. Alternatively, providing 35–40 mL/kg for people aged 16–30 years, 30–35 mL/kg for healthy adults, 30 mL/kg for those 55–65 years old, and 25 mL/kg for those over 65 years can also meet fluid needs. Lastly, a less commonly used practice bases fluid recommendations on nitrogen and energy intake by providing 1 mL/kcal + 100 mL/g nitrogen consumed.[42] Table 7–22 summarizes these ways to estimate daily fluid requirements.[42]

Inactivity

A sedentary lifestyle promotes constipation. Inactivity is often the culprit of such problems in the elderly or those confined to bed. Nutrition

Table 7–22. Selection of ways to determine adequate fluid intake.

Observe Color of Urine

- Clear or light yellow indicates adequate hydration
- Dark yellow or orange or pungent smelling urine indicates dehydration

Cups per Day

- Ideal goal is 64 oz or eight 8-oz cups per day

Based on Energy Intake

- 1 mL fluid per kcal ingested

Based on Body Weight

- Age 16–30 years, give 35–40 mL/kg/day fluid
- Healthy adults, give 30–35 mL/kg/day fluid
- Adults aged 55–65 years, give 30 mL/kg
- Adults >65 years, give 25 mL/kg
- Congestive heart failure or renal disease, give 25 mL/kg
- Infection or draining wounds, give 35 mL/kg

Based on Nitrogen and Energy Intake

- 1 mL/kcal + 100 mL/g nitrogen (g protein divided by 6.25 = g nitrogen)

Fluid Balance Method

- Urine output + 500 mL per day

Data from Academy of Nutrition and Dietetics, 2012.

prescriptions for constipation should include recommendations to participate in daily physical activity when appropriate. While the mechanism of physical activity promoting motility is not entirely understood, a helpful mantra for those with constipation is, "Get moving to get things moving."

Additional Approaches

Traditional nutrition interventions for constipation involve increasing fiber in the diet, increasing fluid intake throughout the day, manipulating medication routines if necessary, and promoting regular physical activity. Including probiotics and prebiotics daily may prove helpful in some situations, as can the use of bulk-forming agents such as psyllium, calcium polycarbophil, or methylcellulose. It is important to note that those who are reliant on laxatives may not respond to fiber treatment.

▪ Intestinal Gas

As is the case with constipation, the presence of gas and flatulence may be caused either by an underlying condition or as a result of a separate therapeutic medication or treatment. Foods and agents that cause gas vary greatly between individuals; and because of the highly individualized nature of such a condition, there is not one blanket diet therapy that will be beneficial for all who experience this uncomfortable GI problem.

Gas can be caused by one of two things: from the swallowing of air or from the breakdown of certain undigested foods by colonic bacteria. The best nutrition advice for gas and flatulence is also the simplest: avoid the offending food or foods. Gas-causing foods include simple sugars, starches, and fiber.[43] The simple carbohydrates that are known to be gas inducing and their sources can be found in Table 7–23. Most starches give off gas as they are broken down in the large intestine; rice is the only starch known to not cause gas.[44] Dietary fiber can contribute to gas. Soluble fiber, found in foods such as oat bran, beans, peas, and most fruit, is not digested by the body, but rather fermented by bacteria in the colon, where it can cause gas. Insoluble fiber is less likely to cause gas as it passes unchanged through the intestines and is not fermented by colonic bacteria. Most fiber-containing foods have a combination of soluble and insoluble fibers. Slowly increasing fiber intake by a few grams per day and assuring adequate fluid intake alongside increasing fiber can help minimize gas associated with higher fiber intakes.

The use of products such as Beano® or Bean-zyme® provides alpha-galactosidase, which works to decrease the amount of undigested carbohydrate going into the large intestine and, in turn, reduces gas production. Table 7–24 contains a list of potentially gas-producing foods that may warrant ingestion of such an enzyme-containing product before eating.

Table 7–23. Simple sugars that can cause gas.

Simple Carbohydrates That Cause Gas	Dietary Sources
Fructose	Also called fruit sugar Found in onions, artichokes, pears, and wheat May be added as a sweetener in some drinks
Lactose	Also called milk sugar Found in milk products and processed foods that have milk foods in them Causes gas in people with low levels of lactase, the enzyme required to break down lactose
Raffinose	Found in dried beans such as kidney, garbanzo, and black beans Found in lesser amounts in cabbage, Brussels sprouts, broccoli, asparagus, and whole grains
Sorbitol	Sugar found in many fruits such as apples, pears, peaches, and prunes May be added as an artificial sweetener in diet and sugar-free foods

Table 7–24. Foods that may produce gas.

Grains	Vegetables	Beans
Bagels	Beets	Black-eyed peas
Barley	Broccoli	Bog beans
Breakfast cereals	Brussels sprouts	Broad beans
Granola	Cabbage	Chickpeas
Oat bran	Cauliflower	Lentils
Pasta	Corn	Lima beans
Rice bran	Cucumbers	Mung beans
Rye	Leeks	Peanuts and peanut butter
Sorghum	Lettuce	Pinto beans
Wheat bran	Onions	Red kidney beans
Whole-wheat flour	Parsley	Seed flour (sesame, sunflower)
Whole-grain breads	Peppers, sweet	Soybeans and soy milk

Reprinted with permission from Beano®. Available at: http://www.beanogas .com/Smart_Problem.aspx.

An additional precaution that can be taken to reduce gas is to reduce the swallowing of air. Chewing foods slowly, avoiding drinking straws, chewing gum, and assuring proper denture fit all can minimize the swallowing of air. For food-based gas reduction, advise those with gas to eat small, frequent meals, and to avoid high-fat fried foods and carbonated beverages. Regular physical activity may also help alleviate gas. The use of lactase enzyme supplements such as Lact-Aid™ may be useful in those whose gas is caused by lactose intolerance.

▪ Diarrhea

As is the case with many other GI maladies, diarrhea is often a sign or symptom of another problem. Diarrhea affects nutritional status as it may cause rapid weight loss, dehydration, electrolyte abnormalities, and acid-base imbalance, and it can also be indicative of a malabsorptive disorder. Diarrhea is defined as the presence of loose, watery stools passed at least three times per day. Diarrhea can also be defined as >200 g/day of stool weight passed by an adult. Acute diarrhea is less than 2 weeks in duration, persistent diarrhea lasts for 2–4 weeks, and chronic diarrhea occurs for more than 4 weeks.[45]

Identifying the etiology and treating the underlying cause of diarrhea is the primary goal of treatment. If infectious diarrhea is present, antibiotic therapy becomes the primary treatment. While the cause of diarrhea can be attributed to many things, foods that may be related to diarrhea include beans and legumes, high-fiber foods, high-fat foods, alcohol, lactose, fructose, caffeine, and sorbitol.[46] Clear liquids are not recommended for diarrhea because of their high osmolality, which increases the likelihood of these foods drawing water into the lumen of the intestine and further exacerbates diarrhea. Keeping a food and symptom diary may help identifying problem foods likely to trigger diarrhea.

Dietary management of diarrhea involves restoring normal fluid, electrolyte, and acid-base balance. Other goals include slowing gut motility, thickening the consistency of the stool, repopulating the gut with normal flora, and the eventual stimulation of the GI tract without exacerbating symptoms. Table 7–25 contains practical applications of these dietary recommendations for the management of diarrhea.[46]

Probiotics and Prebiotics for Diarrhea Treatment

An emerging area of interest in the treatment of diarrhea involves the use of probiotic- and prebiotic-containing foods. Probiotic and prebiotic foods support the growth and repopulation of healthy gut flora. These agents are theorized to assist with diarrhea management by promoting water and electrolyte absorption in the colon, improving mucosal defense in the GI tract, or possibly reducing the growth of harmful bacteria. Sources of probiotics include yogurt or dairy containing acidophilus, lactobacilli, and/or bifidobacteria, as well as tempeh, miso, kim chi, or Kefir®. The variety of strains of bacteria used in different products, alongside the difficulty inherent in maintaining the organisms' viability,

Table 7-25. Dietary recommendations for managing diarrhea.

Restore Normal Fluid, Electrolyte, and Acid-Base Balance
Use oral rehydration solutions such as Pedialyte™, Resol™, Ricelyte™, CeraLyte™, and Rehydralyte™
Decrease Gastrointestinal Motility
Avoid clear liquids and foods high in simple carbohydrates (lactose, sucrose, or fructose) Avoid sugar alcohols (sorbitol, xylitol, and mannitol) Avoid caffeine Avoid alcohol Avoid high-fiber and gas-producing foods
Thicken Consistency of Stool
Banana flakes, apple powder, or other pectin sources can be added to foods for adults
Repopulate GI Tract with Normal Flora
Prebiotic and probiotic supplementation may help diarrhea, but current recommendations do not include dosing information
Stimulate GI Tract by Introduction of Solid Food Without Exacerbating Symptoms
Choose low-fiber, low-fat, lactose-free foods initially Reintroduce lactose if no evidence of lactose-intolerance

Data from Academy of Nutrition and Dietetics, 2012; Duro and Duggan, 2007; Steffen R, Gyr K. Diet in the treatment of diarrhea: from tradition to evidence. Clin Infect Dis 2004;39:472–473.

has made it challenging to enact or recommend universal dosing recommendations. However, recommending foods that contain probiotics and prebiotics, such as yogurt, Kefir, and cheese, is appropriate.[47]

Another dietary tool that has historically been used for diarrhea management is the BRAT diet. BRAT stands for bananas, rice, applesauce, and toast (or tea). While no scientific evidence exists to suggest its efficacy, these foods are mild in nature and are considered safe for diarrhea management, although in long term they are nutritionally inadequate.[48]

Low-residue foods have traditionally been the first solid foods reintroduced for a person who has been experiencing diarrhea. A low-residue diet is one that is low in fiber and food components that would otherwise contribute bulk in the large intestine. Again, despite a dearth in scientific evidence, proving the effectiveness of a low-residue diet, use of low-residue refined grains, such as white rice, white flour, or other bread products made from white or refined flour, may help

Table 7–26. Foods not to consume for people with diarrhea.

Dairy
Whole milk, cream, half-and-half, full-fat condiments, yogurts with dried fruit or nuts
Meat and Protein
Fried meats, high-fat lunch meats such as salami or bologna, hot dogs, sausage, nuts, and chunky nut butters
Grains
Whole grains such as barley and oats, whole-wheat breads, and popcorn
Vegetables
All raw vegetables except lettuce, fried vegetables, cruciferous vegetables such as cauliflower, cabbage, broccoli and Brussels sprouts, and corn or potato skins
Fruits
Any raw fruit except for bananas and melons, any dried fruit, canned fruit in heavy syrup, and fruit sweetened with sorbitol or prune juice
Avoid canned fruit juices; they are hyperosmolar and aggravate diarrhea
Fats
Limit added fats
Beverages
Avoid any caffeine-containing beverages, alcohol, beverages sweetened with sorbitol and limit those with high-fructose corn syrup to 12 oz per day

Data from Academy of Nutrition and Dietetics, 2012; World Gastroenterology Organisation (WGO). WGO practice guideline: acute diarrhea. Munich, Germany: WGO; 2008:28 pages.

mitigate diarrheal exacerbations. Soft, canned, and strained fruits and vegetables are beneficial, as are tender, well-cooked meats made without added fat, decaffeinated beverages, and low-fat or nonfat dairy foods (provided that lactose intolerance is not an issue). Foods that are not recommended with diarrhea are listed in Table 7–26.[46]

■ Malabsorption

Malabsorption refers to the body's inability to properly absorb carbohydrate, fat, or protein. Fat malabsorption is characterized by steatorrhea, the presence of fat in the stool. Steattorhea is defined as stool fat excretion of greater than six of dietary fat intake.[49] While most malabsorptive disorders are associated with steatorrhea, the primary carbohydrate malabsorptive condition, lactose intolerance, is not. Protein malabsorption does not occur independently, but as a result of other diseases.

Fat Malabsorption

The complex nature of fat digestion, transport, and absorption makes it a prime candidate for dysfunction. The goal of diet therapy for fat malabsorption is to prevent exacerbation of symptoms and steatorrhea. When fat in the stool is present, fat restriction in the diet is indicated. For people with steatorrhea, limiting fat to less than 50 grams per day is generally recommended. Foods to be avoided include fried and high-fat foods, such as whole-milk dairy, added fats and oils, and high-fat cuts of meat or luncheon meat. The use of medium-chain triglyceride (MCT) oil supplements can help meet calorie and fat needs, as MCTs are absorbed directly into the body's circulatory system and do not involve the usual intricacies of long-chain triglyceride digestion and absorption.

Carbohydrate Malabsorption

Lactose intolerance is the most commonly observed type of carbohydrate malabsorption. Lactose is the simple sugar found in milk and dairy products. Individuals with minimal or insufficient amounts of lactase enzyme lack the ability to efficiently digest and absorb the milk sugar lactose. Lactose intolerance can be primary or secondary in nature. With primary lactase deficiency, a genetic deficit of lactase exists. Risk factors for lactose intolerance tend to cluster with ethnicity. Those of Asian, Latino, African or African-American, American Indian, or Ashkenazi Jewish descent are at increased risk for primary lactose intolerance.[50] Secondary lactase deficiency can arise as a side effect of gastrointestinal diseases, from diarrhea, or from a prolonged period without GI stimulation.

While exacerbation of lactose intolerance and its resultant symptoms vary from person to person, a number of dietary approaches can help increase tolerance of lactose-containing foods. This is of particular importance for those with increased calcium needs related to risk for osteoporosis and osteopenia. Table 7–27 outlines a number of ways in which a lactose intolerant person might increase tolerance of lactose-containing foods and achieve optimal calcium intake.

Protein Malabsorption

Amino acid or protein digestion and absorption abnormalities are rarely observed in the clinical setting. Rather, protein malabsorption tends to be a result of another disease, or cluster of conditions or diseases. Protein malabsorption is also called protein-losing enteropathy, and it results in the loss of protein in the stool, lowered serum levels of protein, and the presence of peripheral edema resulting from reduced oncotic pressure. Treatment for protein malabsorption depends on the malabsorbed nutrient of concern and the treatment of the underlying disease.

■ Celiac Disease

Celiac disease is an autoimmune disease also called gluten-sensitive enteropathy, or celiac sprue. In celiac disease, gluten ingested from the diet causes damage in the absorptive areas of the small intestine,

Table 7-27. Increasing calcium intake in lactose intolerance.

Choose small portions of lactose-containing foods such as ¼ cup milk or ½ oz cheese
Choose foods that are naturally lower in lactose such as hard cheeses or yogurt
Include one dairy food per day and gradually increase the amount as tolerated
Drink milk or eat dairy foods in combination with other foods, but not by themselves
Consume lactose-containing foods several hours apart from each other
Heating milk may improve tolerance such as in soups or hot chocolate made with milk
Take lactase tablets such as Lactase™ before eating dairy foods
Eat aged cheeses that are naturally lower in lactose than processed cheeses
Yogurt contains bacteria that breaks down lactase and may be better tolerated
Buttermilk is a fermented dairy food that also may be more well tolerated

resulting in villus atrophy. Gluten is the protein found in wheat, rye, and barley. The only therapeutic approach to managing celiac disease is the maintenance of a gluten-free diet. While estimations of the prevalence of celiac disease vary between populations, higher rates are traditionally seen among Caucasians and those of European descent. Prevalence rates of celiac disease in the United States are thought to be 1:133 in the general population, and as high as 1:22 for those who have a first-degree relative (parent, sibling, or child), and who also has celiac disease.[51] Emerging evidence also supports the notion that individuals with other autoimmune conditions (eg, type 1 diabetes, Crohn's disease) may also be at higher risk of developing celiac disease.[52]

Symptoms of celiac disease vary widely and can range from general irritable bowel complaints to constipation and diarrhea. Some people are asymptomatic or have non-GI symptoms such as itchy skin or infertility. If a person has celiac disease and has been undiagnosed for a long period of time, initial symptoms may be those of vitamin and mineral deficiencies. It is estimated that up to 97% of people with celiac disease are undiagnosed, and the average time from onset of symptoms to diagnosis is 12–14 years.[53,54] Although biopsy of the small intestine remains the gold standard in celiac disease diagnosis, people with celiac disease generally have above average levels of particular antibodies. Testing for elevated levels of antitissue transglutaminase antibodies (tTGA) or antiendomysium antibodies (EMA) can provide initial results pointing toward celiac disease. It is important to inform those suspecting celiac disease that they should not intentionally avoid gluten-containing foods before undergoing such antibody tests, as false negatives will result with exclusion of gluten in the period immediately preceding testing.

Nutritional Implications of Celiac Disease

The progression of celiac disease can lead to deficiencies of iron, calcium, and folate, as these nutrients are absorbed in the initial parts of the small intestine. Secondary lactose intolerance exists as a result of damage to the intestine, but tolerance may improve alongside the gut healing that accompanies a gluten-free diet. Those with active lactose intolerance related to celiac disease are advised to follow a lactose-reduced diet, with most needing a calcium supplement with vitamin D to meet bone health needs.

Damage incurred further down the intestinal tract can cause carbohydrate malabsorption from secondary lactose intolerance, as well as difficulties with absorption of fat and the fat-soluble vitamins A, D, E, and K.[55] Although absorbed in the proximal part of the small intestine, vitamin B_{12} deficiency may be also be of concern in celiac disease, particularly in cases of severe malabsorption.[56] Vitamin B_{12}-rich foods are those of animal origin: liver, eggs, dairy, meat, poultry, and seafood. Supplementation of vitamin B_{12} may be indicated in those with low intakes of vitamin B_{12}-containing foods, and certainly for those following strict vegan diets that do not contain animal foods.

The Gluten-Free Diet

The only therapy for celiac disease is the maintenance of a life-long gluten-free diet. Upon initial diagnosis of celiac disease, many patients are overwhelmed by the perceived magnitude of dietary changes that they are required to adopt for ultimate health. Focusing on the foods that "can't" be part of the diet quickly disheartens even the most motivated newly diagnosed individuals. Rather, practitioners should be encouraged to highlight the variety of naturally occurring gluten-free foods that can be included and enjoyed as part of a well-balanced diet. While this does involve initial education regarding gluten-containing and gluten-free foods, with a little creativity and willingness to try new or not-so-familiar grains and food items, most people with celiac disease can comfortably adapt to the gluten-free realities of their nutrition requirements.

People with celiac disease should avoid eating wheat, rye, and barley and their derivative or associated ingredients. The term "gluten" has been used to describe the storage proteins found in wheat, rye, and barley, although this is technically incorrect as gluten only comes from the endosperm of wheat. Regardless, the storage proteins in wheat, rye, and barley can trigger allergy and reaction in celiac disease and, as such, should be eliminated from the diet. While it may initially seem manageable to simply avoid these three types of foods, the extent of gluten-containing ingredients and foods in the food environment is dramatically more complex and widespread. Upon initial inspection, gluten seems to be everywhere: in condiments, thickening agents, and almost every packaged and processed food. Careful reading of ingredient lists and a focus on homemade, whole ingredients, as opposed to reliance on packaged and prepared foods, can help minimize unwanted gluten in the diet. Increasing familiarity with gluten-free flours and naturally gluten-free grains can help assure adequate carbohydrate and micronutrient intake.

Because of the high-sugar, high-fat, high-calorie, and high-carbohydrate content of many packaged and prepared gluten-free foods (eg, cakes, cookies, breads, and crackers), people with celiac disease should be cautioned that excessive intake of these foods will likely lead to weight gain. A more appropriate approach to gluten-free meal planning minimizes the use of gluten-free processed, packaged, and prepared foods and instead encourages whole grains, fruits, vegetables, low-fat or nonfat dairy, lean sources of protein, and naturally gluten-free sources of carbohydrate. Table 7–28 contains lists of foods in each food group that are allowed, not allowed, and should be questioned when preparing a well-balanced gluten-free diet.[55] The table is provided courtesy of Shelley Case, author of the *Gluten Free Diet: A Comprehensive Resource Guide*, and is an excellent resource for anyone following a gluten-free diet.

■ Irritable Bowel Syndrome

IBS refers to the group of disorders characterized by bloating, cramping, diarrhea, and constipation. IBS is a functional bowel disorder (FBD) associated with bowel discomfort and abdominal pain that occurs alongside changes in bowel habits. IBS is diagnosed using the Rome III criteria demonstrating at least 3 months, with onset at least 6 months previously, of recurrent abdominal pain or discomfort, associated with two or more of the following: improvement of pain with defecation, onset associated with a change in frequency of stool, or onset associated with a change in form (appearance) of stool. It is estimated that IBS affects 9–22% of the United States population.[57] The widely variable range of symptoms and the highly individualized nature of the condition make it one of the most frustrating GI disorders to either experience as a patient or attempt to treat as a practitioner.

Proposed theories for the underlying cause of IBS extend from involvement of estrogen hormones in menstruating women to genetic contributors, bacterial overgrowth, food allergies and food intolerances, and infection or inflammation. Regardless of the cause of IBS, practitioners must be sensitive to, and aware of, potential food-based contributors and nutrition-related approaches to treatment. The nutrition assessment for IBS should identify any problems swallowing, the presence of nausea or vomiting, constipation, diarrhea, heartburn, or any other symptoms that interfere with normal food ingestion. Additional attention should be paid to high-fat foods, lactose, fructose, caffeine, sorbitol, and alcohol, which may exacerbate GI discomfort.

Thorough questioning of regular food, meal, alcohol, and other beverage intake patterns, and the use of 24-hour recall or food frequency questionnaire data may help the practitioner identify offending or trigger foods or beverages. Questioning about supplement use or reliance on laxatives or motility agents can also yield insightful information about the IBS patient. Encourage patients to keep a food and symptom journal to track the types and quantities of foods and beverages consumed, along with GI symptoms and emotional or life

Table 7–28. The gluten-free diet.

Milk and Dairy		
Foods Allowed	**Foods to Question**	**Foods not Allowed**
Milk, cream, most ice creams, buttermilk, plain yogurt, cheese, cream cheese, processed cheese, processed-cheese foods, and cottage cheese	Flavored yogurt, frozen yogurt, cheese sauces, cheese spreads, seasoned (flavored) shredded cheese or cheese blends	Malted milk, ice cream made with ingredients not allowed
Breads, Baked Products, and Other Items		
Foods Allowed	**Foods to Question**	**Foods not Allowed**
Made with amaranth, arrowroot, buckwheat, corn bran, corn flour, cornmeal, cornstarch, flax, legume flours (bean, garbanzo, or chickpea, Garfava™, lentil, pea), mesquite flour, millet, Montina™ flour (Indian ricegrass), nut flours (almond, chestnut, and hazelnut), potato flour, potato starch, pure uncontaminated oat products (oat flour, oat groat, and oatmeal), quinoa, rice (black, brown, red, white, and wild) rice bran, rice flours (brown, glutinous, sweet, and white), rice polish, sago, sorghum flour, soy flour, sweet potato flour, tapioca (cassava, manioc), taro, and teff	Items made with buckwheat flour	Items made with wheat bran, wheat farina, wheat flour, wheat germ, wheat-based semolina, wheat starch, durum flour, gluten flour, graham flour, atta, bulgur, einkorn, emmer, farro, kamut, spelt, barley, rye, triticale, commercial oat products (oat bran, oat flour, oat groats, and oatmeal)
Hot Cereals		
Puffed amaranth, cornmeal, cream of buckwheat, cream of rice (brown, white), hominy grits, pure, uncontaminated oatmeal[a], quinoa, rice flakes, soy flakes, soy grits	Rice and soy pablum	Cereals made from wheat, rye, triticale, barley, and commercial oats
Cold Cereals		
Puffed (amaranth, buckwheat, corn, millet, and rice), rice crisps or cornflakes (with no barley malt extract or barley malt flavoring), rice flakes, and soy cereals	Rice and corn cereals	Cereals made with added barley malt extract or barley malt flavoring

(Continued)

Table 7–28. The gluten-free diet. (*Continued*)

Pastas		
Macaroni, spaghetti and noodles made from beans, corn, lentils, peas, potato, quinoa, rice, soy, and wild rice	Buckwheat pasta	Pastas made from wheat, wheat starch, and other ingredients not allowed (eg, orzo)
Rice		
Plain (eg, basmati, black, brown, jasmine, red, white, and wild)	Seasoned or flavored rice mixes	
Miscellaneous		
Corn tacos, rice tortillas, and teff tortillas	Corn tacos, rice tortillas, and teff tortillas	Wheat flour tacos and tortillas, matzoh, matzoh meal, matzoh balls, couscous, and tabbouleh
Plain rice crackers, rice cakes, and corn cakes	Multi-grain or flavored rice crackers, rice cakes, and corn cakes	
Gluten-free communion wafers	Low-gluten communion wafers	Regular communion wafers

Meat and Other Proteins		
Foods Allowed	**Foods to Question**	**Foods not Allowed**
Plain, fresh, or frozen	Deli or luncheon meats (eg, bologna, salami), wieners, frankfurters, sausages, pate, meat and sandwich spread, frozen burgers (meat, fish, and chicken), meatloaf, ham (ready to cook), dried meats (eg, beef jerky), seasoned/flavored fish in pouches, imitation fish products (eg, surimi), meat substitutes, and meat product extenders	Canned fish in vegetable broth containing hydrolyzed wheat protein, frozen turkey basted or injected with hydrolyzed wheat protein, frozen or fresh turkey with bread stuffing, frozen chicken breasts containing chicken broth (made with ingredients not allowed), meat, poultry, or fish breaded in ingredients not allowed

(*Continued*)

Table 7–28. The gluten-free diet. (*Continued*)

Eggs		
Fresh, liquid, dried, or powdered	Flavored egg products (liquid or frozen)	
Others		
Dried beans (black, garbanzo, etc)	Baked beans	
Plain nuts and seeds (chia, flax, sesame, pumpkin, and sunflower)	Seasoned or dry roasted nuts, seasoned pumpkin or sunflower seeds; nut butters (almond, peanut)	
Plain tofu	Flavored tofu, tempeh, and miso	Fu, seitan

Fruits and Vegetables		
Foods Allowed	**Foods to Question**	**Foods not Allowed**
Fruits		
Fresh, frozen, and canned fruits and juices	Dates, fruits with sauces	
Vegetables		
Fresh, frozen, and canned vegetables and juices	Vegetables with sauces, French-fried potatoes cooked in oil also used for gluten-containing products, French fries (various shapes)	Scalloped potatoes (containing wheat flour), battered deep-fried vegetables

Additional Foods and Food Groups		
Foods Allowed	**Foods to Question**	**Foods not Allowed**
Soups		
Homemade broth, gluten-free bouillon cubes, cream soups, and stocks made from ingredients allowed	Canned soups, dried soup mixes, soup bases, and bouillon cubes	Soups made with ingredients not allowed, bouillon cubes containing hydrolyzed wheat protein

(*Continued*)

Table 7–28. The gluten-free diet. (*Continued*)

Fats		
Butter, margarine, lard, shortening, vegetable oils, and salad dressings with allowed ingredients	Salad dressings, suet, baking and cooking spray	Salad dressing made with ingredients not allowed
Desserts		
Ice cream, sherbet, whipped toppings, whipping cream, milk puddings, custard, gelatin desserts, cakes, cookies, pies, and pastries made with allowed ingredients, gluten-free ice cream cones, wafers, and waffles	Cake icings and frostings	Bread pudding, ice cream made with ingredients not allowed (eg, cookie crumbs), cakes, cookies, muffins, pies, and pastries made with ingredients not allowed, ice cream cones, wafers, and waffles made with ingredients not allowed
Sweets		
Honey, jam, jelly, marmalade, corn syrup, maple syrup, molasses, sugar (brown and white), and icing sugar (confectioner's)	Honey powder	
Gluten-free licorice, marshmallows	Hard candies, Smarties®, chocolates, and chocolate bars	Licorice and other candies made with ingredients not allowed
Snack Foods		
Plain popcorn, nuts, soy nuts, potato chips, and corn chips	Seasoned (flavored) potato chips, corn chips, nuts and soy nuts, and wasabi peas	Potato chips with ingredients not allowed
Gluten-free pizza		Pizza made with ingredients not allowed

(*Continued*)

Table 7–28. The gluten-free diet. (*Continued*)

Beverages		
Foods Allowed	**Foods to Question**	**Foods not Allowed**
Coffee and Tea		
Tea, instant or ground coffee (regular or decaffeinated), cocoa, and soft drinks	Flavored and herbal teas, flavored coffees, coffee substitutes, and hot chocolate mixes	Cereal and malt-based beverages (eg, Ovaltine – chocolate malt and malt flavor)
Liquor		
Distilled alcoholic beverages (eg, bourbon, brandy, gin, rum, rye whiskey, scotch whiskey, vodka, and liqueurs), wine	Flavored alcoholic beverages (eg, coolers, ciders, and Caesar vodka beverage)	
Beer		
Gluten-free beer, ale, and lager		Beer, ale, and lager derived from barley
Other Beverages		
Most nondairy beverages made from nut, potato, rice, and soy		Nondairy beverages (nut, potato, rice, and soy) made with barley malt extract, barley malt flavoring, or oats

Condiments, Sauces and Baking Ingredients		
Foods Allowed	**Foods to Question**	**Foods not Allowed**
Condiments and Sauces		
Ketchup, relish, plain prepared mustard, pure mustard flour, herbs, spices, salt, pepper, olives, plain pickles, tomato paste, vinegars (apple cider, balsamic, distilled white, grape or wine, rice, and spirit), gluten-free soy sauce, gluten-free tamari sauce, gluten-free teriyaki sauce, and other sauces and gravies made with allowed ingredients	Specialty prepared mustards, prepared mustard flour, mustard pickles, Worcestershire sauce, salsa, curry paste, and seasoning mixes	Malt vinegar, soy sauce (made from wheat), teriyaki sauce (made with soy sauce containing wheat), and other sauces and gravies made with wheat flour and/ or hydrolyzed wheat protein

(*Continued*)

Table 7–28. The gluten-free diet. (*Continued*)

Baking Ingredients		
Plain cocoa, pure baking chocolate, carob chips and powder, chocolate chips, baking soda, cream of tartar, coconut, monosodium glutamate (MSG), vanilla, pure vanilla extract, artificial (synthetic, imitation) vanilla extract, vanillin, yeast (active dry, autolyzed, Baker's, nutritional, and torula), xanthan gum, and guar gum	Baking powder	Brewer's yeast

[a]Unless specifically indicated to be gluten free oat product.

Adapted from Case, 2010. Reproduced with permission.

events that may trigger reactions. The standard timeframe for such recordkeeping is usually 3 days, preferably capturing 2 weekdays and 1 weekend day of food intake, GI symptoms, and emotional or other lifestyle contributors.

Once an understanding of the individual's IBS triggers and symptoms has been established, nutrition intervention involves normalizing dietary patterns, eliminating culprit foods, gradually increasing dietary fiber intake, utilizing bulking agents if needed, and considering the use of prebiotics and probiotics (although current research does not substantiate dosage recommendations). Table 7–29 outlines considerations for nutrition intervention in the individual with IBS.[58]

Probiotics and Prebiotics Use in IBS Treatment

Probiotics and prebiotics are selectively fermented compounds that are considered beneficial for gut health in that they help restore balance in the intestinal microflora. While numerous studies have evaluated the use of probiotics and prebiotics for IBS, challenges in interpretation of this research persist due to the numerous types of, and differences in, strains used in supplementation. Inability to assure the viability of these strains further compounds the problem. The Academy of Nutrition and Dietetics endorses that the most consistent literature supports the use of the following:

- *Lactobacillus rhamnosus* GG and *Lactobacillus casei* DN-114001 in the treatment of rotavirus in children and traveler's diarrhea
- *Saccharomyces boulardii, Lactobacillus acidophilus, Lactobacillus rhamnosus* GG, and *Lactobacillus casei* DN-114001 for the treatment of antibiotic-associated diarrhea

Table 7–29. Nutrition interventions for IBS.

Normalize Eating Patterns
Discourage grazing, focus on small, frequent, low-fat meals and snacks at prescribed times with well-balanced meal planning to assure adequacy of all nutrients
Eliminate Culprit Foods
Identify food allergies and intolerances with special attention to fructose, caffeine, alcohol, lactose, sorbitol, and raffinose (sugar found in beans, cabbage, Brussels sprouts, whole grains, and other vegetables)
Keep a Food Diary
Track food intake, times of meals and snacks, quantities, and preparation methods as well as related or associated GI symptoms and other emotional, environmental, or activity-related contributors
Increase Fiber
Slowly increase fiber intake to 25–35 grams per day as tolerated with simultaneous increase of fluid
Try Bulking Agents
Bulking agents may improve constipation in certain individuals, although widespread efficacy has not been recognized[58]
Consider Probiotics and Prebiotics
Despite lack of universally agreed-upon dosing recommendations, the use of prebiotics and probiotics—especially in yogurt, Kefir, and cheeses—may help in some IBS cases

- *Bifidobacterium animalis* DN-173 010 (*Bifidus regularis*) is most commonly used in products promoting relief for IBS[46]

The establishment of reliable, specific dosage recommendations will not be possible until further studies are conducted using consistent regimens. In the meantime, supplements that provide access to the aforementioned strains are readily available and may be useful for certain consumers. Practitioners are encouraged to recommend food-based products that contain probiotics and prebiotics; these include yogurt, Kefir, and cheeses.[47]

FODMAPs Approach to IBS Management

Another emerging approach to dietary management of IBS and other functional gut disorders is implementation of a low-FODMAPs diet. FODMAPs stands for Fermentable, Oligosaccharides, Disaccharides, Monosaccharides And Polyols, a group of short-chain carbohydrates that are poorly absorbed by the human gut. These compounds produce osmotic effects and have gas-producing capabilities that can set off bowel-related symptoms. The human body does not have the enzyme required to break down oligosaccharides (including fructo-oligosaccharides (FOS) and inulin), resulting in their total inability to be absorbed. Polyols are only partly absorbed, and absorption rates vary among individuals. Some, but not all, individuals may also experience malabsorption with the presence of fructose and lactose in the gut.[59] It is important to note that the presence of FODMAPs in the diet does not necessarily result in higher rates of IBS-related symptoms, and FODMAPs are not the cause of functional bowel disorders. The approach to minimizing FODMAPs represents a dietary approach to helping manage IBS symptoms, provided that all FODMAPs, not just some, are addressed.

The primary dietary sources of FODMAPs are found in foods with fructose in excess of glucose, honey, apples, and pears; fructans in wheat, rye, onion, and garlic; galactans in cabbage and legumes; lactose in milk and milk products; and polyols such as sorbitol and mannitol in stone fruits (eg, plums, cherries, mangos, peaches, apricots, and nectarines), mushrooms, and certain artificial sweeteners.[60] Referring candidates to a registered dietitian trained in developing a low-FODMAPs diet may be an efficacious dietary approach to minimizing IBS-related symptoms.

- ### Inflammatory Bowel Disease: Crohn's Disease and Ulcerative Colitis

Inflammatory bowel disease (IBD) is an autoimmune disorder characterized by chronic inflammation of the gastrointestinal tract. IBD is a syndrome that encompasses two distinct diseases: ulcerative colitis (UC) and Crohn's disease (CD). These two diseases are similar in nature, but distinguished from one another by their symptoms, GI involvement, biopsy, and antibody testing. Global rates of IBD are the highest in North America, the United Kingdom, and Europe. Ashkenazi Jews have twice the risk for IBD as do Israeli-born, Sephardic, or Oriental Jews. Ulcerative colitis and Crohn's disease are most likely to afflict those aged 15–30 years, with a second peak occurring between 60 and 80.[61] Cigarette smoking doubles the risk of Crohn's, but has a lesser effect on the development of UC.

With IBD, susceptible individuals experience inflammatory damages in the GI tract that result in abdominal pain, diarrhea, and nausea and/or vomiting. Ulcerative colitis generally afflicts the lower bowel, with particular involvement in the colon and rectum. Crohn's disease is not characterized by continuous inflammation; rather, the disease "skips" around the GI tract and can affect any portion of the gut and bowel. Those with IBD are at risk for extraintestinal conditions, including osteopenia and osteoporosis, dermatitis, rheumatologic conditions, ocular symptoms, hepatobiliary complications, and kidney stones. Complications of Crohn's disease can include bowel obstruction, perforation and resection, fistulas, abscesses, and steatorrhea. In the most severe cases, toxic megacolon and intestinal rupture can occur.[62]

Table 7–30. Nutrition concerns in a person with inflammatory bowel disease (IBD).

Nutrients	Deficiencies and Concerns
Energy	Insufficient intake, loss of appetite, and fear of abdominal pain following meals
Protein	Increased protein needs from GI losses caused by inflammation or catabolism when infection or abscesses are present
Fluid and electrolytes	Short bowel syndrome may cause fluid losses
Iron	From blood loss, inadequate intake
Magnesium and zinc	Intestinal losses, particularly with short bowel syndrome
Calcium and vitamin D	Long-term steroid use and reduced intake of dairy foods with lactose-restricted diet
Vitamin B_{12}	Surgical resection of stomach resulting in intrinsic factor loss or resection of terminal ileum, the primary site of vitamin B_{12} absorption
Folate	Medications used to treat IBD may result in lower levels

Data from Academy of Nutrition and Dietetics, 2012; Hou JK, Abraham B, El-Serag H. Dietary intake and risk of developing inflammatory bowel disease: a systematic review of the literature. Am J Gastroenterol 2011;106(4):563–573.

The presence of IBD dramatically increases nutrition risk. Between 60 and 75% of patients with Crohn's disease are considered to be malnourished.[63] In children with IBD, an increased risk for insufficient bone mass and stunting exists. Table 7–30 outlines the potential nutrient deficiencies and concerns for a person with IBD[62]:

The role of diet therapy in IBD management is to correct nutritional deficiencies, reduce disease-related inflammation, and establish nutrient adequacy in the diet. People with IBD often avoid foods or have particular food aversions that lead to insufficient nutrient intake. The use of a food diary for people with IBD is helpful for practitioners attempting to detect and identify nutritional inadequacies. When determining energy needs, adult calorie levels are usually set at 25–35 kcal/kg, but this may vary depending upon the severity of disease, weight status, and nutritional deficiencies.

From a micronutrient standpoint, practitioners are encouraged to use the dietary reference intake (DRI) levels as baseline recommendations, while acknowledging that a person with IBD may need higher levels of vitamins and minerals. The vitamins of particular concern include vitamin B_{12}, folate, thiamin, riboflavin, niacin, vitamin C, vitamin E, vitamin D, and vitamin K. Minerals that may be needed in higher amounts include iron (related to blood loss), zinc, magnesium, selenium, and potassium. The use of omega-3 fatty acids, glutamine, and prebiotics may also be helpful considerations in nutritional management of IBD.[62]

Nutrition intervention for active CD includes bowel rest with nutrition initially provided via total parental nutrition (TPN) or enteral feedings. (See Chapter 11 for more information on nutrition support.) TPN is the preferred route of nutrition support in the presence of fistulas; however, in other arenas, TPN has not been shown to be more beneficial than enteral feedings for treating active IBD.[62] For enteral nutrition, formulas that are elemental or peptide-based are preferred. Refeeding syndrome is common in IBD, and precautions to avoid refeeding should be taken into consideration when determining nutrition support or dietary regimens.

In the recovery period following exacerbations, the diet is slowly progressed to a low-fat, low-fiber, high-protein, high-calorie meal plan with small, frequent meals. A low fiber restriction is recommended only during acute flare-ups or in the presence of strictures.[64] Previous diet therapy for IBD included adherence to a low-residue diet. Current recommendations do not include low-residue foods or diets due to the lack of data demonstrating their efficacy. Vitamin or mineral supplements that may be required in the active IBD and recovery phases include vitamin D, zinc, calcium, magnesium, folate, vitamin B_{12}, and iron.

During remission, the nutritional goal is to maintain weight and to replenish nutrient stores. Persons with IBD may find prebiotic and probiotic supplements to be helpful[65]; furthermore, they may also benefit from omega-3 fatty acid and glutamine supplementation.[66] Increasing antioxidant intake (from food-based sources) and avoiding foods that are high in oxalate are also recommended. Table 7–31 lists high oxalate foods to be avoided in IBD remission. Table 7–32 contain lists of foods recommended to include and to avoid with Crohn's disease and ulcerative colitis.[67]

▪ Diverticular Disease

In both the developed and developing parts of the world, rates of diverticular disease are rising alongside the increased reliance on, and consumption of, processed and packaged foods. Diverticular disease includes diverticulosis (the presence of many small individual outpouches in the colon called diverticulum) and diverticulitis (inflammation of the diverticula that causes severe abdominal pain). Proposed risk factors for the development of diverticulosis include having a history of constipation, low fiber intake, high intakes of red meat, presence of obesity, and lack of physical activity.[67] It is estimated that 10% of Americans aged 40 years and older have diverticulosis and that one-quarter of those will develop diverticulitis.[68]

Table 7–31. High-oxalate foods to avoid with IBD.

Drinks	Chocolate drink mixes, soy milk, Ovaltine, instant iced tea, and fruit juices of fruits from this table
	Black tea, dark beer, cocoa, soy drinks
	Adequate fluid intake helps prevent all types of kidney stones
Fruits	Blackberries, blueberries, carambola, concord grapes, currants, dewberries, elderberries, figs, fruit cocktail, gooseberry, kiwi, lemon peel, lime peel, orange peel, raspberries, rhubarb, canned strawberries, tangerines
Vegetables	Beans (wax, dried), beets and beet greens, chives, collard greens, eggplant, escarole, dark greens of all kinds, kale, leeks, okra, parsley, rutabagas, spinach, Swiss chard, tomato paste, watercress, zucchini, potatoes (baked, boiled, fried), summer squash
Breads, cereals, and grains	Amaranth, barley, white corn flour, fried potatoes, fruitcake, grits, soybean products, sweet potatoes, wheat germ and bran, buckwheat flour, All-Bran cereal, graham crackers, pretzels, and whole-wheat bread
Meat and proteins	Dried beans, peanut butter, soy burgers, and miso Reduce all animal protein, including meat, eggs, and fish
Desserts and sweets	Carob, chocolate, and marmalades
Fats, oils, nuts, and seeds	Nuts (peanuts, almonds, pecans, cashews, and hazelnuts), nut butters, sesame seeds, tahini, and poppy seeds
Miscellaneous	Black pepper (more than 1 tsp), soy sauce, and parsley

Data from Academy of Nutrition and Dietetics, 2012; http://www.upmc.com/patients-visitors/education/nutrition/pages/low-oxalate-diet.aspx.

From a dietary standpoint, fiber is the most important nutritional component in the prevention of the development of diverticula, and both soluble and insoluble fibers are involved here. Soluble fiber, which absorbs water, adopts a soft, gel-like texture in the intestinal tract. Insoluble fiber, which is not absorbed, passes through the intestine unchanged and contributes to stool bulk. Manipulating both the texture and bulk of the stools by increasing total dietary fiber in the diet helps to maintain bowel regularity and prevents the development of diverticula.[69]

While the importance of dietary fiber in the prevention of diverticular disease cannot be overstated, it is important to note that the diet therapy for the treatment of diverticulosis differs dramatically from that of diverticulitis. With diverticulosis, the goal is to prevent the development of inflammation and progression to diverticulitis. Diet therapy for diverticulosis includes a high-fiber diet, with 6–10 grams of fiber per

Table 7–32. Recommended foods for IBD.

Recommended Foods for Crohn's Disease and Ulcerative Colitis
Dairy
Buttermilk Evaporated, skim, powdered, or low-fat milk Smooth, nonfat, or low-fat yogurt Low-fat or reduced-fat cheese Low-fat ice cream or sherbet Choose lactose-free products if lactose intolerance present Choose yogurt with live, active cultures — see ingredient list on yogurt products
Proteins
Tender, well-cooked meats, poultry, fish, eggs, and soy prepared without added fat Smooth nut butter
Grains
Bread, bagels, rolls, crackers, cereals, and pasta made from white or refined flour
Vegetables
Most well-cooked vegetables without seeds Potatoes without skin Lettuce Strained vegetable juice Choose grain foods with less than 2 grams fiber per serving
Fruits
Fruit juice without pulp (except prune juice) Ripe banana or melons Most canned, soft fruits Peeled apples Choose canned fruit in juice or light syrup
Fats and Oils
Limit to less than 8 teaspoons per day
Beverages
Water Decaffeinated coffee Caffeine-free tea Soft drinks without caffeine Very sweet juices or beverages with sugar or high-fructose corn syrup may make diarrhea worse in some people

Data from Academy of Nutrition and Dietetics, 2012; http://www.ccfa.org/resources/diet-and-ibd.html.

Table 7-33. Diet therapies for diverticulosis and diverticulitis.

Diverticulosis Diet Therapy	Diverticulitis Diet Therapy
High-fiber diet of 6–10 grams of dietary fiber above standard 20–35 grams per day levels	NPO with bowel rest until bleeding and diarrhea resolve
Consider use of a fiber supplement with insoluble fiber to help meet needs	Advance to clear liquid diet
Probiotic foods (kefir, yogurt, and miso) may be helpful	Advance diet as tolerated, consider use of supplements to meet nutrition needs
No need to avoid nuts, seeds, corn, and popcorn	Initiate a low-fiber diet until inflammation and bleeding no longer of concern
Increase fluid intake alongside increasing fiber intake	When acute phase subsides, progress to high-fiber, high-fluid diet
	Probiotic foods may be helpful

day encouraged *above* the standard 20- to 35-gram recommendations. Recall that the average North American eats only about 13–15 grams of fiber per day.[41] A fiber supplement consisting primarily of insoluble fiber may be helpful in meeting needs. In addition to assuring a high fiber intake, diverticulosis management may also be aided by the use of probiotic and prebiotic foods, although, again, current research does not substantiate recommended dosage amounts.[67] In the initial phase of diverticulitis, an NPO diet order with bowel rest is advised until bleeding and diarrhea resolve. The diet is then progressed to a clear liquid diet, and may require oral nutritional supplementation to help achieve optimal nutrition status. A low-fiber therapy is initially recommended until the inflammation and bleeding associated with diverticulitis are no longer a risk. After the acute episode has resolved, dietary fiber intake should gradually be increased along with water intake to the diverticulosis diet levels (6–10 grams above 20- to 35-gram recommendations). One recommended regimen is to advance the diet by 5 grams of fiber per week until the goal is obtained.[69] Table 7–33 outlines the diet therapy recommendations for the treatment of diverticulosis versus diverticulitis.

The Low-Residue Diet

Historically, clinicians would advocate for the use of a low-residue diet in the treatment of diverticulosis. As a review, residue refers to the indigestible matter of food that remains in the GI tract and contributes to the bulk of stools. A low-residue diet restricts foods such as nuts, seeds, corn, and popcorn, under the premise that these items can enter, block, or irritate an existing diverticulum and potentially cause diverticulitis.

Table 7–34. List of low-fiber foods for use in resolving diverticulitis.

Beef, poultry, and fish	Milk
Bread, white	Nut butters, smooth
Cheese, all types	Pasta, white
Cottage cheese	Peaches, canned
Cream of wheat, instant	Pears, canned
Egg	Pudding or tapioca
Fruit juice	Rice, white
Green beans, canned	Soy, rice, or almond milk
Ice cream	Spinach
Lactose-free milk	Tofu
Lettuce	Tuna, canned
Mashed potatoes	Yogurt or soy yogurt

Data from Academy of Nutrition and Dietetics, 2012; http://www.mayoclinic
.com/health/diverticulitis-diet/my00736.

There is no scientific evidence to support the recommendation of a low-residue diet, which is also low in fiber, for the treatment of diverticulosis. In fact, the opposite appears to be true: increasing dietary fiber can actually help reverse the pathophysiology of diverticular disease. The only justification for recommendation of a low-fiber diet is during acute phase attacks of diverticulitis. Table 7–34 contains a list of low-fiber foods to be initiated with diet progression during resolving diverticulitis.[67]

■ Intestinal Surgery

Intestinal or bowel diversion surgeries are required when disease or injury necessitate the removal or rest of the large and/or small intestines. In these cases, diet therapy depends upon the type of surgery and the extent of bowel involvement. Decline in, or loss of, function throughout the gut elicits changes in the motility of food, the absorption of nutrients, and the handling and disposal of waste products. The Academy of Nutrition and Dietetics recommends considering three primary questions before determining diet therapy for bowel diversion surgeries:

- Is the ileocecal valve present?
- How much bowel is left?
- What sections of the bowel are left?

The Ileocecal Valve

The ileocecal valve is responsible for regulating the movement of GI contents from the small intestine into the large intestine. In its absence motility rates increase, which, in turn, results in decreased nutrient absorption. Removal of the ileocecal valve also contributes to difficulties in ostomy and fluid management.

Sections and Length of Bowel Remaining

With regards to nutrient absorption, the small intestine is the most crucial part of the anatomy. Removal of the jejunum and the ileum most dramatically impacts nutrient absorption. The jejunum is more adaptive, and its removal is slightly less problematic from a nutrition standpoint. Removal and resection of the terminal ileum, and loss of the ileocecal valve, severely impact nutritional status and often necessitate long-term reliance on total parenteral nutrition (TPN, see Chapter 11). Removing all or part(s) of the large intestine has a less dramatic, yet not ignorable effect on nutritional status. The colon is responsible for the reabsorption of water and electrolytes. Its removal also affects the body's ability to appropriately metabolize soluble fiber to short-chain fatty acids.

For those who have undergone recent bowel resections, successes with diet therapy are particularly time sensitive. Early initiation of oral feeding, preferably within 1 day postop, helps maximize optimal nutrition outcomes. The presence of an ileus will necessitate an NPO diet, with reliance on TPN for nutrition. Enteral nutrition is indicated for those who are unable to meet nutrition needs by mouth, or if feeding access can be obtained distal to a fistula. In an optimal situation, an oral diet is initiated shortly after surgery. In the first phase, a clear liquid diet is prescribed. Clear liquid diets are inadequate to meet long-term human nutrition needs, and upon obtaining tolerance with the clear liquid diet, the patient's diet should be advanced as soon as possible. Advancement progresses from liquids to a low-residue diet, then to a bland diet, with between four and six small feedings per day. Avoiding tough, fibrous meats, vegetables such as corn, peas and spinach, dried fruits and fruit skins, seeds, and popcorn helps prevent incomplete digestion that can cause stoma obstruction. These foods should be avoided in the first 6–8 weeks following surgery.[30]

Micronutrient concerns following bowel diversion surgery include vitamins K and B_{12}. Vitamin K is synthesized by the gut and absorbed throughout the small and large intestines. Adequate vitamin B_{12} absorption requires normal transit time, so removal of the ileocecal valve and its associated effect on transit time will compromise vitamin B_{12} status. Additionally, vitamin B_{12} absorption requires utilization of receptors in the ileum, so the resection of the ileum generally leads to reliance on vitamin B_{12} supplementation. Bile absorption also occurs in the ileum, and its removal may result in fat malabsorption, compromising fat-soluble vitamin status (vitamins A, D, E, and K).

■ Ileostomy and Colostomy

Ileostomies divert the ileum to a stoma and bypass the colon, rectum, and anus. Colostomies involve the removal of the rectum and

Table 7-35. Diet therapy for colostomy and ileostomy management.

Practices To Be Avoided That Cause Swallowing of Air and Gas Formation:	Foods To Be Added That Help Decrease Odor	Foods To Be Added That Help Thicken the Stool
• Chewing gum • Drinking out of straws • Smoking • Chewing tobacco • Eating quickly (eat small bites of food and chew thoroughly)	• Buttermilk • Parsley • Yogurt • Kefir • Cranberry juice	• Banana flakes • Applesauce • Pectin • Pasta • Potatoes • Cheese

Data from Willcutts et al., 2005.

diversion of the colon to a stoma. In both instances, a pouch collects stool and waste products. For colostomies, the amount of the colon that has been resected and the location of the stoma along the GI tract affect the type of fecal matter produced. Fecal matter further along the colon produces a firmer, less watery stool. With an ileostomy, the output is more liquid.

Diet therapy for colostomy centers around providing food choices that will decrease the risk of obstruction, maintain normal fluid and electrolyte balance, reduce excessive fecal output, and minimize the likelihood of gas and flatulence.[70] The diet for a postoperative colostomy should be individualized, although most begin with clear liquids. The diet progresses to a low-fiber diet, avoiding odor-causing and gas-producing foods, as well as foods that may cause obstruction or diarrhea. Table 7-35 contains nutrition interventions for colostomy and ileostomy management.[71]

The typical output for a colostomy is between 200 and 600 milliliters per day. Initially, fluid outputs may be greater from residual disease, or in the adaptation phase. This increases fluid and electrolyte needs, although pre-existing conditions such as renal disease or congestive heart failure may also alter fluid needs. Individual fluid needs can be determined by providing 1 mL/kcal, or 30–35 mL/kg body weight in an average, healthy weight adult.

With ileostomies, there is a watery, less-formed stool, with output averages of 1200 L/day in the beginning, reducing to about 600 mL/day after adaptation. Vitamin B_{12} often needs to be supplemented, and in the presence of short bowel syndrome, vitamin D deficiency also becomes a concern. Foods that cause GI side effects are generally to be avoided with ileostomy, and these include beans, legumes, high-fiber foods, high-fat foods, and products containing lactose, caffeine, and sorbitol. Other diet therapy considerations include minimizing gas and flatulence, reducing excessive fecal output, maintaining normal fluid and

Table 7-36. Nutrition considerations for ileostomies.

Diet Progression	Monitor for	Encourage More	Restrict Foods High in Oxalate
• Begin with clear liquids • Progress to a low-fiber diet • Consume small, frequent meals and maintain adequate hydration • Limit fluid intake if output levels are high	• Symptoms of lactose intolerance • Symptoms of fat malabsorption	• Sodium intake to offset losses	• Grains—wheat bran, wheat germ, and whole-wheat flour • Meats and protein—beans, tofu, and nuts • Vegetables—beets, dark leafy greens, and sweet potatoes • Beverages—beer, cocoa, instant tea, and instant coffee • Miscellaneous—carob, chocolate

electrolyte balance, decreasing the risk of obstruction, and preventing the development of oxalate kidney stones. Table 7–36 contains nutrition considerations for ileostomies.

Enteral and/or parenteral nutrition support may be required following a colectomy, and should be considered when the patient's nutrition needs cannot be met by oral intake. The Academy of Nutrition and Dietetics' Evidence Analysis project recommends the use of enteral nutrition over TPN if the patient is hemodynamically stable with a functioning GI tract. If enteral nutrition is indicated, it should be started within 24–48 hours following surgery.[72] There is no evidence to suggest that immune-enhancing enteral nutrition products are more beneficial than are standard products. See Chapter 11 for more nutrition support information.

■ Short Bowel Syndrome

Short bowel syndrome (SBS) refers to a cluster of problems that result when more than half of the small intestine has been removed. SBS may occur when the remaining part of the functional small intestine is less than 200 centimeters.[73] Causes of SBS include Crohn's disease, bowel injury, and trauma, as well as cancer and cancer treatments (ie, radiation injury). Because the small intestine is the primary site of digestion and nutrient absorption, the removal of half or more of its surface area dramatically impacts nutritional status. The primary symptoms of SBS are related to large volumes of watery diarrhea with cramping, bloating, heartburn, weakness, and fatigue, all of which may contribute to unintended weight loss and suboptimal nutrition status. As with other bowel conditions, the degree of nutrient malabsorption depends upon the site and length of intestinal removal. With the involvement of the duodenum, iron absorption is impaired. In the jejunum, carbohydrate, protein, fat, and vitamin absorption are all affected. In the ileum, bile acids and vitamin B_{12} absorption are the primary nutrition concerns.

In the immediate postoperative phase, patients are dependent on parenteral nutrition while often experiencing large volumes of diarrhea and difficulties with fluid and electrolyte management. Reliance on TPN is generally from 7 to 10 days following enterectomy.[74] In the weeks and months following surgery, the small intestine begins to experience the initial stages of adaptation, whereby the inner lumen of the small intestine has the ability to increase in length and diameter. In this phase, enteral nutrition is initiated. It is believed that enteral nutrition and the secretions stimulated with the initiation of nutrition support enhance and promote mucosal adaptation.[75] Once nutrition status has been stabilized, the transition to an oral diet can begin. Throughout the recovery phase, a combination of TPN, enteral nutrition, and oral diet and supplementation may be indicated to meet nutrition needs. Calorie needs should be estimated at 25–35 kcal/kg/day, and protein needs are 1.0–1.5 g/kg/day.[76] The timeframe to achieve full intestinal adaptation is estimated to be 1–2 years.

With less than 100 centimeters of ileal resection, malabsorption of bile salts causes fluid shifts in the colon and large volumes of watery diarrhea. Resection of more than 100 centimeters of the ileum compromises bile salt availability and leads to malabsorption of fats and fat-soluble vitamins. In these cases, a low-fat diet utilizing medium-chain triglycerides is indicated. Medium-chain triglycerides are more easily absorbed than are the longer-chain triglycerides that are prevalent in the typical diet. Caution should be taken with the low-fat diet approach, as fat can and should serve as a valuable source of calories. Over-restriction of fat can result in inadequate energy intake. Risk also exists for the development of oxalate kidney stones, as unabsorbed fatty acids bind to calcium and reduce calcium's absorption while promoting the absorption of oxalate. Calcium supplements are utilized to promote higher levels of serum calcium while binding oxalate.[77] Carbohydrates are another macronutrient concern in the SBS patient. Over-emphasis on carbohydrate or consumption of a high-carbohydrate, low-fat diet can promote bacterial overgrowth and excessive gas, flatulence, abdominal pain, and diarrhea.

Patients with jejunostomies or ileostomies are encouraged to adhere to a higher-fat diet with macronutrient distribution of approximately 20–30% carbohydrate, 20–30% protein, and 50–60% fat. For those with an intact colon, a higher-carbohydrate diet is appropriate. The macronutrient distribution would then be approximately 50–60% carbohydrate, 20–30% protein, and 20–30% fat. Micronutrients of concern include the fat-soluble vitamins and minerals, sodium, magnesium, iron, zinc, selenium, and calcium, as these are all lost when large volumes of diarrhea are present.[30] Table 7–37 outlines other nutrition recommendations for a patient with short bowel syndrome.[62,75]

Table 7–37. Diet therapy for short bowel syndrome.

Foods to Avoid
Highly sweetened beverages and candies (increases osmotic load in intestine)
Drinking beverages with meals; instead space fluid between meals
Lactose-containing products if lactose intolerance is present
High foods in those prone to oxalate stone formation (see Table 7–31)
Alcoholic or caffeinated beverages
Sugar-free foods with sugar alcohols mannitol, xylitol, and sorbitol, if not tolerated

Foods to Include
Small, frequent meals
Oral rehydration solution if at risk for dehydration
Medium-chain triglyceride supplements if fat malabsorption present
Vitamin and mineral supplements when indicated
Soluble fiber supplements that may promote intestinal adaptation

Data from Academy of Nutrition and Dietetics, 2012; Tilg, 2008.

References

1. National Institutes of Health, U.S. Department of Health and Human Services. Opportunities and Challenges in Digestive Diseases Research: Recommendations of the National Commission on Digestive Diseases. Bethesda, MD: National Institutes of Health; 2009.

2. Everhart J. The Burden of Digestive Diseases in the United States. Bethesda, MD: National Institute of Diabetes and Digestive and Kidney Diseases, U.S. Dept of Health and Human Services; 2008.

3. Cherry D, Hing E, Woodwell D, Rechsteiner E. National Ambulatory Medical Survey: 2006 Summary. Hyattsville, MD: National Center for Health Statistics; 2008.

4. Mahan L, Escott-Stump S. Krause's Food & Nutrition Therapy. 12th ed. St. Louis, MO: Saunders Elsevier; 2008.

5. Wardlaw G, Smith A. Contemporary Nutrition. 8th ed. New York, NY: McGraw Hill; 2011.

6. Smith J, Groff J, Gropper S. Advanced Nutrition and Human Metabolism. 5th ed. Belmont, CA: Wadsworth; 2008.

7. Atkinson J, Wu A. Salivary gland dysfunction: causes, symptoms, treatment. J Am Diet Assoc 1994;125:409–415.

8. Eisbruch A. Reducing xerostomia by IMRT: what may, and may not, be achieved. J Clin Oncol 2007;25(31):4863–4864.

9. Academy of Nutrition and Dietetics. (2012). Xerostomia Treatment. Retrieved January 19, 2013, from Nutrition Care Manual: http://www.nutritioncaremanual.org

10. Academy of Nutrition and Dietetics. (2012). Dysphagia. Retrieved January 19, 2013, from Nutrition Care Manual: http://www.nutritioncaremanual.org

11. McCallum S. The national dysphagia diet: implementation at a regional rehabilitation center and hospital system. J Am Diet Assoc 2003;103(3): 381–384.

12. McCullough G, Pelletier C, Steele C. National dysphagia diet: what to swallow? The ASHA Leader. 2003.

13. Academy of Nutrition and Dietetics. (2012). Renal. Retrieved January 19, 2013, from Nutrition Care Manual: http://www.nutritioncaremanual.org

14. Academy of Nutrition and Dietetics. (2011). Collaboration for Modified Texture Diets; Nutrition Intervention in: Unintended Weight Loss in Older Adults. Retrieved January 19, 2013, from Evidence Analysis Library: http://andevidencelibrary.com

15. Nelms M. Disease of the upper intestinal tract. In: Nelms M, Sucher K, Lacey K, Long Roth S, eds. Nutrition Therapy & Pathophysiology. Belmont, CA: Wadsworth; 2011:352.

16. Academy of Nutrition and Dietetics. (2012). Gastroesophageal Reflux Disease. Retrieved January 19, 2013, from Nutrition Care Manual: http://www.nutritioncaremanual.org

17. Hasler W. Nausea, Vomiting and Indigestion. Harrison's Principles of Internal Medicine. 17th ed. New York, NY: McGraw Hill; 2006.

18. Barak N, Ehrenpreis E, Harrison J, Sitrin M. Gastro-oesophageal reflux disease in obesity: pathyophysiological and therapeutic considerations. Obes Rev 2002;3:9–15.

19. Ramakrishnan K, Salinas R. Peptic Ulcer Disease. Am Fam Physician 2007;76(7):1005–1012.

20. Chey W, Wong B. American College of Gastroenterology guideline on the management of *Helicobacter pylori* infection. Am J Gastroenterol 2007;102(8):1808–1825.

21. Makola D, Peura D, Crowe S. *Helicobacter pylori* infection and related gastrointestinal diseases (review). J Clin Gastroenterol 2007;41(6): 548–558.

22. Schafer T. (2012). For Patients. Retrieved May 6, 2012, from The American College of Gastroenterology: http://www.acg.gi.org/patients/gihealth/peptic.asp

23. Academy of Nutrition and Dietetics. (2012). Peptic Ulcer Disease. Retrieved January 19, 2013, from Nutrition Care Manual: http://www.nutritioncaremanual.org

24. Yang Y, Lewis J, Epstein S, Metz D. Long-term proton pump inhibitor therapy and risk of hip fracture. JAMA 2006;296:2947–2953.

25. O'Connell M, Madden D, Murray A, Heaney R, Kerzner L. Effects of proton pump inhibitors on calcium carbonate absorption in women; a randomized control trial. Am J Med 2005;117(7):778–781.

26. Wang V, Burakoff R. Disorders of Gastric & Small Bowel Motility. Current Diagnosis & Treatment: Gastroenterology, Hepatology & Endoscopy. New York, NY: McGraw Hill; 2009.

27. Academy of Nutrition and Dietetics. (2012). Gastric Surgery. Retrieved January 19, 2013, from Nutrition Care Manual: http://www.nutritioncaremanual.org

28. Brolin R, Gorman J, Gorman R, Petschenik A, Bradley L, Kenler H, et al. Are vitamin B-12 and folate deficiency clinically important after roux-en-y gastric bypass? J Gastrointest Surg 1998;2:436–442.

29. O'Donnell K. Small but mighty: selected micronutrient issues in gastric bypass patients. Pract Gastroenterol 2008;32(5):37–48.

30. Nelms M. Diseases of the lower intestinal tract. In: Nelms M, Sucher K, Lacey K, Long Roth S, eds. Nutrition Therapy & Pathophysiology. Belmont, CA: Wadsworth; 2011:424.

31. Academy of Nutrition and Dietetics. (2012). Constipation. Retrieved January 19, 2013, from Nutrition Care Manual: http://www.nutrition caremanual.org

32. American Dietetic Association. International Dietetics and Nutrition Terminology (IDNT) Reference Manual. 3rd ed. Chicago: American Dietetic Association; 2010.

33. Standards of Practice Task Force of the American Society of Colon and Recal Surgeons. Practice parameters for the evaluation and managment of constipation. Dis Colon Rectum 2007;50(12):2013–2022.

34. Institute of Medicine. Dietary Reference Intakes for Energy, Carbohydrate, Fiber, Fat, Fatty Acids, Cholesterol, Protein, and Amino Acids. Washington, DC: National Academies Press; 2005.

35. Alaimo K, McDowell M, Briefel R, Bischof A, Caughman C, Loria C, et al. Dietary intake of vitamins, minerals, and fiber of persons ages 2 months and over in the United States: third National Health and Nutrition Examination Survey, Phase 1, 1988-1991. Advance Data from Vital and Health Statistics 1998.

36. Tan K, Seow-Choen F. Fiber and colorectal diseases: separating fact from fiction. World J Gastroenterol 2007;13(31):4161–4167.

37. Marlett J, Cheung T. Database and quick methods of assessing typical dietary fiber intakes using data for 228 commonly consumed foods. J Am Diet Assoc 1997;97(10):1139–1151.

38. Bonnema A, Kolberg L, Thomas W, Slavin J. Gastrointestinal tolerance of chicory inulin products. J Am Diet Assoc 2010;110(6):865–868.

39. Storey D, Lee A, Bornet F, Brouns F. Gastrointestinal responses following acute and medium term intake of retrograded resistant maltodextrins, classified as type 3 resistant starch. Eur J Clin Nutr 2007;61(11):1262–1270.

40. Stewart M, Nikhanj S, Timm D, Thomas W, Slavin J. Evaluation of the effect of four fibers on laxation, gastrointestinal tolerance and serum markers in healthy humans. Ann Nutr Metab 2010;56(2):91–98.

41. American Dietetic Association. Position of the American Dietetic Association: health implications of dietary fiber. J Am Diet Assoc 2008; 108(10):1716–1731.

42. Academy of Nutrition and Dietetics. (2012). Fluid Requirements. Retrieved January 19, 2013, from Nutrition Care Manual: http://www .nutritioncaremanual.org

43. Shepherd S, Parker F, Muir J, Gibson P. Dietary triggers of abdominal symptoms in patients with irritable bowel syndrome: randomized placebo-controlled evidence. Clin Gastroenterol Hepatol 2008;6(7):765–771.

44. National Digestive Diseases Information Clearing House. (2008, January). Digestive Diseases. Retrieved March 28, 2011, from Gas in the Digestive System: http://digestive.niddk.nih.gov/ddiseases/pubs/gas/

45. Camilleri M, Murray JA. Diarrhea and constipation. In: Fauci A, Braunwald E, Kasper D, Hauser S, Longo D, Jameson J, et al., eds. Harrison's Principles of Internal Medicine. 17th ed. New York: McGraw Hill; 2008 [chapter 40]. Retrieved July 11, 2013, from http://www.accessmedicine.com/content.aspx?aID=9112979

46. Academy of Nutrition and Dietetics. (2012). Diarrhea. Retrieved January 19, 2013, from Nutrition Care Manual: http://www.nutritioncaremanual.org

47. Douglas L, Sanders M. Probiotics and prebiotics in dietetics practice. J Am Diet Assoc 2008;108(3):510–521.

48. Duro D, Duggan C. The BRAT diet for acute diarhea. Pract Gastroenterol 2007;60–68.

49. Binder HJ. Disorders of absorption. In: Fauci A, Braunwald E, Kasper D, Hauser S, Longo D, Jameson J, et al., eds. Harrison's Principles of Internal Medicine. 17th ed. New York: McGraw Hill; 2008. [chapter 288]. Retrieved July 11, 2013, from http://www.accessmedicine.com/content.aspx?aID=9112979

50. Academy of Nutrition and Dietetics. (2012). Lactose Intolerance. Retrieved January 19, 2013, from Nutrition Care Manual: http://www.nutritioncaremanual.org

51. Fasano A, Berti I, Gerarduzzi T, Not T, Colletti R, Drago S, et al. Prevalence of celiac disease in at-risk and not-at-risk groups in the United States: a large multicenter study. Arch Intern Med 2003;163(3):286–292.

52. Barera G, Bonfanti R, Viscardi M, Bazzigaluppi E, Calori G, Meschi F, et al. Occurrence of celiac disease after onset of type 1 diabetes: a 6-year prospective longitudinal study. Pediatrics 2002;109(5):833–838.

53. Canadian Celiac Association. (2009). Resource Guide for Medical Professionals. Retrieved March 29, 2011, from Diagnosing Celiac Disease: http://www.celiacguide.org/diagnosis.html#Recognizing

54. Cranney A, Zarkadas M, Graham I, Butzner J, Rashid M, Warren R, et al. The Canadian celiac health survey. Dig Dis Sci 2007;52(4):1087–1095.

55. Case S. Gluten-Free Diet: A Comprehensive Resource Guide. Regina, Saskatchewan: Case Nutrition Consulting, Inc; 2010.

56. Case S, Kaplan C. Gluten-Free Guidance: Practical Tips for Dietitians and their Celiac Patients. Today's Dietitian; March 2003:44–49.

57. Podovei M, Kuo B. Irritable bowel syndrome: a practical review. South Med J 2006;99(11):1235–1242.

58. Quartero A, Meineche-Schmidt V, Muris J, Rubin G, de Wit N. Bulking agents, antispasmodic and antidepressant medication for the treatment of irritable bowel syndrome. Cochrane Database Systemic Reviews 2005:CD003460.

59. Gibson P. Food intolerance in functional bowel disorders. J Gastroenterol Hepatol 2011;26(Suppl 3):128–131.

60. Barrett J, Gibson P. Development and validation of a comprehensive semi-quantitative food frequency questionnaire that includes FODMAP intake and glycemic index. J Am Diet Assoc 2010;110(10):1469–1476.

61. Friedman S, Blumberg RS. Inflammatory bowel disease. In: Fauci A, Braunwald E, Kasper D, Hauser S, Longo D, Jameson J, et al., eds. Harrison's Principles of Internal Medicine. 17th ed [chapter 289]: http://www.accessmedicine.com/content.aspx?aID=2883197.

62. Academy of Nutrition and Dietetics. (2012). Inflammatory Bowel Disease. Retrieved January 19, 2013, from Nutrition Care Manual: http://www.nutritioncaremanual.org

63. Krok K, Lichenstein G. Nutrition in Crohn's disease. Curr Opin Gastroenterol 2003;19(2):148–153.

64. Eiden K. Nutritional considerations in inflammatory bowel disease. Pract Gastroenterol 2003;27(5):33–54.

65. Gassull M, Mañé J, Pedrosa E. Macronutrients and bioactive molecules: is there a specific role in the management of inflammatory bowel disease. J Parenter Enteral Nutr 2005;29(4 Suppl):S179–S182.

66. Campos F, Waitzberg D, Teixeira M, Mucerino D, Kiss D, Habr-Gama A. Pharmacological nutrition in inflammatory bowel diseases. Nutr Hosp 2003;18(2):57–64.

67. Academy of Nutrition and Dietetics. (2012). Diverticular Conditions. Retrieved January 19, 2013, from Nutrition Care Manual: http://www.nutritioncaremanual.org

68. Bogardus SJ. What do we know about diverticular disease? a brief overview. J Clin Gastroenterol 2006;40(Suppl 3):S108–S111.

69. Tarleton S, DiBaise JK. Low-residue diet in diverticular disease: putting an end to a myth. Nutr Clin Pract 2011;26(2):137–142.

70. Academy of Nutrition and Dietetics. (2012). Bowel Surgery. Retrieved January 19, 2013, from Nutrition Care Manual: http://www.nutritioncaremanual.org

71. Willcutts K, Scarano K, Eddins C. Ostomies and fistulas: a collaborative approach. Pract Gastroenterol 2005;29(11):63–79.

72. Academy of Nutrition and Dietetics. (2011). Initiation of EN. Retrieved January 19, 2013, from Evidence Analysis Library: http://andevidencelibrary.com

73. O'Keefe S, Buchman A, Fishbein T, Jeejeebhoy K, Jeppesen P, Shaffer J. Short bowel syndrome and intestinal failure: consensus definitions and overview. Clin Gastroenterol Hepatol 2006;4(1):6–10.

74. Buchman A. (2004). Medical and Surgical Management of Short Bowel Syndrome. Available at: http://www.medscape.com/viewarticle/474629_3. Medscape General Medicine .

75. Tilg H. Short bowel syndrome: searching for the proper diet. Eur J Gastroenterol Hepatol 2008;20(11):1062–1064.

76. Buchman A, Scolapio J, Fryer J. AGA technnical review on short bowel syndrome and intestinal transplantation. Gastroenterology 2003;124(4):1111–1134.

77. McQuaid KR. (2011). Chapter 15. Gastroinestinal Disorders. Current Medical Diagnosis & Treatment 2011: http://www.accessmedicine.com/content.aspx?aID=6395.

8

Blood and Bones: Nutrition in Musculoskeletal Disorders, Rheumatic Disease, and Anemias

This chapter covers nutritional management of disorders of the blood and the bones, from osteoporosis to nutritional anemias and rheumatic conditions. While not every disorder or disease of the musculoskeletal and hematological systems has nutritional implications, for those that do, the basic food and nutrition guidelines and evidence-based diet therapies that exist are presented here.

Osteoporosis

Osteoporosis is often called a silent disease. Gradually or rapidly declining bone loss may go unnoticed for years or decades until its silence is loudly interrupted by a fracture. Based on information from the National Health and Nutrition Examination Survey III (NHANES III), the National Osteoporosis Foundation estimates that 10 million Americans have osteoporosis, with an additional 33.6 million who have low bone density of the hip.[1] Furthermore, half of all Caucasian women and one-fifth of Caucasian men can expect to have an osteoporosis-related fracture at some point in their lifetime. The significance of osteoporosis-related fractures cannot be understated, particularly with regards to hip fractures, as:

- Hip fractures are associated with a 10–20% excess mortality within 1 year of fracture;
- Those with hip fractures have a 2.5-fold increased risk of future fractures;
- Twenty percent of hip fracture patients will need long-term nursing home care; and
- Only 40% will return to their prefracture level of independence.[2]

Osteoporosis-related fractures of the vertebrae can lead to complications involving back pain, loss of height, and kyphosis (the curving of the spine that leads to a hunchback or slouching posture). Kyphosis results in postural changes that can impede activity such as bending and reaching, and impair nutritional status due to associated abdominal pain and distention, constipation, reduced appetite, and early onset of satiety. In addition to these physical limitations, osteoporosis represents a massive economic burden for our healthcare system. The US Surgeon General estimates that osteoporosis-related fractures cause more than 432,000 hospital admissions, 2.5 million medical office visits, and 180,000 nursing home admissions each year. Demographic shifts and the aging of the population lead to further estimation that the number of hip fractures and their economic impact will perhaps double, or even triple, by the year 2040.[3]

■ Risk Factors

There are two primary types of bone cells: osteoblasts, which promote bone-building; and osteoclasts, which break down bone. During infancy, childhood, puberty, and other periods of growth, the activity of osteoblasts outpaces that of osteoclasts. Bone mass declines when the bone-breakdown rate of the osteoclast bone cells exceeds that of the bone-building osteoblasts, and this usually occurs in postmenopausal women and men over the age of 65 years. Figure 8–1 shows the comparison of a normal, healthy bone with that of an osteoporotic bone. The osteoporotic bone is structurally weakened as a result of its significantly lower mass.

Most bone growth is completed by 20 years of age, although some bone can continue to be laid down between 20 and 30 years of age. The National Osteoporosis Foundation estimates that 85–90% of adult bone mass has been established by the age of 18 years in females, and by the age of 20 years in males, with bone mass declining at varying rates after that. In premenopausal females, estrogen works to maintain bone health. With loss of this bone-protecting hormonal factor, many

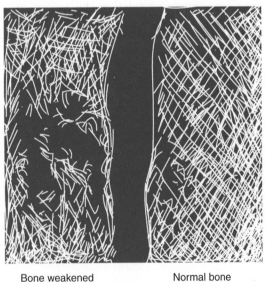

Bone weakened   Normal bone
by osteoporosis

Figure 8–1. Osteoporotic bone compared to normal bone.

Table 8–1. Osteoporosis risk factors.

Female gender
White/Caucasian race
Postmenopausal women
Older adults
Small-framed body size and/or low body weight
Low-calcium diet
Physical inactivity
Alcohol intake of more than 2 drinks per day
Dementia
Estrogen deficiency at onset before age 45 years
Frailty and recent falls

Data from Centers for Disease Control and Prevention, 2011; Academy of Nutrition and Dietetics, 2012.

females experience an accelerated rate of bone loss during and after menopause. Males lose bone mass with age as well, although it tends to be more gradual, and may be related to lowered testosterone levels.[3]

While osteoporosis can afflict both men and women, of the 10 million Americans who are estimated to have osteoporosis, 80% are women.[4] Being of Northern European or Asian descent increases risk, while African and Hispanic descent is associated with lower risk. Increasing age, low BMI, frailty, and having a family history of osteoporosis are also considered osteoporosis risk factors. Lifestyle factors that influence osteoporosis risk include smoking, history of eating disorders, excessive alcohol consumption, physical inactivity, and a diet low in calcium and vitamin D. Medication usage patterns can also mediate osteoporosis risk as chronic thyroid hormone dependence weakens bones, diuretic use increases urinary calcium loss, and corticosteroid therapy can also contribute to weakened bones. Table 8–1 contains a summary of lifestyle and genetic osteoporosis risk factors.[5,6]

The presence of any one of a number of medical conditions can also increase osteoporosis risk. These conditions and diseases are outlined in Table 8–2.[6]

■ Diagnosis

Bone mineral density (BMD) is articulated in grams per square centimeter. Bone density can be measured using a variety of techniques, with dual-energy x-ray absorptiometry (DEXA) being the most widely

Table 8-2. Conditions and medications that increase osteoporosis risk.

Conditions that Increase Osteoporosis Risk		
AIDS/HIV	Gaucher's disease	Multiple myeloma
Amyloidosis	Hemochromatosis	Multiple sclerosis
Ankylosing spondylitis	Hemophilia	Parenteral nutrition
Anorexia nervosa	Hyperparathyroidism	Pernicious anemia
Celiac disease	Hypogonadism	Rheumatoid arthritis
COPD	Idiopathic scoliosis	Schizophrenia and other major mood disorders
Congenital porphyria	Inflammatory bowel disease	Spinal cord transsection
Cushing's syndrome	Liver disease	Stroke
Diabetes	Lymphoma and leukemia	Thalassemia
Female athlete triad	Malabsorption syndromes	Thyrotoxicosis
Gastrectomy	Mastocytosis	Tumor secretion of PTH-related peptide
Medications that Increase Osteoporosis Risk		
Anticoagulants (heparin)	Cancer chemotherapy drugs	Lithium
Anticonvulsants	Glucocorticoids (and adrenocorticotropic hormone [ACTH])	Methotrexate
Cyclosporine A and tacrolimus	Gonadotropin-releasing hormone agonists	Thyroxine

Data from Academy of Nutrition and Dietetics, 2012; http://www.niams.nih.gov/Health_Info/Bone/Osteoporosis/osteoporosis_hoh.asp.

accepted. DEXA scan results are expressed as T-scores, representing the number of standard deviations below normal peak bone density. One standard deviation is equivalent to 10–15% of the BMD value expressed in g/cm^2. The T-score reading is based on a population of healthy women aged 30 years and above from the same ethnic background. Table 8–3 contains a list of indications for BMD testing as recommended by the National Osteoporosis Foundation.[2]

The World Health Organization criteria are most often used to diagnose low BMD, osteopenia, and osteoporosis. Table 8–4 defines the DEXA T-score readings and their relationship to BMD diagnosis.[7]

Table 8-3. Who should have bone mineral density testing?

Women aged 65 years and older and men aged 70 years and older, regardless of clinical risk factors
Younger postmenopausal women and men aged 50-69 years about whom you have concern based on their clinical risk factor profile
Women in the menopausal transition if there is a specific risk factor associated with increased fracture risk such as low body weight, prior low-trauma fracture, or high-risk medication
Adults who have a fracture after age 50 years
Adults with a condition (eg, rheumatoid arthritis) or taking a medication (eg, glucocorticoids in a daily dose ≥5 mg prednisone or equivalent for ≥3 months) associated with low bone mass or bone loss
Anyone being considered for pharmacologic therapy for osteoporosis
Anyone being treated for osteoporosis, to monitor treatment effect
Anyone not receiving therapy in whom evidence of bone loss would lead to treatment

Data from National Osteoporosis Foundation, 2010.

Because the WHO criteria are based on a reference group of women, their effectiveness for use in a male population has been questioned. Current recommendations for osteoporosis diagnosis in males are outlined in Table 8–5.[6]

Bone densitometry is a covered benefit for qualified participants under Medicare Part B, as part of the Bone Mass Measurement Act. Bone mass measurement is covered once every 24 months, or more often if medically necessary. A Medicare beneficiary is qualified and considered to be at risk for osteoporosis if he meets one of five criteria.

Table 8-4. WHO DEXA T-score result diagnostic criteria.

Bone Mineral Density	DEXA T-Score Results
Normal bone mineral	−1 and greater
Osteopenia	−1 to −2.4
Osteoporosis	−2.5 and less
Severe osteoporosis	−2.5 and one or more fragility fractures

Data from World Health Organization, 2004.

Table 8–5. Osteoporosis diagnosis recommendations in males.

Male Age Group	T-Score for Osteoporosis Diagnosis
Males aged 65 + years	−2.5 and less
Males 50–64 years of age	−2.5 and less if other risk factors exist
Males aged less than 50	Do not diagnose osteoporosis using bone densitometry alone; clinical diagnosis is made if secondary causes of low bone density exist and are supported by low BMD scores Z-scores, not T-scores, should be used in men under 50 years of age (and premenopausal women and children)
Males aged less than 20	No densitometric criteria for diagnosing osteoporosis in males (and females) less than age 20 If Z-scores are −2.0 or less (using pediatric database of age-matched controls), can say "low bone density for chronologic age" if applicable

Data from Academy of Nutrition and Dietetics, 2012; The Writing Group for the ISCD Position Development Conference. Diagnosis of osteoporosis in men, premenopausal women, and children. J Clin Densitometry 2004;7(1):17–26.

Determining baseline BMD is important but may be more useful when obtained earlier in life and, more specifically, prior to menopause in females. It is well established that BMD declines during and after menopause, and it is helpful to know what baseline levels were prior to the decline in BMD associated with menopause. To put it plainly: if BMD falls off a cliff after menopause, it would be nice to know how high that cliff was prior to menopause! In order to determine the rate of bone loss during and after menopause, encourage early BMD testing when appropriate. Table 8–6 details the criteria for Medicare qualification for bone mass measurement.[8]

- ## Nutritional Management and Mitigation of Osteoporosis

While medication remains the primary form of treatment of osteoporosis, reducing fracture risk involves a combination of medication, weight-bearing exercise regimens, and a diet that is adequate in calcium and vitamin D. The use of weight-bearing exercise and dietary interventions can help to slow the rate of bone loss, but they do not function as effective, standalone therapies for increasing bone density. The nutrients of concern in bone health intervention include calcium, vitamin D, protein, and sodium. Low intake levels of calcium and vitamin D contribute to weakened bones. Inadequate or excessive intake levels of protein, alongside excessive sodium intake, increase the likelihood

Table 8–6. Bone mass measurement qualification criteria for medicare beneficiaries.

Medicare Qualification for Bone Mass Measurement
Beneficiary meets at least 1 of these 5 criteria:
A woman whose doctor is treating her for estrogen deficiency and is at risk for osteoporosis based on her medical history or other findings
A person with vertebral abnormalities as demonstrated by an x-ray
A person receiving steroid treatments
A person with hyperparathyroidism
A person taking an osteoporosis drug

Data from Centers for Medicare and Medicaid Services.

of urinary calcium excretion, which in turn increases osteoporosis risk and related fractures.

Calcium Intake and Recommendations

The DRI values are a set of recommendations developed by the Institute of Medicine's Food and Nutrition Board. The DRIs include an RDA for calcium intake for males and females over 1 year of age. Adult calcium RDA values are 1000–1200 milligrams of calcium per day.[9] The National Osteoporosis Foundation maintains that intake levels exceeding 1200–1500 milligrams of calcium per day are not beneficial and may increase the risk of kidney stones and cardiovascular disease. Table 8–7 contains the DRIs for calcium.[9]

DRI values for calcium for infants aged 0–12 months are adequate intake (AI) levels; the AI for life-stage and gender group is believed to cover the needs of all healthy individuals in the groups, but lack of data or uncertainty in the data prevents being able to specify with confidence the percentage of individuals covered by this intake.

Dairy foods are the most concentrated sources of dietary calcium. Milk, both powdered and liquid, and milk products such as yogurt, cheese, and kefir are all good sources of calcium. There are many non-dairy sources of calcium as well, although they generally contain less calcium per serving than do dairy foods. Canned salmon with bones, fortified ready-to-eat breakfast cereals, dark green leafy vegetables, almonds, sesame seeds, tofu set with calcium sulfate, clams, and soybeans are good nondairy sources of calcium. Tables 8–8 and 8–9 summarize dairy and nondairy food sources and their calcium content per serving size.[10]

In North America, calcium intake rates generally fall below recommended levels, especially for females and older adults.[11,12] Escalating intakes of sodas and other sweetened beverages, as well as high rates

Table 8–7. Dietary reference intakes: recommended dietary allowances for calcium.

0–6 months old	200 mg	6–12 months old	260 mg
1–3 years old	700 mg	4–8 years old	1000 mg
	Males	Females	Pregnant and Lactating Females
9–13 years old	1300 mg	1300 mg	
14–18 years old	1300 mg	1300 mg	1300 mg
19–30 years old	1000 mg	1000 mg	1000 mg
31–50 years old	1000 mg	1000 mg	1000 mg
51–70 years old	1000 mg	1200 mg	
>70 years old	1200 mg	1200 mg	

DRI values for calcium for infants aged 0–12 months are adequate intake (AI) levels; the AI for life-stage and gender group is believed to cover the needs of all healthy individuals in the groups, but lack of data or uncertainty in the data prevents being able to specify with confidence the percentage of individuals covered by this intake.

Data from Institute of Medicine, 2010.

of lactose intolerance among certain ethnic and racial groups, are likely contributors to substandard calcium intake. Approximately 75–80% of the calcium consumed in American diets comes from dairy products. Table 8–10 demonstrates a practical method for estimating an individual's daily calcium intake.

Calcium Supplements

Encouraging dietary sources of calcium is a recommended first-line approach to preventing calcium-deficiency-related disorders. Utilization of supplements should be considered when adequate dietary intake of calcium is not possible. Two of the most common types of calcium supplements contain calcium carbonate and calcium citrate. Calcium carbonate, which is the least expensive calcium supplement, should be taken with meals, as calcium carbonate requires acid from the digestive process to help make the calcium more soluble and readily absorbed. Calcium citrate supplements may be taken with or without food. Table 8–11 contains information about calcium supplements.

People taking calcium supplements who are also taking iron supplements should avoid taking these together, as these two minerals interfere with each other's absorption. Calcium from supplements is best absorbed when taken in amounts of 500 milligrams or less at a time.

Table 8-8. Dairy foods and calcium content.

Dairy Food	Serving Size	Calcium (mg)	Calories
Plain low-fat yogurt	8 oz	415	143
Romano cheese	1.5 oz	452	165
Swiss cheese, pasteurized, processed	2 oz	438	189
Fruit low-fat yogurt	8 oz	338	243
Swiss cheese	1.5 oz	336	162
Ricotta cheese, part skim	½ cup	335	170
American cheese, pasteurized, processed cheese food	2 oz	387	187
Provolone cheese	1.5 oz	321	149
Mozzarella cheese, part-skim	1.5 oz	333	108
Cheddar cheese	1.5 oz	307	171
Fat-free (skim) milk	1 cup	299	83
Muenster cheese	1.5 oz	305	156
1% (low-fat) milk	1 cup	305	102
1% (low-fat) chocolate milk	1 cup	290	158
2% (reduced fat) milk	1 cup	293	122
2% (reduced fat) chocolate milk	1 cup	272	190
1% (low-fat) buttermilk	1 cup	284	98
Whole-chocolate milk	1 cup	280	208
Whole milk	1 cup	276	146
Ricotta cheese, whole milk	½ cup	255	214
Blue cheese	1.5 oz	225	150
Mozzarella cheese, whole milk	1.5 oz	215	128
Feta cheese	1.5 oz	210	112

Data from Nelms, 2011; US Department of Agriculture, Agricultural Research Service, 2012.

The tolerable upper intake level (UL) for calcium is 2500 mg/day for adults aged 19–50 years, and 2000 mg/day for those aged 51 years and above. Consumers should be advised to avoid consumption of calcium in excess of the UL due to the potential for adverse health outcomes.

Table 8-9. Nondairy foods and calcium content.

Nondairy Food	Serving Size	Calcium (mg)	Calories
Fortified ready-to-eat breakfast cereal, various	1 oz	236-1043	88-106
Silk, plain soy milk	1 cup	299	100
Sardines, Atlantic, in oil, drained	3 oz	325	177
Tofu, firm, prepared w/ calcium sulfate	½ cup	253	88
Pink salmon, canned with bones	3 oz	241	117
Collard greens, cooked from frozen	½ cup	178	31
Molasses, blackstrap	1 tablespoon	172	47
Spinach, cooked from frozen	½ cup	145	32
Soybeans, green, cooked	½ cup	130	127
Turnip greens, cooked from frozen	½ cup	125	24
Ocean perch, Atlantic, cooked	3 oz	29	82
Oatmeal, instant, fortified	1 packet	99-110	97-157
White beans, canned	½ cup	96	149
Kale, cooked from frozen	½ cup	90	20
Okra, cooked from frozen	½ cup	68	27
Soybeans, mature, cooked	½ cup	88	149
Blue crab, canned	3 oz	77	71
Beet greens, fresh, cooked	½ cup	82	19
Chinese cabbage, fresh, cooked	½ cup	79	10
Clams, canned, drained solids	3 oz	55	121
Dandelion greens, fresh, cooked	½ cup	74	17
Rainbow trout, farmed, cooked	3 oz	26	143

Data from Nelms, 2011; US Department of Agriculture, Agricultural Research Service, 2012.

Table 8-10. Practical method for estimating individual daily calcium intake.

Step 1			
Food Item	**Servings Per Day**	**Approximate Calcium Per Serving (mg)**	**Calcium (mg)**
Milk (8 oz)	_____ ×	300	= _____
Yogurt (6 oz)	_____ ×	300	= _____
Cheese (1 oz or 1 cubic in.)	_____ ×	200	= _____
Orange juice, calcium fortified (1 cup)	_____ ×	350	= _____
Breakfast cereals, fortified (1 cup)	_____ ×	200 −1000; calcium content varies; check labels	= _____
Step 2			
Total amount of calcium (mg) from above + 250 mg for nondairy sources = total calcium			
Total calcium (mg)			

Table 8-11. Calcium supplements.

Calcium Supplements	Brands	Requires HCl for Absorption?	Meals or Not?	Calcium Content
Calcium carbonate	• Caltrate • Tums and other antacids • Viactiv • OsCal	Yes	Take with meals	Most supplements contain 500-600 mg calcium
Calcium citrate	• Citracal • Citracal Liquitab	No	Can be taken with or without meals	Most supplements contain 200-300 mg calcium

Table 8–12. Vitamin D content of various foods.

	Serving size	Amount: mcg	Amount: IU
Vitamin-D Fortified Foods			
Milk	1 cup (8 oz)	3.2 mcg	124 IU
Soy milk	1 cup (8 oz)	Varies; 2.9 mcg	Varies; 119 IU
Yogurt	1 cup (8 oz)	0.2 mcg	5 IU
Margarine, with added vitamin D	1 tablespoon	1.5 mcg	60 IU
Fortified orange juice	1 cup (8 oz)	Varies; 3.5 mcg	Varies; 140 IU
Foods Naturally High in Vitamin D			
Cod liver oil	1 tablespoon	34 mcg	1360 IU
Hard-boiled egg	1 egg	1.1 mcg	44 IU
Fatty fish (tuna, mackerel, and salmon)	3-4 oz	12.3 mcg	493 IU

Data from US Department of Agriculture, Agricultural Research Service, 2012.

Vitamin D Intake and Recommendations

Vitamin D plays three important roles in increasing blood concentration levels of calcium and phosphorus: (1) it increases their absorption in the gut; (2) it promotes reabsorption by the kidneys; and (3) it stimulates osteoclast formation and subsequent bone resorption.[13] Vitamin D deficiency is associated with rickets in children and osteomalacia in adults. Naturally occurring food sources of vitamin D are limited; however, some vitamin D is provided by cod liver oil, fatty fish, egg yolks, fortified milk and margarine, yogurt, and juices. Milk is fortified with vitamin D at a level of 100 IU (2.5 micrograms) per cup, which equates to 25% daily value (%DV) for a healthy adult following a 2000-calorie diet. Table 8–12 contains information about the naturally occurring and fortified vitamin D content of various foods.[10]

Vitamin D Supplements

Because of the scarcity of naturally occurring sources of vitamin D, most people are unable to achieve recommended intake levels, and as such, supplemental vitamin D is often indicated. The American Academy of Pediatrics recommends that all children receive 400 IU of vitamin D, beginning in the first few days of life.[14] This is an increase from previous recommendations that called for 200 IU per day, beginning in the first 2 months of life. Vitamin D supplementation is of particular importance for exclusively breastfed infants, as breast milk is not naturally high in vitamin D.

Table 8-13. Dietary reference intakes for vitamin D.

0-6 months old	10 mcg/day or 400 IU/day	6-12 months old	10 mcg/day or 400 IU/day
1-3 years old	15 mcg/day or 600 IU/day	4-8 years old	15 mcg/day or 600 IU/day
	Males	**Females**	**Pregnant and Lactating Females**
9-13 years old	15 mcg/day = 600 IU	15 mcg/day = 600 IU	
14-18 years old	15 mcg/day = 600 IU	15 mcg/day = 600 IU	15 mcg/day = 600 IU
19-30 years old	15 mcg/day = 600 IU	15 mcg/day = 600 IU	15 mcg/day = 600 IU
31-50 years old	15 mcg/day = 600 IU	15 mcg/day = 600 IU	15 mcg/day = 600 IU
51-70 years old	15 mcg/day = 600 IU	15 mcg/day = 600 IU	
>70 years old	20 mcg/day = 1200 IU	20 mcg/day = 1200 IU	

Data from Institute of Medicine, 2010.

Vitamin D status is measured by analyzing the concentration of serum 25-hydroxyvitamin D or 25(OH)D. This represents both dietary vitamin D intake and that which is synthesized by the body (Table 8–13). The Institutes of Medicine now suggest that vitamin D deficiency risk increases at serum 25(OH)D levels below 30 nmol/L (12 ng/mL).[9] There are some populations that will be potentially at risk for vitamin D inadequacy at serum 25(OH)D levels in the range of 30–50 nmol/L (12–20 ng/mL). With regards to establishing adequacy levels, generally all persons are considered to have adequate vitamin D levels when serum 25(OH)D levels are at least 50 nmol/L (20 ng/mL).[9] Varying levels of sun exposure at different latitudes and skin color can affect vitamin D activation potential. The darker one's skin is, the more is sun exposure that is needed to synthesize vitamin D.

Protein and Sodium

The role of animal protein and the degree to which it may or may not affect urinary calcium excretion levels is not entirely understood. Some studies indicate that an increased level of bone loss occurs in people who have high animal protein intake,[15] while other studies demonstrate increasing bone density in light of high protein intake.[16] In general, a

Table 8–14. National Osteoporosis Foundation's clinician's recommendations for postmenopausal women and men aged 50 years and older.

Calcium	At least 1200 mg per day
Vitamin D	800–1000 IU per day with supplements if necessary for those aged 50 years and older
Exercise	Weight-bearing and muscle-strengthening exercises regularly
Smoking	Smoking cessation
Alcohol	Avoid excessive intake
BMD Testing	Women aged 65+ and men aged 70+
	Those who have had a fracture
	Postmenopausal women and men aged 50-69 years when concern exists based on risk factor profile

Data from National Osteoporosis Foundation, 2010.

lower-sodium diet is recommended to promote optimal bone and overall health. Excessive sodium intake increases urinary calcium losses, which negatively impacts bone health.

■ Summary Recommendations

As a nutrition prescription for the prevention of osteoporosis and osteopenia, the Academy of Nutrition and Dietetics states, "(a) diet with moderate-to-low-sodium intake, adequate protein, calcium and vitamin D . . . with five servings of fruits and vegetables each day to supplement adequate amounts of potassium, magnesium and vitamins C and K . . . is beneficial for bone health."[6] A variety of weight-bearing, balance, and flexibility exercises should be regularly undertaken to optimize bone health. Avoiding excessive alcohol, tobacco smoke, and inactivity should also be encouraged. Individuals who have established osteoporosis or osteopenia are advised to receive fall-prevention training. Table 8–14 contains the National Osteoporosis Foundation's summary Clinician's Recommendations for Postmenopausal Women and Men Age 50 and Older.[2]

Rheumatic Disease

According to the Centers for Disease Control and Prevention (CDC), in 2009 50 million adults in the United States reported some form of diagnosed arthritis, rheumatoid arthritis, gout, lupus, or fibromyalgia. Osteoarthritis is the most common form of arthritis, with 27 million American adults currently enduring this painful condition. While patients and clients are often seeking diet-based therapies for the treatment of various rheumatic diseases, it is important for practitioners to understand the relationship between overweight and obesity and the development of some of these conditions, as well as the lack of established diet therapies for their treatment. Of those with doctor-diagnosed arthritis, 66% of diagnosed adults were overweight (BMI >25) or obese (BMI >30).[17] Particularly with regards to osteoarthritis and gout, advanced practice nursing professionals must be comfortable discussing weight realities and counseling on weight loss if and when necessary (see Chapter 3).

▪ Osteoarthritis

As mentioned, the relationship between diet and osteoarthritis tends to be weight-related. Just as two-thirds of the United States' population is overweight or obese, two-thirds of those diagnosed with osteoarthritis are also overweight or obese. Overweight and obesity are situations that put additional pressure and stress on already deteriorating cartilage in the joints and bones. Weight loss of just 11 pounds (5 kg) has been shown to reduce the risk of developing knee osteoarthritis in women by 50%, especially for those women who are more than 10% above their ideal body weight.[18]

The advanced practice nurse is encouraged to discuss weight loss options with overweight and obese persons who are also diagnosed with osteoarthritis. Despite the wealth of diet products, treatments, and supplements that claim to alleviate osteoarthritis pain, the majority are at best questionable, and almost all are lacking in any scientific efficacy. It is never fun to be the bearer of bad news, but for those with osteoarthritis, even those who are not obese or not overweight, the Academy of Nutrition and Dietetics maintains that, "(c)urrently, there is insufficient evidence to support specific recommendations for particular nutrients, foods, or eating plans in the treatment of osteoarthritis."[6]

For overweight and obese individuals with osteoarthritis, an individualized meal plan that limits excessive calories and promotes weight loss is recommended. There are no individual foods or nutrients that should be avoided with osteoarthritis. Regular physical activity within the limits of the individual's capabilities and pain thresholds, possibly in conjunction with physical therapy if indicated, should be adopted to promote weight loss.

Osteoarthritis can impact nutritional status by limiting a person's ability to open jars and food packages, and to cut foods in preparation and at the table. If arthritis affects the mandibular joint of the jaw, it can impede chewing. An increasingly narrow selection of food intake caused by any of these conditions can negatively influence nutritional status, particularly in older adults. Conducting a 24-hour recall or reviewing a client's daily food journal can provide practitioners with insight into the potential for nutrient deficiencies caused by inadequate food intake from osteoarthritic limitations.

What Does the Evidence Say?: Glucosamine and Chondroitin Use for Osteoarthritis

Glucosamine and chondroitin sulfate are by far the most widely used dietary supplements for the treatment of osteoarthritis. Glucosamine is a natural part of human cartilage and other connective tissue. Chondroitin sulfate is a type of complex carbohydrate that works to retain water in cartilage. Despite the fact that annual global sales of glucosamine and chondroitin supplements for joint pain relief are approaching 1 billion dollars,[19] the efficacy of these products has been questioned.

To settle the record on whether or not these supplements aid in alleviating arthritis-related joint pain, two sections of the National Institutes of Health (NIH) funded the Glucosamine/chondroitin Arthritis Intervention Trial (GAIT). GAIT was funded by The National Center for Complementary and Alternative Medicine (NCCAM) and the National Institute of Arthritis and Musculoskeletal and Skin Diseases (NIAMS). In the GAIT trial, participants were randomized to one of five treatment groups: glucosamine by itself, chondroitin sulfate by itself, glucosamine and chondroitin combination, celecoxib (a prescription drug used to manage OA pain), or placebo. The study was double-blinded and conducted at 16 study center sites around the United States. The GAIT analyzed a sample size of 1583 patients aged 40 years or older with knee pain who received treatment for a 24-week period. The primary outcome measure was a 20% or more reduction in knee pain between the beginning and end of the study.

Upon completion of the study, researchers determined that there was no significant difference in pain reduction in any of the treatment groups and placebo. For those reporting mild OA pain, taking glucosamine and chondroitin sulfate together or independently did not yield a statistically significant reduction in pain. Some evidence suggested that for those reporting moderate-to-severe knee pain, glucosamine and chondroitin in combination could effectively reduce pain; however, as the study was not specifically designed to address this particular subgroup, additional research is needed to determine the true value of recommending such a therapy.[20]

So, what is the bottom line for glucosamine and chondroitin supplementation in OA? While glucosamine and chondroitin do not appear to be harmful when used to treat OA-related joint pain, there is no conclusive evidence to suggest that anything beyond the placebo effect is at work in pain reduction.

■ Rheumatoid Arthritis

As with osteoarthritis, rheumatoid arthritis can limit an individual's physical abilities to obtain food. Twisted hands and puffy joints, stiffness, inflammation, pain, and limited range of motion can lead to disability that leads to suboptimal nutritional status. The individual may no longer be able to shop independently or prepare

Table 8-15. Nutrition interview questions for an individual with rheumatoid arthritis.

Taste aberrations	Do foods taste differently to you now than they used to?
	Are there foods you don't eat because of how they taste to you?
Dry mouth	Do you ever feel like your mouth is too dry to eat certain foods?
	What foods do you avoid because of dryness in your mouth?
	How much water per day do you drink?
Nausea	Do you feel nauseous more often than you used to?
	What foods seem to increase nausea in you?
	What foods are more well tolerated when you are nauseous?
Selective food intake	Are there foods you are avoiding because of your RA?
	What foods do you think are associated with RA flare-ups?
Supplements	Do you take any vitamin, mineral, or herbal supplements for RA?
	Are there any therapies such as acupuncture or meditation that you use to help with RA?
Weight	How much do you weigh?
	How much did you weigh a year ago?
	What is your goal weight?

food, or safely chew or swallow. Changes in taste, dryness of the nasal mucosa, and loss of appetite further compound the nutritional problems. When addressing nutritional status in a person with rheumatoid arthritis, special attention should be paid to current versus usual weight, eating habits, and overall energy intake. Table 8–15 contains a variety of questions that you might consider including in your patient interview.

The nutrition recommendations for an individual with RA do not differ dramatically from those for many other patient populations. If inadequate intake is leading to compromised nutritional status, a good approach is to, "make every bite count." Encourage nutrient-dense, low-saturated-fat, and low-*trans*-fat food choices. Keep in mind that patients with severe RA and chronic inflammation are likely experiencing an elevated metabolic rate. As such, they will require greater calorie and protein intake to meet their nutritional needs. Inability to obtain these needs results in unintended weight loss and can lead to the cachectic appearance often seen in those with RA.

Table 8–16. Diet therapy for an individual with rheumatoid arthritis.

Meal pattern	Encourage a variety of foods
Fat intake	Limit total fat and saturated and *trans* fats
Calcium	Encourage calcium-containing foods
Omega-3 fatty acids	Include dietary sources of omega-3 fatty acids from fish sources such as herring, mackerel, and salmon
Vitamin C	Choose foods rich in vitamin C such as citrus fruits, dark green leafy vegetables, strawberries, and tomatoes
Vitamin E	Choose foods rich in vitamin E such as whole grains, nuts and seeds, plant oils, and dark green leafy vegetables
Zinc	Choose foods rich in zinc such as meats, fish, poultry, grains, and vegetables

Encouraging small, frequent meals with calorie and protein-rich options is advisable. If indicated, try high-calorie, high-protein supplements between meals to enhance nutrient intake. If an individual consumes alcohol, recommend that it be taken in moderation. Keep simple sugars to a minimum, and limit processed foods and sweets, as they often displace other more nutritious food sources. Table 8–16 contains a summary of nutrition recommendations for an individual with RA.

What Does the Evidence Say?: Diet and Rheumatoid Arthritis

There are no special foods, supplements, or nutrition therapies that can cure rheumatoid arthritis or alleviate its symptoms. According to the Academy of Nutrition and Dietetics:

"Currently, there is little evidence to support the recommendation of any specific nutrients, foods, or nutrition therapies in the treatment of rheumatoid arthritis. However, depending on the extent and severity of their RA and any existing comorbid conditions, such as osteoporosis, heart disease, or anemia of chronic disease, an eating plan that includes fruits, vegetables, nuts and seeds, whole grains, calcium-rich foods, with appropriate amounts of lean protein, and plenty of fluids at an energy level that will promote a desirable weight will help maintain a proper nutritional status."[21]

- Gout

Gout is among the most painful types of inflammatory arthritis and tends to be most common in men. Gouty flare-ups occur when uric

Table 8-17. Nutrition interview considerations for an individual with gout.

Frequency and source of animal food intake
Frequency and source of dairy foods intake
Frequency and source of fruit and vegetable intake
Frequency and source of alcohol intake, especially beer
Use of vitamin, mineral, herbal, or dietary supplements
Frequency, type, and dose of medications

acid crystals deposit in body tissues and fluids. Risk of gout increases with obesity, excessive alcohol consumption (three or more drinks per day), hypertension, diuretic use, and dependence on a high-purine and high-animal-food diet.[22] When addressing the nutritional status of an individual with gout, it is advisable to question the person's frequency and dietary sources of animal foods, including meat and dairy. Also consider fruit and vegetable intake, alcohol (beer in particular), and use of medications and supplements. Inadequate fluid intake, excessive animal protein intake, and excessive alcohol intake all can exacerbate gout. Table 8–17 contains nutrition interview considerations for an individual with gout.

Nutrition intervention for gout should address hyperlipidemia, diabetes, and hypertension if also present. The goal is to lower uric acid concentrations in the blood by reducing animal-based food intake and eliminating alcohol. Alcohol, particularly beer, is of utmost importance, given that it increases uric acid levels in those prone to gout, when consumed by itself or in conjunction with a purine-rich meal.[23] Table 8–18 contains a list of very high purine, moderately high purine, and low-purine foods.[24] The very high and moderately high purine foods should be avoided or severely limited in the diet of a person prone to gout. Foods that are low in purines should be encouraged in place of the very high and moderately high purine foods. Table 8–19 offers dietary recommendations during acute gout attacks and in the periods between gouty flare-ups.[24]

■ Fibromyalgia

Fibromyalgia is a musculoskeletal syndrome characterized by generalized muscle pain, joint stiffness and tenderness, disordered sleep patterns, cognitive and memory problems, and depression and anxiety. It can also include migraine or tension headache, irritable bowel syndrome, GERD, and other bladder and pelvic pain syndromes. While the disorder is often misunderstood and perhaps generally unrecognized, it is estimated to affect 2–4% of the population, and disproportionately

Table 8-18. Foods that are low in purines, moderately high in purines, or very high in purines.

Food Group	Low-Purine Foods	Moderately High Purine Foods	Very High Purine Foods
Beverages	Water, juice, carbonated drinks, tea, coffee, and cocoa		Alcohol and beer
Breads and cereals	Breads, pasta, rice, cakes, cornbread, and popcorn	Oatmeal – limit to 2/3 cup per day, wheat bran, wheat germ (limit to ¼ cup per day, dry)	
Condiments	Salt, herbs, olives, pickles, relishes, and vinegar		Bakers and brewer's yeast
Dairy foods	All dairy foods; low-fat or nonfat is recommended		
Fats and oils	All types except gravies and sauces made with meat		Gravies and sauces made with meat
Fruits	All fruits		
Protein foods	Eggs, nuts, and peanut butter	Meat and poultry, crab, lobster, oysters (limit to 1-2, 2-3 oz servings/day), dried beans, peas, and lentils (limit to 1 cup cooked daily)	Anchovies
			Sardines
			Herring
			Mussels
			Tuna
			Codfish
			Scallops
			Trout and haddock (remove fish skin)
			Bacon
			Organ meats (liver, kidney, brain, heart)
			Tripe
			Sweetbreads
			Wild game, goose

(Continued)

Table 8–18. Foods that are low in purines, moderately high in purines, or very high in purines. (*Continued*)

Food Group	Low-Purine Foods	Moderately High Purine Foods	Very High Purine Foods
Soups	Made without meat	Meat or fish-based soups, broths, bouillons	
Vegetables	All vegetables except moderate-purine vegetables	Asparagus, cauliflower, spinach, mushrooms, and green peas; limit all to no more than ½ cup per day	
Miscellaneous	Sugar, sweets, and gelatin		Mincemeat pie

Data from Academy of Nutrition and Dietetics, 2012; http://www.upmc.com/patients-visitors/education/nutrition/pages/low-purine-diet.aspx.

so in women.[25] There is no diagnostic test, blood test, or muscle biopsy that can be done to confirm fibromyalgia; rather, diagnosis is made based on symptoms. Additionally, there is no one cure for fibromyalgia, and treatment must be individualized to manage this chronic condition.

While some people with fibromyalgia may experience alleviation of pain or tenderness with the exclusion of certain foods, there is no specific diet therapy that has been conclusively shown to relieve

Table 8–19. Nutrition recommendations for acute gout attacks and between gouty flare-ups.

Food Group	During Acute Attack	Between Gouty Flare-ups
Fluid	Drink 8–16 cups/day—at least half should be water	Drink 8–16 cups/day—at least half should be water
Alcohol	Avoid	Avoid
Animal foods	Limit animal foods and limit meat, fish, or poultry to 4–6 oz/day	Maintain a well-balanced meal plan; can contain animal protein
Protein	Eat only a moderate amount, use low-fat or nonfat dairy foods, tofu, eggs, and nut butters	Eat a moderate amount of protein; avoid high-protein diets

Data from Academy of Nutrition and Dietetics, 2012.

Table 8-20. Nutrition interventions for managing xerostomia (dry mouth).

Avoid alcohol
Avoid caffeine
Use a cool mist humidifier at night
Increase fluid to help chewing and swallowing
Limit sucrose (sugar)-containing foods and carbohydrates that are sticky and increase dental caries risk
Rinse mouth with water and baking soda (1/2-1 tablespoon in 8 oz water) while awake
Avoid mouthwashes that contain alcohol
Brush teeth with very soft bristled toothbrush
Sip on liquids or suck ice chips throughout the day
Trial tart foods that may stimulate saliva flow
Drink through a straw

Academy of Nutrition and Dietetics, 2012; Kogut and Luthringer, 2005.

fibromyalgia symptoms. Low-calorie exclusion diets may result in weight loss, which may be implicated in reported reduction of pain. Despite anecdotal stories claiming that MSG can increase pain in people with fibromyalgia, no clear evidence exists to support this relationship.[26] Additionally, there is no clear evidence that adopting a vegan or vegetarian diet reduces pain in fibromyalgia.

- Sjögren's Syndrome

Sjögren's syndrome is an autoimmune disease that affects the secretory glands, resulting in reduced moisture and dry mouth and dry eyes. It can also impact nerves, the thyroid glands, joints, and organs such as the lungs, muscles, kidneys, liver, pancreas, stomach, and the brain. Individuals with Sjögren's syndrome are at increased risk for dysphagia and xerostomia. Xerostomia (dry mouth) is caused by decreased saliva production. There is no diet therapy indicated for the treatment of Sjögren's. Table 8-20 outlines a number of xerostomia management tips to help minimize discomfort associated with dry mouth.[24,27]

Lupus

Systemic lupus erythematosus (SLE or lupus) is an autoimmune disease characterized by widespread inflammation and tissue damage. The exact causes of SLE are not understood, but they are believed to be associated with genetic makeup, environmental conditions, and hormonal factors. Approximately nine in 10 cases affect women, with blacks and possibly Hispanics, Asians, and Native Americans being more affected than Caucasians.[28] Individuals with lupus may also have other comorbid autoimmune conditions such as Sjögren's syndrome that may impact nutritional status.

There is no specific diet therapy for the treatment of lupus; however, in one published literature review of the link between diet and SLE, Brown and colleagues found that excessive calories, protein, fat (particularly from saturated and omega-6 polyunsaturated sources), zinc, and iron may have a negative or aggravating effect. Dietary indicators that may improve outcomes include vitamin E, vitamin A (from beta-carotene sources), selenium, omega-3 fatty acids from fish oil, evening primrose oil, flaxseed, and calcium plus vitamin D.[29] In an animal study, Leiba et al also found that reducing calories and protein and restricting fat led to significant improvements in mice's lifespan. Including eicosapentaenoic acid (EPA) and docosahexaenoic acid (DHA), the type of omega-3 fatty acids found in fish and fish oils, decreased inflammatory components in the same animal population.[30]

Anemias

Anemia is characterized by blood's inability to transport adequate oxygen to the body. Nutritional anemias can be macrocytic (large celled), microcytic (small celled), or hemolytic (when blood cell destruction outpaces replacement). Macrocytic anemias result in large, immature blood cells. These macrocytes result from inability to form new cells and DNA. Macrocytic anemias can be caused by deficiencies in vitamin B_{12}, folate (folic acid), thiamin, or vitamin B_6. Microcytic anemias are more often the result of impaired heme synthesis, and cause the body to inadequately transport, absorb, store, and use iron. Microcytic anemias can also be exacerbated by deficiencies in protein, iron, vitamin C, vitamin A, vitamin B_6, copper, or manganese.[31] While anemias can be genetic in origin, caused by disease states or drug toxicity, some anemias arise from insufficient nutrient intake, particularly of vitamin B_{12}, iron, and folic acid.

■ Iron Deficiency Anemia

Iron deficiency is the most common micronutrient deficiency, impacting almost 2 billion people around the world.[32] Because iron needs are increased during periods of growth, pregnant women and children are at increased risk for developing iron deficiency. Approximately 20% of perinatal mortality and 10% of maternal mortality in the developing world can be attributed to iron deficiency. While anemia is the end point of a chronic, long-term deficiency of iron, iron deficiency by itself can perpetuate a cycle of poverty, in that iron-deficient children demonstrate delayed cognitive function and iron-deficient adults experience decreased work capacity. In its most severe form, iron deficiency can lead to mental retardation.

Table 8–21. Recommended dietary allowances for iron.

	Life Stage	Iron Needs (mg/day)
Infants	6–12 months	11
Children	1–3 years	7
	4–8 years	10
Males	9–13 years	8
	14–18 years	11
	19–30 years	8
	31–50 years	8
	51–70 years	8
	>70 years	8
Females	9–13 years	8
	14–18 years	15
	19–30 years	18
	31–50 years	18
	51–70 years	8
	>70 years	8
Pregnant women	14–18 years	27
	19–30 years	27
	31–50 years	27
Lactating women	14–18 years	10
	19–30 years	9
	31–51 years	9

Data from Institute of Medicine, 2001.

The risk for developing iron deficiency can be mediated by a number of factors, and inadequate dietary iron intake is a common cause of deficiency. Poor absorption, GI problems, periods of growth, increased blood volume (eg, during pregnancy), and other chronic conditions all can contribute to iron deficiency. Table 8–21 outlines iron needs for males versus females in various life stages.[33]

Dietary Sources of Iron

There are two primary sources of dietary iron: heme iron and nonheme iron. Heme iron is found in animal foods, such as meat, fish, and poultry.

Table 8-22. Factors that limit iron absorption.

	Found in...
Oxalates	Chocolate, spinach, rhubarb, beet greens See Table 7–31 for a full list of high-oxalate foods
Phytic acid, phytates	Whole grains, bran, unleavened bread, soybeans, and soy products
Tannins	Tea, coffee, and some grains
Excessive dietary fiber	High-fiber foods such as bran cereals and fiber-fortified granola bars
Vegetarian diets	Low in or devoid of heme-iron
Very low calorie diets	Inadequate calorie diets are often low in iron

Nonheme iron comes from plant-based foods, including dark green leafy vegetables. Heme iron is more well absorbed than nonheme iron; however, the rate at which a person's body can absorb iron depends on a number of factors. For individuals with chronically low iron stores, such as in those with vegetarian diets devoid of heme-based iron, iron absorption is greater. Well-nourished individuals with adequate iron stores can be expected to absorb 5–10 % of dietary iron, whereas those who have iron deficiency will absorb upward of 20–30% of dietary iron.[34] Vitamin C is known to enhance iron absorption. Individuals at risk for iron deficiency anemia should consider complementing the iron-rich foods in their diet with vitamin C-containing foods. For example, to maximize iron utilization from an iron-fortified cereal, consume the cereal along with a serving of vitamin C-rich citrus fruit or a small glass of orange juice.

Iron absorption is compromised in the presence of substances that chelate iron. These include oxalates, phytates, and tannins. Table 8–22 includes these compounds and other factors, along with their dietary sources, that inhibit iron absorption. Table 8–23 provides tips for

Table 8-23. Tips for enhancing iron absorption.

Vitamin C increases iron absorption—include vitamin C with all iron-containing foods
Look for iron-fortified cereals with >25% daily value for iron per serving
Choose meat, fish, and poultry at meals to increase heme-iron intake
Avoid excessive coffee and tea
Cook with cast-iron cookware to increase absorption from foods cooked in iron pans

Table 8–24. Iron-containing foods.

Food	Amount	Iron (mg)
100% iron fortified ready-to-eat cereal	3/4 cup	18
Grits, instant, dry	½ cup	6
Cream of Wheat	½ cup	5.2
Oatmeal, instant	½ cup	5
Soybeans, cooked	½ cup	4.4
White beans, canned	½ cup	3.9
Lentils	½ cup	3.3
White rice	1/3 cup	3
Spinach	½ c cook, 1 c raw	3
Beef tenderloin	3 oz	3
Baked beans	1/3 cup	3
Veggie or soy burger	1 patty	2.9
Soy milk	1 cup (8 oz)	2.7
Chickpeas	½ cup	2.5
Kidney beans	½ cup	2.5

Data from Academy of Nutrition and Dietetics, 2012; US Department of Agriculture, Agricultural Research Service, 2012.

enhancing iron absorption, and Table 8–24 contains a list of foods that have at least 2 milligrams of iron per serving.[10,34]

Iron Supplements

Even individuals who work consciously to increase dietary iron intake may fall far short of actual iron needs. A typical 3-ounce serving of steak might only have 2–3 milligrams of iron. For an iron-deficient person seeking to consume 50–60 milligrams of elemental iron per day, he or she would have to consume more than 3 pounds of meat per day to obtain the desired amount of iron from foods alone! Thankfully, iron supplements are among the most affordable and effective nutrient supplements available on the market.

Taking an iron supplement along with ascorbic acid (vitamin C) enhances iron absorption from the supplement. Ferrous iron (ie, ferrous sulfate) is the most readily absorbable type of iron, and should be used preferentially over ferric forms of iron. Elemental iron dosages should be in the range of 50–200 milligrams for adults and 6 mg/kg body weight in children. A typical 300-milligram tablet of ferrous sulfate has 50–60 milligrams of oral elemental iron. Supplemental iron is usually administered to an iron-deficient person for 3–5 months, given three times daily.

An individual who absorbs 10–20 milligrams of iron per day can expect to triple red blood cell production rates and promote a rise in hemoglobin concentration of 0.2 g/dL per day, with effects being seen somewhere between day 4 of treatment up to the second or third week of supplementation.[35] Even after normal hemoglobin levels are achieved, iron supplementation should continue for 3–5 months to maximize iron stores.[34] An individual who fails to respond to oral forms of supplemental iron may need to be considered for parenteral administration. Common causes of persistently low hemoglobin levels in light of oral iron supplementation include noncompliance to supplementation due to GI side effects, reduced iron absorption related to malabsorption from steatorrhea, hemodialysis, celiac sprue, or bleeding that may be taking place at a rate that is faster than blood cell replacement.

Supplemental iron is best absorbed on an empty stomach, but this can also cause irritation of the GI tract. GI pain from iron supplements can be minimized by taking iron supplements with food, although this will decrease absorption rates. Iron supplements should be considered for individuals who are unable to obtain adequate iron from dietary sources alone. Those at risk for inadequate dietary iron intake include strict vegetarians and vegans, adherents to very low calorie diets, and people with very high fiber, coffee, and/or tea intake.

Though cheap and rather rapidly effective, iron supplementation is not without its drawbacks. High intakes of iron supplements or iron-containing medications are common causes of childhood poisoning and iron toxicity. The FDA mandates that all iron supplements must carry a warning reading, "WARNING: Accidental overdose of iron-containing products is a leading cause of fatal poisoning in children under 6 years of age. Keep this product out of reach of children. In case of accidental overdose, call a doctor or poison control center immediately."

Individuals with the iron overload condition hemochromatosis must closely monitor iron and vitamin C intakes because of the role that vitamin C plays in accelerating iron absorption. Hemochromatosis affects nearly one in 250 people of Northern European descent.[36] Those who receive frequent blood transfusions may also be at risk for iron overload and are advised to avoid iron supplementation.

The DRI committee has set a UL for iron, and this is the level if surpassed increases risk of toxicity. The upper level for iron for people aged 0–13 years is 40 mg/day and 45 mg/day for those aged 14 years and older.[33]

■ Megaloblastic Anemias

The megaloblastic anemias are characterized by large, immature, irregularly shaped red blood cells. These anemias are caused by deficiencies in folate and/or vitamin B_{12} (also called cyanocobalamin).

Pernicious Anemia

Pernicious anemia is the manifestation of clinically evident vitamin B_{12} deficiency caused by inadequate intrinsic factor. Vitamin B_{12} requires intrinsic factor for optimal absorption. In pernicious anemia, the parietal cells that secrete intrinsic factor are destroyed through an autoimmune mechanism. In this manner, inadequate intrinsic factor production for a prolonged period of time leads to vitamin B_{12} deficiency. Protracted vitamin B_{12} deficiency, in turn, can cause irreversible nerve damage.

Older adults are at risk for developing pernicious anemia due to declining intrinsic factor production as a function of aging, a variety of gastric or intestinal disease states, or inadequate dietary vitamin B_{12} intake in the diet. It is estimated that pernicious anemia affects 1–2% of all older adults. While pernicious anemia is most often treated with intramuscular vitamin B_{12}, a very small percentage of vitamin B_{12} can be absorbed despite the absence of intrinsic factor, implying that high doses of oral vitamin B_{12} may also be an effective treatment modality in pernicious anemia.[37]

Vitamin B_{12} Deficiency

In addition to intrinsic factor-related pernicious anemia, vitamin B_{12} deficiency can also be caused by inadequate intake. The only foods that contain appreciable amounts of vitamin B_{12} are animal products; as such, strict vegetarians and vegans are at increased risk for vitamin B_{12} deficiency and should be supplementing with vitamin B_{12}. The vitamin B_{12}-intrinsic factor compound is absorbed in the terminal ileum; thus, any insult, injury, or resection of this part of the gut can result in vitamin B_{12} deficiency. Atrophic gastritis affects 10–30% of older adults and causes reduced levels of hydrochloric acid secretion, which also impedes vitamin B_{12} absorption. Disorders or diseases of the stomach and small intestine, such as celiac disease and Crohn's disease, can also result in the body's inability to absorb adequate amounts of vitamin B_{12} (see Chapter 7).

Vitamin B_{12} and folic acid work synergistically; as such, high supplemental intakes of folic acid may mask vitamin B_{12} deficiency and can exacerbate the megaloblastic anemia and make the cognitive symptoms worse. The UL for folic acid from fortified foods and supplements is set at 1000 mcg/day for adults over the age of 19 years to help prevent the masking of vitamin B_{12} deficiency from folic acid.[37] Vitamin B_{12} deficiency can be treated with vitamin B_{12} injections, as this route circumvents potential barriers to direct absorption. Oral vitamin B_{12} supplementation can be an effective treatment in those who are able to absorb vitamin B_{12}.

Folate Deficiency Anemia

Megaloblastic anemia can also be caused by folate deficiency. The word "folate" is derived from *folium*, the Latin word for leaf. Dark green leafy vegetables are among the richest dietary sources of folate. Folic acid is the synthetic form of folate found in fortified foods, folic acid dietary supplements, multivitamins, and prenatal vitamins. Inadequate folate intake or folic acid deficiency causes impaired cell division and red blood cell and other protein synthesis.

■ Sickle Cell Anemia

Sickle cell disease (SCD) affects 90,000–100,000 Americans, disproportionately affecting those whose ancestors came from sub-Saharan Africa, Spanish-speaking regions of the Western Hemisphere, Saudi Arabia, India, and the Mediterranean countries. In the United States, SCD occurs in about 1 of every 500 Black or African-American births and in 1 out of every 36,000 Hispanic-American births.[38]

The SCD process causes weight loss and increases calorie and protein needs. Resting energy expenditure (calorie needs) may be 6–22% higher, and protein turnover rates are 44–100% higher in the sickle cell population. Those with SCD require a high-calorie, high-protein diet and may need as much as 120–150% of the recommended daily allowance for calories and protein.[34] Children with SCD experience impaired growth, delayed puberty, insufficient fat stores, muscle wasting, and inadequate protein stores.

General nutrition recommendations for SCD involve maintaining a well-balanced diet with adequate fluid intake. Energy and fat-dense foods can help restore lost weight. Adding cream, butter, whole milk, sugar, full-fat condiments and dressings, gravies, and sauces to foods can bulk up the calorie content of meals and snacks. A high-calorie nutrition liquid supplement consumed between meals is also helpful for providing additional calories and promoting weight gain. Additional, specific nutrition considerations and accommodations may need to be made for improper growth rates, constipation, hypercholesterolemia, and diabetes. Table 8–25 contains a list of micronutrient deficiencies that have been associated with SCD.[34,39]

Maintaining adequate fluid status is of utmost importance in SCD, as dehydration can cause a pain crisis. Those with SCD should minimize their intake of alcohol and caffeinated beverages such as colas, coffee, and tea because of the dehydrating nature of alcohol and caffeine. Factors that further increase fluid needs include having a fever, vomiting, diarrhea, exercising and excessive perspiration, hot weather, and pain crises, and precautions should be taken to ensure adequate fluid during these periods.

Table 8–25. Potential micronutrient deficiencies in sickle cell disease.

Magnesium	Vitamin B_{12}
Zinc	Folate
Iron	Riboflavin
Vitamin E	Vitamin C
Vitamin D	Vitamin A
Vitamin B_6	

Data from Academy of Nutrition and Dietetics, 2012, Hyacinth et al., 2010.

References

1. National Osteoporosis Foundation. America's Bone Health: The State of Osteoporosis and Low Bone Mass in Our Nation. Washington, DC: National Osteoporosis Foundation; 2002.

2. National Osteoporosis Foundation. Clinician's Guide to Prevention and Treatment of Osteoporosis. Washington, DC: National Osteoporosis Foundation; 2010.

3. US Department of Health and Human Services. Bone health and osteoporosis: a report of the Surgeon General. 2004.

4. National Osteoporosis Foundation. (n.d.). National Osteoporosis Foundation. Retrieved October 1, 2011, from Fast Facts: http://www.nof.org/node/40

5. Centers for Disease Control and Prevention. (2011, April 6). Nutrition for Everyone: Basics. Retrieved October 1, 2011, from Calcium and Bone Health: http://www.cdc.gov/nutrition/everyone/basics/vitamins/calcium.html

6. Academy of Nutrition and Dietetics. (2012). Osteoporosis. Retrieved January 19, 2013, from Nutrition Care Manual: http://www.nutritioncare manual.org

7. World Health Organization. WHO Scientific Group on the Assessment of Osteoporosis at Primary Healthcare Level. Geneva, Switzerland: World Health Organization; 2004.

8. Centers for Medicare & Medicaid Services. (n.d.). Medicare Preventive Service Bone Mass Measurement Information. Retrieved October 1, 2011, from Bone Mass Measurements: http://www.medicare.gov/navigation/manage-your-health/preventive-services/bone-mass-measurement.aspx?A spxAutoDetectCookieSupport=1

9. Institute of Medicine. Dietary Reference Intakes for Calcium and Vitamin D. Washington, DC: National Academies Press; 2010.

10. Nelms M. Diseases of the musculoskeletal system. In: Nelms M, Sucher K, Lacey K, Long Roth S, eds. Nutrition Therapy & Pathophysiology. Belmont, CA: Wadsworth Cengage; 2011:783.

11. US Department of Agriculture, Agricultural Research Service. (2012). USDA National Nutrient Database for Standard Reference, Release 25. Retrieved January 31, 2013, from Nutrient Data Laboratory Home Page: http://www.ars.usda.gov/ba/bhnrc/ndl

12. Mangano K, Walsh S, Insogna K, Kenny A, Kerstetter J. Calcium intake in the United States from dietary and supplemental sources across adult age groups: new estimates from the National Health and Nutrition Examination Survey 2003-2006. J Am Diet Assoc 2011;111(5):687–695.

13. Ma J, Johns R, Stafford R. Americans are not meeting current calcium recommendations. Am J Clin Nutr 2007;85(5):1361–1366.

14. American Academy of Pediatrics. Prevention of Rickets and Vitamin D Deficiency in Infants, Children and Adolescents. American Academy of Pediatrics; 2008.

15. Sellmeyer D, Stone K, Sebastian A, Cummings S. A high ratio for dietary animal protein to vegetable protein increases the rate of bone loss in elderly men and women. Am J Clin Nutr 2001;73:118–122.

16. Dawson-Hughes B, Harris S. Calcium intake influences the association of protein intake rates of bone loss in elderly men and women. Am J Clin Nutr 2002;(75):773–779.

17. Centers for Disease Control and Prevention. (2010, October 8). Prevalence of Doctor-Diagnosed Arthritis and Arthritis-Attributable Activity Limitation - United States, 2007-2009. Morbidity and Mortality Weekly Report (MMWR), 59(39), pp. 1261–1265.

18. Felson D, Zhang Y, Anthony J, Naimark A, Anderson J. Weight loss reduces the risk for symptomatic knee osteoarthritis in women. The Framingham Study. Ann Intern Med 1992;116(7):535–539.

19. Silbert J. E. Dietary glucosamine under question. Glycobiology 2009; 19(6):564–567.

20. National Institutes of Health: National Center for Complementary and Alternative Medicine. (2008, October). Backgrounder: Questions and Answers: NIH Glucosamine/chondroitin Arthritis Intervention Trial Primary Study. Retrieved October 16, 2011, from http://nccam.nih.gov/research/results/gait/qa.htm

21. Academy of Nutrition and Dietetics. (2012). Osteoarthritis. Retrieved January 19, 2013, from Nutrition Care Manual: http://www.nutritioncaremanual.org

22. Choi H, Atkinson K, Karlson E, Curhan G. Obesity, weight change, hypertension, diuretic use, and risk of gout in men. Arch Intern Med 2004; 363:1277–1278.

23. Choi H, Atkinson K, Karlson E, Willett W, Curhan G. Alcohol intake and risk of incident gout in men: a prospective study. Lancet 2004; 363(9417):1277–1281.

24. Academy of Nutrition and Dietetics. (2012). Gout. Retrieved January 19, 2013, from Nutrition Care Manual: http://www.nutritioncaremanual.org

25. American College of Rheumatology. (2010, May). From Practice Management: Fibromyalgia: http://www.rheumatology.org/practice/clinical/patients/diseases_and_conditions/fibromyalgia.asp

26. Geenen R, Janssesns E, Jacobs J, van Staveren W. Hypothesis - dietary glutamate will not affect pain in fibromyalgia. J Rheumatol 2004;31(4): 785–787.

27. Kogut V, Luthringer S. Appendix C. Nutrition impact symptoms and interventions. In: Nutritional Issues in Cancer Care. Pittsburgh, PA: Oncology Nursing Society; 2005;348–349.

28. Pisetsky D, Buyon J, Manzi S. Systemic lupus erythematosus. In: Klippel J, Crofford L, Stone J, Weyand C, eds. Primer on the Rheumatic Disease. Atlanta, GA: Arthritis Foundation; 2001 [chapter 17].

29. Brown A. Lupus erythematosus and nutrition: a review of the literature. J Ren Nutr 2000;10(4):170–183.

30. Leiba A, Amital H, Gershwin M, Shoenfeld Y. Diet and lupus. Lupus 2001;10(3):246–248.

31. Heuberger RA. Diseases of the hematological system. In: Nelams M, Sucher K, Lacey K, Long Roth S, eds. Nutrition Therapy & Pathophysiology. Belmont, CA: Wadsworth Cengage; 2011:569.

32. World Health Organization. The World Health Report: Chapter 4, Childhood and maternal undernutrition. World Health Organization; 2001.

33. Institute of Medicine. Dietary Reference Intakes for Vitamin A, Vitamin K, Arsenic, Boron, Chromium, Copper, Iodine, Iron, Manganese, Molybdenum, Nickel, Silicon, Vanadium, and Zinc. Washington, DC: National Academies Press; 2001.

34. Academy of Nutrition and Dietetics. (2012). Anemia. Retrieved January 19, 2013, from Nutrition Care Manual: http://www.nutritioncaremanual.org

35. National Institutes of Health: Office of Dietary Supplements. (2007). Dietary Supplement Fact Sheet: Iron.

36. Burke W, Cogswell M, McDonnell S, Franks A. Public health strategies to prevent the complications of hemochromatosis. In: Khoury MJ, Thomson WB, eds. Genetics and Public Health in the 21st Century: Using Genetic Information to Improve Health and Prevent Disease. Cary, NC: Oxford University Press; 2000.

37. National Institutes of Health: Office of Dietary Supplements. (2011). Dietary Supplement Fact Sheet: Vitamin B12.

38. Centers for Disease Control and Prevention. (2011, September 16). Data & Statistics. Retrieved January 31, 2013, from Sickle Cell Disease: http://www.cdc.gov/ncbddd/sicklecell/data.html

39. Hyacinth HI, Gee BE, Hibbert JM. The role of nutrition in sickle cell disease. Nutr Metab Insights 2010;3:57–67.

9

Nutrition in Hepatobiliary, Pancreatic, and Kidney Disease

Hepatitis

Hepatitis is the result of inflammation of liver tissue that can be caused by alcohol toxicity, a virus, medication, or fatty deposits. Acute hepatitis is that which occurs for a period of 0–6 months, whereas chronic hepatitis lasts for longer than 6 months.[1] Liver disease resulting from hepatitis is characterized by progression through three stages: inflammation, fibrosis, and cirrhosis (scarring of the liver cells). While acute hepatitis rarely causes permanent liver disease, the presence of hepatitis B and C, in addition to the continued consumption of alcohol, can induce chronic disease. Regardless of the originating virus, impaired nutritional status in hepatitis occurs as a combination of inadequate food intake and the progressive, infectious process. Nutritionally, glucose, protein, and fat metabolism are disrupted alongside electrolyte imbalances and improper nutrient absorption.[2] The physiological changes seen with hepatitis include weight fluctuations and loss of muscle mass, ascites and/or edema, jaundice, dark urine and/or light-colored stools, fatigue or loss of stamina, difficulty tolerating food as evidenced by nausea, vomiting, anorexia and dysgeusia (altered taste perception), and various vitamin and mineral deficiencies.

The goal of nutrition therapy in hepatitis is to help the individual reach and maintain a healthy body weight while encouraging adequate intakes of macronutrients (fat, carbohydrate, and protein) and micronutrients (vitamins and minerals). Those with acute hepatitis may struggle with achieving adequate caloric intake due to early satiety, fatigue, and loss of appetite, and may require additional supplemental sources of calories in addition to meals. Estimated energy needs for hepatitis are baseline needs (at dry weight) plus 20%; alternatively, some patients will require 30–35 kcal/kg/day. Protein needs are likely to be in the 1.0–1.2 g/kg/day range.[3,4] Protein restriction is rarely indicated in acute or chronic hepatitis, as both conditions may actually increase protein needs in order to promote liver cell regeneration. Protein restrictions may be required in people with end-stage cirrhotic liver disease who experience difficulty in the management of their portal systemic encephalopathy.[3] Additional nutrition therapy recommendations for hepatitis include a 2000 milligram sodium restriction in the case of fluid retention, four to six small, frequent meals to promote adequate intake and mitigation of muscle mass loss, and a low-fat diet with no more than 30% of calories from fat in cases of steatorrhea.[5]

Alcoholic Liver Disease and Nutrition for Alcoholism

Alcoholic liver disease is characterized by three disorders: fatty liver, alcoholic hepatitis, and cirrhosis. Fatty liver is present in more than 90% of chronic and binge drinkers,[6] but it can exist in individuals who do not consume or abuse alcohol. In the nonalcohol-related cases, the condition is referred to as nonalcoholic steatohepatitis (NASH). Individuals with alcoholic hepatitis and coexisting cirrhosis have a 60% death rate at 4 years.[6] Cirrhosis is the 12th leading cause of death in the United States.[7] The treatment of alcoholic liver disease is predicated on absolute abstinence from alcohol.

A chronic abuser of alcohol is likely to be malnourished and at risk for inadequate intake of all essential nutrients. The inflammation associated with long-term alcohol abuse leads to inflammation of the gastrointestinal tract and inadequate secretion of digestive enzymes. Because of its toxic nature, alcohol manages to disrupt the normal metabolism and absorption of fat-soluble vitamins, thiamin, and folic acid. Additionally, alcohol exacerbates urinary excretion of vitamin B_6 and folate.[8] Chronic alcoholics have increased needs for nearly all nutrients, and a recommended schedule of oral nutritional supplementation for these individuals is provided in Table 9–1.[9]

Calorie needs for individuals who chronically abuse alcohol should be 30–35 kcal/kg body weight, and protein is given at 1–2 grams protein/kg of body weight.[10] These intake guidelines are based on ideal body weight, rather than current weight, if those two numbers differ significantly. Table 9–2 outlines additional macronutrient adjustments to be made in the cases of hepatitis, hepatic cirrhosis, hepatic encephalopathy, and acute pancreatitis.[10]

In addition to micronutrient supplementation, other nutrition therapies may be indicated in the treatment of the chronic abuser of alcohol:

- *Sugar*—moderate or discontinue sugar intake. Some recovering alcoholics crave sugar and replace alcohol with sugar, essentially swapping addictive behaviors. Lowering sugar intake levels can decrease alcohol cravings and reduce relapse potential.[10]
- *Caffeine*—moderate or discontinue caffeine intake. Caffeine is addictive and many alcoholics will not be able to consume even modest amounts of caffeine, even as little as the equivalent of one to two servings per day.
- *Macronutrients*—moderate fat intake, acknowledging that recovering alcoholics tend to gain weight and turn to food in the absence of alcohol. Encourage high-fiber sources of carbohydrate and lean protein sources.
- *Multivitamin*—supplementation regimen of that in Table 9–1 is recommended, including a typical multivitamin.
- *Meal patterning*—encourage small, frequent meals with three small meals and one to three snacks with no more than 4–5 waking hours between food intake.

Table 9-1. Nutrition supplements recommended for chronic abusers of alcohol.

Thiamin	• 50-100 mg for 7-14 days • Should be given to all alcoholics because prevalence of deficiency is high and assessing deficiency is difficult
Folic acid	• 1 mg (1000 mcg) daily
Riboflavin	• Amount in typical multivitamin
Vitamin B_6	• 1-3 mg as part of multivitamin • Use of large amounts should be avoided because of toxicity risk
Vitamin B_{12}	• 6-12 mg as part of a multivitamin
Vitamin C	• 175-500 mg/day
Vitamin A	• Amount in typical multivitamin • May be given only for clear cases of deficiency because of potential for hepatotoxicity
Vitamin D	• 200-500 IU because of decreased bone density, bone mass, and susceptibility to fractures
Vitamin E	• 10-50 IU as part of a multivitamin
Iron	• Standard amount in multivitamin for premenopausal women • For men and postmenopausal women, multivitamin with no iron may be the safest route; potential for overload, additional iron therapy restricted unless clearly deficient
Magnesium	• 100-400 mg/day if magnesium deficiency suspected or confirmed • With severe magnesium deficiency, parenteral replacement may be necessary
Selenium	• 5-50 mcg daily
Zinc	• Amount available in multivitamin zinc levels may not respond to supplementation, and zinc toxicity may occur with large dose supplementation • Zinc replacement should only be given for night blindness

Data from Markowitz et al., 2000.

- *Fluids*—fluid restriction is indicated in the cases of edema, ascites, and hepatic encephalopathy; rehydration is necessary for alcoholics who experience dehydration from vomiting, diarrhea, or diuresis.
- *Nutrition support*—for individuals unable to meet their nutrition needs by mouth, or whose guts are unable to tolerate nutrition, nutrition support may be indicated. Oral feedings are preferred, but

Table 9–2. Nutrient considerations and modifications for hepatic diseases.

Calories	Protein	Carbohydrate	Fat	Notes
General alcoholic nutrition guidelines				
30–35 kcal/kg	1–2 g/kg		<30% calories	
Hepatitis				
30–35 kcal/kg	1.5–2 g/kg	6–8 g/kg	<30% calories	
Hepatic cirrhosis				
30–35 kcal/kg	1–2 g/kg		<30% calories MCT may be better tolerated Limit fat if steatorrhea	May need to restrict fluid and sodium with ascites or edema
Hepatic encephalopathy				
At least 1800 calories per day to minimize muscle catabolism	Modest protein if protein-sensitive hepatic encephalopathy (0.6–0.8 g/kg or 20–30 g/day and gradually increase by 0.2/kg body weight/day until 40–50 g/day) HBV protein, space throughout day	50% calories from carbohydrate to reduce protein catabolism	30% calories from fat	Possible fluid and sodium restriction
Acute pancreatitis				
NPO, enteral nutrition, and/or TPN may be required				

Data from Academy of Nutrition and Dietetics, 2012.

if not attainable, in the presence of a functioning gut, tube feeding is preferred over TPN. Tube-feeding formulas should be high in protein (nitrogen) and may contain enhanced branched-chain amino acids, milk protein, and medium-chain triglycerides (MCTs).

The Academy of Nutrition and Dietetics offers additional tips for sober meal planning[10]:

- Consume frequent meals and snacks, skipping no more than 5 waking hours between meals or snacks.
- Take healthful snacks that travel well, low-sugar protein bars, nuts, cheese, yogurt, sunflower seeds, whole grain crackers, fruits, and vegetables.
- Push fluid intake, aiming for at least eight glasses of fluid per day.
- Eat breakfast: include protein foods such as eggs, meat, yogurt, cottage cheese, peanut butter, or milk.
- Avoid anything prepared with alcohol, food and drinks with caffeine, fast food, and high-sugar foods.
- Eat with sober friends, "Isolation and secrecy were part of your addiction: socialization is an important part of recovery."

Cirrhosis

Cirrhosis is the permanent scarring of the liver tissue caused by disease that results in disruption of blood flow to the organ. Causes of cirrhosis include alcoholism, hepatitis B, hepatitis C, autoimmune hepatitis, NASH, biliary cirrhosis, chronic viral hepatitis, and inherited metabolic liver disease (hemochromatosis, Wilson's disease, and cystic fibrosis).[11] For people with cirrhosis, common feeding-related complaints include anorexia, early satiety, nausea and/or vomiting, abdominal bloating, gas or distention, altered taste perception, constipation or diarrhea, and fatigue.

The nutrition therapy for cirrhosis includes sodium restriction (usually 2000 milligrams or less per day), four to six small, frequent meals and snacks, modest protein intake for cirrhosis patients with protein-sensitive hepatic encephalopathy (0.8–1.2 g/kg protein per day), no more than 30% of calories from fat, and fluid restriction for those with hyponatremia. If serum sodium falls under 128 mEq/L, restrict total fluid to 1200–1500 mL/day. If sodium levels are more severe (less than 125 mEq/L), restrict fluid to 1000–1200 mL/day.[5]

All individuals with cirrhosis are advised to avoid high-salt foods such as canned soups, meats, cheeses, and processed and packaged foods. One practical application for sodium reduction is to avoid foods with more than 300 milligrams of sodium per serving. If ascites is present, limit salt intake to ≤2000 milligrams of sodium per day. Care should be taken to minimize foods that may trigger foodborne illness, such as unpasteurized juices and cider, raw milk or dairy foods, unpasteurized cheeses and salad dressings, raw or undercooked meat, poultry, fish, game, and seafood, raw tofu, raw or undercooked eggs, unwashed produce, and all raw vegetable sprouts (alfalfa, radish, mung, and bean).[5]

Liver Transplantation

The approach to nutritional management of liver transplantation applies to both the pre-and postoperative transplantation state. In the preop state, nutritional status tends to decline, and the focus is on minimizing the effects of malnutrition and controlling ascites. In the postoperative state, protein catabolism, side effects of medication, surgical stress, and high blood sugar all can negatively impact nutritional status. Underweight, poor nutrient absorption, inadequate intake, impaired GI function, food-medication interactions, and involuntary weight loss all may persist.

Calorie needs in the postop period are estimated to be baseline plus 15–30%, while protein needs are 1.5–2.0 g/kg/day.[12] Hyperglycemia management should be conducted by reducing simple sugar intake and encouraging that 50–60% of calories come from carbohydrates, with an emphasis on increasing fiber-containing foods. Calcium supplements and a multivitamin are recommended to promote optimal bone health and to meet baseline micronutrient needs. Postoperative liver transplant recipients are advised to drink 8–12 cups of fluid per day, as fluid losses are experienced from drains, the nasogastric tube, stool output, and urine. Table 9–3 contains a list of foods that should not be eaten by the transplant recipient, and Table 9–4 contains a list of foods that are recommended for a transplant patient who has a stabilized weight and a relatively good appetite.[13]

Table 9–3. Foods to be avoided by transplant recipients.

Alcohol (or consult with healthcare practitioner to determine if low levels are safe)
Grapefruit or grapefruit juice (if taking cyclosporine or prograf because grapefruit interferes with drug metabolism)
Raw or undercooked meat, poultry, seafood, eggs, or products that contain raw/undercooked eggs (homemade Caesar salad dressing, raw cookie dough, homemade eggnog)
Unpasteurized (raw) milk or soft cheese made from unpasteurized (raw) milk such as feta, Brie, Camembert, blue-veined, queso fresco
Unpasteurized juice or cider
Fresh sprouts: alfalfa, radish, mung, and bean
Spoiled or moldy food or those past "use by" date
Unwashed fresh vegetables, including lettuce and salads
Hot dogs, deli meats, and luncheon meats that have not been reheated to 165°F
Unpasteurized, refrigerated pâtés or meat spreads

Data from Academy of Nutrition and Dietetics, 2012; www.fda.gov/downloads/Food/ResourcesForYou/.../UCM312793.pdf.

Table 9–4. Foods that are appropriate for transplant recipients with good appetites.

Food Group	Recommended Foods for Transplant Recipients
Dairy	All milk and cheese should be pasteurized
	Hard cheeses, processed cheeses, cream cheese, and mozzarella
	Soft cheeses that are clearly labeled as being "made from pasteurized milk"
Meat and poultry	Previously cooked seafood heated to 165°F
	Canned fish and seafood
	Seafood cooked to 145°F
	Skinless chicken and turkey
	Extra-lean, fresh beef, and pork
	Dry beans and peas
	Unsalted nuts
	Tofu
	Egg whites
	Canned or shelf-stable pâtés or meat spreads
Eggs	Pasteurized eggs
Fruits	Unsweetened canned and frozen fruit (except grapefruit and pomegranate)
	Unsweetened juice in small amounts
	Unsweetened dried fruits
Vegetables	Wash all fresh vegetables, including lettuce and salad
	Unsalted canned or frozen vegetables, cooked vegetables
	Unsalted vegetable juices
	Cooked sprouts
Grains	Whole-grain breads
	Whole-grain pastas, rice, or brown wild rice
	Whole-grain, unsweetened cereals
Fats and oils	Olive oil
	Canola oil
	Trans-fat-free margarine
	Nonfat or low-fat salad dressing
Seasonings	Fresh or dried cooking herbs
	Onion or onion powder (not onion salt)
	Garlic or garlic powder (not garlic salt)
	Salt-free and sodium-free seasonings

Data from Academy of Nutrition and Dietetics, 2012; www.fda.gov/downloads/Food/ResourcesForYou/.../UCM312793.pdf.

Gallstones

Diseases of the biliary system may involve a variety of conditions that affect either the anatomy or the function of the gallbladder. The gallbladder is a pear-shaped organ that acts as the storage mechanism for bile; bile is produced in the liver and aids in the digestion of fats in the small intestine. When bile becomes concentrated in the gallbladder, stones are formed. The mere presence of these stones (8% are cholesterol stones and 20% are pigment stones) may not cause symptoms, but they do become problematic if they block the bile ducts, resulting in inflammation, infection, or pancreatitis.

When blockages do become symptomatic, the recommended therapy is surgical removal of the gallbladder (cholecystectomy). Even without a gallbladder, individuals will produce enough bile in the liver to digest a modest amount of fat. Following cholecystectomy, individuals do not have to maintain a fat-free diet, although they are advised to minimize fat, consuming less than 30% of calories from fat. When the gallbladder has been removed, bile will flow from the liver directly into the small intestine, and can cause softer and more frequent stools in approximately 1% of people.[14]

Risk factors for gallbladder disease and stones include being female, especially if pregnant, on hormone therapy, or using birth control. Risk of gallbladder disease is high in the following populations:

- Individuals over the age of 60 years
- Native Americans and Mexican Americans
- Obese individuals
- Those with a history of rapid or significant weight loss or on very low calorie diets
- People with high fat and sugar intakes
- Individuals with sedentary lifestyles
- Patients receiving long-term parenteral nutrition
- Females receiving hormone therapy and taking birth control pills or clofibrate.[15]

Bile is released from the gallbladder into the intestines, where it plays a role in fat digestion. When gallstones are present, bile cannot be released and fat cannot be digested. Therefore, the recommended nutrition therapy is the adoption of a low-fat diet given in small, frequent feedings spread throughout the day. The diet should provide no more than 30% of calories from fat, which equates to no more than 67 grams of fat for a 2000-calorie diet (2000 calories × 30% ÷ 9 calories per gram of fat = 67 grams). Individuals are advised to choose foods that are low in fat and to avoid high-fat greasy or fried foods, foods with strong odors, and those that cause gas (eg, cauliflower, cabbage). A good rule of thumb is to choose foods that contain no more than 3 grams of fat per serving.

The fluid needs for gallbladder disease are similar to that of the healthy population: provide 1 milliliter of fluid per calorie consumed. Adjust fluid intake with increased fluid losses, fever, or diarrhea. Acute attacks are associated with obstruction and necessitate inactivity of the gallbladder, with an NPO diet and complete bowel rest until symptoms subside.[16] Parenteral nutrition should only be initiated if the patient is unable to take any nutrients by mouth or by tube feeding for more than 10 days. As symptoms subside and once oral diet tolerance has been established, advance the diet to low-fat liquids. Disruptions in fat digestion alter absorption of fat-soluble vitamins and may require supplemental forms of vitamins A, D, E, and K.

Pancreatitis

Pancreatitis can be acute or chronic in nature. The most common causes of acute pancreatitis include gallstones (30–60%), alcohol (15–30%), and hypertriglyceridemia (1.3–3.8%).[8] The risk for inducing acute pancreatitis is seen when triglyceride levels surpass the 1000 mg/dL threshold. The most common cause of chronic pancreatitis is alcoholism in adults and cystic fibrosis in children. Genetic defects may cause up to 15% of chronic pancreatitis cases.[17]

The recommended nutrition therapy for acute pancreatitis has changed in recent years. Whereas oral feeding has traditionally been withheld until pain and symptoms subside, current recommendations advise immediate refeeding to maximize optimal outcomes and to shorten hospital stay time. In one recent prospective, randomized, controlled, double-blind clinical trial, there was no demonstrated difference in symptom relapse in patients with mild pancreatitis who were advanced to a solid food diet, as opposed to a clear liquid or lower-calorie solid food diet.[18] The fat content of the transitional diet should be moderated if steatorrhea and abdominal pain persist.

Fluids are given at roughly 1 mL/kcal/day and should be given intravenously in the NPO patient. The use of pancreatic enzyme supplementation may be required in those who progress to chronic pancreatitis. If oral feedings cannot be established or tolerated, and in the case of severe pancreatitis, early initiation of nutrition support is advised. Tube feeding should be initiated within 24–48 hours at a starting rate of 25 mL/hour, advancing to goal calories of 25 calories/kg within the first 24–48 hours. Low-fat and elemental formulas cause the least amount of pancreatic stimulation; however, small-peptide formulas that give 70% of the fat as MCTs (and which may stimulate the pancreas slightly more than the low-fat formulas) are better absorbed.[8] Parenteral nutrition is recommended only following unsuccessful enteral nutrition attempts or for those who have been NPO for 5 days or more.[19] The parenteral solution should provide goal calories of 25 kcal/kg with fat giving 15–30% of total calories, and fat adjustments made on an individual basis with attention given to steatorrhea or other signs of malabsorption.[8]

The goals of nutrition therapy for chronic pancreatitis are to prevent additional damage to the pancreas, stave off further acute inflammatory attacks, minimize pain, manage steatorrhea, correct malnutrition, and prevent unintentional weight loss while promoting modest weight gain toward appropriate weight levels. Meals should be low in fat and spaced out in small increments over the day. Pancreatic enzymes taken with each meal or snack help improve digestion and absorption. Fat provides a concentrated source of calories and should be included, as tolerated, to help meet energy needs but without exacerbating steatorrhea (if it exists).

Additional vitamin supplementation is recommended for pancreatitis in those with a history of alcoholism. Water-soluble forms of the fat-soluble vitamins A, D, E, and K are recommended. Other daily supplements to be included are thiamin at 100 milligrams by mouth, folate at 1000 micrograms by mouth, and a general multivitamin.[5] In some cases, parenteral administration of vitamin B_{12} may be indicated.[8]

Chronic Kidney Disease and Dialysis

Chronic kidney disease (CKD) is characterized by a permanent and progressive loss of kidney function resulting in declining glomerular filtration rate (GFR), decreasing creatinine clearance, and elevated serum creatinine concentration.[20,21] CKD is defined as a reduction in kidney function with estimated GFR (eGFR) <60 mL/minute/1.73 m² for a period of 3 months or longer and/or evidence of kidney damage, including persistent albuminuria, defined as >30 milligrams of urine albumin per gram of urine creatinine.[22] The National Kidney Foundation has established five stages of CKD that are listed in Table 9–5.[23]

At Stage 5 kidney disease, the kidney cannot sustain life, and renal replacement therapy is now indicated, as either dialysis or transplantation.[23] Chronic renal failure refers to the irreversible reduction in the number of nephrons and generally corresponds to CKD Stages 3–5.

The National Kidney Foundation estimates that more than 20 million Americans have CKD and that millions of others are at elevated risk for developing it.[24] Those at increased risk for developing CKD include individuals with diabetes, hypertension, and a family history of the

Table 9–5. Five stages of chronic kidney disease.

Stage 1	Kidney damage with normal or elevated GFR (GFR ≥90 mL/minute/1.73 m²)
Stage 2	Kidney damage with mild decrease in GFR (GFR 60-89 mL/minute/1.73 m²)
Stage 3	Moderate decrease in GFR (30-59 mL/minute/1.73 m²)
Stage 4	Severe decrease in GFR (15-29 mL/minute/1.73 m²)
Stage 5	Also referred to as end-stage renal disease (ESRD) or kidney failure; occurs when the GFR is less than 15 mL/minute/1.73 m²

Data from National Kidney Foundation, 2002.

disease. African Americans, Hispanics, Pacific Islanders, Native Americans, and older individuals are also at increased risk. In the United States, African Americans make up 13% of the general population, but they represent 32% of those with kidney failure. This is due in large part to the disproportionately high rates of diabetes and high blood pressure among African Americans, the two leading causes of kidney failure in this population. Hispanic people are also increasingly being diagnosed with kidney disease. The National Kidney Foundation estimates that since the year 2000, the number of Hispanics with kidney failure has increased by more than 70%. Hispanics are one and a half times more likely to be diagnosed with kidney failure than non-Hispanics.[25]

The primary nutrition therapies for the management of CKD are focused on avoiding and reversing protein-calorie malnutrition (PCM), providing adequate dietary protein, and moderating dietary potassium, phosphorus, sodium, dietary calcium, and fluid intake.[20] There are no specific nutrition guidelines that have been established for CKD Stages 1 and 2. At these stages nutrition therapy should center on managing comorbid conditions such as diabetes, hypertension, or cardiovascular disease. In Stages 3 and 4, the goals are to prevent malnutrition, provide enough protein to maintain muscle mass and serum proteins, individually attend to abnormalities in vitamin and mineral absorption and utilization, as well as promote blood lipid normalization.

In nondialysis CKD, with declining GFR, the nutrition complications that may be seen include malnutrition, metabolic acidosis from reduced acid (hydrogen ion) excretion, hyperkalemia, mineral imbalance, bone disorders (involving calcium, phosphorus, and vitamin D status), and anemia due to impaired erythropoiesis and low iron stores. These complications are in addition to cardiovascular disease and dyslipidemia, which are also typically present in CKD.[22]

Unique nutrition, food, and feeding issues may need to be considered in those on maintenance dialysis. For hemodialysis (HD), concerns about adequate intake arise due to meals that may be missed because of the treatment schedule, multiple medication usage, concurrent illness, psychosocial issues, lack of energy required to prepare meals, loss of appetite, or uremia. For peritoneal dialysis (PD), pressure of the dialysate leads to an increased feeling of fullness. In this case, encourage small, frequent feedings, or promote eating when drained, before inflow of next exchange starts. There is also potential in the PD patient for weight gain caused by dextrose from dialysate, and these individuals may also experience elevated triglyceride levels.[20]

■ Energy Needs

In CKD Stages 1–4, the Academy of Nutrition and Dietetics has set forth calorie guidelines based on age. For individuals less than 60 years old, give 35 kcal/kg body weight per day. For those aged 60 years and older, 30–35 kcal/kg body weight per day is recommended. When calculating calorie needs and protein needs, the National Kidney Foundation

Kidney Disease Outcomes Quality Initiative (K/DOQI) Nutrition Guidelines say an adjusted body weight should be used for those who are overweight, obese, or underweight. The equation for adjusted body weight (ABW) is, ABW = edema-free body weight + [(standard body weight – edema-free body weight) × 0.25]. The standard body weight is derived from the NHANES II standard body weight (SBW) tables for 50th percentile, in kilograms shown in Table 9–6.[26,27] The Academy of Nutrition and Dietetics cautions that, "(a)lthough data [in these tables] is validated and standardized and uses a large database of ethnically-diverse groups, data is provided only on what individuals weight, not what they should weigh in order to reduce morbidity and mortality."[28] The patient's edema-free body weight should be adjusted when he or she is <95% or >115% of standard body weight.[29] Table 9–7 shows a sample calculation on how to determine adjusted body weight in both an obese and an underweight subject.

■ Protein

A low-protein diet or protein restriction is indicated in the predialyzed CKD patient. Low-protein diets reduce nitrogenous waste and mitigate the effects of hyperphosphatemia, metabolic acidosis, hyperkalemia, and other electrolyte disorders. Low protein intake levels may also slow the rate of progression to renal failure and delay the onset of dialysis.[30] For Stages 1–4 CKD, protein should be limited to 0.6–0.8 g/kg, with 50% or more of the protein coming from high biological value (HBV) sources. HBV sources of protein include those that come from animal foods, also called complete proteins. Table 9–8 contains a list of HBV protein sources.

The Academy of Nutrition and Dietetics' Evidence Analysis project states, with "strong/conditional" evidence, that "0.7 g dietary protein per kg of body weight per day, ensuring adequate calorie intake, can slow GFR decline and maintain stable nutrition status in adult nondiabetic patients with CKD" and (with "fair/conditional" evidence) that adults with diabetic nephropathy should have 0.8–0.9 grams of protein per kilogram of body weight per day, acknowledging that providing 0.7 g/kg/day may lead to hypoalbuminemia.[28]

In those undergoing maintenance HD or PD, protein restrictions are not indicated, and protein intakes should be higher than in the healthy population. Protein recommendations for HD and PD are ≥1.2 g/kg/day and ≥1.2–1.3 g/kg/day, respectively; both PD and HD protein sources should be at least 50% HBV in nature. When assessing protein needs, use the NHANES II standard body weight tables to adjust for body weight in those who are <95% or >115% of standard body weight.

■ Potassium

Potassium needs and restrictions are determined in HD and PD by the individual's degree of kidney function, their serum potassium levels, and the drug therapy they are following. Hyperkalemia can be avoided by the adoption of a low-potassium diet. The Academy of Nutrition and

Table 9-6. Standard body weight tables based on NHANES II weight table, 50th percentile in kilograms.

Males	25-54 years			54-74 years		
Height (in)	Small	Medium	Large	Small	Medium	Large
62	64	68	82	61	68	77*
63	61	71	83	62	70	80
64	66	71	84	63	71	77
65	66	74	79	70	72	79
66	67	75	84	68	74	80
67	71	77	84	69	78	85
68	71	78	86	70	78	83
69	74	78	89	75	77	84
70	75	81	87	76	80	87
71	76	81	91	69	84	84
72	74	84	91	76*	81	90
73	79*	85	93	78*	88	88
74	80*	88	92	77*	95	89
Females	**25-54 years**			**54-74 years**		
Height (in)	Small	Medium	Large	Small	Medium	Large
58	52	63	86	54	57	92
59	53	66	78	55	62	78
60	53	60	87	54	65	78
61	54	61	81	56	64	79
62	55	61	81	58	64	82
63	55	62	83	58	65	80
64	57	62	79	60	66	77
65	60	63	81	60	67	80
66	58	63	75	68	66	82
67	59	65	80	61*	72	80
68	62	67	76	61*	70	79
69	63*	68	79	62*	72*	85*
70	64	70	76	63*	73*	85*

Note: The clinician's judgment should be used in assigning these weights. Some categories are based on a small sample size of patients or estimated (*) by linear regression equation.

Data from Frisancho, 1984; McCann, 2009.

Table 9–7. Using standard weight tables to determine adjusted body weight for overweight and underweight individuals with CKD.

What is the equation?	Adjusted body weight (ABW) = edema-free body weight + [(standard body weight − edema-free body weight) × 0.25]
When do you adjust body weight?	When individual is <95% or >115% of standard body weight
What is the standard body weight?	See the information in Table 9-6 for NHANES II standard body weight references by gender, age, height, and frame size
Overweight example: patient is female, 53 years old, medium-framed, 62" tall, and weighs 167 pounds (76 kg)	Nonedema weight is 76 kg; standard weight for female, 25–54 years, medium-framed, 62" tall, 61 kg 76 ÷ 62 × 100 = 123% SBW, adjust weight ABW = 76 + [(61 − 76) × 0.25] ABW = 72.25 kg = 159 pounds
Underweight example: patient is male, 70 years old, small-framed, 69" tall, and weighs 110 pounds (50 kg)	Nonedema wt is 50 kg; standard weight for male, 54–74 years, small-framed, 69" tall, 75 kg 50 ÷ 75 × 100 = 67% SBW, adjust wt ABW = 50 + [(75 − 50) × 0.25] ABW = 56.25 kg = 124 pounds

Dietetics recommends restricting potassium to 2–3 g/day in HD and 3–4 g/day in PD, although individual levels should be adjusted based on serum potassium levels. As seen in Table 9–9, many fruits, vegetables, and other plant-based foods are high in potassium and should be eaten rarely or in moderation by those on HD or PD.[31] Table 9–10 contains a

Table 9–8. Sources of high biological value (HBV) protein.

Eggs
Milk
Cheese
Yogurt
Meat
Fish
Poultry

Table 9–9. High-potassium foods to limit to no more than 1 serving/day.

High-Potassium Foods (>200 mg/serving) – No More than 1 Serving/day		
Fruits	**Vegetables**	**Other Foods**
Apricots, raw (2 medium), dried (5 halves)	Acorn squash	Bran/bran products
Avocado (1/4 whole)	Artichoke	Chocolate (1.5–2 ounces)
Bananas (1/2 whole)	Bamboo shoots	Granola
Cantaloupe	Baked beans	Milk (all types, 1 cup)
Dates (5 whole)	Butternut squash	Molasses (1 tablespoon)
Dried fruits	Refried beans	Nutrition supplements: use only under direction of provider or dietitian
Grapefruit juice	Beets, fresh then boiled	Nuts and seeds (1 ounce)
Honeydew	Black beans	Peanut butter (2 tablespoons)
Kiwi (1 medium)	Broccoli, cooked	Salt substitutes: Lite Salt®, Nu-Salt®
Mango (1 medium)	Brussels sprouts	Salt-free broth
Nectarine (1 medium)	Chinese cabbage	Snuff/chewing tobacco
Orange (1 medium)	Carrots (raw)	Yogurt
Orange juice	Dried beans and peas	Whole grains
Papaya (1/2 whole)	Greens, except kale	
Pomegranate (1 whole)	Hubbard squash	
Pomegranate juice	Kohlrabi	
Prunes	Legumes (lentils)	
Prune juice	Mushrooms, canned	
Raisins	Parsnips	
	Potatoes, white, and sweet	
	Pumpkin	
	Rutabagas	
	Spinach, cooked	
	Tomatoes/tomato products	
	Vegetable juices	

Data from National Kidney Foundation, 2013.

Table 9–10. Low-potassium foods that are appropriate in moderation for kidney disease.

Low-Potassium Foods – portion is ½ cup unless otherwise noted Eating more than 1 portion makes low-potassium food a higher-potassium food		
Fruits	**Vegetables**	**Other Foods**
Apples (1 medium)	Alfalfa sprouts	Rice
Apple juice	Asparagus (6 spears)	Noodles and pasta
Applesauce	Beans, green or wax	Bread, not whole grain
Apricots canned in juice	Cabbage, green and red	
Blackberries	Carrots, cooked	Cake, angel, yellow
Blueberries	Cauliflower	Coffee (limit to 8 oz)
Cherries	Celery (1 stalk)	Pies without chocolate or high-potassium fruit
Cranberries	Corn, fresh (1/2 ear), frozen (1/2 cup)	Cookies without nuts or chocolate
Fruit cocktail	Cucumber	Tea (16 oz)
Grapes	Eggplant	
Grape juice	Kale	
Grapefruit (1/2 whole)	Lettuce	
Mandarin oranges	Mixed vegetables	
Peaches, fresh (1 small), canned (1/2 cup)	Mushrooms, fresh	
Pears, fresh (1 small), canned (1/2 cup)	Okra	
Pineapple	Onions	
Pineapple juice	Parsley	
Plums (1 whole)	Peas, green	
Raspberries	Peppers	
Strawberries	Radish	
Tangerine (1 whole)	Rhubarb	
Watermelon (limit to 1 cup)	Water chestnuts, canned	
	Watercress	
	Yellow squash	
	Zucchini squash	

Data from National Kidney Foundation, 2013.

Table 9–11. How to leach potassium from high-potassium potatoes, sweet potatoes, carrots, beets, and rutabagas.

1. Peel and place the vegetable in cold water so they won't darken
2. Slice vegetable to 1/8 inch thickness
3. Rinse in warm water for a few seconds
4. Soak for a minimum of 2 hours in warm water; use 10 times the amount of water to the amount of vegetables; if soaking longer, change the water every 4 hours
5. Rinse under warm water again for a few seconds
6. Cook vegetables with 5 times the amount of water to the amount of vegetables

Note that leaching does not remove all potassium; must still limit intake.

Data from National Kidney Foundation, 2013.

list of low-potassium foods that may be utilized more regularly with HD or PD.[31] For HD or PD patients who are insistent on eating some high-potassium vegetables such as potatoes, sweet potatoes, carrots, beets, or rutabagas, they can follow the procedure outlined in Table 9–11 to leach potassium from their vegetables and lower the overall potassium content during preparation. Table 9–12 explains how to leach potassium from high-potassium squash, mushrooms, cauliflower, and frozen greens.

■ Phosphorus

The goal of CKD management of phosphorus is to keep phosphorus levels within the normal range: <4.5 mg/dL for predialysis, and between 3.5–5.5 mg/dL when on dialysis. For CKD, dietary phosphorus restrictions and the use of phosphorus binders may be indicated if serum

Table 9–12. How to leach potassium from high-potassium squash, mushrooms, cauliflower, and frozen greens.

1. Allow frozen vegetables to thaw to room temperature and drain
2. Rinse fresh or frozen vegetables for warm water for a few seconds
3. Soak for a minimum of 2 hours in warm water; use 10 times the amount of water to the amount of vegetables; if soaking longer, change the water every 4 hours
4. Rinse under warm water again for a few seconds
5. Cook the usual way, but with 5 times the amount of water to the amount of vegetables

Note that leaching does not remove all potassium; must still limit intake.

Data from National Kidney Foundation, 2013.

Table 9–13. High-phosphorus foods to limit or avoid in CKD.

Beverages	Organ meats
Ale	Oysters
Beer	Sardines
Chocolate drinks	Vegetables – Dried Beans and Peas
Cocoa	Baked beans
Drinks made with milk	Black beans
Dark colas	Chick peas (garbanzo beans)
Canned iced teas	Kidney beans
Dairy Products	Lentils
Cheese	Lima beans
Cottage cheese	Northern beans
Custard	Pork 'n beans
Ice cream	Split peas
Milk	Soy beans
Pudding	Other Foods
Cream soups	Bran cereals
Yogurt	Brewer's yeast
Protein	Caramels
Carp	Nuts
Crayfish	Seeds
Beef liver	Wheat germ
Chicken liver	Whole-grain products
Fish roe	

Data from National Kidney Foundation, 2013.

phosphorus levels are elevated. The National Kidney Disease Education Program (NKDEP) maintains that no level of restriction has yet been determined for nondialysis CKD. Other resources suggest that optimal serum phosphorus levels can be aided with a daily dietary phosphorus restriction of 800–1000 mg/day. Foods that are high in phosphorus include colas, eggs, dairy foods, nuts, beans, and meat. Table 9–13 contains a list of high-phosphorus foods, and Table 9–14 contains lower-phosphorus alternatives of higher-phosphorus foods.[32]

Table 9-14. Lower-phosphorus alternatives for high-phosphorus foods.

High-Phosphorus Foods – Instead of	Phosphorus (mg)	Low-Phosphorus Foods – Try	Phosphorus (mg)
8 ounce milk	230	8 ounce nondairy creamer or 4 oz milk	100 115
8 ounce cream soup made with milk	275	8 ounce cream soup made with water	90
1 ounce hard cheese	145	1 ounce cream cheese	30
½ cup ice cream	80	½ cup sherbet or 1 popsicle	0
12 ounce can cola	55	12 ounce can of ginger ale or lemon soda	3
½ cup lima or pinto beans	100	½ cup mixed vegetables or green beans	35
½ cup custard or pudding made with milk	150	½ cup pudding or custard made with nondairy creamer	50
2 ounce peanuts	200	1½ cup light salt/ low-fat popcorn	35
1½ ounce chocolate bar	125	1½ ounce hard candy, fruit flavors, or jelly beans	3
⅔ cup oatmeal	130	⅔ cup cream of wheat or grits	40
½ cup bran cereal	140-260	½ cup nonbran cereal, shredded wheat, rice cereals, or corn flakes	50-100

Data from National Kidney Foundation, 2013.

Patients are advised to read ingredient lists and look for "phos" to identify foods with phosphate additives; these phosphate additives may be absorbed more efficiently than food-based sources. Limiting whole grains may help if further phosphorus reduction is needed. When the GFR drops below 20–30 mL/minute, the dietary restriction of phosphorus rarely suffices to reach target levels, and the use of phosphorus binders (also called phosphate binders) is then incorporated.[33] Phosphate binders must be taken with food in order to effectively control serum phosphorus levels. Calcium acetate and calcium carbonate are common calcium-containing phosphate binders that may be used for people with CKD. Using phosphate binders with calcium citrate is not advised for CKD patients; calcium citrate may increase aluminum absorption, and excessive accumulation of aluminum can cause bone disease.[34]

▪ Calcium

People with CKD have higher calcium needs than those with healthy kidney function, although at this time there are no established calcium intake recommendations for nondialysis CKD.[22] The goal for serum calcium levels is to maintain within normal range of 8.5–10.2 mg/dL. Serum calcium levels tend to be lower in CKD because of metabolic alterations with vitamin D, lowered absorption levels in the intestine, and higher serum phosphorus levels.

At the very time when calcium needs are elevated, the foods that are the best dietary sources of calcium (ie, the dairy foods) are usually restricted due to their phosphorus levels. Calcium supplements may help individuals meet their calcium needs, and these should be taken between meals, on an empty stomach, or at bedtime, and not in amounts exceeding 500 mg per dose. Calcium intake from all foods, supplements, and phosphate binders should not exceed 2000 milligrams per day.[29]

▪ Sodium and Fluid

In CKD Stages 1–4, fluid needs are determined by medical status, and fluid restriction is usually not indicated. For those on HD, fluid intake is recommended to be urine output plus 1000 mL per day. For PD, fluid intake is prescribed only to maintain balance.[20,27] Sodium intake levels of >3–4 g/day can cause edema, hypertension, and congestive heart failure. Limiting sodium intake to <1 g/day can lead to hypotension and volume depletion. CKD patients approaching HD may benefit from a restriction of 2 grams/day, and those on HD or PD often require fluid restrictions of 1.5–2 g/day.[33] The *Dietary Guidelines for Americans, 2010* say to limit sodium intake to 1500 milligrams a day or less for people with kidney disease.[35]

▪ Other Nutrients

Those undergoing maintenance dialysis may also be deficient in vitamin D, folic acid, B vitamins and vitamin C, zinc, and iron.[36] Because of the restrictions on protein and (possibly) potassium in CKD Stages 1–4, average DRI intakes of other micronutrients may be suboptimal. Uremia and alterations in nutrient absorption further compound the metabolism of these vitamins, including vitamin D, folic acid, vitamin B_6, and vitamin C. Vitamin D monitoring and supplementation should be individualized as per the K/DOQI Bone Disease Management Guidelines, available at: http://www.kidney.org/professionals/kdoqi/guidelines_commentaries.cfm#guidelines.

In general, a renal water-soluble vitamin is prescribed to meet the DRI for some of these potentially deficient nutrients. Note that general multivitamins are contraindicated in renal disease. Renal-specific multivitamins contain a greater proportion of water-soluble vitamins, the ones CKD patients are more likely to be deficient in. These include vitamin B_1 (thiamin), B_2 (riboflavin), B_3 (niacin), B_6, B_{12}, folic acid, pantothenic acid, biotin, and a small amount of vitamin C.[37]

Table 9–15 contains a summary of general nutrition recommendations for CKD and for dialyzed patients (on HD or PD).[20,22,23,27,38,39] The tables following the Kidney Transplantation section, Tables 9–16 to 9–31, contain specific nutrition recommendation guidelines from the Academy of Nutrition and Dietetics' Evidence Analysis Library's

Table 9–15. Summary of nutrition recommendations for various degrees of kidney disease.

	CKD Not on Dialysis	HD	PD
Calories	<60 years: 35 kcal/day, or 23–35 kcal/kg Overweight adults with CKD and diabetes, not on dialysis: 1780–1823 kcal/day ≥60 years: 30–35 kcal/kg/day	<60 years: 35 kcal/kg/day ≥60 years: 30–35 kcal/kg/day	<60 years: 35 kcal/kg/day ≥60 years: 30–35 kcal/kg/day Including dialysate calories
Protein	0.6–0.75 g/kg/day – may be difficult for adherence 0.8 g/kg/day in nondiabetic 1.0 g/kg/day in diabetic ≥50% HBV protein 0.8–0.9 g protein/kg if diabetic nephropathy present	≥1.2 g/kg/day ≥50% HBV protein	≥1.2–1.3 g/kg/day ≥50% HBV protein
Potassium	Unrestricted unless serum level ↑ Restrict when serum level 5.0 mEq/L or higher <2.4 g/day for Stages 3-4 CKD	2–3 g/day Adjust based on serum levels	3–4 g/day Adjust based on serum levels

(Continued)

Table 9–15. Summary of nutrition recommendations for various degrees of kidney disease. (*Continued*)

	CKD Not on Dialysis	HD	PD
Phosphorus	800–1000 mg/day or 10–12 mg phosphorus per gram protein when serum phosphorus >4.6 mg/dL or PTH ↑	800–1000 mg/day when serum phosphorus >5.5 mg/dL or PTH ↑	800–1000 mg/day when serum phosphorus >5.5 mg/dL or PTH ↑
Sodium	<2.4 g/day	1–3 g/day	2–4 g/day. Monitor fluid balance
Calcium	N/A for CKD. Not >2 g/day with binder load in Stages 3–4	≤2 g/day. Include binder load	≤2 g/day. Include binder load
Fluid	None; determined by medical status, blood pressure control, physical findings, and alterations in UOP	UOP + 1000 mL	Maintain balance
Supplement	B-complex. Vitamin C. Individualize: vitamin D (if 25-hydroxyvitamin D level less than 30 ng/mL), iron (oral or IV supplementation if serum ferritin below 100 ng/mL and transferrin saturation below 20%), zinc	Vitamin C: 60–100 mg/day. Vitamin B$_6$: 2 mg/day. Folate: 1 mg/day. Vitamin B$_{12}$: 3 mcg/day. Vitamin E: 15 IU/day. Zinc: 15 mg/day. Individualize: iron and vit D	Vitamin C: 60–100 mg/day. Vitamin B$_6$: 2 mg/day. Folate: 1 mg/day. Vitamin B$_{12}$: 3 mcg/day. Thiamin: may need 1.5–2 mg/day because of dialysis losses. Vitamin E: 15 IU/day. Zinc: 15 mg/day. Individualize: iron and vitamin D

Data from Academy of Nutrition and Dietetics, 2012; National Kidney Foundation, 2003; National Kidney Foundation, 2002; National Kidney Disease Education Program, 2011; Academy of Nutrition and Dietetics, 2010; McCann, 2009; Academy of Nutrition and Dietetics, 2011.

Table 9–16. Academy of Nutrition and Dietetics' Evidence Analysis Library, protein recommendations in CKD.

Who?	CKD w/o DM, no HD/PD, eGFR <50 mL/minute/1.73 m²	CKD w/o DM, no HD/PD, eGFR < 20 mL/minute/1.73 m²	CKD with diabetic nephropathy	Adult kidney transplant recipients w/ adequately functioning allograft
Protein Intake Recs	0.6–0.8 g/kg/day	0.3–0.5 g/kg/day	0.8–0.9 g/kg/day	0.8–1.0 g/kg/day
Evidence Grade	Strong, Conditional	Strong, Conditional	Fair, Conditional	Consensus, Conditional
Note	0.7 g/kg/day, ensuring adequate calorie intake, can slow GFR decline and maintain stable nutrition status	Additional keto acid analogs and vitamin or mineral supplementation needed to maintain adequate nutrition status on this very low protein-controlled diet	Providing protein at 0.7 g/kg/day may result in hypoalbuminemia	Adequate, but not excessive, protein intake supports allograft survival and minimizes impact on comorbid conditions

Data from Academy of Nutrition and Dietetics, 2010.

Table 9–17. Academy of Nutrition and Dietetics' Evidence Analysis Library, energy recommendations in CKD.

Who?	Adults with CKD, including postkidney transplant after surgical recovery
Energy Intake Recs	23–35 kcal/kg/day
Evidence Grade	Fair, Imperative
Note	Individualize kcal needs based on weight status and goals, age, gender, level of physical activity, and metabolic stressors

Data from Academy of Nutrition and Dietetics, 2010.

Nutrition Practice Guideline on Chronic Kidney Disease, published at www.andevidencelibrary.com and copyrighted by the Academy of Nutrition and Dietetics.[40]

The following tables contain specific nutrition therapy recommendations based on the Academy of Nutrition and Dietetics' Evidence Analysis Library's Evidence-Based Nutrition Practice Guideline on Chronic Kidney Disease published at www.andevidencelibrary.com and copyrighted by the Academy of Nutrition and Dietetics.[28]

Table 9–18. Academy of Nutrition and Dietetics' Evidence Analysis Library, phosphorus recommendations in CKD.

Who?	Adults with CKD Stages 3–5	Adult kidney transplant recipients exhibiting hypophosphatemia
Phosphorus Intake Recs	Low-phosphorus diet: 800–1000 mg phosphorus or 10–12 mg phosphorus per gram of protein	High-phosphorus intake from diet or supplements to replete serum phosphorus as needed
Evidence Grade	Strong, Conditional	
Note	CKD patients have a predisposition for mineral and bone disorders Phosphorus control is cornerstone for treatment and prevention of secondary hyperparathyroidism, renal bone disease, and soft tissue calcification	Hypophosphatemia is common in postkidney transplant

Data from Academy of Nutrition and Dietetics, 2010.

Table 9–19. Academy of Nutrition and Dietetics' Evidence Analysis Library, phosphate binder adjustments CKD.

Who?	Adults with CKD Stages 3-5
Phosphate Binder Adjustment Recs	Dose and timing of phosphate binders should be individually adjusted to the phosphate content of meals and snacks to achieve desired serum phosphorus levels
Evidence Grade	Strong, Conditional
Note	Serum phosphorus levels are difficult to control with dietary restrictions alone

Data from Academy of Nutrition and Dietetics, 2010.

Table 9–20. Academy of Nutrition and Dietetics' Evidence Analysis Library, total elemental calcium recommendations in CKD.

Who?	Adults with CKD Stages 3-5 and postkidney transplant
Elemental Calcium Intake	Do not exceed 2000 mg per day (total from dietary calcium, calcium supplementation, and calcium-based phosphate binders)
Evidence Grade	Consensus, Conditional
Note	CKD patients have predisposition for mineral and bone disorders

Serum calcium concentration is the most important factor regulating PTH secretion affecting bone integrity and soft tissue calcification |

Data from Academy of Nutrition and Dietetics, 2010.

Table 9–21. Academy of Nutrition and Dietetics' Evidence Analysis Library, vitamin D recommendations in CKD.

Who?	Adults with CKD Stages 3-5 and postkidney transplant
Vitamin D	Supplement to maintain adequate levels of vitamin D if serum level of 25-hydroxyvitamin D is less than 30 ng/mL (75 nmol/L)
Evidence Grade	Consensus, Conditional
Note	CKD patients have a predisposition for mineral and bone disorders, as well as other conditions that may be affected by insufficient vitamin D. Sufficient vitamin D should be recommended to maintain adequate levels of serum vitamin D.

Data from Academy of Nutrition and Dietetics, 2010.

Table 9–22. Academy of Nutrition and Dietetics' Evidence Analysis Library, iron supplementation recommendations in CKD.

Who?	Adults with CKD and postkidney transplant
Iron	Oral or IV iron administration if serum ferritin is below 100 ng/mL and TSAT is below 20%
Evidence Grade	Consensus, Conditional
Note	CKD patients have a predisposition for anemia. Sufficient iron should be recommended to maintain adequate levels of serum iron to support erythropoiesis.

Data from Academy of Nutrition and Dietetics, 2010.

Table 9–23. Academy of Nutrition and Dietetics' Evidence Analysis Library, vitamin B_{12} and folic acid recommendations in CKD.

Who?	Adults with CKD and postkidney transplant
Vitamin B_{12} and Folic Acid	Vitamin B_{12} and folic acid supplementation if the MCV is over 100 ng/mL and serum levels of these nutrients are below normal values
Evidence Grade	Consensus, Conditional
Note	CKD patients have a predisposition for anemia and all potential causes should be investigated.

Data from Academy of Nutrition and Dietetics, 2010.

Table 9–24. Academy of Nutrition and Dietetics' Evidence Analysis Library, vitamin C for treatment of anemia in CKD

Who?	Adults with CKD and postkidney transplant who are anemic
Vitamin C	DRI for Vitamin C for those who are anemic
Evidence Grade	Consensus, Conditional
Note	Insufficient evidence to recommend use of vitamin C > DRI
	DRI for vitamin C: 90 mg/day for males aged 19+ years; 75 mg/day for females aged 19+ years; 85 mg/day for pregnant females aged 19+ years; 120 mg/day for lactating females aged 19+ years; note that smokers have vitamin C needs above those of the nonsmoking population

Data from Academy of Nutrition and Dietetics, 2010.

Table 9–25. Academy of Nutrition and Dietetics' Evidence Analysis Library, L-carnitine for treatment of anemia recommendations in CKD.

Who?	Adults with CKD and postkidney transplant who are anemic
L-carnitine	Do not recommend L-carnitine supplementation
Evidence Grade	Consensus, Conditional
Note	Insufficient evidence to recommend use of L-carnitine in the management of anemia in adults with CKD including postkidney transplant.

Data from Academy of Nutrition and Dietetics, 2010.

Table 9–26. Academy of Nutrition and Dietetics' Evidence Analysis Library, medical nutrition therapy for diabetes care to manage hyperglycemia to achieve a target HbA1c of approximately 7%.

Who?	Adults with diabetes and CKD, including postkidney transplant
A1C goal	Implement medical nutrition therapy for diabetes care to manage hyperglycemia to achieve a target A1c of approximately 7%
Evidence Grade	Strong, Conditional
Note	Intensive treatment of hyperglycemia, while avoiding hypoglycemia, prevents diabetic kidney disease (DKD) and may slow progression of established kidney disease

Data from Academy of Nutrition and Dietetics, 2010.

Table 9–27. Academy of Nutrition and Dietetics' Evidence Analysis Library, sodium in CKD recommendations.

Who?	Adults with CKD, including postkidney transplant, Stages 1-5
Sodium	Less than 2.4 grams per day
Evidence Grade	Fair, Imperative
Note	Adjust based on blood pressure, medications, kidney function, hydration status, acidosis, glycemic control, catabolism, and GI issues (including vomiting, diarrhea, and constipation).

Data from Academy of Nutrition and Dietetics, 2010.

Table 9–28. Academy of Nutrition and Dietetics' Evidence Analysis Library, fish oil/omega-3 fatty acid in CKD.

Who?	Adults with CKD, including postkidney transplant
Fish oil or omega-3 fatty acids	Conflicting evidence regarding effectiveness: research reports that renal outcomes were inconsistent among patients with IgA nephropathy who received fish oil supplementation. Insufficient evidence to support fish oil therapy to improve renal function and patient or graft survival for kidney transplant patients
Evidence Grade	Fair, Conditional
Note	Evidence does support benefit of fish oil supplementation in reducing oxidative stress and improving lipid profile in adults with CKD, including postkidney transplant.

Data from Academy of Nutrition and Dietetics, 2010.

Table 9–29. Academy of Nutrition and Dietetics' Evidence Analysis Library, physical activity recommendations in CKD.

Who?	Adults with CKD, including postkidney transplant
Physical activity	Increase frequency or duration of physical activity as tolerated (if not contraindicated)
Evidence Grade	Fair, Conditional
Note	Studies report that physical activity may minimize the catabolic effects of protein restriction and improve quality of life.

Data from Academy of Nutrition and Dietetics, 2010.

Table 9–30. Academy of Nutrition and Dietetics' Evidence Analysis Library, multivitamin supplementation in CKD.

Who?	Adults with CKD, including postkidney transplant with no known nutrient deficiency (biochemical or physical)
Multivitamin	Recommend or prescribe multivitamin preparation for those who may be at higher nutritional risk due to poor dietary intake
Evidence Grade	Consensus, Conditional
Note	Sufficient vitamin supplementation should be recommended to maintain indices of adequate nutritional status.

Data from Academy of Nutrition and Dietetics, 2010.

Table 9-31. Academy of Nutrition and Dietetics' Evidence Analysis Library, potassium in CKD.

Who?	Adults with CKD Stages 3–5, including postkidney transplant who exhibit hyperkalemia
Potassium	Intake less than 2.4 grams per day
Evidence Grade	Fair, Conditional
Note	Adjust based on serum potassium level, blood pressure, medications, kidney function, hydration status, acidosis, glycemic control, catabolism, and GI issues.

Data from Academy of Nutrition and Dietetics, 2010.

▪ Nutrition Support

When adequate caloric intake cannot be established by PO feedings alone, nutrition support is indicated. If the gut is functional, enteral nutrition should be initiated. The formulas used in CKD treatment are energy-dense, with low-to-moderate amounts of protein that meet protein needs but do not provide excessive calories from protein. Commonly used formulas for patients with CKD Stage 5 on dialysis include Nepro® (Abbott Nutrition) and Novasource® Renal (Nestle). Nepro contains 1.8 calories/mL, and Novasource Renal provide 2.0 calories/mL; both products contain 18% of calories from HBV protein.

There are also renal-specific formulas for nondialyzed CKD patients. Abbott makes the formula Suplena® for people with Stages 3 and 4 CKD, and this formula is low in protein, potassium, phosphorus, and sodium. Suplena provides 1.8 calories/mL and 10% of calories from protein. The comparable product from Nestle is called Renalcal®; it provides 2.0 calories/mL and 7% of calories from protein.

Practitioners who are managing the nutrition support of a dialyzed individual should take into account the patient's dialysis schedule, as feeding rates and the number of hours of infusion may need to be adjusted around the dialysis treatments. For those managing enteral feedings for PD patients, they are advised to provide fewer calories from the formula, taking into account the calories provided from the absorbed energy of the dialysate. For those unable to tolerate enteral feedings, total parenteral nutrition (TPN) may be indicated. The contents of the TPN bag should be tailored and are dependent upon the individual's renal replacement therapy, GFR, stress level, metabolic state, nitrogen balance, and electrolyte levels.[27]

▪ Nutrition Referrals

The Academy of Nutrition and Dietetics recommends referring newly dialyzed patients to a registered dietitian (RD) 3–4 weeks after the initial encounter, or as necessary. Every dialysis center employs a renal dietitian who has additional training specific to the nutritional management of kidney disease.

Medicare also covers medical nutrition therapy (MNT) with an RD for beneficiaries with diabetes (types I or II, fasting blood glucose >125 mg/dL on 2 tests) and for those with nondialysis kidney disease (GFR 13–50 mL/minute/1.73 m^2). The "nondialysis" kidney disease part of Medicare's nutrition coverage is because dialysis centers provide nutrition therapy via their renal dietitians. Renal dietitians at dialysis centers generally follow up with each patient every month, reviewing their clinical data and lab work, evaluating the diet, addressing behavioral outcomes, and adjusting goals as necessary.

Acute Kidney Injury

Acute kidney injury (AKI), formerly called acute renal failure (ARF), occurs when kidney function abruptly declines and the kidneys suddenly lose their ability to clear nitrogenous wastes. The new terminology for AKI, used primarily in published literature, was established to assist health professionals with considering the disease as a spectrum of injury rather than a single condition.[40] The Acute Kidney Injury Network (AKIN), an international interdisciplinary group of adult and pediatric nephrologists and critical care physicians and other practitioners working in the realm of AKI, has proposed a revised set of consensus recommendations standardizing the terminology, diagnostic criteria, and staging of AKI.

The AKIN diagnostic criteria for AKI is, "an abrupt (within 48 hours) reduction in kidney function currently defined as an absolute increase in serum creatinine of >0.3 mg/dl (>25 micromole/L), a percentage increase of 50% or a reduction in urine output (documented oliguria of <0.5 ml/kg/hr for >6 hours)." AKI occurs commonly in 5–7% of hospitalized patients and in approximately 30% of patients admitted to the intensive care unit.[41] Mortality rates for AKI are high, with death occurring in 40% of nonsurgical patients who have severe AKI, to as many as 80% undergoing surgery, and 20% of those with noncatabolic conditions.[29]

The three stages of AKI are prerenal, intrarenal, and postrenal. Prerenal azotemia is the most common form of AKI. It occurs when an underlying situation impairs necessary blood flow to the kidney and decreases GFR. This may be the result of volume depletion, hypotension and shock, congestive heart failure, renal vasoconstrictions, or renal artery occlusion. In the intrarenal stage, parts of the kidney, such as the tubule, interstitium, glomerulus, or the vasculature, are damaged, which may be precipitated by hypertension, infection-related interstitial inflammation, acute tubular necrosis or interstitial nephritis, nephrotoxicity, or intrarenal obstruction. In the postrenal stage, crystals, protein deposits, or malignant tumor infiltrates obstruct the flow of urine.

Because of its hypercatabolic nature, malnutrition is a primary complication of AKI. Further nutritional implications seen with acute kidney failure include a rapid decrease in urine output, electrolyte imbalances such as hyperkalemia and hyperphosphatemia, acidosis, fluid disturbances, impaired glucose utilization, and the accumulation of metabolic waste products.[20] Individual nutrient requirements are dictated by the type of renal replacement therapy, if present, as well as nutritional status, metabolic state, and extent of hypercatabolism.

Exact energy needs are difficult to determine, but calories are generally given at 30 kcal/kg recommended body weight for those with no or mild catabolism, at 35 kcal/kg recommended body weight for moderate catabolism, and at 35–50 kcal/kg recommended body weight for severe catabolism, burns, or sepsis. Indirect calorimetry can help determine energy requirements and will be roughly 130% of the calculated basal energy expenditure.[20] Protein needs vary from 0.6 g/kg in the nondialyzed individual to 2.0 g/kg for burns/sepsis; protein needs are also estimated using kilograms of recommended body weight. Providing adequate protein promotes a decrease in negative nitrogen balance and promotes recovery from AKI. Continuous renal replacement therapy (CRRT) removes amino acids and proteins and, as such, dictates a minimal protein intake of 1.5 kg/kg recommended body weight per day. Carbohydrates should constitute roughly 60% of calorie needs and should not exceed 4–5 mg/kg/minute/day in those receiving parenteral nutrition.[42] The remainder of the calories (20–35%) should be provided by fat.

In the absence of edema, sodium intake is recommended at 1.1–3.3 grams per day, and sodium intake levels should mirror those of urinary losses.[43] Potassium is also individualized and should be 2.0–3.0 g/day. Hyperkalemia and hyperphosphatemia are seen during AKI, but hypokalemia and hypophosphatemia may occur with refeeding syndrome due to the intracellular shift of potassium and phosphorus as the anabolic response takes place. Serum magnesium, calcium, and phosphorus may also need to be provided via oral supplementation. Because loss of magnesium, calcium, phosphorus, and potassium are often seen with CRRT, these serum minerals require close monitoring.[44] Table 9–32 summarizes nutrient recommendations for patients with AKI,[20,45] and Table 9–33 provides a vitamin and mineral supplementation regimen for individuals who are on CRRT.[46] Note that water-soluble vitamin needs in AKI are higher due to losses from dialysis, inadequate oral intake, potential drug-nutrient interactions, and overall higher nutrient needs.[36]

Further nutrition prescription recommendations from the Academy of Nutrition and Dietetics are outlined in Table 9–34.[47]

Table 9–32. Nutrient recommendations for acute kidney injury.

Extent of Catabolism	None or Mild	Moderate	Severe	Burn or Sepsis
GFR (mL/minute)	5-10	—	—	—
Urea nitrogen appearance	4-5 g N/day	5 g N/day+	5 g N/day+	5 g N/day+
Dialysis	None	As needed	HD/PD	CRRT
Calories per kg recommended wt	30	35	35-50	35-50
Protein (g/kg recommended wt per day)	0.6-1.0	1.0-1.2	1.2-1.8	1.5-2.0
Carbohydrates as % of kcal	60	60	60	60
Fat as % of kcal	35	20-30	20-30	20-30

Data from Bajpai, 1998; Academy of Nutrition and Dietetics, 2012.

Table 9–33. Vitamin and mineral supplementation in acute kidney injury on CRRT.

Vitamin or Mineral Supplement for AKI	Dose
Vitamin A	Avoid as supplement
Thiamin (vitamin B_1)	1.5 mg/day
Riboflavin (vitamin B_2)	1.5-1.7 mg/day
Niacin (vitamin B_3)	20 mg/day
Vitamin B_6 (pantothenic acid)	5-10 mg/day
Vitamin B_{12}	4 mcg/day
Folic acid	1 mg/day
Vitamin C	60-125 mg/day
Vitamin E	10 IU/day
Vitamin K	4 mg/week
Biotin	150-300 mcg/day
Zinc	20 mg

Data from Marin and Hardy, 2001.

Table 9–34. Nutrition prescription for acute kidney injury.

Protein	0.8–1.2 g/kg body weight noncatabolic, no dialysis
	1.2–1.5 g/kg body weight with catabolic and/or initiation of dialysis
Calories	25–35 kcal/kg body weight
	Depends on stress/status of nutrition
	Depends on kcal from CRRT if present
Sodium	2.0–3.0 g/day
	Individualize based on blood pressure and edema
	Replace losses in diuretic phase
Potassium	2.0–3.0 g/day
	Replace losses in diuretic phase
Phosphorus	8–15 mg/kg
Calcium	Maintain serum value within normal limits
Fluid	500 mL + urine output
	Depends on urinary sodium, total fluid output including urine and modality of dialysis (if present)
Vitamins and minerals	Provide DRI, adjust depending on level of catabolism

Data from Byham-Gray and Wiesen, 2004.

■ Nutrition Support

If nutrition support is indicated, and if the gut is functional, enteral nutrition is preferred over parenteral to help maintain and preserve gut function, promote possible immune enhancement, and lower the likelihood of bacteremia and infection.[48] Gastroparesis is a common problem in AKI and, if present, small bowel enteral access may be preferred over gastric access.

High-calorie, high-protein formulas are indicated for the hypercatabolic patient, and additional protein needs may be met with modular protein products added to the enteral formula. For those fed via parenteral nutrition, formulation is tailored to the individual's underlying illness, catabolic state, and current nitrogen balance. CRRT promotes protein losses of approximately 15 g/day, and this affects individual protein needs.[49] Highly concentrated solutions of 20% amino acids, 50–60% dextrose, and 20–30% lipids are advised to reduce overall volume from TPN, with trace elements being administered two to three times per week.[50]

Nutritional complications of TPN administration in the AKI patient include hyperglycemia (count calories from CRRT as part of intake; use insulin when needed), electrolyte imbalances, elevated triglycerides, difficulty with ventilator weaning if overfeeding causes increased carbon dioxide production, and increased risk of infection.[20] Refeeding syndrome is a consequence of rapidly reintroducing nutrition into the system of a malnourished individual and may be seen with oral or enteral feeds, causing intolerance to glucose, fluid disruptions, and hypophosphatemia, hypokalemia, and hypomagnesemia. Potassium, magnesium, calcium, and phosphate all should be closely monitored in potential refeeding cases.[20]

Kidney Transplantation

Increasing rates of obesity and diabetes are resulting in more individuals with ESRD who may eventually require kidney transplantation. In 2008, there were more than 11,300 deceased-donor kidney transplants and almost 6000 living-donor transplants done in the United States. As of 2011, over 87,000 individuals were awaiting kidney transplants, and more than 2000 were waiting for kidney and pancreas transplants.[51] Transplant surgery increases metabolic demands and nutritional requirements. The recommended nutrition therapies are split and differ between the acute phase (transplantation to 8 weeks postop), and the chronic phase (starting at the ninth week after transplantation).

Calories are given at 30–35 calories per kilogram in the acute phase and adjusted to assist with healthy weight maintenance in the chronic phase. The elevated protein needs required in the acute phase (1.3–1.5 g/kg of standard or adjusted body weight) decline in the chronic phase (1.0 g/kg) with stricter limitations (if chronic graft dysfunction present). Over time, low-fat protein sources should be adopted to help mitigate risk for dyslipidemia, diabetes, obesity, and cardiovascular disease. Hyperglycemia is problematic in the post-transplant state due to the reliance on corticosteroids and other medications that elevate blood sugar. Simple and refined sugars should be minimized and replaced with high-fiber carbohydrate sources such as fruits, vegetables, and whole grains.

A low-fat diet is indicated due to the prevalence of cardiovascular disease in kidney transplant recipients. Fat should constitute 25–35% of calories, and saturated fatty acids should be limited to no more than 7% of calories.[29] This equates to 56–78 grams of fat and no more than 16 grams of saturated fat for an individual stabilized on a 2000-calorie per day diet.

The amount of fluid output dictates fluid needs in kidney transplantation. With reduced urine output, limit fluid intake to urine output plus 500 mL/day. For those with very high urine output, such as that which occurs immediately following a living-donor transplant, replace fluid at a level slightly less than urine output. For example, 80% of urine output could be replenished as fluid, helping to reduce urine output levels to within normal limits. In the longer term, those kidney transplant recipients who are experiencing good graft function should drink 8–12 cups of fluid per day.[52]

Kidney Stones

Urolithiasis refers to stones that occur in the urinary tract and may also be referred to as urinary tract stone disease or nephrolithiasis. Nephrolithiasis, more commonly known as kidney stones, affects approximately 5% of the US population.[53] The most common types of stones are calcium phosphate, struvite, uric acid, cysteine, and calcium oxalate; calcium oxalate is the most prevalent type of kidney stone.[54] Risks for developing kidney stones include insufficient fluid intake, urinary tract blockage, gout, recurrent urinary tract infections, chronic bowel infection, or intestinal bypass or ostomy surgery.[55]

Fluid intake is by far the most important nutrition concern in preventing and reducing risk for formation of kidney stones. Increased fluid intake helps prevent all types of stones from forming. Fluid intake recommendations are 12–16 cups per day to produce urine output volume of at least 2.5 liters per day.[54] Protein should be consumed at 0.8–1.0 g/kg body weight per day. Sodium intake should be moderate, maximum of 2300 milligrams per day, and high doses of vitamin C and vitamin D supplements should be avoided as they contribute to stone formation.

It was previously believed that high calcium intake precipitated stone formation; however, the prevailing theory now is that high-calcium foods such as dairy foods work to prevent stone formation, possibly due to the notion that lowering dietary calcium intake would increase oxalate excretion. Because calcium binds oxalate in the gut, including moderate amounts of calcium can help reduce oxalate excretion. Calcium intake levels should be at 800 mg/day for men and 1200 mg/day for women. For those at risk of forming calcium oxalate stones, oxalate should be limited to 40–60 mg/day.[20]

The Academy of Nutrition and Dietetics recommends maintaining a low-sodium, low-oxalate meal plan with plenty of fluids for those at risk for developing calcium oxalate stones. While there are long, exhaustive lists available detailing foods that contain oxalates, the foods that have been shown to increase urinary oxalate excretion are beets, chocolate, cocoa, nuts, spinach, rhubarb, almonds, and wheat bran.[29,53] Table 9–35 contains a list of high-oxalate foods that should be avoided or eaten infrequently in urolithiasis, and Table 9–36 contains information about high-sodium foods to be avoided.[20]

Table 9–35. High-oxalate foods to avoid or eat infrequently in urolithiasis.

Avoid Foods High in Oxalate	
Apricots (dried)	Leeks
Beans	Legumes (lentils, dried peas and beans)
Beer	Marmalades
Beets	Nuts and nut butters
Berries	Oranges
Bran cereals	Parsley
Buckwheat flour	Peanut butter
Carob	Poppy seeds
Chocolate	Rhubarb
Coffee	Rutabagas
Colas	Soy foods, miso, tofu
Cranberries	Sweet potatoes
Currants	Tea
Eggplant	Tofu
Escarole	Tomato paste
Figs	Watercress
Greens (spinach, mustard, kale, collards, Swiss chard)	Wheat bran and what germ
	Whole wheat bread
Kiwi	Zucchini

Data from Academy of Nutrition and Dietetics, 2012.

Table 9–36. High-sodium foods to avoid in urolithiasis.

Salt, salt seasonings, and MSG
Soy sauce and other salty condiments or sauces
Salted crackers, popcorn and other packaged snack foods
Vegetables prepared in brine such as pickles, sauerkraut
Cured and processed meats, including cold cuts and smoked fish
Condensed or canned soups that are made by adding more water

Data from Academy of Nutrition and Dietetics, 2012.

References

1. Longo D, Fauci A, Kasper D, Hauser S, Jameson J, Loscalzo J. Chronic hepatitis. In: Longo D, Fauci A, Kasper D, Hauser S, Jameson J, Loscalzo J, eds. Harrison's Principles of Internal Medicine. 18th ed. New York, NY: McGraw-Hill; 2012 [chapter 306].

2. Florez D, Aranda-Michel A. Nutritional management of acute and chronic liver disease. Semin Gastroinest Dis 2002;13(3):169–178.

3. Cordoba J, Lopez-Hellin J, Planas M, et al. Normal protein diet for episodic hepatic encephalopathy: results of a randomized study. J Hepatol 2004;41(1):38–43.

4. Hasse J, Weseman B, Fuhrman M, Loeffer M, Francisco-Ziller N, DiCecco S. Nutrition therapy for end-stage liver disease: a practical approach. Support Line (DNS Publication) 1997;19(4):8–15.

5. Academy of Nutrition and Dietetics. (2012). Liver, Gallbladder, and Pancreas Diseases. Retrieved January 21, 2013, from Nutrition Care Manual: http://www.nutritioncaremanual.org

6. Mailliard M, Sorrell M. Alcoholic liver disease. In: Longo D, Fauci A, Kasper D, Hauser S, Jameson J, Loscalzo J, eds. Harrison's Principles of Internal Medicine. 18th ed. New York, NY: McGraw-Hill; 2012 [chapter 307].

7. CDC National Center for Injury Prevention and Control. (2010, June 1). WISQARS Leading Causes of Death Reports, 1999-2007. Retrieved April 4, 2012, from 12 Leading Cuases of Death, United States 2007, All Races, Both Sexes: http://webappa.cdc.gov/cgi-bin/broker.exe

8. Sucher K, Mattfeldt-Beman M. Diseases of the liver, gallbladder, and exocrine pancreas. In: Nelms M, Sucher K, Lacey K, Long Roth S, eds. Nutrition Therapy & Pathophysiology. Belmont, CA: Cengage Wadsworth; 2011 [chapter 16].

9. Markowitz J, McRae A, Sonne S. Oral nutritional supplementation for the alcoholic patient: a brief overview. Ann Clin Psychiatry 2000;12(3):153–158.

10. Academy of Nutrition and Dietetics. (2012). Alcoholism. Retrieved January 21, 2013, from Nutrition Care Manual: http://www.nutritioncaremanual.org

11. Bacon B. Cirrhosis and its complications. In: Longo D, Fauci A, Kapser D, Hauser S, Jameson J, Loscalzo J, eds. Harrison's Principles of Internal Medicine. 18th ed. New York, NY: McGraw-Hill; 2012 [chapter 308].

12. Stickel F, Inderbitzin D, Candina D. Role of nutrition in liver transplantation for end-stage chronic liver disease. Nutr Rev 2008 Jan;66(1):47-54. PMID: 18254884.

13. Academy of Nutrition and Dietetics. (2012). Organ Transplant. Retrieved January 21, 2013, from Nutrition Care Manual: http://www.nutrition caremanual.org

14. National Digestive Diseases Information Clearinghouse (NDDIC). (2007, July). Retrieved April 5, 2012, from Gallstones: https://vpn.ucsf.edu/ddiseases/pubs/gallstones/,DanaInfo=digestive.niddk.nih.gov+index.aspx

15. Academy of Nutrition and Dietetics. (2012). Gallbladder. Retrieved January 21, 2013, from Nutrition Care Manual: http://www.nutrition caremanual.org; Academy of Nutrition and Dietetics. (2012). Bladder and

Urinary Tract Disease. Retrieved January 21, 2013, from Nutrition Care Manual: http://www.nutritioncaremanual.org

16. Kalloo A, Kantsevoy S. Gallstones an biliary disease. Prim Care 2001;28: 591–606.

17. Hartmann D, Felix K, Ehmann M. Protein expression profiling reveals distinctive changes in serum proteins associated with chronic pancreatitis. Pancreas 2007;35:334–342.

18. Moraes J, Felga G, Chebli L, et al. A full solid diet as the initial meal in mild acute pancreatitis is safe and result in a shorter length of hospitalization. J Clin Gastroenterol 2010;44(7):517–522. PMID: 20054282.

19. McClave S, Martindale R, Vanek V, et al. Guidelines for the provision and assessment of nutrition support therapy in the adult critically ill patient: Society of Critical Care Medicine (SCCM) and American Society for Parenteral and Enteral Nutrition (ASPEN). JPEN J Parenter Enteral Nutr 2009;33(3):277–316.

20. Academy of Nutrition and Dietetics. (2012). Kidney Disease. Retrieved January 21, 2013, from Nutrition Care Manual: http://www.nutritioncare manual.org

21. Bargman J, Skorecki K. Chronic kidney disease. In: Longo D, Fauci A, Kasper D, Hauser S, Jameson J, Loscalzo J, eds. Harrison's Principles of Internal Medicine. 18th ed. New York, NY: McGraw-Hill; 2012 [chapter 280].

22. National Kidney Disease Education Program. (2011). Chronic Kidney Disease (CKD) and Diet: Assessment, Management, and Treatment – Treating CKD Patients Who Are Not on Dialysis, An Overview Guide for Dietitians. National Institutes of Health, National Institute of Diabetes and Digestive and Kidney Diseases. National Kidney Disease Education Program.

23. National Kidney Foundation. K/DOQI clinical practice guidelines for chronic kidney disease: evaluation, classification, and stratification. Am J Kidney Dis 2002;39(2 suppl 1):S1–S266.

24. CDC. (2012, November 5). National Chronic Kidney Disease Fact Sheet 2010. Retrieved January 21, 2013, from Diabetes Public Health Resource: http://www.cdc.gov/diabetes/pubs/factsheets/kidney.htm

25. National Kidney Disease Education Program. (2012, July 10). Race, Ethnicity and Kidney Disease. Retrieved January 21, 2013, from Learn About Kidney Disease: http://nkdep.nih.gov/learn/are-you-at-risk/race-ethnicity.shtml

26. Frisancho A. New standards of weight and body composition by frame size and height for assessment of nutritional status of adults and the elderly. Am J Clin Nutr 1984;40:808–819.

27. McCann L. Pocket Guide to Nutrition Assessment of the Patient with Chronic Kidney Disease. New York, NY: National Kidney Foundation Council on Renal Nutrition; 2009.

28. Academy of Nutrition and Dietetics. (2011). Chronic Kidney Disease: Evidence-Based Nutrition Practice Guidelines - Executive Summary of Recommendations. Retrieved January 21, 2013, from Evidence Analysis Library: http://andevidencelibrary.com

29. Lacey K, Nahikian-Nelms M. Diseases of the renal system. In: Nelms M, Sucher K, Lacey K, Long Roth S, eds. Nutrition Therapy & Pathophysiology. Belmont, CA: Cengage Wadsworth; 2011 [chapter 18].

30. National Kidney Foundation. K/DOQI clinical practice guidelines for nutrition in chronic renal failure. Am J Kidney Dis 2000;35(6):S1–S104.

31. National Kidney Foundation. (2013). Potassium and Your CKD Diet. Retrieved January 31, 2013, from A to Z Health Guide: http://www.kidney.org/atoz/content/potassium.cfm

32. National Kidney Foundation. (2013). Phosphorus and Your CKD Diet. Retrieved January 31, 2013, from A to Z Health Guide: http://www.kidney.org/atoz/content/phosphorus.cfm

33. Watnick S, Dirkx T. Kidney disease. In: McPhee S, Papadakis M, Rabow M, eds. Current Medical Diagnosis & Treatment 2012. New York, NY: McGraw-Hill; 2012 [chapter 22].

34. Cannata-Andia J, Fernandez-Martin J. The clinical impact of aluminium overload in renal failure. Nephrol Dial Transplant 2002;17(suppl 2):9–12.

35. US Department of Agriculture and US Department of Health and Human Services. Dietary Guidelines for Americans, 2010. 7th ed. Washington, DC: US Government Printing Office; 2011.

36. Kopple J, Massry S. Nutrition Management of Renal Disease. Philadelphia, PA: Lippincott Williams & Wilkins; 2004.

37. National Library of Medicine. (2010, September). Daily Med. Retrieved April 9, 2012, from NEPHROCAPS: http://dailymed.nlm.nih.gov/dailymed/drugInfo.cfm?id=24001

38. National Kidney Foundation. K/DOQI guidelines on bone metabolism and disease in chronic kidney disease. Am J Kidney Dis 2003;42(4 suppl 3):S1–S201.

39. Academy of Nutrition and Dietetics. (2010). Chronic Kidney Disease (CKD) Evidence-Based Nutrition Practice Guideline. Retrieved January 21, 2013, from Evidence Analysis Library: http://andevidencelibrary.com

40. The Renal Association. Clnical Guidelines: Acute Kidney Injury. Hampshire, England: The Renal Association; 2011.

41. Waikar S, Bonventre J. Acute kidney injury. In: Longo D, Fauci A, Kasper D, Hauser S, Jameson J, Loscalzo J, eds. Harrison's Principles of Internal Medicine. 18th ed. New York, NY: McGraw-Hill; 2012 [chapter 279].

42. Rosmarin D, Wardlaw G, Mirtallo J. Hyperglycemia associated with high, continuous infusion rates of TPN dextrose. Nutr Clin Pract 1996;11:151–156.

43. ASPEN Board of Directors and The Clinical Guidelines Task Force. Guidelines for the use of parenteral and enteral nutrition in adult and pediatric patients. JPEN 2002;6(suppl 1):78SA–80SA.

44. Klein C, Moser-Veillon P, Schweitzer A. Magnesium, calcium, zinc, and nitrogen loss in trauma patients during continuous renal replacement therapy. JPEN 2002;26:77–92.

45. Bajpai S. Nutrition in acute renal failure. Renal Nutr Forum 1998;17(4):1–7.

46. Marin A, Hardy G. Practical implications of nutritional support during continuous renal replacement therapy. Curr Opinion Clin Nutr Metab Care 2001;4(3):219–225.

47. Byham-Gray L, Wiesen K. A Clinical Guide to Nutrition Care in Kidney Diseases. Chicago, IL: American Dietetic Association; 2004.

48. Fiaccadori E, Maggiore U, Giacosa R, et al. Enteral nutrition in patients with acute renal failure. Kidney Int 2004;65(3):999–1008.

49. Barco K. Total parenteral nutrition for adults with renal failure in acute care. American Dietetic Association Renal Practice Group Renal Nutrition Forum 2003;22(2):4–12.

50. Wooley J, Btaiche I, Good K. Metabolic and nutritional aspects of acute renal failure in critically ill patients requiring continuous renal replacement therapy. Nutr Clin Pract 2005;20:176–191.

51. National Institute of Diabetes and Digestive and Kidney Diseases. (2012, February 15). National Kidney & Urologic Diseases Information Clearinghouse (NKUDIC). Retrieved April 10, 2012, from Kidney and Urologic Disease Statistics for the United States: http://kidney.niddk.nih.gov/kudiseases/pubs/kustats/

52. Blue L. Adult kidney transplantation. In: Hasse J, Blue LS. Comprehensive Guide to Transplant Nutrition. Chicago, IL: American Dietetic Association; 2002:44–57.

53. National Institute of Diabetes and Digestive and Kidney Diseases (NIDDK). (2010, September 2). National Kidney & Urologic Diseases Information Clearinghouse (NKUDIC). Retrieved April 11, 2012, from Kidney Stones in Adults: http://kidney.niddk.nih.gov/kudiseases/pubs/stonesadults/

54. Asplin J. Hyperoxaluric calcium nephrolithiasis. Endocrinol Metab Clin North Am 2002;31(4):927–929.

55. Hess B. Nutritional aspects of stone disease. Endorinol Metab Clin North Am 2002;31(4):1017–1030.

10

Skin, Surgery, and Stress: Nutrition in Metabolic Stress, Cancer, and HIV/AIDS

Nutrition Needs for the Metabolically Stressed, Critically Ill Patient

Starvation and metabolic stress both cause deviations in normal nutrient metabolism and alter individual nutrient needs. The chronically starved, hypometabolic patient with mild metabolic stress experiences a reduction in resting metabolic rate of somewhere between 10 and 30%.[1] This reduction in resting metabolic rate is the body's response to lowered energy intake that leads to a decrease in overall energy needs. In starvation, with the absence of adequate fuel (glucose) from carbohydrate, the body makes alterations to utilize fat as a primary source of fuel. Lipolysis, the process of breaking down of fat for fuel, occurs as the body is adapting to conserve lean muscle mass and to prevent valuable protein loss in the absence of adequate intake. Unless this process is interrupted with the gradual resumption of normal nutrition, the chronically starved individual will eventually develop anorexia and/or cachexia.

In the metabolically stressed patient, malnutrition occurs when infection, traumatic injury, sepsis, or chronic inflammatory illness increase nutrient needs beyond the individual's ability to meet those needs. In metabolic stress, nutrient needs are so high that they are often unable to be met with oral intake alone, and in these cases, nutrition support becomes an integral component of treatment. This chapter will focus on hypermetabolic states that increase nutrient needs and will cover the recommended dietary therapies to help offset the metabolic effects that increase energy expenditure and nutrient needs, raise the risk of protein-energy malnutrition, and impair proper nutrient utilization or GI function.

- ■ Nutrition Assessment

Obtaining an accurate weight is of key importance when assessing a critically ill patient. Regular weight documentation tracks fluid and hydration status and is useful for monitoring the effectiveness of restorative nutrition therapies. Because patients are often unable to communicate during critical illness, family members may be useful in helping to determine usual body weight and explain recent weight fluctuations, which can help determine the percent of body weight lost or gained prior to hospitalization. Family members can also shed light on recent and long-term food intake patterns and provide diet and nutrition history information to elucidate the patient's present nutrition status.

Determining Energy Needs

Calorie needs are elevated in metabolic stress. As compared to the healthy state, resting energy expenditure (REE) in sepsis may increase by 50–80% (and can include urinary nitrogen excretion loads of up to 30 grams per day due to muscle catabolism and impaired protein synthesis).[2] Indirect calorimetry is the preferred method for determining energy needs for critically ill patients. Indirect calorimetry has been shown to be more accurate than energy estimations made from predictive equations (see Chapters 3 and 11 for more information on indirect calorimetry and predictive equations).[3] Critically ill patients should be allowed to rest for 30 minutes prior to the measurement of resting metabolic rate.[3]

In the event that predictive equations are used (when indirect calorimetry is unavailable), the Academy of Nutrition and Dietetics Evidence Analysis Project suggests that the Penn State equations are accurate more often than are other equations in both nonobese and obese critically ill patients. The Evidence Analysis Project's Critical Illness Workgroup also recently concluded that the Ireton-Jones (1992) equation and the Penn State equations are the most accurate in obese, critically ill patients.[3] Table 10–1 contains information about these selected prediction equations.[4] Evidence-based guidelines recommend against the use of the Harris-Benedict and Fick equations for determining resting metabolic rate in the critically ill, as they do not provide adequate prediction accuracy. Furthermore, the Mifflin-St. Jeor equation is not appropriate in critical illness as it was designed for healthy people. Despite a lack of extensive validation work on the Swinamer equation, the expert panel of the Critical Illness workgroup recommends that this equation should also be listed among the prediction equations that could be chosen from, and as such, it is also listed in Table 10-1.

In the case of critical illness and obesity (BMI >30), the American Society for Parenteral and Enteral Nutrition (A.S.P.E.N.) recommends permissive underfeeding (hypocaloric feeding) with enteral nutrition (EN). Permissive underfeeding may be associated with lower mortality rates than targeted feedings.[5] In permissive underfeeding, calories should not exceed 60–70% of target energy requirements, or 11–14 kcal/kg actual body weight per day (approximately 22–25 kcal/kg ideal body weight per day).[6] Adult ideal body weight can be calculated using the Hamwi method, giving 106 pounds for a 5-feet-tall male, with 6 additional pounds added for every inch over 5 feet. For females, ideal body weight starts at 100 pounds for 5 feet and five additional pounds for every inch over 5 feet. To determine ideal body weight in adults who are under 5 feet tall, a general rule of thumb adjustment is to subtract 2.5 pounds for every inch under 5 feet in females (retaining 100 pounds for 5 feet starting point) and 3 pounds for every inch under 5 feet in males (retaining 106 pounds for 5 feet starting point).

Table 10–1. Selected prediction equations for use when indirect calorimetry is unavailable.

Penn State, 2003b (Penn State Equation)

Can be used to predict resting metabolic rate (RMR) for patient of any age with BMI <30 or patients who are <60 years with BMI >30

RMR = (Mifflin × 0.96) + (V_e × 31) + (T_{max} × 167) − 6212

See below for Mifflin, V_e is minute volume in L/min, T_{max} is maximum body temperature (in Celsius) in last 24 hours

Penn State, 2010 (Modified Penn State Equation)

Can be used to predict resting metabolic rate (RMR) for patient >60 years and BMI >30

RMR = (Mifflin × 0.71) + (V_e × 64) + (T_{max} × 85) − 3085

See below for Mifflin, V_e is minute volume in L/min, T_{max} is maximum body temperature (in Celsius) in last 24 hours

Mifflin-St Jeor (to be used in Penn State equations)

Men: RMR = (9.99 × weight) + (6.25 × height) − (4.92 × age) + 5

Women: RMR = (9.99 × weight) + (6.25 × height) − (4.92 × age) − 161

Weight is in kg, height is in cm, age is in years

Swinamer, 1990

REE = (945 × body surface area) − (6.4 × age) + (108 × temperature) + (24.2 × respiratory rate) + (817 × V_T) − 4349

Body surface area in m^2, age in years, temperature in Celsius, respiratory rate in breaths per minute, V_T is tidal volume in liters per minute

Ireton-Jones, 1992

Spontaneously breathing = 629 − (11 × age) + (25 × weight) − (609 × obesity factor)

Ventilator dependent = 1925 − (10 × age) + (5 × weight) + (281 × sex factor) + (292 × trauma factor) + (851 × burn factor)

Age in years, weight in kg, obesity: present = 1, absent = 0, sex: male = 1, female = 0, trauma: present = 1, absent = 0, burn: present = 1, absent = 0.

Data from Walker and Heuberger, 2009; Academy of Nutrition and Dietetics. (2012). Equations. Retrieved June 8, 2013, from Nutrition Care Manual: http://www.nutritioncaremanual.org

Determining Protein Needs

Protein needs are heightened during critical illness, but to what degree they are elevated remains undetermined. Protein needs are generally assumed to be in the 1.5–2.0 g/kg/day range for metabolically stressed patients. A.S.P.E.N. guidelines lump protein needs in the 1.2–2.0 g/kg/day range for those with BMI <30, and acknowledge that protein needs may be even higher in cases of burns or multitraumas.[6]

The RDA for healthy adults for protein is 0.8 g/kg/day.[7] General guidelines suggest increasing protein to 1.0–1.1 g/kg/day in minor surgery, 1.2–1.5 g/kg/day for major surgery, and 1.5–2.0 g/kg/day for burn patients. For a critically ill, obese adult patient, protein should be provided at a level ≥2 g/kg ideal body weight per day if BMI is 30–40, and ≥2.5 g/kg ideal body weight per day if BMI ≥40.[6]

Determining Fluid Needs

Fluid needs in critical care are individualized based on factors that include volume depletion, degree of endothelial injury and capillary leak, and varying levels of cardiac and renal function.[3] General fluid guidelines are estimated at 30 mL/kg/day, but hypovolemia, renal status, and cardiac function all necessitate individualization of therapy. It is unlikely that enteral formulas alone will meet fluid needs, and additional water via oral, intravenous, or enteral routes is most often required to meet needs.

▪ Nutrition Support

The timely initiation of aggressive nutrition support helps maximize outcomes in critically ill patients. In patients with a functioning gut, early initiation of EN helps to maintain gut integrity, reduces oxidative stress, and regulates systemic immunity.[8] Gastric access is preferred, but if stomach feedings are not tolerated, duodenal or jejunal access is appropriate when gastric residuals are ≥200 mL on two or more occasions, despite the use of prokinetic agents.[6]

The head of bed should be elevated 45 degrees to prevent aspiration in patients receiving tube feedings. Formulas should be high in protein and low in total fat, with at least 25% of fat coming from medium-chain triglyceride (MCT), and the formula should contain at least 100% DRI of vitamins and minerals as well as adequate amounts of soluble dietary fiber.[9] The Academy of Nutrition and Dietetics makes limited recommendations regarding immunonutrition formulas. The Canadian guideline, guidelines from ASPEN, and European Society for Parenteral and Enteral Nutrition all give more favorable recommendations for these types of formulas based on more recent research findings.[6,9-11]

In critical care nutrition support, the primary goal is to introduce early enteral feeds (within 24–48 hours of hospitalization) in those who are not anticipated to start oral feedings within 3–5 days. Feeds are started at 10–30 mL/hour and then gradually advanced to goal rates within the next 48–72 hours.[9] A.S.P.E.N. guidelines recommend achieving 50–65% of goal nutrition intake by the end of the first week. After the end of 7–10 days, if enteral feeds are insufficient to meet total calorie needs, the practitioner may consider initiating supplemental parenteral nutrition (PN).

Nutrition support and the tolerance of EN or total parenteral nutrition (TPN) must be closely monitored. Complications of nutrition support may be gastrointestinal in nature, may increase the risk of aspiration, and can result in fluid imbalances or hyperglycemia. Diarrhea is the most common complication of EN and may occur as a result of medication, use of hypertonic solutions, or antibiotic use that kills beneficial bacteria.[9] The primary approach to managing diarrhea with EN should be review of the medication list. Initiation of soluble fiber may also be beneficial.

Aspiration risk is minimized by elevating the head of the bed and by treating residuals observed on two separate occasions at >250 mL (when used with promotility agents). Blue dye should not be added to EN solutions to detect aspiration, as the risks of blue dye use outweigh any perceived benefits.[9] If fluid overload occurs, adjust formula by selecting an alternate regimen with different concentration. See Chapter 11 for more information about managing hyperglycemia and preventing refeeding syndrome in nutrition support patients.

Nutrition Needs for the Burn Patient

The nutrition needs for burn patients differ from that of other critically ill populations. To start, the burn patient is generally in good health prior to hospitalization, whereas those hospitalized with other critical illnesses may be preceded by long periods of declining health and nutrition status. Burns initiate a hypermetabolic, catabolic response that can double or triple metabolic rates and can cause up to 20% loss of body protein in the first 2 weeks following the burn injury.[2,12,13] The overarching goals of nutrition therapy for the burn patient are to give adequate calories and protein without overfeeding, to prevent weight loss of more than 10% of admit weight, and to supplement with vitamins and minerals as necessary.[14]

- ▪ Nutrition Assessment

Due to their extremely high nutrition needs, burn patients are often on complex nutrition regimens that may involve oral, enteral, and parenteral feeds. Generally, those with burns of less than 20% total body surface area (TBSA) can meet their elevated nutrient needs with a high-calorie, high-protein meal plan consisting of frequent meals and snacks. Those with greater TBSA burns who are meeting less than 75% of nutrition needs for 3 days or longer with by mouth feedings may require supplemental EN.

While calorie counts are often unreliable in many clinical settings, a calorie count may be a useful tool in assessing whether or not a burn patient is meeting his or her daily goals.[15] Initiating nocturnal tube feeds may help supplement inadequate daytime oral intake. For those with minimal oral intake, enteral feeds may be needed to provide 100% of nutrition needs. In these cases, start EN at 20–40 mL/hour, monitor for tolerance, and advance to goal within 24–48 hours.[14] See Chapter 11 for more information on nutrition support.

Determining Energy Needs

Although energy needs are higher with burns, care should be taken to avoid overfeeding. Indirect calorimetry is preferred in the burn unit as it measures both energy expenditure and energy requirements. The indirect calorimetry results should be increased by 20–30% when dressing changes, surgical procedures, physical or occupational therapy, or routine nursing procedures are taking place, as these activities increase energy expenditure and, in turn, calorie needs.

Predictive equations may be used to determine energy needs if indirect calorimetry is not available. For burns that cover more than 20% of TBSA, give 25–30 cal/kg, or basal energy expenditure times a factor of 1.3–1.4. Other ways to estimate calorie needs are to multiply the Harris-Benedict equation by a stress factor of 1.5, or to use the Curreri equation (an equation designed specifically for estimating calorie needs in burn patients).[14] These equations may be useful, but they have been shown to yield results that differ significantly from indirect calorimetry estimations.[16] Table 10–2 reviews the Harris-Benedict equation and introduces the Curreri formula.

Table 10–2. Predictive equations for estimating calorie needs in burn patients.

Harris-Benedict Equation
Men: RMR = 66 + (13.75 × weight) + (5.0 × height) − (6.8 × age)
Women: RMR = 655 + (9.6 × weight) + (1.7 × height) − (4.7 × age)
Weight is in kg (actual body weight), height is in cm, and age is in years
Multiply times stress factor of 1.5 for burns
Curreri Formula
(25 kcal × kg body weight) + (40 kcal × % TBSA)
For burns covering ≥50% TBSA, use a maximum value of 50%

Academy of Nutrition and Dietetics. (2012). Burns. Retrieved January 22, 2013 from Nutrition Care Manual: http://www.nutritioncaremanual.org

Table 10-3. Tips for increasing protein.

Stir nonfat dry milk powder into whole milk, soups, and stews, and add to hot or cold cereal

Use milk in place of water in recipes when applicable and in oatmeal or hot cereal

Add meat and cheese in soups, casseroles, canned spaghetti sauce, pasta dishes, or vegetables

Add cheese in sandwiches and soups, on top of vegetables or on toast

Try cottage cheese or regular or Greek yogurt mixed with fruit and high-protein cereals

Spread peanut or nut butter on toast, fruit, or celery

Use eggs in salads, sandwiches, and casseroles—the protein is in the egg white

Sprinkle nuts and seeds on salads, mix in yogurt, or snack on between meals

Try canned beans in chili, soups, casseroles, or salads

Determining Protein Needs

Protein needs in burn patients are given at a range of 1.5–2.5 g/kg/day.[2,14] If TBSA is less than 10%, or if an individual is obese, give 1.2 g/kg/day protein.[14] Protein should make up roughly 20–25% of total calories.[15] The number of grams of protein per day should be calculated, and then ascribed to the preferred meal pattern. Spread protein intake out over meals and snacks throughout the day, focusing on high biological value protein such as that found in animal and soy protein. Table 10–3 contains ideas on how to increase protein intake for burn recovery, and Table 10–4 contains recipes for five different high-calorie, high-protein shakes.[17]

Determining Fluid Needs

Burns covering more than 10% TBSA increase fluid needs, and the Parkland formula is recommended for determining fluid needs in these cases. The Parkland formula figures that the total fluid required during the first 24 hours = (% body burn) × (body weight in kg) × 4 mL. With this amount, give half the total amount in the first 8 hours (from the time of burn), give one-fourth of the total amount over the second 8 hours, and administer the final fourth of the total over the third 8 hours.[18] Burns may precipitate widespread loss of fluid into the extravascular body compartments and cause acute kidney injury. This affects 25% of people with ≥10% TBSA.[19] For those who have advanced to oral intake and are not receiving IV fluids, closely monitor fluid intake and urine output to assess adequacy of hydration status.

Table 10–4. High-calorie, high-protein fortified recipes.

Fortified Recipe	Ingredients	Directions	Nutrition Information
Chocolate Almond Milkshake (10 servings)	• 5 cups half and half • 2½ quarts chocolate ice cream • 10 packages chocolate instant breakfast mix • 5 caps full of almond extract	• Blend all ingredients in a blender or food processor until smooth	• Per 1 cup serving • 575 calories • 33 g fat • 55 g carbohydrate • 14 g protein
Cheddar Cheese Soup (10 servings)	• ½ cup margarine • ¼ cup onion, chopped • 1 quart chicken broth • 1 quart evaporated milk • 2 teaspoons Worcestershire sauce • 1 quart cheddar cheese, grated	• Melt margarine in pan on stovetop • Add onions and cook until translucent • Add chicken broth and evaporated milk • Bring to a high simmer on medium heat • Add Worcestershire sauce and cheddar cheese • Stir until cheese is completely melted	• Per 1 cup serving • 402 calories • 31 g fat • 13 g carbohydrate • 17 g protein

Reproduced with permission from Cassens and Eck Mills, 2012, and www.flavorfulfortifiedfood.com.

▪ Nutrition Support

When less than 75% of nutrition needs are met by oral intake after 3 days, initiate nutrition support in conjunction with continued oral trials and meals. EN is indicated in those with ≥20% TBSA and simultaneous mechanical ventilation.[14] EN is preferred over PN, as infectious complications are more likely with PN.[2] Standard enteral formulas are usually sufficient, although added protein from modular sources may occasionally be required to meet individual protein needs. PN should be initiated in burns for reasons similar to that of other disease states. If NPO status is anticipated to last more than 7 days, if more than 70% of the bowel has been resected, if enterocutaneous fistulas are present, if bowel rest is needed for more than 7 days, or if for any other reason EN is not indicated, then the parenteral route is appropriate.[6]

Table 10–5. Shriners burn hospital micronutrient supplementation schedule for burn patients >3 years old, >40 pounds with >20% TBSA.

Multivitamin	1 per day
Vitamin C (ascorbic acid)	500 mg twice a day Give in enteral feeding, as orally administered may cause nausea and vomiting
Vitamin A	10,000 IU once a day
Zinc sulfate	220 mg once a day Give in enteral feeding, as orally administered may cause nausea and vomiting

Data from Mayes et al., 1997.

■ Supplements

Micronutrient needs are elevated in burn patients due to a combination of metabolic changes and losses from the wound site. If oral intake is inadequate, consider between meal liquid nutrition supplements as an additional source of calories and protein. The effects of arginine supplementation are not entirely clear: they appear to be helpful for trauma and surgery situations, but detrimental in sepsis situations.[6,20] Table 10–5 outlines the supplementation regimen used at Shriners Burn Hospital for burn patients aged 3 years and older.[21]

Nutrition Before and After Surgery

Presurgical malnutrition is a marker for poor surgical outcomes.[22] A patient who is malnourished prior to surgery typically requires longer hospital stays, has more nutrition-related complications during and following his or her hospital stay, and is likely to experience a greater number of infections and poor health outcomes.[23] Therefore, a central preoperative goal is to help assure that the patient achieves the greatest nutritional potential going into surgery. This may mean postponing any noncritical surgeries in order to help the patient retain or achieve improved nutrition status.

Proper assessment in the preoperative state helps establish accurate baseline nutrition measurements. Serum albumin levels, in both the preoperative and postoperative states, have been shown to be a better predictor of surgical outcome than other indicators.[24-26] Other useful pre- and postoperative measures include weight fluctuations and C-reactive protein (CRP).[27,28]

In the immediate postoperative state, the sooner the patient can be fed, whether by enteral, parenteral, or oral routes, the better the postoperative recovery process is likely to be.[29,30] If adequate oral intake cannot be established, EN should be initiated, provided the gut is capable of tolerating the formula. If NPO status is anticipated for a period of longer than 5 days, the practitioner should initiate TPN to meet recovery nutrition needs. Care should be taken to maintain good blood sugar control before, during, and after surgery. Prior to surgery, a patient's fasting blood glucose goal should be <180 mg/dL, and those with elevated blood sugar levels should be treated with sliding scale insulin both before and after surgery.[31,32]

Nutrition needs are heightened following surgery. Energy needs can be estimated using REE multiplied by an appropriate activity and injury factor, although indirect calorimetry, as with other critical illness conditions, is the preferred method for determining energy requirements. Protein needs are elevated in the postoperative, recovery state. Generally used protein intake levels for surgery are 1.0–1.1 g protein/kg/day for minor surgery, and 1.2–1.5 g protein/kg/day for major surgery.

Nutrition in Wound Care

A pressure ulcer is defined as "a localized injury to the skin and/or underlying tissue usually over a bony prominence, as a result of pressure or pressure in combination with shear."[33] Malnutrition is frequently associated with the development of pressure ulcers. Published in 2009, results from the National Nursing Home Survey indicate that 11% of nursing home residents have pressure ulcers and that 20% of nursing home residents with recent weight loss also have pressure ulcers.[34] Additional risks for the development of pressure ulcers include high initial severity of illness, history of recent pressure ulcer, significant weight loss, oral eating difficulties, and use of catheters and positioning devices.[35]

▪ Nutrition Assessment

The Wound, Ostomy, and Continence Nurses Society (WOCN) Guidelines for Prevention and Management of Pressure Ulcers stress upon the importance of adequate nutrient, protein, and fluid intake for the optimal healing of pressure ulcers.

Determining Energy Needs

The primary goal of energy provision in wound healing is to provide adequate energy to maintain or regain lost weight.[36] The WOCN *Guidelines* recommend that calorie intake levels should be 35–50 kcal/kg/day.[37] Other general recommendations for pressure ulcers are 30–35 kcal/kg/day, and *the National Pressure Ulcer Advisory Panel* recommends increasing energy level to 35–40 kcal/kg for those who are underweight or at risk of losing weight.[38]

Determining Protein Needs

The primary goal of protein provision in wound care is to provide adequate protein for positive nitrogen and to spare the breakdown of lean body mass.[36] The RDA for protein for healthy adults is 0.8–1.0 g/kg/day, while other data suggest higher levels at 1.0–1.2 g/kg/day for elderly patients.[7,39] *The WOCN Guidelines* recommend that for people with wounds, protein be given in the 1.2–1.8 g/kg body weight per day range. *The National Pressure Ulcer Guidelines* recommend giving 1.25–1.5 g/kg/day.[40] Other studies have suggested increasing protein intake up to 2.1 g/kg body weight per day; however, care must be taken to account for dehydration that may occur with this high level of protein.[41]

Determining Fluid Needs

Fluid intake should be adjusted based on fluid losses, including loss from the wounds, vomiting, diarrhea, edema, and medication use. One approach to estimating fluid needs is to provide 30 mL/kg body weight per day, with a minimum of 1500 mL given per day.[42] *The National Pressure Ulcer Guidelines* recommend giving at least 1 mL/kcal per day, and the recommended nutrition and fluid guidelines from this organization are listed in Table 10–6.[40] Another approach is to use the Holiday-Segar formula for maintenance fluid requirements, outlined in Table 10–7.[43]

Vitamin and Mineral Supplementation in Wound Care

A standard multivitamin/mineral supplement should be given if vitamin and mineral deficiencies are present or suspected.[44] In the absence of deficiencies, increasing supplementation has not been shown to lower risk of pressure ulcers or to help promote pressure ulcer wound healing.[45] Select a multivitamin with mineral supplement that provides as close to 100% DRI for as many vitamins and minerals as possible.

The effect of zinc has been studied extensively with regards to wound healing. One study of 1815 long-term care facility residents found that

Table 10–6. Nutrition and fluid recommendations from *the International Pressure Ulcer Guidelines.*

Calories	30–35 kcal/kg/day
Protein	1.25–1.5 g/kg/day
Fluid	1 mL/kcal/day

Data from European Pressure Ulcer Advisory Panel and National Pressure Ulcer Advisory Panel, 2009.

Table 10-7. Holliday-Segar formula for maintenance fluid requirements by weight.

Weight (kg)	Water (mL per day)	Water (mL per hour)
0–10 kg	100 per kg	4 per kg
11–20 kg	1000 + 50 per kg for each kg over 10	40 + 2 per kg for each kg over 10
More than 20 kg	1500 + 20 per kg for each kg over 20	60 + 1 per kg for each kg over 20

Data from Holliday and Seger, 1957; Academy of Nutrition and Dietetics. (2012). Burns. Retrieved January 22, 2013 from Nutrition Care Manual: http://www.nutritioncaremanual.org

supplementing with zinc in amounts of more than 40 mg/day (as compared to no zinc or smaller doses) actually significantly increased the odds that pressure ulcers would form (after controlling for age, sex, severity of comorbidities, weight loss, diabetes, EN support, and dose and type of zinc supplement used). This may be due to the potential that zinc supplementation interferes with copper absorption in the GI tract.[46] The Academy of Nutrition and Dietetics recommends that if a confirmed or suspected zinc deficiency exists, give $ZnSO_4$ 220 milligrams (50 milligrams of elemental zinc) two times per day, for no longer than 2–3 weeks (to prevent copper deficiency).[36] To date, there has been no conclusive evidence that zinc supplementation promotes wound healing in those who are not zinc deficient.[47]

Arginine and glutamine are two conditionally essential amino acids whose roles have been studied in wound healing. At this time there are no significant data to support therapeutic recommendations for doses of arginine or glutamine in wound healing, although many commercially available nutrition supplements for wound patients contain extra amounts of these amino acids.

Nutrition in Pulmonary Stress

- Nutrition in Acute Respiratory Distress Syndrome

Pulmonary stress initiates a hypermetabolic, catabolic state. Even in an overweight individual with acute respiratory distress syndrome (ARDS), weight loss should be prevented.[48] A secondary goal of ARDS nutrition therapy is to prevent overfeeding, as overfeeding leads to excessive CO_2 production, which further depresses respiratory function. Protein needs in ARDS and acute lung injury (ALI) are estimated to range from 1.5 to 2.0 g/kg body weight per day.[49] Fluid needs are normal for ARDS and ALI, unless another underlying condition dictates a fluid restriction.

There is not a generally agreed-upon consensus regarding the use of immune-enhancing formulas in an enterally fed patient with ARDS and ALI. A number of studies suggest that these patients should receive enteral formulas enriched with dietary fish oil containing eicosapentaenoic acid, borage oil containing gamma-linolenic acid, and higher levels of antioxidant vitamins.[50-52] The Academy of Nutrition and Dietetics' evidence analysis project on the topic states the opposite, maintaining that,

> *"Immune-enhancing enteral nutrition is not recommended for routine use in critically ill patients in the intensive care unit. Immune-enhancing enteral nutrition is not associated with reduced infectious complications, length of stay, reduced cost of medical care, days on mechanical ventilation, or mortality in moderately to less severely ill intensive care unit patients. Their use may be associated with increased mortality in severely ill intensive care unit patients, although adequately-powered trials evaluating this have not been conducted. For the trauma patient, it is not recommended to routinely use immune-enhancing enteral nutrition, as its use is not associated with reduced mortality, reduced length of stay, reduced infectious complications or fewer days on mechanical ventilation."[48]*

▪ Nutrition in Chronic Obstructive Pulmonary Disease

Underweight and unintentional weight loss are common problems for people with chronic obstructive pulmonary disease (COPD). Individuals with COPD who are underweight experience compounded nutrition-related problems, as their condition greatly increases energy requirements. The work required for breathing in COPD may be 10–20 times that of a person with normal lung function. Energy expenditure is elevated as the body works harder to breathe, combats chronic infection, and experiences altered metabolism. Energy expenditure is also affected by participation in pulmonary rehabilitation exercise programs, which can lead to increased fatigue at mealtime, further decrease intake, and increase weight loss. Risk for COPD-related death doubles with weight loss, and BMI of <20 kg/m^2 may be seen in up to 30% of individuals with COPD. Energy needs are even higher during COPD exacerbation. The most accurate way to determine caloric needs in these patients is through the use of indirect calorimetry.

Feeding goals for COPD focus on achieving maximum nutrition with minimal effort and fatigue. Encourage patients to eat slowly, biting and chewing methodically, and breathing deeply while they eat. Put utensils down between bites in order to pace intake. Select foods that are easy to chew and prepare, nutritionally dense, and opt for five or six small meals per day. Drink liquids between meals or at the end of meals to conserve valuable space in the stomach for food. Sit upright while eating and avoid lying down immediately after meals in order to reduce pressure on the lungs.

While the calorie needs are significantly higher in the COPD population, the distribution of macronutrients does not differ much from that

Table 10–8. Nutrition intervention strategies for COPD.

Liberalize diet to encourage oral intake within the parameters of medical priorities
Provide small, frequent, mini-meals, and snacks to help compensate for shortness of breath and reduced oxygen supply to GI tract
Choose foods that are easy to chew, swallow, and digest
Utilize easy-to-prepare whole grains, fruits, and vegetables to achieve fiber intake goals
Include nutrient-dense nutrition supplements or shakes between meals to meet calorie goals
Supplement diet with vitamin/mineral supplement
Exercise appropriate sitting posture and practice sequencing of breathing to increase ease of swallowing and eating
Discourage elimination of milk from the diet; milk is unrelated to mucus production despite common beliefs otherwise

Data from Academy of Nutrition and Dietetics, 2012.

of healthy people. Specific vitamin and mineral considerations involve vitamin C and sodium. As with other smokers, people with COPD who smoke have increased vitamin C needs of 35 mg/day above the healthy, nonsmoking population. This means that male adult smokers need 125 milligrams of vitamin C per day and female adult smokers need 105 milligrams of vitamin C total per day.[53] For people with cor pulmonale and fluid retention, consider limiting both sodium and fluid. If on diuretic therapy, the COPD patient should increase dietary potassium intake. Individuals with COPD are advised to undergo bone mineral density screening, as they are at increased risk for developing osteoporosis.[48] By far, the greatest challenge in nutrition care for COPD, especially in underweight people, is consuming adequate calories. Table 10–8 contains a list of helpful nutrition intervention strategies for people with COPD to maximize intake.[48]

- ■ Nutrition in Cystic Fibrosis

Cystic fibrosis (CF) is a chronic, genetic disease that affects roughly 30,000 Americans.[54] The majority of CF cases are diagnosed in child-hood, and more than 70% are diagnosed by the age of 2 years. Advances in medicine have increased the mean survival age of a person with CF to the late 30s.[55] The pathophysiology of CF causes thick mucus secretions to accumulate in the lungs, digestive tract, and other areas of the body. CF secretions obstruct the pancreas and interfere with enzymatic production. In turn, this impedes normal digestion and impairs nutrition status. In addition to digestive difficulties, individuals with CF also do

Table 10-9. Fat-soluble vitamin supplementation schedule by age for cystic fibrosis.

	0-12 months	1-3 years	4-8 years	>8 years
Vitamin A (IU/day)	1500	5000	5000-10,000	10,000
Vitamin D (IU/day)	400	400-800	400-800	400-800
Vitamin E (IU/day)	40-50	80-150	100-120	200-400
Vitamin K (mg/day)	At least 0.3 mg			

Data from Yankaskas et al., 2004; Borowitz et al., 2002.

not appropriately absorb the fat-soluble vitamins A, D, E, and K, and thickened secretions disrupt liver function and can cause liver damage.

Pancreatic damage causes loss of islet cells and leads to cystic fibrosis related diabetes (CFRD). CFRD has features of both type 1 and type 2 diabetes in that people with CFRD do not produce enough insulin, and they also experience insulin resistance. When screening CF patients for CFRD, test casual blood sugar levels every visit. In those with a casual (random) blood glucose <126 mg/dL, no further inquiry is needed. If casual blood glucose is >126 mg/dL, test a fasting blood glucose; and, if that is >126 mg/dL on two separate occasions, or if a second casual blood sugar is >200 mg/dL, diagnose as CFRD.[56] Once CFRD has been established, short-acting insulin should be used prior to meals and snacks to accommodate liberalized carbohydrate intake (Table 10-9).[57,58]

Nutritional management of CF involves the use of high-fat and high-calorie foods to help maintain ideal weight. Due to increased energy needs and fat malabsorption, fat may constitute as much as 35-40% of total calories in CF, as opposed to 25-35% recommended for the healthy population. For CF patients who are underweight or with a BMI <19 or BMI in <10th percentile for children, aggressive EN support is indicated in addition to oral feedings. Use tube feedings nocturnally to supplement daytime oral meal and supplement intake. Formulas should be nutrient and calorie dense, and will require pancreatic enzyme replacement to be administered before and after feeding. Table 10-10 contains a list of other recommendations for general nutrition principles in CF.[48]

Nutrition complications in CF include hypernatremia due to excessive sodium losses through sweat. A high-salt diet is indicated for all people with CF, as is adequate fluid intake. Dehydration can cause distal intestinal obstruction syndrome, increased risk for kidney stones, and acute renal failure in those on nephrotoxic medications.[48] Other physical manifestations of malnutrition in CF include edema, hair loss, skin rash, and night blindness. Those with malabsorption are at heightened risk for developing zinc deficiency. Test zinc levels to look for zinc deficiency, but suboptimal zinc levels may also be suspected with acrodermatitis enteropathica

Table 10-10. Nutrition recommendations for cystic fibrosis.

Eat three meals and two or three snacks per day
Use pancreatic enzyme and vitamin supplementation
Use high-fat foods and additives as part of an unrestricted diet
Supplement with nutrient-dense oral formulas between meals for extra calories
Promote a variety of fresh and whole fruits, vegetables, grains, and legumes for vitamins and minerals
Give extra salt to replace sodium lost in sweat; particularly important during exercise, hot weather, or with fever
Optimize bone health with calcium, vitamin D, and vitamin K
Supplement with MCT fats if indicated

Data from Academy of Nutrition and Dietetics, 2012; Stallings VA, Stark LJ, Robinson KA, Feranchak AP, Quinton H. Clinical Practice Guidelines on Growth and Nutrition Subcommittee; Ad Hoc Working Group. J Am Diet Assoc 2008;108(5):832–839.

(severe diaper rash), anorexia, and delayed growth. In these cases, start zinc supplementation when deficiency is suspected.[48] The use of pancreatic enzyme treatments can promote malabsorption of fat-soluble vitamins (vitamins A, D, E, and K) and may require supplementation of these vitamins. Further calcium, vitamin D, and vitamin K supplementation, along with weight-bearing exercise, can help prevent bone disease.

Calorie needs are higher due to elevated REE and nutrient malabsorption seen in CF. The energy needs in CF are 1.2–2 times higher than the DRI for age in those who are not growing at normal rates and who are experiencing malabsorption, and they are even higher during pulmonary exacerbations. For those with inadequate growth rates, use the following procedure to estimate calorie needs[48]:

1. Calculate basal metabolic rate using World Health Organization equations:

   - Females aged 10–18 years: 12.2(kg) + 746
   - Males aged 10–18 years: 17.5(kg) + 651
   - Females aged 18–30 years: 14.7(kg) + 496
   - Males aged 18–30 years: 15.3(kg) + 879
   - Females aged 30–60 years: 8.7(kg) + 829
   - Males aged 30–60 years: 11.6(kg) + 879

2. Select the appropriate activity coefficients:

   - Confined to bed: 1.3
   - Sedentary: 1.5
   - Active: 1.7

3. Add disease coefficient to activity coefficient and multiply times BMR

   - Forced expiratory volume in 1 second (FEV1) >80%: [BMR × (AC + 0)]
   - Moderate lung disease FEV1 40–79%: [BMR × (AC + 0.2)]
   - Severe lung disease FEV1 <40: [BMR × (AC + 0.3 − .05)]

4. Calculate total calorie needs estimated from expenditure, taking into account the level of steatorrhea:

   - If pancreatic sufficient (demonstrated by patient on enzymes with coefficient of fat absorption greater than 93% of intake), daily energy requirement equals expenditure
   - If pancreatic insufficient, calculate the coefficient of fat absorption (CFA) as a fraction of fat intake; the daily energy requirement is equal to the daily energy expenditure times (0.93/CFA). (If a stool fat collection is unavailable to determine fraction of fat intake, use approximate value of 0.85 in the calculation.)

Nutrition in Cancer Prevention and Management

■ Nutrition for Cancer Prevention

Despite great strides made in the field of oncology, much remains unknown about the true relationship between diet and the development of certain types of cancer. The World Cancer Research Fund (WCRF) and American Institute for Cancer Research (AICR) maintain that one in three global cancer cases can be prevented, due in large part to changes in diet, weight, and physical activity factors. The WCRF/AICR general cancer prevention guidelines recommend that individuals aim to be a healthy weight throughout life, choose mostly plant foods, limit red meat and avoid processed meat, and be physically active every day in any way for 30 minutes or more.[60]

The *WCRF/AICR's Second Expert Report Food, Nutrition, Physical Activity and the Prevention of Cancer: a Global Perspective* is a comprehensive analysis of the existing literature on diet, physical activity, and cancer. The report summarizes "convincing" and "probable" judgments that link certain factors with the development of particular types of cancer. The authors suggest that there exists "convincing increased risk" of alcohol consumption and the development of cancers of the mouth, pharynx, and larynx, esophagus, colorectal cancer, and both premenopausal and postmenopausal breast cancers. Red meat and processed meat intake show "convincing increased risk" for the development of colorectal cancer, whereas physical activity is linked to "convincing decreased risk" for colorectal cancer. Consumption of fruits and non starchy vegetables garners "probable decreased risk" categorization for cancers of the mouth, pharynx, and larynx, as well as esophageal and stomach cancer. Body fatness shows "convincing increased risk" for esophageal, pancreatic, colorectal, postmenopausal breast cancer, endometrial and kidney cancers. Lactation has been shown to yield convincing decreased risk for both premenopausal and postmenopausal breast cancers. Despite diet and cancer research studies that periodically contradict previous findings, the prevailing recommendation is that a diet high in fruits and vegetables and low in red and processed meats, in conjunction with a physically active lifestyle, appears to be protective against certain types of cancer, and in particular, colorectal cancer.

Health professionals touting the benefits of fruits and vegetables, while warning about the hazards of high red meat and processed meat intakes, has been a hallmark of dietary cancer prevention recommendations for decades. To support this dietary approach, the American Institute for Cancer Research developed a teaching tool called the "New American Plate," which helps consumers put these recommendations into practice. Long before the USDA's MyPlate tool, the New American Plate model emphasized a plate-based approach to promote appropriate portion sizes and ratios of food groups (Figure 10–1). The premise of the New American Plate is that two-thirds or more of the plate should be taken up by vegetables, fruits, whole grains, and beans, with the remaining one-third (or less) comprising animal protein (or nonanimal protein if vegetarian or purposely trying to reduce animal protein consumption).[59]

Despite the earnest efforts of fad diet promoters and supplement salespeople to convince consumers otherwise, there is no one known dietary approach that will outright prevent cancer. Research indicates that the combination of a healthy diet with a physically active lifestyle and maintenance of a healthy weight are the cornerstones of cancer prevention.[60] The WCRF and AICR have outlined 10 general cancer

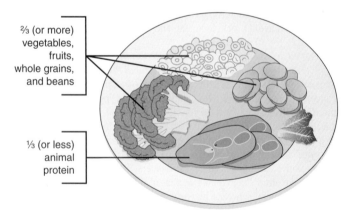

Figure 10–1. The new American Plate. (Data from American Institute for Cancer Research, 2013.)

Table 10–11. Cancer prevention guidelines from the World Cancer Research Fund and American Institute for Cancer Research.

Body fatness	Be as lean as possible within the normal range of body weight
Physical activity	Be physically active as part of everyday life
Foods and drinks that promote weight gain	Limit consumption of energy-dense foods and avoid sugary drinks
Plant foods	Eat mostly foods of plant origin
Animal foods	Limit intake of red meat and avoid processed meat
Alcoholic drinks	Limit alcoholic drinks
Preservation, processing, and preparation	Limit salt intake and avoid moldy cereals (grains) or pulses (legumes)
Dietary supplements	Aim to meet nutritional needs through diet alone
Breastfeeding	Mother should breastfeed when possible
Cancer survivors	Follow the recommendations for cancer prevention

Data from World Cancer Research Fund and American Institute for Cancer Research, 2007.

prevention guidelines based on weight, physical activity, and dietary patterns. One of the most striking inclusions in this list is the recommendation that individuals *not* rely on supplements for cancer prevention. Many patients, and in particular cancer patients, turn to the promise of dietary and herbal supplements to help where traditional medication has failed them. While dietary supplements may be useful in treating established nutrient deficiencies related to poor intake or cancer treatments, they rarely have demonstrated therapeutic effects, and are not a replacement for sound dietary practices or proven medical interventions. The WCRF and AICR cancer prevention guidelines are outlined in Table 10–11.[60]

▪ Nutrition During Cancer Treatment

For individuals who have cancer, nutrition status is affected in various ways depending upon the type of cancer and its treatment modality. Any therapy that interferes with the safe and comfortable ingestion and digestion of food has the potential to disrupt nutritional status. Cancers of the head and neck may result in swallowing difficulty, aspiration, inflamed mucosa, dry mouth, or altered taste and smell. If the esophagus is involved, dysphagia, aspiration risk, GERD, and inflamed mucosa decrease dietary intake. Cancer of the stomach leads to anorexia and early satiety, delayed stomach emptying (gastroparesis), decreased hydrochloric acid production, and impaired intrinsic factor production and vitamin B_{12} absorption. If the intestine is involved, inflamed mucosa and bacterial overgrowth, obstructions, lactose intolerance, nutrient malabsorption, bile insufficiency, and fluid and electrolyte imbalances all are nutritional threats. With pancreatic cancer, nutrition status is affected quickly by deficits in digestive enzyme secretion, bile insufficiency, malabsorption, nutrient deficiencies, and hyperglycemia.

Monitoring weight status helps track nutrition progress or regression with cancer. Maintaining usual body weight or restoring lost body weight is a challenging but important task for cancer patients undergoing invasive treatments that severely impact appetite and intake. If weight loss occurs, explore what underlying causes may be precipitating the observed weight loss. Consider that depression, surgery, diarrhea, nausea, changes in smell or taste, sensitivity to temperature of foods, or anxiety all may be causing weight loss.

Cancer patients who experience a weight loss of greater than or equal to 10% of their usual body weight experience shorter rates of survival with cancer than do their well-nourished counterparts. Weight loss should be documented over time, and in general, nutrition risk increases with weight loss of 5% of usual body weight over 1 month, and/or 10% realized over a period of 6 months.[61] To calculate percent weight loss, subtract current weight from usual weight, divide the difference by usual weight, and multiply the result by 100.

Determining Energy Needs

There are no validated predictive equations that accurately estimate energy needs in cancer. As seen in other instances, indirect calorimetry remains the preferred and most accurate method for obtaining energy needs for cancer patients.[62] In the absence of indirect calorimetry, these general guidelines may be used to estimate calorie needs: 25–35 kcal/kg body weight for nonambulatory or sedentary adults, and 30–35 kcal/kg for slightly hypermetabolic patients, to promote weight gain, during the first month following allogeneic hematopoietic stem cell transplant or for an anabolic patient, and 35 kcal/kg in hypermetabolism or the severely stressed, those with graft-versus-host disease or malabsorption, and for people receiving 75% or more of calories from TPN. For those with elevated calorie needs, Table 10–12 offers high-calorie, high-protein recommendations for meeting increased needs.

Determining Protein Needs

Alongside a reduction in muscle protein synthesis, protein turnover rates increase in cancer. Evidence-based guidelines state that protein needs are elevated beyond the standard 0.8 g/kg RDA for those with head and neck cancer, in those undergoing radiation therapy, and in those with hematological malignancies undergoing allogeneic hematopoietic stem cell transplants. Protein needs are 0.8–1.0 g/kg for normal maintenance, 1.0–1.2 g/kg for nonstressed patients with cancer,

Table 10–12. High-fat, high-calorie ideas to increase intake in cancer.

Add oils, butter, or margarine to foods, soups, and casseroles
Sauté vegetables and meats in oil
Use full-fat condiments such as mayonnaise or salad dressings and cream cheese
Try half and half and cream, whole milk
Snack on nuts, cheese, and eggs, or add high-fat meats to menu items
Drink oral supplements between meals
Consume beverages between meals to increase calorie intake from foods at meals

1.2–1.5 g/kg for those undergoing treatment, 1.5–2.0 g/kg for stem cell transplant, and 1.5–2.5 g/kg for those with protein-losing enteropathies or wasting.[63,64] Protein should be limited to 0.5–0.8 g/kg with hepatic or renal compromise, when blood urea nitrogen (BUN) is approaching 100 mg/dL, or in light of elevated ammonia levels.[65] Track serum proteins such as albumin, prealbumin, and transferrin to monitor nutrition status. CRP may also be a useful biomarker, as it is sensitive to inflammation and may serve as a precursor to cachexia.

- **■ Management of Nutrition-Related Treatment Side Effects**

Cancer treatment can be as vicious to the body as the disease itself. Side effects from chemotherapy or radiation treatments that alter nutrition include nausea and vomiting, constipation, inflammation of the mucosa and mouth (mucositis and stomatitis), smell and taste alterations (dysgeusia), dry mouth (xerostomia), early satiety, and cancer cachexia-anorexia syndrome. The following sections offer suggestions for alleviating these side effects that have the potential to impair optimal nutrient intake.

Nausea and Vomiting

For managing nausea and vomiting associated with cancer treatment, aim to eat six to eight small meals and snacks per day, spread out over the day, in lieu of three larger meals. Some people find that ingesting bland, dry foods such as saltines before getting out of bed in the morning may minimize nausea and vomiting. Stay away from foods that have strong odors; many find that cold foods are more well tolerated than hot-temperature and spicy foods.

Fried foods, greasy foods, and high-fat foods all may trigger nausea and vomiting. Sipping on juices, sports drinks, ginger ale, or clear soda throughout the day will help avoid dehydration while also providing calories. Prolonged vomiting can induce dehydration; during bouts of vomiting, sip on clear liquids as much as possible, aiming to drink an additional ½–1 cup of liquid for each episode of vomiting. Sucking on hard candies can help alleviate nausea. People with cancer who are experiencing nausea and vomiting should work to create a peaceful eating place that is devoid of distractions, and one that is well ventilated to prevent accumulation of food and cooking odors.[66]

Diarrhea and Constipation

If cancer treatment is causing constipation, the same guidelines for minimizing constipation in the healthy population are recommended. Those with constipation should work to increase fluid intake, whole grains, and fiber intake from fruits, vegetables, and legumes. Increasing physical activity can also help alleviate constipation, although exercise may be contraindicated or overly exhausting during treatment. When necessary, consider a bulking agent or an over-the-counter fiber supplement. However, be mindful that fiber-containing foods may be filling and may reduce overall intake. As such, patients should be closely monitored to ensure they are ingesting sufficient calories and not losing weight.

For diarrhea, investigate what may be making diarrhea worse. Medication adjustments or removal of certain supplements may help alleviate diarrhea. Limiting juices, particularly those with sorbitol, can help decrease diarrhea. Foods or beverages that contain sugar alcohols (such as mannitol, sorbitol, and xylitol) will likely make diarrhea worse. On the other hand, sipping on low-sugar, clear liquids can help rehydrate. During active diarrhea, encourage fluid intake of at least one cup of fluid for each loose bowel movement. Provide intravenous fluids if dehydration risk is imminent, and recommend antidiarrheal medications when appropriate. Probiotic supplements may be helpful in those whose diarrhea is related to altered microflora counts from antibiotic use. General dietary precautions in diarrhea are to avoid foods with excess fat, lactose, and simple sugars in them.[63] Chapter 7 contains more information about GI disorders and nutrition.

Mucositis and Stomatitis

Both mucositis (inflammation of the mucus membrane of the mouth or GI tract) and stomatitis (inflammation of the mouth) inhibit the cancer patient's ability to achieve optimal nutrient intake. Those with inflammation of the oral cavity should avoid known irritants such as tobacco, alcohol, spicy foods, and coarse or acidic foods such as tomatoes, oranges, or other citrus foods that aggravate the tissues. Cold-temperature foods may be more well tolerated than hot-temperature foods. Likewise, soft, moist foods may be better than dry, rough, or coarse foods. Sucking on ice chips or popsicles can help numb the mouth area and reduce discomfort during mealtimes. The use of topical and/or systemic analgesics may also be helpful in pain management. The Academy of Nutrition and Dietetics recommends supplementation with zinc at levels of 220 milligrams two to three times per day to help improve mucositis and taste changes that occur with radiation therapy.[63]

Table 10-13. Potential supplements for use in cancer-related mucositis.

Glutamine	May reduce mucositis during cancer therapies
	10 g glutamine 3-4 times per day
	For sore mouth: swish around mouth for 1-2 minutes, swallow
	Not for use with compromised renal or liver function
Chamomile	Believed to have anti-inflammatory, antibacterial, and antifungal properties
	Safe when consumed in food; inexpensive
	Not definitely shown to alleviate pain when compared to placebo
Capsaicin	Substance derived from hot pepper plant
	Known analgesic properties
	Postulated that repeat administration of capsaicin desensitizes and inactivates sensory neurons, giving pain relief
Honey	Ameliorating potential for severity of mucositis for patient undergoing radiation
	20 mL pure honey 15 minutes before, 15 minutes after, and 6 hours postradiation therapy
	Topical application had slight reduction in grade 3-4 mucositis with 54% maintaining or gaining weight

Data from Coghlin Dickson et al., 2000; Rogers, 2001; Berger et al., 1995; Surh and Lee, 1995; Biswal et al., 2003.

Table 10-13 contains a list of other potentially helpful supplements used in managing mucositis.[67-71]

Taste and Smell Alterations

Cancer treatment often disrupts the normal taste and smell of foods. Foods that used to be preferred may become repellent during chemotherapy or radiation. Metallic tastes are particularly heightened during certain cancer treatments. If oral nutrition supplements are consumed, avoid drinking them from a metal can or container; instead, transfer the liquid supplement to a plastic cup, or drink it through a straw to avoid contact with the metallic vessel. Consider plastic utensils if metallic ones are bothersome. Chilled foods tend to be more well tolerated than hot foods. If foods are too sweet, consider adding sour sauces, lemon, or salt to decrease the sweetness. Marinate meats, which are high in mineral content, in fruit juice or sweet wine to disguise any potential bitter or metallic tastes. If red meats are too bitter to be palatable, consider poultry, fish, and vegetarian sources of protein as nutrient-dense alternatives.[63]

Encourage people undergoing cancer treatment to avoid eating their favorite foods unless they are feeling well; consuming favorite foods during times of illness will cause the person to associate that formerly favorite food with being sick, and will slowly (or quickly) decrease the pleasure that was previously associated with eating those favorite foods.

Dry Mouth (Xerostomia)

While dry mouth (xerostomia) may be precipitated by chemotherapy agents and radiation of the oral cavity, other factors may also contribute, including Sjögren's syndrome, dehydration, alcohol, tobacco, medication use, poor oral hygiene, graft-versus-host disease, and the physiology of aging.[72] Oral care protocol should be used to prevent xerostomia: rinse mouth with water and baking soda (1/2–1 tablespoon in eight ounces of water) every 2 hours while awake, avoid mouthwashes that contain alcohol, and brush teeth with very soft head baby toothbrush.

Maintaining good oral hygiene and using a cool mist humidifier over night may help prevent dry mouth. Avoid tobacco, alcohol, and caffeine because they all lead to further dryness. Encourage increased fluid intake and constant sipping of water throughout the day. Other pharmacological agents that may be given prior to radiation to prevent dry mouth include saliva substitutes or artificial saliva that moisten the oral mucosa and facilitate ease of speaking, swallowing, and chewing foods.[63] Additionally, reduce intake of sucrose-containing foods and carbohydrates in the diet that will stick to the teeth and, in turn, increase the risk of cavities.

Nutrition in HIV/AIDS

It is estimated that there are 1.18 million people currently living with HIV infection in the United States. Of these, it is likely that 20% have undiagnosed infection.[73] Each year in the United States, approximately 500,000 people are infected with HIV. With advances in medicine that have led to the widespread use of highly active antiretroviral therapy (HAART) drugs, people with HIV/AIDS are experiencing longer lifespans. As a result, those with HIV/AIDS are increasingly more likely to succumb to the same nutritional pitfalls of chronic diseases that afflict the noninfected population than they are to experience nutrition-related side effects of the HIV/AIDS condition. As such, nutrition therapy with HIV/AIDS should concentrate on the realities of existing comorbidities that are typically seen in noninfected aging groups, such as dyslipidemia, cardiovascular disease, hypertension, stroke, renal and liver disease, and diabetes.

Lipodystrophy syndrome is common in HIV infection and is characterized by high plasma triglycerides, total cholesterol, and apolipoprotein B seen in conjunction with hyperinsulinemia and hyperglycemia. In lipodystrophy syndrome, subcutaneous fat is lost in the limbs and facial region, but is redeposited in the abdomen, dorsocervical, and breast areas. Lipodystrophy affects 33–75% of those with HIV infection who are receiving combination antiretroviral therapy (cART), and approximately 20% of people with HIV-associated lipodystrophy also meet the diagnostic criteria for the metabolic syndrome. See Chapter 5 for nutrition therapy for metabolic syndrome.[74]

Calorie needs are determined using many of the same factors that are relevant to the noninfected population: age, gender, disease state, nutrient status, presence or absence of opportunistic infections, inflammation, medication, or comorbidities. REE may be 5–17% higher in some cases of HIV, but the energy expenditure rates of HIV patients are often similar to that of healthy individuals.[75]

Calorie distribution guidelines in HIV are similar to those for general health. The majority of calories should come from carbohydrate (45–65%), and the diet should be moderate in fat and protein (20–35% and 10–35% of calories from these macronutrients, respectively) and should contain at least 14 grams of fiber per every 1000 calories consumed. High-fat diets should be avoided as they are associated with increased fat deposition (obesity) and insulin resistance. Because of the risk for hyperlipidemia in HIV infection, a diet low in saturated and total fats, and one that includes omega-3 fatty acids should be used to help lower triglyceride levels and possibly raise HDL levels. No more than 7% of calories should come from saturated fat, with minimal or less than 1% of calories from *trans* fat and less than 200 milligrams of cholesterol per day.

The biochemical changes seen with HIV/AIDS lead to anemias, depleted visceral protein stores, protein catabolism, oxidative stress, disruption in carbohydrate metabolism, dyslipidemia, bone mineral density losses, and alterations in micronutrient absorption.[76] Physiological changes that occur with the disease process may negatively impact gut health. The Academy of Nutrition and Dietetics' evidence analysis project on HIV recommends that infected individuals who struggle with diarrhea and malabsorption should increase their intake of soluble fiber, electrolyte-containing beverages, and medium-chain triglycerides (MCTs). The project also recommends avoiding or strictly limiting those foods that make the diarrhea worse.[75] MCT oils, because they are absorbed more rapidly than long-chain fats, produce fewer stools, lighter weight stools, and stools that promote fat absorption. As such, MCT oils are commonly recommended for HIV patients experiencing chronic diarrhea.

Low CD4 cell counts are linked to increased rates of opportunistic infections. Maintaining food safety standards is especially important for people with low CD4 cell counts and, in particular, those with CD4 levels less than 200 cells/mm^3.[75] Fluid needs go up with diarrhea, vomiting, and fever.

Regular physical activity should be encouraged for HIV positive people in whom exercise is not contraindicated. Constant or interval aerobic physical activity, resistance exercise, or a combination of both, performed for at least 20 minutes per session and no less than three times per week, is safe for people with HIV. Participating in activity may also elicit improvements in a patient's endurance, strength, cardiopulmonary fitness, and lower depressive symptoms.[75]

References

1. Heimburger D. Malnutrition and nutritional assessment. In: Longo D, Fauci A, Kasper D, Hauser S, Jameson J, Loscalzo J, eds. Harrison's Principles of Internal Medicine. 18th ed. New York, NY: McGraw-Hill; 2012 [chapter 75].

2. Barbour J, Barbour E, Hermann V. Surgical metabolism & nutrition. In: Doherty G, ed. Current Diagnosis & Treatment: Surgery. 13th ed. New York, NY: McGraw-Hill; 2010 [chapter 10].

3. Academy of Nutrition and Dietetics. (2012). Critical Illness. Retrieved January 22, 2013, from Nutrition Care Manual: http://www.nutritioncaremanual.org

4. Walker R, Heuberger R. Predictive equations for energy needs for the critically ill. Respir Care 2009;54(4):510–521.

5. Arabi Y, Tamim H, Dhar G, Al-Dawood A, Al-Sultan M, Saakijha M, et al. Permissive underfeeding and intensive insulin therapy in critically ill patients: a randomized controlled trial. Am J Clin Nutr 2011;93(3): 569–577.

6. McClave S, Martindale R, Vanek V, McCarthy M, Roberts P, Taylor B, et al. Guidelines for the provision and assessment of nutrition support therapy in the adult critically ill patient: Society of Critical Care Medicine (SCCM) and American Society for Parenteral and Enteral Nutrition (A.S.P.E.N.). JPEN 2009;33(3):277–316.

7. Institute of Medicine. Dietary Reference Intakes for Energy, Carbohydrate, Fiber, Fat, Fatty Acids, Cholesterol, Protein, and Amino Acids (Macronutrients). Washington, DC: National Academies Press; 2005.

8. Heyland D, McClave S. Nutrition in the critically ill. In: Hall J, Schmidt G, Woods L, eds. Principles of Critical Care. 3rd ed. New York, NY: McGraw-Hill; 2005 [chapter 11].

9. Academy of Nutrition and Dietetics. (2012). Recommendations Summary: Critical Illness (CI). Retrieved January 22, 2013, from Evidence Analysis Library: http://andevidencelibrary.com

10. Heyland D, Dhaliwal R, Drover J, Gramlich L, Dodek P. Canadian clinical practice guidelines for nutrition support in mechanically ventilated, critically ill adult patients. JPEN J Parenter Enteral Nutr 2003;27(5):355–373.

11. Kreymann K, Berger M, Deutz N, Hiesmayr M, Jolliet P, Kazandjiev G, et al. ESPEN guidelines on enteral nutrition: intensive care. Clin Nutr 2006; 25:210–223.

12. Rodriguez N, Jeschke M, Williams F, Kamolz L, Herndon D. Nutrition in burns: Galveston contributions. JPEN J Parenter Enteral Nutr 2001;35(6):704–714.

13. Chan M, Chan G. Nutritional therapy for burns in children and adults. Nutrition 2009;25:261–269.

14. Academy of Nutrition and Dietetics. (2012). Burns. Retrieved January 22, 2013, from Nutrition Care Manual: http://www.nutritioncaremanual.org

15. Mayes T, Gottschlich M. Burns. In: Matarese L, Gottschlich M, eds. Contemporary Nutrition Support Practice. Philadelphia, PA: WB Saunders Co; 2003:595–615.

16. Dickerson R, Gervasio J, Riley M, Murrell J, Hickerson W, Kudsk K, et al. Accuracy of predictive methods to estimate resting energy expenditure of thermally injured patients. JPEN J Parenter Enteral Nutr 2002;26:17–29.

17. Cassens D, Eck Mills L. Flavorful Fortified Food: Recipes to Enrich Life. La Habra, CA: Cassens Associates and Dynamic Communication Services; 2012.

18. Gomella L, Haist S. Fluids and electrolytes. In: Gomella L, Haist S, eds. Clinician's Pocket Reference: The Scut Monkey. 11th ed. New York, NY: McGraw-Hill; 2012 [chapter 9].

19. Walkar S, Bonventre J. Acute kidney injury. In: Longo D, Fauci A, Kasper D, Hauser S, Jameson J, Loscalzo J, eds. Harrison's Principles of Internal Medicine. 18th ed. New York, NY: McGraw-Hill; 2012 [chapter 279].

20. Zaloga G, Siddiqui R, Terry C, Marik P. Arginine: mediator or modulator of sepsis? Nutr Clin Pract 2004;19:201–215.

21. Mayes T, Gottschlich M, Warden G. Clinical nutrition protocoles for continuous quality improvements in the outcomes of patients with burns. J Burn Care Rehabil 1997;18:365–368.

22. Hill G, Blackett R, Pickford I, Burkinshaw L, Young G, Warren J, et al. Malnutrition in surgical patients. An unrecognised problem. Lancet 1977; 26:1(8013):682–692.

23. Detsky A, Baker J, O'Rourke K, Johnston N, Whitwell J, Mendelson R, et al. Predicting nutrition-associated complications for patients undergoing gastrointestinal surgery. J Parenter Enteral Nutr 1987;11:440–446.

24. Ryan A, Hearty A, Prichard R, Cunningham A, Rowley S, Reynolds J. Association of hypoalbuminemia on the first postoperative day and complications following esophagectomy. J Gastrointest Surg 2007;11(10):1355–1360.

25. Gibbs J, Cull W, Henderson W, Daley J, Hur K, Khuri S. Preoperative serum albumin level as a predictor of operative mortality and morbidity: results from the National VA Surgical Risk Study. Arch Surg 1999;134(1): 36–42.

26. Goldwasser P, Feldman J. Association of serum albumin and mortality risk. J Clin Epidemiol 1997;50(6):693–703.

27. Warschkow R, Tarantino I, Folie P, Beutner U, Schmied B, Bisang P, et al. C-reactive protein 2 days after laparoscopic gastric bypass surgery reliably indicates leaks and moderately predicts morbidity. J Gastrointest Surg 2012 Jun;16(6):1128–1135.

28. Balciunas M, Bagdonaite L, Samalavicius R, Griskevicius L, Vuylsteke A. Pre-operative high sensitive C-reactive protein predicts cardiovascular events after coronary artery bypass grafting surgery: a prospective observational study. Ann Card Anaesth 2009;12(2):127–132.

29. Andersen H, Lewis S, Thomas S. Early enteral nutrition within 24 h of colorectal surgery versus later commencement of feeding for postoperative complications. Cochrane Database Syst Rev 2006;18(4):CD004080.

30. Pruthi R, Chun J, Richman M. Reducing time to oral diet and hospital discharge in patients undergoing radical cystectomy using a perioperative care plan. Urology 2003;62(4):651–655.

31. Schricker T, Meterissian S, Donatelli F, Carvalho G, Mazza L, Eberhart L, et al. Parenteral nutrition and protein sparing after surgery: do we need glucose? Metabolism 2007;56(8):1044–1050.

32. Smiley D, Umpierrez G. Perioperative glucose control in the diabetic or nondiabetic patient. S Med Assoc 2006:580–589.

33. National Pressure Ulcer Advisory Panel (NPUAP) and European Pressure Ulcer Advisory Panel (EPUAP). Prevention and Treatment of Pressure Ulcers: Clinical Practice Guideline. Washington, DC: National Perssure Ulcer Advisory Panel; 2009.

34. Park-Lee E, Caffrey C. Pressure Ulcers Among Nursing Home Residents: United States, 2004. NCHS Data Brief. 2009.

35. Horn S, Bender S, Ferguson M, Smout R, Bergstrom N, Taler G, et al. The National pressure ulcer long-term care study: pressure ulcer development in long-term care residents. J Am Geriatr Soc 2004;52:359–367.

36. Academy of Nutrition and Dietetics. (2012). Wound Care. Retrieved January 22, 2013, from Nutrition Care Manual: http://www.nutritioncaremanual.org

37. Wound, Ostomy, and Continence Nurses Society (WOCN). Guidelines for Prevention and Managment of Pressure Ulcers. Glenview, IL: Wound, Ostomy, and Continence Nurses Society; 2003.

38. Clark M, Schols J, Benati G, Jackson P, Engfer M, Langer G, et al. Pressure ulcers and nutrition: a new European guideline. J Wound Care 2004;13:267–272.

39. Campbell W, Crim M, Young V, Joseph L, Evans W. Effects of resistance training and dietary protein intake on protein metabolism in older adults. Am J Phyiol 1995;268:E1143–E1153.

40. European Pressure Ulcer Advisory Panel and National Pressure Ulcer Advisory Panel. Prevention and treatment of pressure ulcers: quick reference guide. Washington, DC: National Pressure Ulcer Advisory Panel; 2009.

41. Mathus-Vliegen E. Old age, malnutrition and pressure sores: an ill-fated alliance. J Gerontol 2004;59A(4):355–360.

42. Chernoff R. Effects of age on nutrient requirements. Clin Geriatric Med 1995;11(4):641–651.

43. Holliday M, Seger W. The maintenance need for water in parenteral fluid therapy. Pediatrics 1957;19(5):823–832.

44. Bergstrom N, Bennett M, Carlson CE. Pressure Ulcer Treatment. Clinical Practice Guidelines. No. 15. Rockville, MD: US Department of Health & Human Service, AHCPR Pub. No. 95-0653; 1994.

45. Reddy M, Gill SS, Kalkar SR, et al. Treatment of pressure ulcers: a systematic review. JAMA 2008;300(22):2647–2662.

46. Beckman N, Houston S, Hentges D, Boudreau FM, Bender S, Voss A. Oral zinc supplementation, pressure ulcer development, and healing in long-term care residents. Exp Biol 2002;A975.

47. Wilkinson E, Hawke C. Oral zinc for arterial and venous ulcers (Cochrane Review). The Cochrane Library (202).

48. Academy of Nutrition and Dietetics. (2012). Pulmonary. Retrieved January 22, 2013, from Nutrition Care Manual: http://www.nutritioncaremanual.org

49. Schwartz D. Pulmonary failure. In: Matarese L, Gottschlich M, eds. Contemporary Nutrition Support Practice: A Clinical Guide. Philadelphia, PA: WB Saunders; 1998:395–408.

50. Singer P, Theilla M, Fisher H, Fibstein L, Grozovski E, Cohen J. Benefit of an enteral diet enriched with eicosapentaenoic acid and gamma-linolenic acid in ventilated patients with acute lung injury. Crit Care Med 2006;34:1033–1038.

51. Pontes-Arruda A, Aragao A, Albuquerque J. Effects of enteral feeding with eicosapentaenoic acid, gamma-linolenic acid, and antioxidants in mechanically ventilated patients with severe sepsis and septic shock. Crit Care Med 2006;34:2325–2333.

52. Gadek J, DeMichele S, Karlstad M, Pacht E, Donahoe M, Albertson E, et al. Effect of enteral feeding with eicosapentaenoic acid, gamma-linolenic acid, and antioxidants in patients with acute respiratory distress syndrome. Enteral Nutrition in ARDS Study Group. Crit Care Med 1999;27:1409–1420.

53. Institute of Medicine. Dietary Reference Intakes for Vitamin C, Vitamin E, Selenium, and Carotenoids. Washington, DC: National Academies Press; 2000.

54. American Lung Association. State of Lung Disease in Diverse Communities 2010.

55. Cystic Fibrosis Foundation. (2012). What You Need to Know. Retrieved May 1, 2012, from About Cystic Fibrosis: http://www.cff.org/AboutCF/

56. Moran A, Hardin D, Rodman D. Diagnosis, screening and management of CFRD: a consensus conference report. J Diabetes Res Clin Pract 1999;45:61–73.

57. Yankaskas J, Marshall B, Sufian B, Simon R, Rodman D. Cystic fibrosis adult care: consensus conference report. Chest 2004;125:1S-39S.

58. Borowitz D, Baker R, Stallings V. Consensus report on nutrition for pediatric patients with cystic fibrosis. J Pediatr Gastroenterol Nutr 2002;35:246–259.

59. American Institute for Cancer Research. (2013). The New American Plate. Retrieved January 31, 2013, from http://www.aicr.org/new-american-plate/

60. World Cancer Research Fund and American Institute for Cancer Research. Second Expert Report: Food, Physical Activity & The Prevention of Cancer. 2007.

61. Ottery F. Supportive nutrition to prevent cachexia and improve quality of life. Semin Oncol 1995;22(suppl 3):98–111.

62. Academy of Nutrition and Dietetics. (2008). Recommendations Summary: Oncology. Retrieved January 22, 2013, from Evidence Analysis Library: http://andevidencelibrary.com

63. Academy of Nutrition and Dietetics. (2012). Oncology. Retrieved January 22, 2013, from Nutrition Care Manual: http://www.nutritioncaremanual.org

64. Hurst J, Gallagher A. Energy, macronutrient, micronutrient, and fluid requirements. In: Elliott L, Molseed LL, McCallum PD, eds. The Clinical Guide to Oncology Nutrition. Chicago, IL: American Dietetic Association; 2006.

65. Cohen D. Neoplastic Disease. In: Nelms M, Sucher K, Lacey K, Roth S, eds. Nutrition Therapy and Pathophysiology. Belmong, CA: Wadsworth; 2011.

66. Eldridge B, Hamilton K. Management of Nutrition Impact Symptoms and Educational Handouts. Chicago: The American Dietetic Association; 2004.

67. Coghlin Dickson T, Wong R, Offrin R, Shizuru J, Johnston L, Hu W, et al. Effect of oral glutamine supplementation during bone marrow transplantation. JPEN J Paren Enteral Nutr 2000;24(2):61–66.

68. Rogers B. Mucositis in the oncology patient. Nurs Clin North Am 2001;36(4):745–759.

69. Berger A, Henderson M, Nadoolman W, Duffy V, Cooper D, Saberski L, et al. Oral capsaicin provides temporary relief for oral mucositis pain secondary to chemotherapy/radiation therapy. J Pain Symptom Manage 1995;10(3):243–248.

70. Surh YJ, Lee S. Capsaicin, a double-edged sword: toxicity, metabolism, and chemopreventive potential. Life Sci 1995;56:1845–1855.

71. Biswal B, Zakari A, Ahmad N. Topical application of honey in the management of radiation mucositis: a preliminary study. Support Care Cancer 2003;11(4):242–248.

72. Strohl R. Stomatitis/xerostomia. In: Camp-Sorell D, Hawkins RA, eds. Clinical Manual for the Oncology Advanced Practice Nurse. Pittsburgh, PA: Oncology Nursing Press, Inc; 2002.

73. Centers for Disease Control and Prevention. HIV Surveillance – United States - 1981-2008. Morbidity and Mortality Weekly Report (MMWR) 60(21):689–693.

74. Fauci A, Lane H. Human immunodeficiency virus disease: AIDS and related disorders. In: Longo D, Fauci A, Kasper D, Hauser S, Jameson J, Loscalzo J, eds. Harrison's Principles of Internal Medicine. New York, NY: McGraw-Hill; 2012 [chapter 189].

75. Academy of Nutrition and Dietetics. (2011). Recommendations Summary: HIV/AIDS. Retrieved January 22, 2013, from Evidence Analysis Library: http://andevidencelibrary.com

76. Academy of Nutrition and Dietetics. (2012). HIV/AIDS. Retrieved January 22, 2013, from Nutrition Care Manual: http://www.nutritioncaremanual.org

11

When Food Won't Do: Nutrition Support

Populations and Medical Conditions as Indicators for Adult Nutrition Support

As the previous chapters in this book have hopefully established, in many medical settings, but particularly in the critical care environment, the importance of evidence-based diet therapy cannot be overstated. Nutrition support in the critically ill population was once regarded as mere adjunctive care to support the patient with exogenous fuels during the catabolic stress response. Today, however, nutrition support is viewed increasingly as a proactive therapy, due in part to our greater understanding of the molecular and biological effects of nutrients in reducing disease severity and complications, reducing length of stay and associated costs in the intensive care unit, and promoting overall favorable patient outcomes.[1,2] Table 11–1 illustrates past nutrition support objectives as they compare to today's more proactive nutrition support stance.[1]

Although a critically ill adult patient does not represent anything close to a homogenous population, many will require nutrition support during the critical care period. Medical and surgical conditions that are appropriate for nutrition support in the critical care setting may include (but are not limited to) sepsis and systematic inflammatory response syndrome (SIRS), trauma, head injury, pancreatitis, respiratory failure, neurological injury, burns, and multiorgan failure.[2]

Catabolic illness alters nutritional needs as well as disrupts fluid balance, leading to an overall reduction in body fat and overall body cell mass, which compounds the complexity of nutrition assessment. A thorough nutritional assessment is indicated with a weight loss of just 10% compared to usual body weight. With an unintentional weight loss of 10–20%, moderate protein-energy malnutrition can occur, with severe malnutrition likely being present when weight loss is greater than 20%. Traditional nutrition assessment tools (eg, albumin, prealbumin, and anthropometry) have not been validated for use in the critical care setting. Consequently, nutritional assessment parameters prior to initiation of nutrition support should be based on the following parameters[1,2]:

- Magnitude of weight loss and/or deviation from usual body weight
- Presence of excess fluid or dehydration
- Delayed expectations for taking in food by the usual oral route

Table 11–1. Nutrition support goals: past and present.

Past Nutrition Support Goals	Present Nutrition Support Goals
Preserve lean body mass	Attenuate the metabolic stress response
Maintain immune function	Prevent oxidative cellular injury
Avert metabolic complications	Favorably modulate the immune response

Data from McClave et al., 2009.

- Previous nutrient intake prior to admission
- Level of disease severity and comorbid conditions
- Function of the GI tract

Energy Assessment

Accurate assessment of energy requirements is crucial for critically ill ICU patients. Chapters 3 and 10 have covered how an advanced practice nurse can set realistic weight goals, and how a clinician can determine energy needs for both a healthy and a critically ill individual. Many of the same principles apply when assessing energy needs in a patient who is on or is about to begin nutrition support, although obtaining accurate weight may be challenging if fluid imbalance or malnutrition prior to admission is an issue.

As a review, remember that indirect calorimetry is the preferred and recommended method for determining resting metabolic rate (RMR), and that indirect calorimetry is more accurate than RMR predictive equations. The Academy of Nutrition and Dietetics Evidence Analysis Project's Critical Illness Workgroup has determined that the Ireton-Jones (1992) and Penn State (2003b, aka the Modified Penn State Equation) equations are the most accurate for use in obese, critically ill patients.[2] Table 10-1 in Chapter 10 contains the Ireton-Jones (1992) and Penn State (2003b) equations, while Table 3–5 in Chapter 3 lists the conditions that are required for an indirect calorimetry measurement to achieve a resting state and an accurate test of RMR. Table 11–2 includes additional conditions required for an indirect calorimetry measurement for a critically ill patient in the ICU setting who is receiving nutrition support.[2]

The "kcal/kg/day" method for determining estimated energy needs has been covered previously in Chapters 3 and 10. When using this method of estimation, the practitioner should use clinical judgment and take into account the patient's weight status and goals, age, sex, level of physical activity, and metabolic stressors, all of which may impact actual

Table 11–2. Optimal conditions for indirect calorimetry measurement to achieve a resting state and an accurate test of RMR for the critically ill patient on nutrition support.

Conditions Affecting RMR	Control of Condition
IV, enteral formula, or parenteral nutrition solution (thermic effect of food [TEF]) *Note: Measuring RMR during the time of the TEF will produce inaccurately high values*	Rate and concentration should remain unchanged during the 24-hour period before and during the RMR measurement; since after a 24-hour equilibration the impact of TEF on RMR is constant, the RMR measurement can proceed
Intermittent enteral feeding >400 kcal per feeding (thermic effect of food [TEF])	Hold feedings for a minimum of 5 hours before measuring RMR (if a 5-hour fast is not clinically feasible, or when <400 kcal is being given, a 4-hour fast is allowed)
Nursing activity or medical procedure (eg, suctioning, wound care, ventilator setting changes, or central venous access)	Allow a 30-minute rest period after procedures to achieve a resting state during RMR measurement
Peritoneal and hemodialysis procedures *Note: Removes CO_2 during treatment and requires a few hours after treatment for acid-base to stabilize*	Measurement should not occur during or <4 hours after treatments
Patients with rapidly changing clinical course (eg, hemodynamic instability, spiking fevers, immediate postoperative status, and ventilator weaning)	RMR measures should be done more frequently
Steady-state interval and measurement duration	For ventilated patients, if a steady state is achieved, then a single measurement is accurate. To achieve a steady state, discard the first 5-minute period with CV = 5% for O_2 consumption and CO_2 production; alternate protocol: 25 minutes in duration if a CV of 10% is achieved (if proper attention is given to achieving resting conditions, ≥80% of RMR measures in ventilator patients will be in steady state). Steady-state measures are improved if the patient is sedated
Nonsteady-state measurement	Interpret results carefully For chronic (eg, patient posturing): higher measures may reflect actual energy expenditure For episodic (ventilator change, nursing intervention, anxiety, coughing, sneezing, and movement): take RMR measurement at another time

Data from Academy of Nutrition and Dietetics, 2003.

Table 11–3. Kcal/kg/day recommended to estimate energy needs for selected health conditions.

Health Condition	Kcal/Kg/Day
Chronic kidney disease and post kidney transplant (after surgical recovery)	23–35 kcal/kg/day
Hematologic malignancies-hematopoietic stem cell transplant (HCT)	30–35 kcal/kg/day 1st month post HCT *(may be higher during acute graft-vs-host disease (GVHD) and/or for patients receiving >75% of total daily energy from PN*
Spinal cord injury rehabilitation	Quadriplegia: 22.7 kcal/kg/day Paraplegia: 27.9 kcal/kg/day

Data from Academy of Nutrition and Dietetics, 2012.

energy needs. Table 11–3 provides the evidence-based kcal/kg/day recommendations for energy estimation for selected health conditions.[2,3]

Enteral versus Parenteral Nutrition

For critically ill patients who are unable to maintain volitional oral intake, early enteral nutrition (EN) support should be initiated to ensure appropriate macro- and micronutrient delivery. Meticulous glycemic control is a secondary yet equally important goal of therapeutic nutrition provision. The quick initiation with proper nutrient distribution has the greatest potential to favorably modulate the stress response to critical illness, and to promote optimal patient outcomes.[1]

The enteral route is the preferred method of nutrition support in the ICU patient who is hemodynamically stable and has a functional gastrointestinal tract. EN support results in less sepsis and fewer infectious complications than parenteral nutrition (PN). EN discourages bacterial translocation by preventing atrophy of the intestinal villi, and helps to maintain a normal gut mucosal barrier. When compared with PN, EN support is safer, is correlated with better patient outcomes, and is associated with significant healthcare savings.[2]

PN should only be used when the GI tract is nonfunctional, as a result of physical (severe bowel syndrome) or physiologic (chronic intestinal pseudo-obstruction) events.[4] If the GI tract is functional, but not accessible due to anatomical or pathophysiologic circumstances, then it is appropriate to use PN. However, due to the variety of surgical and nonsurgical options for placing feeding tubes, these situations rarely occur.[4]

Because of the nonvolitional nature of nutrition support (meaning that the practitioner, not the patient, controls both the nutrient composition and the amount of nutrients provided), it is vital that the practitioner pays close attention to the formulas or solutions that are recommended or ordered for the patient. Different clinical settings will employ the use of different formulas and formularies. In most cases, it will be prudent for the advanced practice nurse to refer nutrition support decisions to the nutrition support team, a multidisciplinary group of practitioners dedicated to promoting best practices for achieving optimal health outcomes through the provision of either EN or PN.

Enteral Nutrition

EN involves delivering nutrients through an enteral access device into a functioning GI tract. EN is reserved for those individuals who are unable to take in adequate nutrients via the oral route. A functioning GI tract is one that has sufficient length and absorptive capacity. Although EN is safer and less complex than PN, serious harm and death can result if not properly initiated and carefully managed.

■ Enteral Access

The main considerations for EN access are the anatomical site and the feeding tube size and diameter. The anticipated length of therapy is the main determinant for the anatomical site that is chosen for EN. If the anticipated length of therapy is for less than 6 weeks, then short-term devices and methods are chosen (ie, nasogastric or nasojejunal tubes); whereas, if reliance on EN is anticipated for longer than 6 weeks, long-term enteral access is used (ie, percutaneous endoscopic gastrostomy or PEG, or percutaneous endoscopic jejunostomy or PEJ).[5] The anatomical site chosen and the age of the patient (adult vs pediatric) will determine the feeding tube length used. The internal diameter of the tube will be an important consideration for ensuring ease of enteral formula flow.[5]

Short-Term Enteral Access

For short-term enteral access, the nasal feeding tubes will most often be selected. Oral feeding tubes may sometimes be used, but generally with less frequency. Placing a gastric feeding tube into the stomach is usually easier than placing an intestinal feeding tube past the stomach into the small bowel; however, in critically ill patients, the risk of aspiration or reduced gastric emptying should be considered, even though research has not shown definitively that small bowel feedings reduce the risk for aspiration.[5]

Placement of the tip of the feeding tube beyond the ligament of Treitz is believed in some cases to reduce the risk of aspiration. Special devices can be used to guide and confirm the bedside placement of nasojejunal (NJ) tubes. Larger-diameter feeding tubes (larger than 10 French) are used for short-term gastric feedings because of their ease of placement and management, and because of their ability to be

Table 11–4. Long-term enteral access.

System Accessed	Procedure
Gastrointestinal	• Percutaneous endoscopic gastrostomy (PEG) • Surgical gastrostomy
Small intestine	• PEG with jejunal extension • Percutaneous endoscopic jejunostomy (PEJ) • Surgical jejunostomy • Needle catheter jejunostomy (rarely done)

used for medication delivery and suctioning. However, because these larger diameter tubes are made from stiffer plastics, they are often more uncomfortable for the patient.

Long-Term Enteral Access

Percutaneous gastric or intestinal access is generally obtained for long-term EN. Where the tube enters the body and where the tip of the tube lies are important components of the EN equation. Table 11–4 lists the types of long-term enteral access for the gastrointestinal and small intestine endpoints.

Small-bore feeding tubes (smaller than 8 French) are usually made from softer silastic or polyurethane, and are used for longer-term enteral access because they are generally more comfortable for the patient. Unfortunately, these tubes can be more difficult to maintain due to their softness and smaller diameter; therefore, attention to proper flushing and maintenance is vital when medications are administered through these feeding tubes.[5]

▪ Initiation and Timing of Enteral Feeds

The critically ill patient who has been adequately resuscitated should begin EN therapy within the first 24–48 hours following injury or admission to the Intensive Care Unit (ICU). Although the timing of EN therapy has not been adequately evaluated in published research, it is known that early initiation of EN reduces infectious complications and may reduce ICU length of stay.[5] Neither the presence nor the absence of bowel sounds, nor evidence of passage of flatus and stool, is required for the initiation of enteral feeding in the ICU patient population. Evidence of bowel motility or resolution of clinical ileus is not required to initiate EN support.[1]

▪ Assessment and Monitoring Parameters

Delivery of Energy

The determination of actual daily EN intake should be a major part of the monitoring plan of the critically ill ICU patient. As mentioned, EN should be started no longer than 48 hours after injury or admission to the ICU. During the first week, 60–70% of the patient's total estimated energy requirements should be routinely administered. Fewer days of mechanical ventilation, fewer infectious complications, and shorter lengths of stay in critically ill patients all have been demonstrated when actual delivery of EN support is approximately 14–18 kcal/kg/day or 60–70% of EN goal in the first week of ICU admission.[5] Levels of EN administration that are lower than this may prevent mucosal atrophy, but are not sufficient to achieve the desired endpoints just mentioned.[1]

The practitioner should be careful to avoid under-delivering prescribed or ordered calories, an unintentional yet common practice in the critical care setting because many other factors are known to interfere with the delivery of the enteral formula. For example, when administering some medications, tube feedings must be turned off 2 hours before and after medication administration. This 4-hour hold drastically reduces the amount of nutrients delivered to a patient receiving a 24-hour EN regimen unless the hourly rates are changed to accommodate for the 4-hour hold. Implementation of enteral feeding protocols should be in place in order to increase the overall percentage of goal calories provided.[1]

Obesity increases the risk of other comorbidities in the ICU setting. These may include insulin resistance, sepsis, infections, deep venous thrombosis, and organ failure. Obese medical ICU and surgical patients achieving greater than 70% of goal intake may have less positive outcomes when compared with individuals who received less EN; therefore, permissive underfeeding or hypocaloric feeding with enteral nutrition is recommended in this population. The goal of EN support for all classes of obesity with a BMI ≥30 should not exceed 60–70% of target energy requirements or 11–14 kcal/kg actual body weight per day (or 22–25 kcal/kg ideal body weight per day).[1]

Even if the patient receiving EN is unable to meet energy requirements at 100% of target goal calories in the initial 7–10 days, the initiation of supplemental parenteral nutrition has not demonstrated any beneficial outcomes. Instead, PN will only add to the medical costs, will not provide additional benefits, will not improve overall outcomes, and may actually be detrimental to the patient. Only after 7–10 days on EN support alone, should supplemental PN be initiated, if meeting 100% of energy requirements is not possible.[1]

Delivery of Protein

Ongoing assessment and monitoring of adequate provision of protein is essential in enteral feeding. Standard enteral formulas tend to have high nonprotein calorie: nitrogen ratios and the use of modular protein supplements may be needed to meet elevated protein needs. Protein requirement in the range of 1.2–2.0 grams/kg actual body weight per day for patients with a BMI of <30 is suggested, with higher needs often required in burn or multitrauma patients. For obese class I and class II patients with a BMI ≥30–<40, protein should be provided in a range of

≥ 2.0 g/kg ideal body weight per day, with ≥ 2.5 g/kg ideal body weight per day for class III (BMI ≥ 40).[1]

Tolerance to Feeding

Patient tolerance to enteral feedings should be monitored on a regular and routine basis. Tolerance is determined by factors that include patient complaints of pain and/or distention, physical examination, passage of flatus and stool, and abdominal x-rays. Unfortunately, for approximately 20% of the infusion time, more than 85% of patients have their feedings discontinued for reasons related to medication distribution and procedures. It is important, though, to recognize that more than 65% of the time, these tube feeding holds are avoidable. About one-third of the time holding the feeds is due to intolerance, of which only half of this is true intolerance. In the other two-thirds of patients, the feeding is stopped due to the patient being NPO for tests and procedures, and the other half of the time due to gastric residual volume (GRV) and tube displacement.[1]

Because ileus may be caused by NPO status, in order to prevent inadequate delivery of nutrients and prolonged periods of ileus, the time period that a person is placed on NPO status should be minimized.[1] In general, only half of the calculated daily nutrient requirements are received by patients on a daily basis, due to under-ordering and inadequate overall delivery of the enteral formula (due to intolerance and/or NPO status).

Gastric residual volume

There is a poor correlation between gastric residual volume (GRV) and gastric emptying.[6] Despite a lack of consensus agreement, nutrition support teams (NSTs) and critical care protocols may reflect a wide range of GRV cut-points for holding EN, and evaluating GRV will likely be a component of critical illness evaluation. If GRV is ≥ 250 mL on two or more consecutive occasions, then the EN should be held. When GRV is <250 mL, holding the EN support may only serve to deliver less EN.

At this time, the impact of GRV on aspiration pneumonia has not been adequately studied, and GRV may not be a useful tool to assess the risk of aspiration pneumonia.[5] In the absence of other signs of intolerance, holding EN for GRV <500 mL should be avoided.[1] When assessing the impact of GRV, it is helpful to think of fluid volume in more visually familiar terms. For example, if an EN formula is infusing at 60 mL/hour, this is the same as 4 tablespoons per hour; 150 mL is equal to 5 fl oz, or slightly more than one-half cup.[7]

Gut ischemia

In patients with inadequate mesenteric perfusion, EN has been associated with hypoxia and may promote the development of small bowel hypoxia and necrosis. Signs of enteral feeding intolerance that could indicate early gut ischemia include abdominal distention, increasing nasogastric tube output or GRV, decreased passage of stool and flatus, hypoactive bowel sounds, and increasing metabolic acidosis and/or base deficiency.[1] The Academy of Nutrition and Dietetics maintains that EN should be held if any of the following occurs[5]:

- A sudden period of hypertension
- A need for increased dosages of pressor agents
- An increased need for ventilator support
- Sudden increases in nasogastric output
- Sudden abdominal distention
- Development of abdominal pain

In order to avoid the risk of gut ischemia, the following guidelines have been suggested by the Academy of Nutrition and Dietetics[5]:

- Feed into the small bowel
- Administer feedings into patients when adequately resuscitated
- Administer feedings when mean arterial pressure can be sustained at ≥70 mm Hg
- Consider use of iso-osmolar formulations
- Advance feedings when tolerance demonstrated

■ Potential Complications

Aspiration

One of the most feared complications of EN is the risk of aspiration that can lead to pneumonia and bacterial colonization of the upper respiratory tract. Contamination with oropharyngeal secretions is more likely to be the culprit than is regurgitation and aspiration of contaminated gastric contents. Criteria that can increase the risk for aspiration include:

- Use of a nasoenteric tube versus intestinal feeding tube
- Endotracheal tube with mechanical ventilation
- Age >70 years
- Reduced level of consciousness (use of sedation and analgesic agents)
- Patient position
- Transport out of ICU
- Poor oral health
- Use of bolus intermittent feeding

The following criteria should be considered when monitoring patients for the potential risk of aspiration:

- *Patient positioning:* If not contraindicated, in order to decrease the risk of aspiration pneumonia and reflux of gastric contents into the esophagus and pharynx, critically ill patients should be placed in a 45-degree head of bed elevation.[5]
- *Continuous infusion:* For high-risk patients or those intolerant to gastric feeding, intermittent or bolus feedings should be replaced with continuous or 24-hour infusion of the formula.[5]
- *Promotility agents:* Studies have shown an association between agents that promote motility (such as metoclopramide and

erythromycin) and increased gastrointestinal transit time, improved feeding tolerance, improved EN delivery, and possibly reduced risk of aspiration. Therefore, if the critically ill ICU patient on EN support experiences repeated high GRV or has a history of gastroparesis, addition of a promotility agent should be considered if there are no other contraindications.[5]

In order to reverse the effects of opioid narcotics that are known to decrease gut motility, narcotic antagonists (such as naloxone and alvimopan) may be added to the enteral feeding in order to reduce GRV, increase the volume of the enteral feeding infused, and decrease the risk of ventilator-associated pneumonia.[1]

Gastric versus small bowel feeding tube placement

For most critically ill patients, EN administered into the stomach is acceptable. However, when the patient is in a supine position or under heavy sedation, placing the feeding tube postpylorically in the small bowel is preferable given this is associated with reduced GRV (and possibly a reduction for the risk of aspiration). For patients with >250 milliliters of GRV, or reflux of formula on two consecutive measurements, small bowel tube feeding placement should be considered. Specific disease states or conditions, such as fistulas, pancreatitis, or gastroparesis, may also warrant small bowel tube feeding placement.[2]

Chlorhexidine mouthwash

The use of chlorhexidine mouthwash twice daily in order to promote optimum oral health may reduce the risk of ventilator-associated pneumonia.[1]

Blue-dye use

The addition of blue dye to enteral formulas is not a sensitive indicator for detecting aspiration and should not be used, since it has been determined that the risk outweighs any perceived benefits.[5] Mitochondrial toxicity and patient death have been associated with blue-dye use.[1]

Gastrointestinal Side Effects
Diarrhea

Monitoring for the potential risk of diarrhea is necessary in order to determine the etiology of diarrhea (infectious or osmotic), and to stop its occurrence. Although most diarrhea is mild and self-limiting, the practitioner should first investigate if medications that cause hyperosmolality, such as hypertonic electrolytes, sorbitol-containing sugar-free elixirs, or broad-spectrum antibiotics that destroy commensal bacteria, are being used.[1]

The overgrowth of pathogenic bacteria, such as *Clostridium difficile*, can lead to colitis and secretory diarrhea; however, bacteria normally account for a large portion of the dry weight of stool, and with the destruction of the commensal bacteria, a loss of the solid mass makes the stool more liquid.[5] The following interventions may be considered to assist with reducing diarrhea with enteral nutrition:

- Use a soluble fiber-containing formula in cases of diarrhea, where hyperosmolar agents and *Clostridium difficile* infection have been ruled out as causes[1]
- Add soluble fiber such as pectin, or insoluble fiber such as psyllium[5]
- Add probiotic or prebiotic supplements[5]
- Use an antidiarrheal agent[5]

Constipation

As is also the case with diarrhea, constipation may be caused by medications. Narcotics are the most common medication classification that will contribute to constipation. Water-soluble dietary fiber-containing formulas can also be helpful in reducing the potential side effect of constipation, along with providing adequate fluid.[5]

Fluid Imbalance

If the EN support fails to be integrated with the infusion or intake of other fluids, there is a potential for fluid overload or deficit. Clinicians should monitor for changes in renal, cardiac, hepatic, and pulmonary status, and appropriate EN support adjustments should be made to avoid fluid imbalances.[5]

Hyperglycemia

Optimal patient outcomes for those on nutrition support in critical care are dependent on good glycemic control. As such, the avoidance of hyperglycemia is crucial. There are several reasons why a critical care patient may become hyperglycemic (other than from having diabetes and/or insulin resistance). These may include glucose intake from nutrition support or other sources, steroid use, gluconeogenesis, and impaired glucose utilization due to inflammation and the stress response.[5]

ASPEN guidelines recommend a blood glucose goal range of 140–180 mg/dL.[8] Despite this recommendation, the optimum level of blood glucose for minimizing mortality risk in the ICU is not generally agreed upon. Tight glycemic control (80 mg/dL–110 mg/dL) does not necessarily decrease mortality risk. It is believed that tight or moderate control (140 mg/dL) of blood glucose reduces length of ICU stay and days on mechanical ventilation.[5]

Refeeding Syndrome

Refeeding syndrome is a spectrum disorder that can range from a variety of mild symptoms, to more severe and life-threatening changes in metabolic and organ function. The patient who has not been fed (or not been fed adequately) for a significant period of time has adapted to starvation by switching to fat-based metabolism. The sudden availability of carbohydrates provided with EN causes insulin secretion and increased requirement of thiamine and minerals such as potassium, magnesium, and phosphorus. Because of the rapid uptake from the bloodstream into the cells, hypophosphatemia, hypokalemia, and hypomagnesemia can occur. Heart failure and edema result from sodium and water retention, and a thiamine deficiency can develop that leads to neurological dysfunction, acidosis, and hyperventilation.[5]

Most cases of refeeding syndrome are mild and result in decreases in serum electrolytes that respond quickly to standard repletion regimens, even when EN regimens are rapidly initiated and advanced. As long as electrolyte deficiencies are corrected, cardiac or other complications are not likely to occur in mild cases, and the initiation of EN is not interrupted. Therefore, it is important that the practitioners aggressively monitor the EN support daily and have repletion protocols in place to avoid changes in electrolytes that may occur from refeeding.[5]

In the more severe cases of refeeding syndrome, it is important that the practitioner identifies the patient who is at highest risk for this condition in order to minimize the associated 25% mortality risk, and to avoid any unnecessary interference in the advancement of the EN feeding in the patient at low risk. Treating refeeding syndrome may involve thiamine supplementation (100 mg/day), aggressive electrolyte replacement, attention to fluid and sodium balance, and slow advancement of feeding. Although treatment of refeeding syndrome appears to conflict with the principles of early enteral feeding in the ICU, it is still possible to initiate early EN feeding, but with lower starting rates and slower advancement than in those not at risk for refeeding.[5]

■ Selection of Appropriate Formulas

There are many different enteral formulas available on the market today, the majority of which are gluten and lactose-free. Enteral formulas are classified as standard (polymeric), elemental (hydrolyzed), and/or specialized (disease-specific). In addition, there are modulated formulas with single nutrients (such as protein powders, oils, and glucose sources) and adjunctive therapies (including arginine, glutamine, or probiotics).[5]

The patient's clinical condition and the nutrition diagnosis will be the best determinants of the appropriate enteral formula. A standard, nutrient-intact enteral formula should be appropriate for most patients requiring EN support and should be the formula of choice, provided that there are no contraindications. Specialized and hydrolyzed formulas are always more expensive than standard formulas, and, in many cases, may be unnecessary. Blenderized enteral formulas are more likely to be used in the home setting.[5]

Standard Formulas

Standard enteral formulas comprise intact nutrients. As mentioned, standard formulas are appropriate for many patients, disease states, and conditions. It is not always necessary, and certainly not cost-effective, to use a specialized formula just because one exists for a given condition. For example, a person with diabetes with good blood sugar control is a perfectly fine candidate for a standard formula and will not necessarily require a diabetic formula. The energy density of standard formulas fluctuates between products and manufacturers, but they generally contain 1.0–2.0 kcal/mL.

Selecting a more calorically concentrated formula (eg, 2.0 kcal/mL) is recommended for patients who need less volume, whereas a less concentrated source of energy (eg, 1.0 kcal/mL) is appropriate for those needing standard fluid and energy requirements because they provide a good amount of water in the formula itself. Somewhere between 70 and 85% of a standard formula will comprise water, contributing quite substantially to total fluid intake of the enterally fed patient.

Standard formulas usually contain 30–60% of calories from carbohydrate, 10–25% of calories from protein, and 10–45% of calories from fat. Table 11–5 lists the common sources of carbohydrate, protein, and fat found in standard formulas. For micronutrients, a standard formula will provide 100% of the adult DRI in a given volume of fluid, usually between 1000 and 1500 mL. The formula manufacturer's nutrition information and accompanying literature will say exactly what volume provides 100% of the DRI. Giving multivitamins or specific vitamin and mineral supplements on top of the 100% DRI being provided by the enteral formula volume is often unnecessary and should be reserved only for use in suspected or diagnosed micronutrient deficiencies, rather than as a general practice.

Table 11–5. Macronutrient sources in standard enteral formulas.

Macronutrient	Sources in Standard Enteral Formula
Carbohydrate Standard formulas generally have 30–60% of calories from carbohydrate	Corn syrup solids Sucrose Fructose Sugar alcohols
Protein Standard formulas generally have 10–25% of calories from protein	Casein Caseinates Soy protein Whey protein Milk protein
Fat Standard formulas generally have 10–45% of calories from protein	Canola oil Corn oil Fish oil Safflower oil Sunflower oil

Elemental (Hydrolyzed) Formulas

Elemental or hydrolyzed formulas represent a way to deliver predigested or hydrolyzed nutrients to a patient via EN. Elemental formulas are appropriate for those with digestive or absorptive pathologies that inhibit the normal and healthy digestive process. Elemental formulas tend to be expensive, are used in rare circumstances, and are infrequently indicated in a stable, long-term tube-fed patient. Table 11–6 lists the macronutrient sources found in elemental formulas.

Specialized Formulas

The enteral products market is full of disease-specific specialty formulas. There are formulas for diabetes, kidney disease, hepatic failure, immunocompromised conditions, wound healing, acute respiratory distress syndrome (ARDS), and chronic obstructive pulmonary disease (COPD). The use of these formulas has not been well established in scientific literature, and research papers on some specialized formulas lack external validity and contain methodological concerns that prevent informed decision-making with regards to their use.[5] In other cases, the only published literature on some disease-specific formulas and adjunct therapies has been sponsored by the same company that is trying to sell and promote the product's use. However, in some situations the use of a specialized formula is indicated, particularly in the critical care setting, and for example, with the unique macronutrient needs of the COPD patient (high-fat, low-carbohydrate diet to reduce respiratory quotient). Formulations of these specialty EN products tend to be in line with the

Table 11–6. Macronutrient sources in elemental (hydrolyzed) formulas.

Macronutrient	Sources in Elemental (Hydrolyzed) Formula
Carbohydrate	Hydrolyzed cornstarch
	Hydrolyzed maltodextrin
	May contain sucrose and/or fructose
Protein	Free amino acids
	Dipeptides and tripeptides
	Some longer oligopeptides
Fat	Combination of long-chain and medium-chain triglycerides

Data from Nestle Healthcare. (2011). Products & Applications. Retrieved May 6, 2012, from Peptide-Based/Amino-Acid Based Elemental: http://www.nestle-nutrition.com/Products/Category.aspx?CategoryId=e37cf8a6-4f8d-44fa-adec-b16cd1860f62 general diet therapy guidelines for oral feedings (eg, renal formulas are lower in phosphorus and potassium as compared to standardized formulas). The practitioner should be cautious in choosing an appropriate formula for the specific patient population and diagnosis. The following information on specialized formulas is provided with the understanding that the use of such specialty products should be considered only when the use of a standard formula has been appropriately ruled out.

Immune-enhancing specialty enteral formulas

Immune-modulating enteral formulas are those that have been enhanced or supplemented with agents such as arginine, glutamine, nucleic acid, omega-3 fatty acids, and antioxidants. In certain critically ill patients in the ICU, adding immune-enhancing pharmaconutrients to the enteral formula improves patient outcomes more than standard enteral formulas. These outcomes may include reduced duration of mechanical ventilation, infectious morbidity, hospital length of stay in the ICU, and cost of medical care.[1] Additionally, it should be noted that there has been no demonstrated impact on mortality in published literature, and in some cases, these immune-enhanced EN formulas may actually increase risk of other side effects.[1]

Immune-modulating formulas vary considerably in their make-up and dosage of individual components, and as a result, the use of these formulas should be limited to a select population of ill ICU patients where improved outcomes have been previously documented without risk. Appropriate candidates who are most likely to show favorable outcomes and those where favorable outcome is least likely are listed in Table 11–7.[1]

Standard enteral formulas should be used in patients who are least likely to have a favorable outcome with the immune-enhancing EN formulas. When the immune-enhancing EN formulas are used, it is important to deliver at least 50–65% of the goal energy requirements, in order to receive the most optimal therapeutic benefit.[1]

Table 11-7. Most favorable versus less-favorable outcomes of ICU patients with use of immune-modulating enteral formulas.

Favorable Outcome Most Likely	Favorable Outcome Least Likely
Major elective GI surgery	Moderate to less severely ill
Trauma with an abdominal trauma index score >20	Severely septic
Burns with body surface area >30%	
Hand and neck cancer	
Mechanical ventilation (not severely septic)	

Data from McClave et al., 2009.

Anti-inflammatory lipid profile enteral nutrition formulas

Anti-inflammatory lipid profile EN formulas are fortified with omega-3 fatty acids in the form of eicosapentaenoic acid (EPA), borage oil (gamma-linoleic acid or GLA), and antioxidants. Compared to the use of a standard enteral formula, use of an anti-inflammatory lipid profile EN formula significantly reduced hospital length of stay in the ICU, duration of mechanical ventilation, sepsis, organ failure, and mortality in patients with ARDS, and severe acute lung injury (ALI).[1]

■ Adjunctive Therapy

Probiotics

Probiotics are microorganisms of human origin that may convey health benefits. The potential gastrointestinal benefits of probiotics are introduced in Chapter 7. Some of the proposed mechanisms by which probiotics may aid in health are by competitively inhibiting pathogenic bacterial growth, blocking epithelial attachment of invasive pathogens, eliminating pathogenic toxins, enhancing the mucosal barrier, or favorably modulating the host inflammatory response.[1] Despite the multiple factors in the ICU that induce rapid and persistent changes in the commensal microbiota, the use of probiotics have not yet demonstrated a consistent, beneficial outcome for the general ICU patient population. Probiotics have been shown to decrease infection in transplantation, major abdominal surgery, and severe trauma.[1]

Antioxidant Vitamins and Trace Minerals

Some studies have demonstrated positive patient outcomes with the use of antioxidant vitamin and trace mineral supplementation, particularly in the cases of burns, trauma, and critical illness requiring mechanical ventilation. The antioxidants with potentially beneficial effects include vitamins C and E and the trace minerals zinc, copper, and selenium.[1] Selenium is the antioxidant that has proven the most likely to positively impact patient outcomes and to reduce mortality in patients with sepsis or shock. Note that the patient's renal status should be carefully assessed prior to supplementing the enteral formula with antioxidants and trace minerals.[1]

Glutamine and Arginine

Glutamine is the most abundant amino acid in the human body, and three-quarters of this is located within the skeletal muscles. Glutamine is a nonessential amino acid in healthy individuals, but during stress states, peripheral glutamine stores deplete quickly, making it a conditionally essential amino acid.[9,10] In stress cases involving sepsis or in tumor-bearing hosts, glutamine becomes preferentially shunted as a fuel source in the direction of visceral organs and tumors, respectively. The glutamine-deficient environment in a stressed individual leads to enterocyte and immunocyte starvation.[11]

Arginine is also a nonessential amino acid, and it has gained favor due to its immune-enhancing qualities, benefits for wound healing, and links to improved survival in animal models of sepsis and injury. Arginine as an enteral additive has shown some promise in critically ill and injured septic patients with regards to its ability to promote nitrogen retention and protein synthesis (whereas isonitrogenous diets did not).[11]

Adding arginine, glutamine, and omega-3 fatty acids to enteral formulas has been studied in some clinical trials, but such fortification does remain a controversial practice.[12,13] While not fully understood or elucidated in the literature, supplemental arginine appears to be beneficial in trauma and surgery patients, but may be harmful in those who are septic.[14] Despite the conflicting and not entirely clear picture regarding the effectiveness or recommended use of added arginine and glutamine in enteral formulas, the Academy of Nutrition and Dietetics Evidence Analysis Project has analyzed the use of these adjunct therapies in enteral feedings. As you can see from the "What Does the Evidence Say" section that follows, the majority of the findings from studies that analyzed glutamine added to enteral formulas do not support its use. Less research has been done regarding arginine.

Supplemental Enteral Glutamine and Critical Illness: What Does the Evidence Say?

Regarding infectious complications: The balance of the evidence does not support the use of supplemental enteral glutamine to reduce infectious complications in adult, critically ill patients (Evidence Grade II, fair)

Regarding ventilator days: Evidence does not support the use of supplemental enteral glutamine to reduce days on mechanical ventilation in adult, critically ill patients (Evidence Grade II, fair)

Regarding impact on cost of care: There have been no studies identified to evaluate supplemental enteral glutamine and cost of care in adult, critically ill patients (Evidence Grade V, not assignable)

Regarding impact on ICU length of stay and hospital length of stay: Evidence does not support the use of supplemental enteral glutamine to reduce length of stay in adult, critically ill patients (Evidence Grade II, fair)

Regarding mortality: Evidence does not support the use of supplemental enteral glutamine to reduce mortality in adult, critically ill patients (Evidence Grade II, fair)[15]

If the practitioner does determine that the use of glutamine as a supplement to enteral formula is indicated, glutamine should be given in two or three divided doses to provide 0.03–0.5 g/kg/day. The glutamine powder should be mixed with water to a consistency that allows infusion through a feeding tube without clogging. Modular glutamine should not be added to an immune-modulated formula already containing glutamine.[1]

Soluble Fiber

Although no differences have been reported in duration of mechanical ventilation, length of hospital stay in the ICU, or multiorgan dysfunction syndrome (MODS), supplementation with soluble fiber in the fully resuscitated, hemodynamically stable, critically ill patient receiving EN has been shown to reduce and possibly improve the side effect of diarrhea.[1] No improvement in the incidence of diarrhea has been shown with the use of insoluble fiber. In patients at high risk for bowel ischemia and severe dysmotility, it is necessary to reduce risk of bowel obstruction by avoiding both soluble and insoluble fibers.[1]

Parenteral Nutrition

The normal processes of ingestion, digestion, and absorption of nutrients are completely bypassed with the infusion of PN. PN uses intravenous catheters to infuse nutritive solutions into the vascular space. PN does not stimulate pancreatic secretions and can be initiated in patients with multiple health circumstances, including pancreatitis, presence of fistulas, GI cancers, recent GI surgery with or without complications, short-bowel syndrome, or findings associated with GI dysfunction, as well as nutrition diagnoses including malnutrition, impaired nutrient utilization, inadequate oral intake, inadequate EN infusion, or inadequate protein-calorie intake.[4]

▪ Parenteral Access

There are several types of vascular access that can be used for infusing PN. The type of vascular access will depend on several factors, including projected length of therapy and osmolarity of the parenteral solution.

Central Venous Catheters

In an acute care setting for short-term infusions, single or multilumen central venous catheters (CVCs) are used and are usually placed in a jugular or subclavian vein.[4]

Peripherally Inserted Catheters

Peripherally inserted central catheters (PICC) lines are threaded up so that the tip lies in the superior vena cava after insertion in the basilic, cephalic, or brachial vein. PICC lines are mainly used in the inpatient settings for short-term PN.[4]

Tunneled Catheters

Commonly used tunneled catheters, accessed externally, include the Broviac, Hickman, and Groshong. These catheters have an antimicrobial cuff that acts to prevent migration or movement of the catheter. Tunneled catheters are used when long-term vascular access is required.[4]

Implanted Port

Like tunneled catheters, implanted ports are used when long-term vascular access is required. Although most commonly used for chemotherapy, they can also be used for PN. Unlike tunneled catheters, implanted ports are entirely internal and are accessed by piercing the skin.[4]

Peripheral Access

With lower osmolarity PN formulas, peripheral access can be used.[4] Peripheral PN (or PPN) is usually infused into veins in the extremities. PPN, as with PN via a central vein, contains dextrose, amino acids, electrolytes, vitamins, and minerals, although it is in a more limited capacity and is intended only for short-term use or supplementation.[16]

▪ Osmolarity of Solution

In order to avoid damage to a vein, the infusion of an extremely hypertonic PN formula with a final dextrose concentration >10% must occur into a large vein.[4]

▪ Initiation and Timing

PN should never be initiated on an emergency basis. Prior to initiating PN at any time, the proper route of access, approach for glycemic management, and optimization of fluids and electrolytes should be considered and carefully planned out. In general, initial PN orders may be written with full volume, but with partial macronutrients, or with partial volume and partial macronutrients. Advancement of PN rates should be determined by the patient's status and their nutritional needs.[4]

During the first 7 days following admission to the ICU, if initiation of EN is not feasible, then no nutrition support should be provided. However, after those first 7 days of hospitalization when EN is not available, PN should be initiated in the patient who has no evidence of protein-calorie malnutrition and who was previously healthy prior to critical illness. The rationale for initiating at this point is that a deterioration of nutritional status will occur beyond 7 days with no nutrition support and may lead to a negative effect on clinical outcome.[1] If the patient admitted to the ICU does have evidence of protein-calorie malnutrition (recent weight loss of >10–15% or actual body weight <90% ideal body weight) and EN is not feasible, then PN should be initiated as soon as possible following adequate resuscitation.[1]

Gastrointestinal Surgery

For the patient undergoing GI surgery (esophagectomy, gastrectomy, pancreatectomy, or other major abdominal procedure) who is an ineligible candidate for EN, PN initiation should follow these recommended guidelines[1]:

- Initiate PN 5–7 days preoperatively in the malnourished patient, and continued into the postoperative period
- Delay in the immediate postoperative period for 5–7 days (should not be initiated in the immediate postoperative period)
- Initiate only if the anticipated duration of therapy is for ≥7 days (PN given for <5–7 days is expected to have no outcome effect and may further increase risks)

Inadequate Enteral Nutrition

Supplemental PN should be initiated in the patient who is unable to reach target energy requirements with EN after 7–10 days. Improved outcome is not likely if supplemental PN is initiated prior to 7–10 days, and may possibly be detrimental.[1]

■ Solution Composition

The PN solution is made up of a complex mixture of macro- and micronutrients. If required, certain medications can also safely be added to the PN solution. Practitioners on a nutrition support team generally defer to the pharmacist for ultimate decisions regarding specialized PN solutions.

Carbohydrate (Dextrose)

Anhydrous dextrose is the form of carbohydrate used in PN solutions,[4] and may provide up to 70% of energy requirements in a typical PN formulation.[17] Normally, carbohydrate in food provides 4.0 kcal/g, but due to its physiochemical properties, the energy contribution of anhydrous dextrose in solution is slightly less, at 3.4 kcal/g. Dextrose solution concentrations range from 5 to 70%, which for 1 liter of solution translates to 50–700 grams of dextrose. In order to avoid damage to the peripheral vein, the final PPN solution should contain no greater than 10% dextrose, and for any concentration greater than 10%, infusion through a large vein is necessary.[4]

The minimum amount of dextrose to be provided with PN is thought to be 100–125 grams of dextrose per day in adults.[4] This minimum amount has been shown to meet central nervous system glucose requirements, and to optimally suppress hepatic gluconeogenesis. The actual upper limit for dextrose in PN solutions should be individualized based on the patient's clinical condition, as well as based on estimates of the individual's oxidation rates of glucose. The body is unable to oxidize glucose any faster than at a rate of 5 mg/kg/min.[4] At faster rates, hepatic steatosis, alterations in liver enzymes and fat synthesis, and pulmonary dysfunction secondary to excessive carbon dioxide production from overfeeding can occur.[17]

Protein (Amino Acids)

Protein in today's PN solutions are composed of crystalline amino acids, as opposed to earlier PN solutions where the protein source was in the form of protein hydrolysates. As with protein from food sources, the energy contribution of the amino acid solutions is 4 kcal/g. Amino acid solution concentrations range from 3 to 15%, thereby providing 30–150 grams of protein in 1 liter of solution.[4]

The nitrogen content of different amino acid solutions may vary slightly from one manufacturer to another, but the differences are slight. In addition, although there are slight variations in amino acid solution composition between manufactures, all standard PN solutions are designed to provide both the essential and nonessential amino acids in appropriate amounts, meaning that in most cases, no manipulation of values will be required by the practitioner.[4]

Specialty amino acid solutions are available, but there is little evidence supporting their use. Despite the lack of evidence, products available on the market include solutions with high amounts of branched-chain amino acids and low amounts of aromatic amino acids for hepatic failure, solutions exclusively containing essential amino acid preparations for use in renal failure, and solutions with high amounts of branched-chain amino acids for use in stress and trauma.[4]

Fat (Lipid)

An emulsion of safflower or soybean oil makes up the intravenous fat solutions available in the United States, ranging in concentration from 10 to 30%. The only access for use of the 30% lipid solution is the three-in-one PN solutions, where the three macronutrients are combined in one solution.[4] Due to the glycerol that is used in the emulsification of these lipid solutions, slight variations in their energy contribution result. Because the emulsifying agent in lipid emulsions is egg phospholipid, use of current lipid emulsions should be avoided in patients who have an egg allergy.

Lipids in food provide 9 kcal/g, whereas intravenous lipid provides 10 kcal/g. The energy content of the different lipid concentrations is also altered by the emulsification process, resulting in differing energy distributions depending upon the percent lipid emulsion selected. Ten percent lipid emulsions give 1.1 kcal/mL, 20% lipid emulsions give 2.0 kcal/mL, and 30% emulsions provide 3.0 kcal/mL.[4] Larger volumes of lipid emulsions are important for reaching the energy goals for patients where decreased carbon dioxide production is desired (eg, in chronic obstructive pulmonary disease), as well as for glucose intolerant patients who have indications for reduced carbohydrate (dextrose) intake. In general, lipid emulsions provide 30–50% of the total PN energy requirements.[17] Note that this is significantly different than the typical oral diet that is generally preferred to provide 25–35% of calories from fat.

The recommended minimum amount of lipid solution in long-term PN to prevent essential fatty acid deficiency (EFAD) is 4% of total energy requirements, or 500 mL of 10% lipids (provided as linolenic acid), infused two to three times per week, or 200 mL daily. If there is a pre-existing EFAD, then 8% of total energy should be supplied by linolenic acid.[17] In the United States, because the only available lipid emulsions contain mostly omega-6 fatty acids (which are implicated as contributing to the inflammatory response), practitioners are cautioned to use intravenous lipids sparingly in critically ill patients. In noncritically ill patients, their use is recommended to be limited to 25–35% of the total energy intake, mirroring that of the standard heart-healthy oral diet recommendations.

Energy from fat can be substituted for energy from glucose in fluid-restricted patients; however, it is recommended that in adults, not more than 60% of total energy of intravenously fat emulsions be administered, with dosing no more than 2.5 g/kg per day. In animal studies, hepatomegaly, splenomegaly, and impaired function of the reticuloendothelial system has been seen with the delivery of lipids at levels consisting of greater than 75% of total energy.[17]

Electrolytes

Sodium, potassium, phosphorus, magnesium, chloride, and acetate are included in standard electrolyte packages. Despite standard formulations and PN protocols, the addition of electrolytes to the PN solution should still be individualized. Sodium, potassium, calcium, and magnesium are ions, and to balance these ions, chloride and acetate are needed. The patient's fluid/electrolyte and acid/base status should ultimately determine how the electrolyte content of the PN solution is adjusted.[4]

Interaction between some electrolytes is known to occur, for example, as is seen with the formation of a precipitate with calcium and phosphorus, which depends on the solution's pH and amino acid composition. The role of the experienced PN pharmacist in helping to avoid these complications cannot be overstated, and the pharmacist should be consulted regarding all micronutrient additives.

Vitamins and Trace Minerals

There are standard adult and pediatric vitamin and trace mineral solutions for PN that are formulated to meet patient's estimated requirements. Practitioners can select solutions that include four trace elements (copper, selenium, zinc, and manganese) or seven trace elements (copper, selenium, zinc, manganese, iodine, molybdenum, and chromium).[4] Therapeutic parenteral iron infusion can cause anaphylaxis; therefore, it is not routinely added to parenteral solutions. Instead, oral iron supplementation is the preferred method for iron supplementation.[17] Before iron supplementation is given parenterally, a test dose should be given under strict medical supervision. Hemosiderosis and cellular damage, or an increased risk of infection with patients who are septic, all can occur with excessive iron infusion.[17]

Historically, the use of vitamin K in PN formulations has been a topic of controversy. In the past, vitamin K was not part of the standard vitamin package in a PN preparation because of its known interaction and contraindication with anticoagulant therapy. Today, it is possible to purchase preparations of multivitamins for PN that either includes or

Table 11–8. Recommended daily trace element supplementation for adult PN formulations.

Trace Element	Recommendation in PN
Chromium	10–15 mcg
Copper	0.3–0.5 mg
Manganese	60–100 mcg
Zinc	2.5–5.0 mg

Data from McClave et al., 2009.

excludes vitamin K.[4] Vitamin K, if it is added, should be added on an individual basis, and on a daily or weekly basis.[17] Iodine is also available in parenteral solutions; however, caution of its use is indicated. Sufficient amounts of iodine may be absorbed cutaneously through use of iodine-containing germicides or through oral supplements.[17] Table 11–8 contains recommended daily trace element supplementation for adult PN formulations.[1]

■ Assessment and Monitoring Parameters

When evaluating the patient's needs for PN, the nutritional assessment is based on a number of factors, including past medical history, alcohol abuse, chronic medication therapy, chronic disease, malnutrition, major organ functioning, clinical status (eg, sepsis, stress, wound healing, surgical repair, and GI loss), and tolerance to the PN solution. Ongoing monitoring is necessary in order to measure the patient's response to the PN support, and also to prevent potential risk and complications. It is crucial that clinical and laboratory monitoring protocols be in place for patients receiving PN.[17]

Delivery of Energy

Just as with EN, the initial energy content of the PN solution and its progression is an important monitoring parameter of PN support. Initially, mild permissive underfeeding of PN at 80% of the assessed energy requirements is indicated as the initial goal dose of the PN feeding. The efficacy of PN is improved with this strategy by decreasing the potential for insulin resistance, infectious morbidity, prolonged duration of mechanical ventilation, and increased hospital stay associated with excessive energy intake.[1]

The calculation of energy is evaluated from the carbohydrate and fat components of the parenteral solution, with the ultimate goal to be sparing of protein. In order to prevent negative energy balance, the practitioner's goal is to provide energy as close to possible to the measured energy expenditure. Should indirect measurement of calorie requirements not be possible for the ICU patient, energy requirements should provide approximately 25 kcal/kg ideal body weight per day, while increasing toward the energy target over the next 2–3 days. The minimum amount of carbohydrate required each day is 2 g/kg of glucose.[18]

Delivery of Protein

Protein requirements usually range from 0.8–2.0 g/kg of ideal body weight per day, and are dependent upon the patient's nutritional status, degree of metabolic stress, disease state, presence of unusual protein losses, and organ function. To determine the adequacy of protein intake, nitrogen balance studies may be used.[17] When evaluating PN prescriptions, it is not unusual to omit the energy contribution of protein, since the main function of the amino acids is to provide for synthesis and repair, thus sparing protein from being used as energy.[17] A balanced amino acid mixture should be infused at approximately 1.3–1.5 g/kg ideal body weight, along with an adequate energy intake.[18]

Tolerance to Infusion

The establishment of tolerance to the dextrose load is an important monitoring parameter. Hyperglycemia and/or glycosuria are proof of glucose intolerance and may require the exogenous administration of insulin, either directly added to the PN solution, or via subcutaneous insulin injection, insulin administered intravenously, or modification of the dextrose composition of the parenteral solution, or a combination of these.[17]

Intravenous administration of fat emulsions can also cause potential adverse reactions, such as fever, chills, oily taste, headache, and respiratory distress. Although these occurrences are rare, they generally occur immediately after initiation and are rate- and dose-dependent. To evaluate for the possibility of side effects, a test dose of 1 mg/minute for 30 minutes can be administered.[17] To assess lipid tolerance, triglyceride levels should be monitored in the fasting state before infusion, and again 4–6 hours after infusion. In individuals with severe hypertriglyceridemia, intravenous administration of lipids is contraindicated. Some bodies recommend 300–350 mg/dL as the upper limits of serum triglycerides considered to be borderline hypertriglyceridemia and that would necessitate discontinuation of IV lipids. Alternative guidelines recommend that acceptable serum triglyceride levels are less than 250 mg/dL 4 hours after lipid emulsion is discontinued and less than 400 mg/dL in continuous lipid infusions. Individuals with serum triglyceride levels >400 mg/dL should have their lipid emulsions held.[19] Supplementation of essential fatty acids is recommended in those patients unable to tolerate intravenous lipid infusions in order to prevent essential fatty acid deficiency.[17]

Management of Fluid and Electrolytes

Daily monitoring of PN includes evaluation of serum electrolytes (sodium, potassium, carbon dioxide, chloride, magnesium, and phosphorus), along with the evaluation of blood urea nitrogen and creatinine levels. For patients who are critically ill and/or at high risk for fluid and electrolyte imbalance, during the first 4 days of PN support, electrolytes should be monitored every 4–6 hours.[4] The requirements for electrolyte and mineral requirements will vary depending upon the patient's organ function, disease process, electrolyte and mineral losses, and individual metabolic profile. Patients who are undergoing anabolic treatments that include wound healing and repair, and protein synthesis or growth, may require additional potassium, phosphorus, and magnesium.[17]

Potassium and phosphorus needs are elevated with excessive GI or urinary losses, some medications, insulin therapy, and aggressive refeeding. Potassium and phosphorus requirements may decrease with renal dysfunction, and potassium requirements may also decrease with increased tissue breakdown, or potassium-sparing therapies. Hypoparathyroidism may decrease the requirements for phosphorus.[17]

The need for calcium may be increased in patients with steatorrhea and diuresis, while needs are decreased in those with renal insufficiency. The need for increased magnesium is required in patients who need refeeding, alcoholics, those who require cisplatin and cyclosporine therapy, and who have increased GI and urinary losses. Requirements for magnesium are decreased with renal failure.[17] Average adult maintenance mineral requirements are outlined in Table 11–9.[17]

In patients on long-term PN, or in patients who are malnourished, chromium deficiencies have been caused by hyperglycemia, insulin resistance, elevated liver enzymes, or decreased lipid clearance; therefore, these patients may require increased chromium supplementation. The daily maintenance requirement for zinc may be greatly increased in patients who have excessive zinc losses due to ostomies, fistulas, or diarrhea.[17]

There is no consensus regarding exact trace mineral (and vitamin) requirements; therefore, proper assessment and monitoring of many of these nutrients is required. The practitioner should also consider that only recent intake and not total body stores may be reflected in serum levels.[17]

Table 11–9. Adult maintenance mineral requirements for consideration in PN.

Sodium	60–150 mEq
Potassium	40–100 mEq
Calcium	4–20 mEq
Phosphorus	7–35 mmol
Magnesium	8–30 mEq

Data from McCrae et al., 1993.

Table 11–10. Estimation of patients' maintenance fluid requirements in PN.

Method A
18–55 years old: 35 mL/kg/day
Young, muscular adults: 40 mL/kg/day
Children weighing >20 kg: 1500 mL + 30 mL/kg above 20 kg
Method B
100 mL for first 10-kg plus
50 mL for second 10-kg plus
20 mL/kg for patients younger than 50 years
15 mL/kg for patients older than 50 years

Data from McCrae et.al., 1993.

Additional fluid to prevent hydration is indicated in patients with excessive fluid losses due to gastrointestinal tubes, diarrhea, wounds, fistulas, or ostomies.[17] For patients with fluid retention disorders, due to renal, hepatic, or cardiac dysfunction, further organ failure and overhydration should be prevented with a more concentrated parenteral solution.[17] There are two ways to estimate adult PN fluid requirements, both are outlined in Table 11–10.[17]

Evaluation of Laboratory Data

Because of the known potential for adverse PN outcomes associated with poor glycemic control, blood glucose should be monitored frequently during the initiation and advancement of PN. The frequency of blood glucose monitoring will depend on whether the patient has a history of poor glycemic control, or a pre-existing diagnosis of diabetes, and if so, the type of diabetes the patient has.[4]

The patient's trauma and stress severity will also determine frequency of blood glucose monitoring. During the first 24 hours of PN administration, the capillary blood glucose should be checked every 4–6 hours, with a decrease in monitoring required as blood glucose results return to acceptable levels. All patients on PN, regardless of severity and blood glucose results, should have capillary blood glucose assessed at least daily. Confirmation with serum glucose should be obtained in the event of abnormal values.[4]

In addition to regular blood sugar monitoring, serum triglycerides, liver function tests, prothrombin time, international normalized ratio (INR), potassium, phosphorus, magnesium, and complete blood count (CBC) should be checked at baseline, and routinely followed during the course of PN administration.[4] Abnormal liver function tests are often observed during PN support. Elevations in liver function tests are most likely to occur around the 2-week mark following PN initiation. Often, liver function tests are elevated postoperatively in patients with sepsis and liver disease, and baseline liver function values should be obtained prior to starting PN.[17] In stable, long-term PN patients, laboratory measurements should be evaluated every 4–6 months, and although the evaluation of serum hepatic transport proteins is often advocated for, it is a costly practice that is not supported in the literature.[4]

Assessment of Physical Findings

A physical examination should be conducted daily during the initiation of PN. Elevated body temperature may be an early indicator of infection. If possible, obtaining a daily weight is desirable in order to get a rough estimate of fluid balance as well as to evaluate for trends.[4]

■ Gastrointestinal Complications

PN is not without risks, and the practitioner should be aware of the short-term and long-term potential complications of PN. Proper management can minimize risks, but daily assessing and monitoring for these potential complications is essential. Short-term PN complications include acalculous cholecystitis (ACC), whereas long-term problems that may arise are PN-associated liver disease (PNALD) and metabolic bone disease.

Acalculous Cholecystitis

Acalculous cholecystitis is gallbladder inflammation that occurs without the presence of gallstones. ACC is a rare, short-term complication of PN infusion. Symptoms of ACC include severe upper-right quadrant pain, fever, nausea and vomiting, and jaundice. Surgical removal of the gallbladder is often necessary. In order to stimulate gallbladder contraction, if possible, it is recommended that oral or enteral feeding be given.[4]

Parenteral Nutrition-Associated Liver Disease

Parenteral nutrition-associated liver disease is the most common long-term complication of PN. Normally, it is common to have elevated liver enzymes during the first few weeks of PN infusion, but these values usually revert to baseline without requiring medical intervention. However, continuous elevations of serum liver enzymes and bilirubin can indicate a high risk for liver disease.

Although the cause of PNALD is not entirely known, potential etiologies are thought to involve overfeeding of total energy, excessive infusion of protein, dextrose, or lipid, and/or inadequate infusion of certain amino acids of fatty acids. Because the true etiology is not known, focusing on reducing the signs and symptoms is the treatment of choice. Limiting lipids and protein to no more than 1 g/kg/day and accurately measuring energy expenditure are priority.[4]

Metabolic Bone Disease

Metabolic bone disease is another long-term complication of PN use, and the development of osteopenia caused by reduced bone mineralization is a risk factor for patients receiving long-term PN. Vitamin D deficiency and hypercalciuria are thought to be causative factors. Ensuring adequate amounts of nutrients that are vital to bone health, such as vitamin D, calcium, phosphorus, magnesium, and vitamin K, is the recommended therapeutic nutrition intervention for osteopenia.[4]

Assuring appropriate aluminum content of all PN infusions is an important monitoring criterion because aluminum can interfere with bone remodeling and growth. Although less of a problem today, aluminum contamination of PN solutions has historically been known to be problematic. Those especially vulnerable to the development of aluminum toxicity are patients with kidney disease and neonates.[4] Additional, nonnutrient-based treatments for the prevention of bone loss include promotion of resistance (weight-bearing) exercises, smoking cessation, and possible addition of medications such as Boniva.[4]

■ Nutrient Complications

Refeeding Syndrome

The refeeding syndrome refers to a group of electrolyte disorders that occur following initiation of PN. Refeeding can include hypophosphatemia, hypokalemia, or hypomagnesemia (singly or in combination), along with the development of edema, cardiac, and respiratory abnormalities. In order to appropriately facilitate management of PN refeeding, the practitioner should have a thorough understanding of the physiology of starvation and feeding, as well as an understanding of the patient population most at risk for this condition. Regardless of risk, the practitioner should carefully monitor electrolytes and replace them as needed in all patients receiving PN. Once refeeding syndrome has been identified, many practitioners advance PN slowly, which has the unfortunate consequence of prolonging the time until optimal nutrient provision occurs. The Academy of Nutrition and Dietetics recommends a more preferable approach that utilizes a briefer initiation time frame, with monitoring and replacement of electrolytes on an as needed basis.[4]

Hyperglycemia

Hyperglycemia is defined as a blood glucose reading of >200 mg/dL occurring on two or more occasions. Hyperglycemia is seen regularly with PN, and most NSTs employ a glycemic protocol that advocates for strict blood sugar management, with special attention paid to the reduction of risk for hypoglycemia. Regardless of practice setting, the practitioner is advised to have a protocol in place that allows for the promotion of moderately strict control of serum glucose during PN support.[1]

Reduced sepsis, reduced ICU length of stay, and lower hospital mortality has been associated with strict glucose control (blood glucose levels between 80 and 110 mg/dL while receiving PN) compared to conventional insulin therapy (maintaining blood glucose levels <200 mg/dL). However, compared to tighter control, keeping glucose levels between 140 and 180 mg/dL has been shown to reduce the risks of hypoglycemia, and the subsequent mortality associated with it. Therefore, serum glucose in the range of 110–150 mg/dL has been accepted as most appropriate during PN support.[1]

Essential Fatty Acid Deficiency

The development of EFAD can occur with long-term use of lipid-free PN. In the short-term, healthy adults have adequate lipid stores to avoid EFAD, but alterations in lipid metabolism, and mobilization and utilization of lipid stores may become altered during acute and chronic illness. To prevent EFAD in patients who are not receiving oral or EN feedings while also on PN, the infusion of a minimum of 500 mL of 10% lipids should be infused two to three times per week.[4]

As a result of poor oral intake, fat malabsorption, administration of lipid-free PN, or noncompliance with a lipid infusion regimen, an EFAD can occur. Signs of EFA deficiency include dry, cracked, scaly skin, hair loss, impaired wound healing, and mild diarrhea.[17]

Carnitine Deficiency

Carnitine, which is normally synthesized in the liver, is involved in fatty acid oxidation and transport of fatty acids across the mitochondrial membrane. Because carnitine is not added in PN solutions, patients on long-term PN, malnourished patients, or those with liver and kidney impairment may suffer a deficiency of carnitine due to an inability to synthesize adequate amounts.[4] A deficiency of carnitine has been linked with hepatic steatosis, muscle weakness, and myopathy.[17]

■ Mechanical Complications

Monitoring for both the potential short-term and long-term mechanical complications is important for the prevention of major undesirable consequences associated with PN. Pneumothorax (perforation of a lung), hemothorax (perforation of a blood vessel), and thrombophlebitis (inflammation of the vein) are the most common of the short-term mechanical complications of PN, typically occurring during the insertion of a PN catheter. It is vitally important to confirm proper catheter tip placement by x-ray, prior to initiation of the PN infusion to prevent these occurrences.[4]

Air embolisms represent another potential mechanical complication of PN. An air embolism is a short-term complication that is potentially life-threatening. It is caused by inadvertent breaks in the tubing or connections or by failing to clamp the catheter during connections. When precipitates form in the catheter tip, an occlusion can occur. Flushing the catheters properly, and formulating the PN solutions to avoid precipitation of nutrients is necessary to prevent catheter occlusions. Both local and systematic catheter infections are also problematic and are serious complications of both short- and long-term PN. Local catheter infections result in the usual signs and symptoms of a localized infection, including warmth, swelling, redness, and temperature elevation. When an exit site infection is diagnosed, the prompt administration of an antibiotic may prevent the need for removal of the long-term catheter; however, short-term CVCs should also be removed.[4]

Systemic catheter infections or catheter-related blood stream infections (CRBSI) are usually diagnosed when patients exhibit fever and shaking chills. CRBSI is often difficult to treat; therefore, it is important that blood cultures be obtained and treatment quickly initiated. If intravenous antibiotic is initiated, it may be possible to maintain the catheter integrity, but often treatment is unsuccessful and the catheter must be removed and replaced with another intravenous device. In order to prevent CRBSI, sterile technique is crucial during all manipulations of the catheter. Appropriate dressings that minimize the risk should be used.[4]

▪ Transitioning to Enteral Feedings

The maintenance of an intact gut mucosal barrier is believed to be dependent on the conditionally essential amino acid glutamine, due to its properties for potentially preventing bacterial translocation across the GI tract, and its function in enterocyte proliferation. However, due to its physical instability at room temperature and the potentially toxic substances (ammonia and glutamate) that can result from this instability, current PN solutions normally do not contain glutamine. The long-term use of PN may result in gut compromise and, in turn, delay the return to EN. As a result, gut stimulation as adjunctive therapy to PN, with the simultaneous administration of an enteral feeding at low volume, is a recommended approach.[17]

As mentioned previously, EN is superior to PN with significant benefits over PN; therefore, the practitioner should aggressively repeat efforts to initiate EN in the stabilized critically ill patient on PN. To compensate for the increase in calories that are delivered via the enteral route as enteral feedings are assumed, the amount of calories delivered by the parenteral route should be reduced accordingly, in order to reduce the risk of overfeeding. As tolerance is seen with the enteral feeding and the volume delivered increased, the parenteral feeding should be reduced but not terminated until the enteral feeding exceeds 60% of targeted energy requirements.[17]

With regards to cost, EN formulas are significantly cheaper than PN formulations (and are also considered to be more cost-effective than PN).[20] However, positive outcomes associated with EN versus PN, both before and during the transition from PN to EN, are still dependent on effective management of patient selection, initiation of feeding, and continuous monitoring during feedings to prevent or mitigate complications.[3]

Summary

Assuring adequate and timely nutrition support in the ICU setting is a major responsibility for the healthcare provider entrusted with this task; thus, understanding the implications and principles of this form of MNT by the practitioner is essential. In a study conducted by Braga et al., EN recommendations by registered dietitians (RDs) resulted in 1.5 fewer hospital days, and improved nutritional status, as indicated by improved albumin compared to physician-prescribed EN.[21] Although a team-based approach to nutrition support is still the preferred mechanism for administering this important component of comprehensive care, in the absence of a nutrition support team, the data from this study indicated that patient care improved when RDs had the authority to write nutrition support orders and provide early nutrition intervention.

In the area of PN, the most costly mode of diet therapy available, studies have shown that in 8–38% of cases, PN was ordered incorrectly as a result of inconsistent knowledge and skill base of physicians.[22] Therefore, the primary healthcare provider, whether it be a physician or advanced practice nurse, who does not have the expertise needed to adequately write nutrition support orders, is providing excellent healthcare when they seek the recommendations of a specialist and/or uses a team approach.

In the late 1960s, with the development of PN, NSTs began to be organized by hospitals in order to allow the delivery of timely, safe, and appropriate cost-effective nutrition support therapy by skilled professionals. NSTs traditionally include a physician, nurse, dietitian and pharmacist; however, NSTs are clearly not possible in all institutions because of financial constraints, lack of physician/provider or administrative support, lack of time, or education/expertise. Whether or not an NST is in place in the institution, it is clear that a patient's nutritional status improves, and the safety and efficacy of care are enhanced when dietitians, nurses, pharmacists, and physicians/advanced practice nurses collaborate as a team to provide expert nutrition support.[23]

References

1. McClave S, Martindale R, Vanek V, McCarthy M, Roberts P, Taylor B, et al. Guidelines for the provision and assessment of nutrition support therapy in the adult critically ill patient: Society of Critical Care Medicine (SCCM) and American Society for Parenteral and Enteral Nutrition (A.S.P.E.N.). JPEN J Parenter Enteral Nutr 2009;33(3):277–316.

2. Academy of Nutrition and Dietetics. (2003). CI: Enteral vs. Parenteral Nutrition 2003. Retrieved January 22, 2013, from Evidence Analysis Library: http://andevidencelibrary.com

3. Academy of Nutrition and Dietetics. (n.d.). Equations. Retrieved January 22, 2013, from Nutrition Care Manual: http://www.nutritioncaremanual.org

4. Academy of Nutrition and Dietetics. (n.d.). Parenteral Nutrition. Retrieved January 22, 2013, from Nutrition Care Manual: http://www.nutritioncaremanual.org

5. Academy of Nutrition and Dietetics. (n.d.). Enteral Nutrition. Retrieved January 22, 2013, from Nutrition Care Manual: http://www.nutritioncaremanual.org

6. Parrish C, McClave S. Checking gastric residual volumes: a practice in search of science. Nutrition Issues in Gastroenterology, Series #(2008, October). 67:33–47.

7. Fessler T. Gastric residuals - understand their significance to optimize care. Today's Dietitian 2010, June;12(5):8.

8. McMahon M, Nystrom E, Braunschweig C, Miles J, Compher C, Directors AS. A.S.P.E.N. clinical guidelines nutrition support of adult patients with hyperglycemia. JPEN J Parenter Enteral Nutr 2013;37(1):23–36.

9. National Cancer Institute. (n.d.). Glutamine. Retrieved January 31, 2013, from NCI Drug Dictionary: http://www.cancer.gov/drugdictionary?cdrid=42298

10. US National Library of Medicine. (2011, February 8). Aminio Acids. Retrieved January 31, 2013, from MedlinePlus: http://www.nlm.nih.gov/medlineplus/ency/article/002222.htm

11. Jan B, Lowry S. Systemic response to injury and metabolic support. In: Brunicardi F, Anderson D, Billiar T, Dunn D, Hunter J, Matthews J, et al., eds. Schwartz's Principles of Surgery. 9th ed. New York, NY: McGraw-Hill; 2010. [chapter 2].

12. Gottschlich M, Jenkins M, Warden G, Baumer T, Havens P, Snook J, et al. Differential effects of three enteral dietary regimens on selected outcome variables in burn patients. JPEN J Parenter Enteral Nutr 1990;14:225–236.

13. Saffle J, Wiebke G, Jennings K, Morris S, Barton R. Randomized trial of immune-enhancing enteral nutrition in burn patients. J Trauma 1997;42:73–82.

14. Zaloga G, Siddiqui R, Terry C, Marik P. Arginine: mediator or modulator of sepsis? Nutr Clin Pract 2004;19:201–215.

15. Academy of Nutrition and Dietetics. (2010). Enteral Glutamine. Retrieved from January 23, 2013, Nutrition Care Manual: http://andevidencelibrary.com

16. Gura K. Is there still a role for peripheral parenteral nutrition. Nutr Clin Pract Dec 2009;24(6):709–717.

17. McCrae J, O'Shea R, Udine L. Parenteral nutrition: hospital to home. J Am Diet Assoc 1993;93(6):664–670, 673.

18. Kreymann G. New developments in clinical practice guidelines. South African J Clin Nutr 2010;23(suppl 1):29–32.

19. Adamkin DH, Gleke KN, Anderws BF. Fat emulsions and hypertriglyceridemia. J Parenter Enteral Nutr 1984;8:563–567.

20. Kattelmann K, Hise M, Russell M, Charney P, Stokes M, Compher C. Preliminary evidence for a medical nutrition therapy protocol. J Am Diet Assoc 2006;106(8):1226–1241.

21. Braga J, Hunt A, Pope J, Molaison E. Implementation of dietitian recommendations for enteral nutrition results in improved outcomes. J Am Diet Assoc 2006;106(2):281–284.

22. Vanek V, Sharnek L, Snyder D, Kupensky D, Rutushin A. Assessment of physicians' ability to prescribe parenteral nutrition support in a community teaching hospital. J Am Diet Assoc 1997;97(8):856–859.

23. DeLegge M, Wooley J, Guenter P, Wright S, Brill J, Andris D, et al. The state of nutrition support teams and update on current models for providing nutrition supoprt therapy to patients. Nutr Clin Pract 2010;25(1):76–84.

12

Nutrition as a Complementary and Alternative Medicine

Nutrition and CAM

The roots of complementary and alternative medicine (CAM) can be traced back to ancient Greek mythology, where tales were told of the healing and poisoning powers of plants and herbs. Even Western medicine, as laid out by Hippocrates, was built on principles that are more in line with CAM than traditional medicine, namely, that the body is to be treated as a whole entity, and not just as a series of parts. Hippocrates noted that there were differences in the severity of disease symptoms, as well as in a person's ability to cope and deal with disease and to mediate healing. He theorized that the human body is endowed with an ability of natural healing that is dependent on rest, a well-balanced diet, fresh air, and cleanliness.[1]

Fast-forwarding through the history of medicine, CAM as a theory and field was also espoused by more modern personalities, such as Florence Nightingale. In addition to being credited as the founder of modern nursing, Florence Nightingale is also recognized as one of the first advocates for holistic nursing. Nightingale's core values of healing, leadership, and global action were very much in line with those of many of today's holistic healthcare practitioners.[2,3] As an advanced practice nurse, you may regularly address, or have at least contemplated the role of holistic or CAM in your practice. Just as interest from the general public in CAM is rising, so are professional approaches to dealing with the more holistic side of human health.

Congress created the Office of Alternative Medicine (OAM) in 1992 with an initial budget[4] of $2 million.[5] In 1999, the OAM became the National Center for Complementary and Alternative Medicine (NCCAM). In 2012, the NCCAM's annual budget grew to $128 million, and since its establishment, OAM and NCCAM have spent $1.6 billion in research studying nontraditional approaches to health and wellness.[5] Despite these growing numbers, advocates of CAM are quick to point out that this money represents only a very small component of the overall healthcare budget.

CAM, as a field, is difficult to define. This is due in part to its broad and changing nature, as well as its divergent interpretations and iterations. The NCCAM definition of CAM is that it encompasses a, "(g)roup of diverse medical and health care systems, practices, and products that are not generally considered part of conventional medicine."[6] The boundaries that exist between CAM and conventional medicine (also called Western medicine) are not absolute, or even clearly defined, but rather amorphous and overlapping. For example, an advanced practice nurse counseling a woman who is trying to become pregnant may consider the use of a number of both conventional medicine and CAM practices to achieve conception. These may consist of recommendations on diet and weight loss or weight gain in both the male and female partners to achieve optimal weight status (diet therapy), use of Clomid (clomiphene) to stimulate ovulation (pharmacotherapy), advice to begin a prenatal vitamin in the event of immediate conception (dietary supplement use), or acupuncture treatment as a method to stimulate fertility (CAM). Today's practitioner should be adequately equipped and ready to deal with the rising public interest in, and reliance on, combination therapies of traditional medicine and CAM approaches to health, wellness, and disease.

■ CAM Classification

In the United States, NCCAM groups CAM practices into the categories of mind and body medicine, manipulative and body-based practices, and natural products. As the name implies, the natural products category includes substances that have their basis in nature, such as foods, vitamins, minerals, botanicals, herbs, and other natural therapies. Probiotics are also included under the CAM "natural products" grouping.

The majority of natural products are sold over the counter as dietary supplements. Despite their technical classification as a dietary supplement, NCCAM does not include practices such as taking a multivitamin to meet daily nutritional requirements, or calcium to promote bone health, technically as CAM. The CAM term "natural products" replaces NCCAM's previous use of the term "biologically based practices," noting that *biologically based* is no longer used, as other CAM modalities also have the potential to exert biologically based effects.[7] Table 12–1 contains a list of the NCCAM's products that are considered CAM natural products.[7]

Table 12–1. CAM natural products, as categorized by the National Center for Complementary and Alternative Medicine (NCCAM).

Dietary supplements
Herbal or botanical products
Traditional medicine formulations
Folk medicines
Homeopathic remedies
Probiotics
Food-based phytochemicals

Data from National Center for Complementary and Alternative Medicine (NCCAM), 2012.

▪ Trends in CAM Use

The 2007 National Health Interview Survey (NHIS) included a comprehensive survey on the use of CAM that gathered information from 23,393 American adults and 9417 children. NHIS findings published in 2008 showed that approximately[8] 38% of adults (roughly 4 in 10) aged 18 years and over, and 12% of children (about 1 in 9), use some form of CAM. CAM use by adults was found to be greatest in women and those with higher income and education levels.[9] Another more recent study put the number of dietary supplement users in the United States at over 50%, and found that the most commonly used dietary supplements are multivitamins/multiminerals, but also noted an increased use of vitamin D, which rarely occurs naturally in food sources.[10]

The NHIS findings indicate that nonvitamin, nonmineral natural products are the most commonly used CAM therapies among American adults. Increases in the use of other therapies such as deep breathing exercises, massage therapy, yoga, and meditation were also noted. Adults were found to most commonly use CAM for musculoskeletal problems such as neck, back, or joint pain. The three most popular natural products used by adults in the 2007 NHIS study included fish oil/omega-3 (reported to be used by 37.4% of all adults using natural products), glucosamine (19.9%), and echinacea (19.8%). The same data were also compiled previously in 2002; Table 12–2 compares the ten most common natural products used by adults in 2002 versus 2007.[9]

Table 12–2. Ten most common natural products among adults, NHIS Data 2002 versus 2007.

Ranking of Most Common Natural Products Used by Adults	2002 NHIS Findings	2007 NHIS Findings
1	Echinacea	Fish oil/omega-3
2	Ginseng	Glucosamine
3	Ginkgo biloba	Echinacea
4	Garlic supplements	Flaxseed oil/pills
5	Glucosamine	Ginseng
6	St. John's wort	Combination herb pills
7	Peppermint	Ginkgo biloba
8	Fish oil/omega-3	Chondroitin
9	Ginger supplements	Garlic supplements
10	Soy supplements	Coenzyme Q-10

Data from US Department of Health and Human Services, 2008.

Trying to quantify the financial impact of rising supplement use rates is about as difficult as strictly defining parameters for CAM practices. The 2007 NHIS study found that adults in the United States spent $33.9 billion out of pocket on the purchase of CAM products, materials, and classes, and direct costs for visits to CAM practitioners. Two-thirds of those costs were for products, materials, and classes, while the remaining one-third was for practitioners. Forty four percent of out-of-pocket costs for CAM, $14.8 billion, was spent on the purchases of nonvitamin, nonmineral, natural products.[11] Other market research analyses suggest that supplement sales are forecasted to reach $15.5 billion per year by 2017,[12] while functional foods and drinks could top $149 billion by 2018.[13] On a global scale, a report from the industry-sponsored Nutrition Business Journal found that the combined contributions of supplement sales, natural and organic foods, functional foods, and natural and organic personal care and household products amounted to over $300 billion in annual sales in 2010.[14]

■ Does CAM Work?

As Oscar Wilde once said, "Everything popular is wrong." CAM is certainly popular, but does it work? This is the subject of much debate, often pitting the evidence- and science-based medicine groups against their holistic and CAM adversaries. The former claim that the practices of the latter lack rigorous scientific rigor. The latter claim the former are too focused on clinical trial outcomes that do not adequately elucidate the complex and multifactorial nature of pathology and the human body.

Some particularly vocal groups and individuals have called for the abolishment of the NCCAM, claiming that taxpayer dollars should not be used to promote "suspect medicine," "studies that lack a sound biological underpinning," and therapies such as homeopathy and Reiki.[15,16] Other criticisms maintain that research money would be better spent on studying the CAM therapies under the umbrella of existing institutes of the NIH, rather than having a center dedicated to CAM.[16] The American Medical Association states, "There is little evidence to confirm the safety or efficacy of most alternative therapies."[17]

Although differing opinions about CAM do and will continue to exist, and regardless of where you fall on the opinion spectrum, most practitioners would argue that there is a frustrating lack of evidence about CAM therapies in general. As an advanced practice nurse answering questions about CAM therapies, you start to wonder if you sound like a broken record, increasingly finding yourself saying, "More research is needed on that diet," "The data on that supplement are not clear," and "No studies have found conclusive evidence to that effect…" But the reality is, much of the time, we truly do not know or do not have enough data to adequately assess whether these CAM therapies are effective, safe, or should be recommended.

Despite the booming human interest in supplements and nutritionals, and the consequent rising global sales numbers, the vast majority of studies regarding these products' use have shown that they have no benefits. A number of studies have demonstrated that echinacea and megavitamin supplementation does not treat the common cold, milk thistle does not treat hepatitis, St. John's wort does not treat depression, garlic does not treat elevated LDL cholesterol, ginkgo does not improve memory, glucosamine with chondroitin does not treat arthritis, and saw palmetto does not treat benign prostatic hypertrophy (BPH).[16,18,19] On top of these primarily negative findings, all too often, any demonstrable benefit that *is* shown can often be explained by, or attributed to, the placebo effect. It is, however, important to note that a study demonstrating a supplement's ineffectiveness is not the same as the study showing the supplement is harmful. This puts practitioners in a challenging predicament: is it ethical to recommend a supplement or CAM therapy that has proven (thus far?) not to be effective, but at the same time has also been proven (thus far?) not to be harmful?

The case of glucosamine/chondroitin and its effect on joint pain provides excellent insight into this conundrum. Glucosamine with chondroitin is used routinely by people for the alleviation of arthritis and joint pain. The Glucosamine/Chondroitin Arthritis Intervention Trial (GAIT) studies have shown, conclusively, that the supplement fairs no better than placebo in providing relief from osteoarthritis pain, no better than placebo in preventing loss of cartilage in knee osteoarthritis, or is any better than celecoxib (Celebrex) or placebo in lowering pain threshold scores.[20-22] The last of these three GAIT studies was published in 2010. And yet, in that same year, one-third of people surveyed who took multiple dietary supplements took a joint health supplement, and sales of glucosamine and chondroitin exceeded $800 million dollars in 2010, showing that just because something is popular does not mean it is right.[23]

In spite of the dearth of conclusive evidence about the efficacy and safety of popular CAM therapies, at the very minimum, it is incumbent upon practitioners to caution about known safety issues regarding harmful CAM practices. This is especially true with regards to the use of herbals and dietary supplements that are contraindicated with certain medication therapies, as well as for those for which contamination events have been reported or have had recalls issued. (For information on dietary supplement recalls, see the *FDA's Dietary Supplement Alerts and Safety Information* website.)

Another consideration is the financial impact that these products have on those with limited and fixed incomes. This is of particular concern in the elderly population, as many dietary supplement companies unscrupulously market their products directly to the elderly, making convincing, yet undeliverable claims about their products' abilities to promote longevity, memory retention, and cognitive function. Many people, regardless of age, are in economic situations where they are already faced with difficult decisions about allocating funds for basic survival needs, healthy foods, and/or prescription medications. This is the very population who *least* needs to be considering whether or not to spend their limited resources on what most often turns out to be ineffective products.

Many practitioners are also increasingly interested in the emerging field of Integrative Medicine. Whereas alternative medicine refers to a CAM therapy that is used *in place* of standard treatments, the National Cancer Institute defines Integrative Medicine as, "an approach that combines treatments from conventional medicine and CAM for which there is some high-quality evidence of safety and effectiveness."[24] Proponents of Integrative Medicine maintain that their approach is not oppositional to traditional medicine, but, rather, that employing and integrating components of naturopathic medicine into more traditional care as part of a comprehensive approach to medical management is ideal.[25]

■ CAM Practitioners

CAM Credentials

To date, there is no standardized or national system for credentialing CAM practitioners across the spectrum of healthcare providers. The US federal government does not regulate CAM or license CAM practitioners.[26] CAM credentialing can vary between states and professions. Some individual disciplines do have their own subspecialty, credentials, and professional organizations for holistic and CAM medicine. The American Holistic Nurses Association is a nonprofit membership association whose mission is to advance holistic nursing through community building, advocacy, research, and education.[27] The Dietitians in Integrative and Functional Medicine are members of a dietetic practice group of the Academy of Nutrition and Dietetics. Licensure of selected types of CAM practitioners is listed in Table 12–3.[6,28]

Tips for Choosing a CAM Practitioner

People turn to CAM for a variety of reasons, primarily to further their own personal pursuit of health, healing, and wellness. They may be disenchanted by or disappointed with results from traditional, Western medicine, or maintain a belief that not one single modality will hold the answers to their medical condition. The NCCAM maintains that the most common reason why people turn to CAM is chronic back pain, but also for relief from neck pain, joint pain, and headache.[7]

Cancer patients and survivors are also likely populations to turn to CAM. The American Cancer Society's studies of cancer survivors have found that most cancer survivors report using CAM therapies. The most often cited uses of CAM are prayer and spiritual practices (61%), relaxation techniques (44%), faith and spiritual healing (42%), and nutrition and vitamin supplementation (40%).[24,29] CAM therapies have also been employed from anywhere by 31–84% of pediatric cancer patients, both in and outside of clinical trials.[24,30]

When considering the selection of a CAM practitioner, it is wise to encourage the patient to ask careful questions about the CAM practitioner, about the proposed therapy, and even about their own personal

Table 12–3. Licensure of selected types of CAM practitioners.

	US States with Licensure	Education	Examination	Continuing Education
Acupuncture	50 state and the District of Columbia	3 years of 1905 hours, including Chinese herbology and clinical practice; some states require training in anatomy, physiology, and pathology	Most states require the NCCAOM written examination, or a state written examination. Some states also require the Practical Examination of Point Location Skills (PEPLS), or a state practical examination	16 states require some continuing education units (CEUs); average is 15 hours per year – note that the information in this section applies to nonphysician acupuncturists
Chiropractic	50 states and the District of Columbia	4–5 years or 4200 hours, including basic medical sciences and clinical experience	All states accept or require the NBCE written examination; 40 states also accept or require the NBCE practical examination	Most states require some CEUs; specific requirements vary widely from state to state
Homeopathy	3 states; licensure as a homeopathic physician is available only to practitioners holding an M.D. or D.O. degree in Arizona, Connecticut, and Nevada	Arizona requires 300 hours of training; Nevada requires 6 months; and Connecticut does not specify training requirements	Each licensing state administers its own oral or written examination	Only Nevada requires CEUs (20 hours per year)

(continued)

Table 12-3. Licensure of selected types of CAM practitioners. (*Continued*)

	US States with Licensure	Education	Examination	Continuing Education
Massage therapy	43 states and the District of Columbia	Training requirements range from 100 to 1000 hours with most states requiring a minimum of 500 hours; some states require graduation from a training program approved by the Commission on Massage Therapy Accreditation (COMTA) or equivalent program, or training in a specific area such as anatomy	Most states that license massage therapists require passing Massage and Bodywork Licensing Examination (MBLEx) or 1 of 2 examinations provided by the National Certification Board for Therapeutic Massage and Bodywork	29 states and the District of Columbia require some CEUs
Naturopathy	15 states and the District of Columbia	4-year postgraduate program, includes natural sciences, clinical sciences, and natural therapeutics	Naturopathic Physicians Licensing Examination (NPLEX) written examination, usually covers basic sciences and clinical examinations in a number of areas	14 states and the District of Columbia require some CEUs; specific requirements vary from state to state

Data from National Center for Complementary and Alternative Medicine, 2011; Eisenberg et al, 2002.

feelings regarding both the practitioner and the therapy. Table 12–4 contains some recommended questions for patients to consider when selecting CAM therapies and practitioners.[31]

Some patients fear that their primary care practitioners will not understand or will disapprove of their use of CAM. Research shows that many people do not disclose their supplement use to their primary care practitioners; but on the other hand, many primary care practitioners fail to ask about supplement use as part of the routine patient interview.[32] It is important for the advanced practice nurse to promote

Table 12–4. Recommended questions for patients to consider when selecting CAM therapies and practitioners.

Questions to Ask the CAM Practitioner
What CAM therapies do you specialize in? What type of CAM do you practice?
What is your CAM training background and CAM qualifications?
How have you previously used CAM to treat other patients similar to me?
How will you work with my primary care provider?

Questions to Ask About the CAM Therapy
Is there research to support the use of this CAM therapy?
What are the risks and side effects of the CAM therapy?
How does this CAM therapy interfere with or support my other medical treatments?
How long will the therapy take and what will it cost?
Under what conditions would you recommend not using this CAM therapy?
Do you have additional resources or recommendations where I can learn more about the CAM therapy?

Questions to Ask Yourself about CAM
Do I feel comfortable with this practitioner and his/her expertise?
Do I like the staff and do they seem supportive of the CAM therapies?
How far am I willing to travel and how much am I willing to pay for this CAM therapy?
Do the potential benefits of this experience outweigh the risks?
Does my insurance cover the cost of CAM?
Does my own independent research support or refute the statements of the practitioner about the proposed therapy?

Adapted from US Department of Health and Human Services, 2005.

discussion about how CAM therapies may be incorporated as part of an integrative medicine approach, should that be the desire of the patient. Talk with patients about how CAM might help them cope, reduce stress, feel better, feel less tired, and deal with symptoms such as pain, or side effects of treatment, like nausea. If the patient decides to go forward with a CAM therapy, talk openly about how it might potentially interfere with treatment or medicines, help the patient interpret data or publications about the practice, refer to qualified CAM professionals when appropriate, and brainstorm about how you will work with the selected CAM practitioner.[31]

▪ Diet Therapy and Pharmacotherapy—Potential Interactions

How Drugs Impact Diet and Nutrition Status

The action of a drug can impact nutrition status. Conversely, the nutrient composition of one's diet has the ability to affect drug action. Dietary supplements can interfere with both nutrient status and drug metabolism. In addition to increasing or decreasing appetite and causing weight changes, drugs can also affect nutrition status by altering the taste and smell of foods (which decreases intake), by upsetting the GI tract (causing nausea, vomiting, constipation, or diarrhea), by altering the absorption of nutrients, or by depleting mineral and vitamin status. Table 12–5 provides examples of ways that medications can potentially impact nutrition status.[33-35]

How Nutrition Status and Diet Impact Drug Therapy

Food intake can also affect drug metabolism. Most drug absorption occurs in the first part of the small intestine, which is also where many nutrients compete for absorption. Foods can affect gastric emptying, with high-fat, high-fiber, and high-protein foods taking longer to digest than do carbohydrate-containing foods. This can impact the absorption of medications that have specification about whether to consume with food or in the absence of food. Taking some drugs on an empty stomach can increase their absorption because those drugs exit the stomach quickly, and go directly to the small intestine. Other drugs require an acidic environment for maximum absorption. Antacids are alkaline (basic) and can reduce the absorption of other drugs that require an acidic environment. There are compounds in foods such as phytates, oxalates, and tannins that interfere with iron, calcium, and other mineral absorption.

Tyramine and monoamine oxidase inhibitor diet

Monoamine oxidase (MAO) is an intricate enzyme system circulated primarily in nervous tissue, liver, and lungs. The enzyme system plays a role in inactivating neurotransmitters such as dopamine, norepinephrine, and serotonin after they have done their part in delivering messages to the brain. Monoamine oxidase inhibitors (MAOIs) block this activity. If the excess neurotransmitters are not destroyed, they

Table 12–5. Ways that drugs can affect nutrition.

Drugs That Alter Taste and Smell of Foods

Elavil (tricyclic antidepressant) reduces salivation, and causes dry mouth and a sour or metallic taste

Biaxin (antibiotic) causes bitter taste in saliva

Tetracycline (antibiotic) reduces natural bacteria in the mouth, leading to yeast overgrowth (candidiasis)

Flagyl (antibiotic) causes metallic taste in the mouth (dysgeusia)

Cisplatin, methotrexate (cancer drugs) may cause esophagitis, glossitis, stomatitis, and dysgeusia

Drugs Can Upset the Gastrointestinal Tract

Many drugs can cause nausea, vomiting, and changes in healthy gut flora

Some drugs alter peristalsis by increasing or decreasing motility rates in the gut

NSAIDs (aspirin, Advil, and Motrin) and naproxen (Aleve) can irritate the stomach and may cause gastric bleeding

Antipsychotics, antidepressants, and antihistamines can reduce emptying of the stomach and transit through the gut, causing constipation

Cipro (antibiotic) allows for bacterial growth, and can cause colitis

Drugs Can Alter Nutrient Absorption

Tagamet (gastric antisecretory) helps post bowel resection patients by lowering gastric acid and lowering flow of food into intestine, but its long-term use can lead to reduced absorption of vitamin B_{12}, thiamin, and iron

Questran (antihyperlipidemic) binds vitamins A, D, E, and K in the intestine and reduces the body's absorption of these vitamins

Colchicine (used for gout) can lead to vitamin B_{12} deficiency and megaloblastic anemia

Alcohol abuse leads to thiamin, vitamin B_{12}, and folic acid metabolism disruption

Laxative abuse can lower mineral absorption, including calcium

Methotrexate used in cancer treatment can reduce intestinal absorption of calcium, and works by inhibiting folic acid metabolism

Drugs Can Deplete Vitamin and Mineral Status

Diuretics reduce sodium levels and can affect potassium, magnesium, and zinc

Spironolactone (potassium-sparing diuretic) misuse and potassium supplements can cause hyperkalemia

Alcohol abuse can deplete potassium, magnesium, and zinc stores

Antacid overuse can cause phosphorus deficiency

Aspirin can cause iron deficiency and blood loss from the stomach or intestine if abused

Coumadin (anticoagulant) stops regeneration of vitamin K

Cancer drugs can lower folate metabolism

Oral contraceptives can reduce riboflavin, vitamin B_6, vitamin B_{12}, and vitamin C

Data from Nelms and Sucher, 2011; Fragakis and Thomson, 2007; Burke et al., 2003.

will build up and accumulate in the brain. MAO breaks down another amine, tyramine. If an MAOI blocks MAO, tyramine levels can also rise. Excess tyramine leads to sudden, occasionally fatal increases in blood pressure. To avoid this life-threatening consequence, those on MAOIs should avoid or limit foods with high levels of tyramine. Table 12–6 contains a list of foods that are high in tyramine that should be avoided and foods that can be eaten in moderation for people on MAOIs.[33,36,37]

Grapefruit and drug interactions

There are many drugs that interact with grapefruit. Compounds in grapefruit called furanocoumarins irreversibly inhibit cytochrome P450 3A4 isoenzymes (3A4) in the intestine's wall. This decreases the presystemic metabolism of the affected drugs for up to 72 hours following grapefruit consumption. During this time, intestinal 3A4 activity can remain impaired, while the body makes more enzymes. Higher amounts of 3A4-metabolized drugs may then enter circulation, leading to an increase in drug levels that can impact therapeutic effect, and cause adverse outcomes or toxicity. The list of medications to avoid or use caution with grapefruit was recently updated and is available at: www.cmaj.ca/content/suppl/2012/11/26/cmaj.../grape-bailey-1-at.pdf.

Dietary Supplements

As defined by the United States Congress in the Dietary Supplement and Health Education Act of 1994 (DSHEA), a dietary supplement is a product (other than tobacco) that is intended to supplement the diet. A supplement contains one or more dietary ingredients (including vitamins, minerals, herbs or other botanicals, amino acids, and other substances) or their constituents; is intended to be taken by mouth as a pill, capsule, tablet, or liquid; and is labeled on the front panel as being a dietary supplement.[38,39]

▪ Industry Regulation

The dietary supplement industry is regulated by the FDA, the Federal Trade Commission (FTC), and individual state governments. Despite its assigned regulatory oversight bodies, critics of the supplement industry often refer to it as an unregulated industry, in that dietary supplements are regulated in a remarkably different fashion than are prescription drugs, foods, and medical devices.[40,41] Under DSHEA, dietary supplements that contain established ingredients (those that were sold in the United States prior to 1994) can be marketed without providing any prior evidence regarding their effectiveness or safety. For new ingredients in supplements, DSHEA requires that manufacturers provide the FDA with evidence about its safety, although critics claim enforcement has been inconsistent.[42,43]

Table 12–6. Tyramine and the MAOI diet.

Food Group	Foods Allowed	Foods to Limit	Foods to Avoid
Beverages	• Milk • Decaffeinated coffee and tea • Carbonated drinks	• Chocolate drinks • Coffee, tea, and other caffeinated drinks • White wine and clear spirits (limit to two 8 oz servings)	• Alcoholic drinks, especially beer, ale, wine (Chianti, burgundy, sherry, vermouth, or sauterne), and nonalcoholic beer and wine • Acidophilus milk
Bread	• Whole-wheat enriched white breads, rolls, crackers, and quick breads	• None	• Cheese breads • Crackers • Sourdough and fresh, homemade, yeast-leavened breads
Cereals	• Cooked and dry cereals	• None	• None
Cheese and dairy	• Cottage cheese, farmer or pot cheese, cream cheese, ricotta cheese, and processed cheese	• Buttermilk (limit to 4 oz), sour cream, yogurt (national brands only limit to 4 oz per day)	• All other cheese: aged cheese, Camembert, cheddar, Gouda, Gruyere, mozzarella, Parmesan, provolone, Roquefort, and Stilton

(continued)

Table 12-6. Tyramine and the MAOI diet. (*Continued*)

Food Group	Foods Allowed	Foods to Limit	Foods to Avoid
Desserts and sweets	• Cakes and cookies • Gelatins • Ice cream and sherbets • Pastries • Puddings • Sugars, hard candies, honey, molasses, and syrups	• Chocolate desserts • Chocolate candies and chocolate syrups	• Cheese-filled desserts and cheesecake • Imported chocolate
Eggs	• All	• None	• Quiche with cheese
Fats	• All	• None	• None
Fruits	• Fresh, frozen, or canned fruits and juices	• None	• Banana peel extract • Overripe and spoiled fruits
Meat, fish, and poultry	• All fresh or frozen meats, fish, or poultry	• Aged meats and frankfurters • Fresh sausage and pepperoni • Canned sardines • Canned meats • Fish roe (caviar) and paté (limit to 1 oz)	• Caviar (more than 1 oz) • Chicken and beef liver • Dried, salted, and pickled fish • Fermented and dry sausages • Salami • Dried meats and meat extracts

Potatoes, starches	• White and sweet potatoes • Grits, pasta, and rice	• None	
Soups	• All cream and broth soups, except those on the "avoid" list	• None	• Soups from Italian broad beans and fava beans • Cheese soup • Soup made with beer or wine • Any soup cubes or meat extract • Packet soups and packaged soups • Miso soup
Vegetables	• All fresh, frozen, canned, or dried vegetables and vegetable juices, except those on the "avoid" list	• None	• Chinese pea pods • Fava beans and Italian broad beans • Sauerkraut • Fermented soybean products, miso, and some tofu products
Miscellaneous	• Salt • Nuts and peanut butter • Spices, herbs, and flavorings	• Soy sauce (limit to ¼ cup) and teriyaki sauce (limit to ¼ cup) • Brewer's yeast	• Marmite (vegetable extracts) • Yeast concentrates • Vitamin supplements with brewer's yeast • Monosodium glutamate (MSG) • All aged products

Data from Nelms and Sucher, 2011; Hall-Flavin, 2013; University of Pittsburgh Medical Center.

Additional criticisms about supplements include variations in potency, as well as a lack of standards that dictate product purity. DSHEA was passed in 1994, and part of the requirements included the establishment of Good Manufacturing Practice (GMP) standards for the dietary supplement industry. The final rule on GMP was not issued by the FDA until 2007, leaving a 13-year gap where dietary supplements essentially self-regulated, leading to discrepancies in product branding, labeling, and complaints of adulteration and contamination.[44]

Health Claims for Supplements

Despite the fact that drugs and supplements are both regulated by the FDA, the degree and types of health claims that can be made on the labels and packaging materials of prescription drugs and dietary supplements differ. Drug manufacturers can claim that their drug will diagnose, cure, mitigate, treat, or prevent a disease. These claims cannot be made for dietary supplements. Rather, a dietary supplement or food product may contain one of three types of claims: a health claim, a nutrient content claim, or a structure/function claim.

The health claims explain the relationship between a food, food component, or ingredient in a dietary supplement, and the reduction in risk of a disease entity or health condition. Nutrient content claims explain the relative amount of a nutrient or dietary component in a product. A structure/function claim explains how a product might affect the body's organs or systems, but it cannot mention any specific disease. Structure/function claims do not require preapproval for use by the FDA, although the manufacturer has to provide the FDA with text of the claim within 30 days of selling the product on the market. Any dietary supplement product that contains an allowable FDA health claim must also include a disclaimer that reads, "This statement has not been evaluated by the FDA. The product is not intended to diagnose, treat, cure, or prevent any disease."[45]

Dietary Supplement Labels

While a manufacturer can decide whether or not to include health claims about the dietary supplement, there is other information that the FDA mandates must be disclosed. General information that has to be included on the supplement packaging includes the name of the product (including the word "supplement," or a statement saying that the product is a supplement), the net quantity of contents, the name and place of business of manufacturer, packer, or distributor, and directions for use.

The supplement must display a Supplement Facts panel (similar in appearance to the Nutrition Facts panel on foods) that lists the serving size, list of dietary ingredients, amount per serving size (by weight), and the percent of daily value (%DV), provided that a DV has been established for that particular nutrient. In the event that the dietary supplement is a botanical, the scientific name of the plant or the common or usual name has to be stated. If the dietary ingredient is a proprietary blend exclusive to the manufacturer, the total weight of the blend and its components must be listed in order of predominance by weight. Any additional nondietary ingredients (fillers, artificial colors, sweeteners, flavors, or binders) also have to be listed in order by weight.[45]

■ Efficacy and Safety

Because of the natural and holistic attributes ascribed to dietary supplements, consumers often do not realize that these products may interact with other medications (or even other supplements), may cause side effects of their own, and even contain potentially harmful ingredients that are not listed on the supplement's label. Furthermore, most supplements have not been tested for safety in pregnant and nursing women, or children.[6] Dietary supplements sold in the United States are not required to be standardized, so consumers cannot be certain that they are consuming products that have been subject to uniform manufacturing practices, standardized recipes, or consistent levels of active ingredients. Federal law does not require that dietary supplements be tested for safety and/or effectiveness prior to their sale.[45]

Avoiding Toxicity

When it comes to dietary supplements, average consumers, including patients, often operate with a mentality that "if a little is good, then more must be better." They may think that a supplement that provides 1000% of the DV for a nutrient is ten times better than the one that provides "just" 100% DV. Higher-than-average intakes of water-soluble vitamin supplements, while they may certainly prove problematic in very high doses, are generally considered to be not as harmful as are high doses of fat-soluble vitamin supplements. The body does not have a storage mechanism for water-soluble vitamins, and you tend to excrete excess amounts of these water-soluble vitamins in your urine (creating in heavy water-soluble vitamin supplement users as what informally may be referred to as "expensive pee"). Fat-soluble vitamins, on the other hand, can build up to toxic levels in the body and, as such, are not recommended to be consumed in high levels.[46] While there is no strict definition for the term megadose, a megadose is generally considered to be one that is significantly higher than the recommended dietary allowance (RDA) for a vitamin or mineral, and as a practice, megadosing should be discouraged.[47]

Practitioners are encouraged to be familiar with and to reference the dietary reference intakes' (DRIs') tolerable upper intake levels (ULs) that have been established for some vitamins and minerals. There are not ULs for all vitamins and minerals, but for those that do exist, people should be cautioned not to exceed the UL. Regularly exceeding the UL for daily intake of a vitamin and/or mineral has been demonstrated to have negative health consequences and may increase the risk for toxicity. The ULs are listed with the DRI tables as part of Appendix A. Encourage patients to also consider the additional vitamin and mineral contributions they may be receiving from substances such as protein powders, drink mixes, and fortified foods such as orange juice and cereal that may also have high levels of certain nutrients. Consuming many of these products, on top of dietary supplements, may put an individual at risk for exceeding the UL.[48,49]

Independent Testing

There are a number of independent testing agencies that provide third-party quality control for dietary supplements in the United States. These independent organizations provide quality testing and allow products that pass the tests to display their seals of approval. These seals indicate that the product was properly manufactured, contains the ingredients that are listed on the label, and does not have harmful levels of contaminants. While the seals may add another layer of confidence for consumers, they are not guarantees that the product is safe or effective. Well-known organizations that offer this type of testing include US Pharmacopeia, ConsumerLab.com, and NSF International.[45]

Other products may tout claims about being "high-potency," "pharmacy-grade," "prescription-strength," "pure," or "natural." Consumers and practitioners are encouraged to remember that these terms mean nothing; they are not legally definable, are nothing more than marketing taglines, and may be downright misleading. Consumers are also misled when they select supplements based on the highest price. Paying more for a supplement or brand-name product is never an assurance that the product is of superior quality. When selecting a multivitamin, a generic product that provides as close to 100% of the daily value for as many vitamins and minerals as possible is usually a safe bet (keeping in mind that it is not possible to provide exactly 100% DV for all micronutrients, as that would cause the size of the pill to be too large to swallow). Table 12–7

Table 12–7. Supplement safety tips for consumers.

Tell your healthcare provider about the supplements you are taking
Research the supplements you are taking and whether they might interact with your prescription drug medications or foods in your diet
Note that "natural" does not mean safe; other supplement terms that are meaningless include "prescription-strength," "high-potency," "pharmacy-grade," and claims about "purity"; more expensive products are not always better
When selecting a multivitamin/mineral supplement, look for one with as close to 100% daily value (100% DV) for as many of the vitamins and minerals as possible
Some dietary supplements can have unwanted effects during surgery; always talk to your doctor and surgeon about supplement use before surgical procedures
Report any adverse effects of supplements directly to the FDA's MedWatch at 1-800-FDA-1088

Data from Academy of Nutrition and Dietetics, 2012; US Food and Drug Administration, 2002; Office of Dietary Supplements, 2011.

Table 12–8. Questions to ask when searching the internet for information on dietary supplements.

Who operates the site?
- Is it run by the government, a university, or a reputable medical or health-related association?
- Does the information appear to be written or reviewed by qualified health professionals, experts in the field, academia, government, or the medical community?

What is the purpose of the site?
- Is the site's purpose to objectively education the public, or is it to sell a product?
- Commercial sites should clearly distinguish scientific information from advertisements.
- The majority of nonprofit and government sites will not contain advertising, and access to these sites and the material they contain will usually be offered for free.

What is the source of the information and is it properly referenced?
- Has the study been reviewed by recognized scientific experts?
- Has it be been published in reputable peer-reviewed scientific journals?
- Does the information say "some studies show…" instead of citing exactly which study is being referenced?
- Was the study paid for by the supplement industry, or the for-profit company?
- How big was the sample size in the study?
- Were the results applicable to the general population?

Is the information current?
- What date was the material written, posted, or updated?
- Is there new research that refutes the findings in the old material?

Is the product making promises that are too good to be true?
- Are the claims being made unlikely or exaggerated?
- Learn to distinguish hype from evidence-based science.
- Be cautious of nonsensical lingo or overly technical jargon intended to confuse you into acceptance.

Adapted from US Food and Drug Administration, 2002.

provides more tips for consumers about supplement safety, and Table 12–8 provides information on how to analyze internet information about dietary supplements.[45,48,50]

Supplement Interactions

From a legal standpoint, dietary supplements differ from plant-derived prescription drugs (eg, morphine, digitalis/digoxin, and atropine) because they are available without a prescription. As an industry, this distinction allows dietary supplements to avoid the FDA proof of efficacy and safety standards that are mandated and required prior to the sale of prescription drugs.[44] Because they can be purchased without a prescription, and are often marketed as being "natural," patients may mistakenly assume that herbals and other dietary supplements are harmless. This is certainly not the case, as botanicals have the potential to contain hundreds of active (as well as inactive) ingredients that may act like drugs, and that present the very real possibility of serious clinical consequences.[51] Products may have differing amounts of active ingredient from brand to brand, or even within brands and between batches. One study analyzed the variations in label information for the ten most commonly purchased herbs. The researchers found that of the 880 products they evaluated, 43% were consistent with a benchmark in ingredients and recommended daily dose, 20% were consistent in ingredients only, and 37% were either found to be inconsistent or with insufficient label information to determine content. With its nod to a recommended "buyer beware" approach in considering these products, the published article was appropriately titled, "Variations in product choices of frequently purchased herbs: caveat emptor."[52]

Even if you have information about the particular supplements that an individual is taking, you will not necessarily have the entire picture about what that could possibly entail. Due to the very complex nature of dietary supplements, coupled with minimal industry regulation, practitioners are hard-pressed to fully understand how individual supplements and herbal medicines may interact with prescribed medication. Practitioners are not expected to know the details about every dietary supplement and the clinical consequences of their use when combined with other therapies; however, practitioners should routinely ask patients about dietary supplement use, research potential interactions on a case-by-case basis, and caution individuals about the potential interactions and consequences of certain supplement use. A good mantra to keep in mind for counseling on potential dietary supplement–drug interactions is, "When in doubt, leave it out." The end of this chapter provides useful resources for the practitioner to reference in considering the very real impact of drug–supplement interactions.

Some known dietary supplement–drug interactions are as follows:

1. St. John's wort (*Hypericum perforatum*), which is an inducer of liver enzymes, and has been known to reduce the blood concentration of medications such as Lanoxin, Mevacor and Altocor (lovastatin), and Viagra (sildenafil).
2. Vitamin E taken with a blood thinner such as Coumadin increases the risk of bleeding, as it interferes with anticlotting capabilities of the medication.
3. Ginseng can also interfere with Coumadin-related bleeding, and influence the bleeding effects of aspirin, NSAIDs such as ibuprofen, naproxen, and ketoprofen, as well as heparin. If combined with MAOIs such as Nardil or Parnate, ginseng can cause headache, difficulty sleeping, hyperactivity, and nervousness.
4. *Ginkgo biloba* has been shown to decrease the effectiveness of anticonvulsant therapies in those who are taking medications for

seizure control, including Tegretol, Equetro or Carbatrol (carbamazepine), and Depakote (valproic acid).

5. Because of its questionable role in immune modulation, echinacea should be avoided by those who are taking immunosuppressant medications (eg, organ transplant recipients), those with immune deficiency disorders (eg, cancer, AIDS), and those with autoimmune disorders (eg, multiple sclerosis, rheumatoid arthritis) and tuberculosis.[44,51,53]

Who May Need a Supplement and Why?

The Academy of Nutrition and Dietetics Evidence Analysis project is quick to point out that most health organizations do not recommend dietary supplements to prevent disease. Rather, most bodies maintain that the focus should be on whole foods and a well-balanced diet as a more preferable route to preventing risk for certain chronic diseases.[48] Despite the many limitations and concerns that surround dietary supplement use, there are certainly conditions where the use of dietary supplements is indicated and warranted. Different life stages, dietary preferences, and disease states or conditions may dictate dietary supplement need. Table 12–9 contains a list of who might need a dietary supplement and why.[45,48,54-57]

Who Should Not Take a Supplement and Why?

In addition to those who are at risk for drug–supplement interactions, there are other groups for whom the use of certain dietary supplements is not indicated. Those taking Niacin/simvastatin to lower cholesterol should avoid antioxidant supplements such as vitamin C, vitamin E, beta-carotene, or selenium, as these have the potential to lower HDL cholesterol levels. Healthy, postmenopausal women and adult men are unlikely to need iron supplements. Those with the iron storage disease hemochromatosis should avoid vitamin C supplements and foods fortified or enriched with vitamin C, as vitamin C is known to enhance iron absorption. Postmenopausal women taking vitamin A supplements should do so primarily in its beta-carotene form, and not retinol, due to the possible negative effects on bone mineral density that retinol can have. Smokers are advised to avoid beta-carotene supplements, as they have been linked to higher rates of lung cancer.[48] The effects of herbal products and many dietary supplements on a pregnant woman and her developing fetus are largely unknown, and as such, pregnant women are advised to avoid herbal products or other supplements, except prenatal vitamins.[58] All individuals who take vitamin or mineral supplements should avoid surpassing the UL. The UL for vitamins and minerals are included with the DRI tables as part of Appendix A.

■ Selected Supplements—Highlight and Lowlights

The scientific community's understanding of the effects of dietary supplementation on our health can best be described as an evolving body of knowledge. Over time, certain supplements have come into, fallen out of, and occasionally reappeared back in popular favor. Vitamin E, for a short while, was panned as a miraculous antioxidant panacea, but quickly became a cautionary tale about the dangers of megadosing. Vitamin D, which, for years, has been routinely fortified into the United States milk supply, is now suddenly a superstar vitamin, with many rushing to ascribe health detriments to its deficiency, and benefits from its supplementation. It is unlikely that we will ever completely understand the need for supplementation (if it exists at all), or truly comprehend its impact on health. In order to best serve our patients and to properly answer their questions about dietary supplements, we can and should stay abreast of the latest research about these products, but also be aware of historical trends and patterns that may portend future applications. The following material is presented as a small sub-section of selected dietary supplements, including historical anecdotes and research summaries that either substantiate or repudiate their clinical use. With the exception of vitamin E, the following dietary supplements are all included on the list of the top ten most commonly purchased dietary supplements, as determined by the evaluation of CAM use section of the 2007 NHIS (see Table 12–9).[9] Vitamin E is included because of its historical importance as a once regularly touted supplement that is now rarely recommended.

Fish Oil

Omega-3 fatty acid supplementation from fish oil is promoted primarily for its positive effects on cardiovascular disease outcomes. The essential fatty acid profile of the typical American diet is one that disproportionately favors omega-6 over omega-3 fatty acids. Omega-6 fatty acid intake is roughly ten times omega-3 fatty acid intake.[59] While a typical American eats plenty of dietary fat, the overarching dietary goal should not be to promote omega-3 fatty acid intake that increases total fat intake, but rather to shift the ratio of omega-6 to omega-3 fatty acids in a more favorable direction (less omega-6 and more omega-3). Primary and secondary prevention studies have shown that omega-3 fatty acid intake, as well as fish and fish oil, is associated with reduced all-cause mortality, as well as a number of CVD outcomes including sudden death, cardiac death, and myocardial infarction. Evidence is strongest for fish and fish oil supplements.[59]

The National Cholesterol Education Program (NCEP) recommends eating two fish meals per week.[60] Similarly, the Academy of Nutrition and Dietetics' Evidence Analysis Library guidelines also recommend consuming dietary sources of omega-3 fatty acids, from two four-ounce servings of fish per week (preferably fatty fish such as mackerel, salmon, herring, trout, sardines, or tuna) and 1.5 grams of plant-based alpha-linolenic acid (from 1 tablespoon canola or walnut oil, 0.5 tablespoon ground flax seed, or <1 tablespoon flaxseed oil) as part of a cardioprotective diet (Evidence grade: Fair, Conditional).[61] For individuals who do not eat food sources of omega-3 fatty acids, 1 gram of EPA

Table 12–9. Who may need a dietary supplement and why?

Group	Why They Might Need a Supplement
Dieters	• Those on very low calorie diets or restrictive diets will benefit from a multivitamin/mineral supplement
Vegans and vegetarians	• Animal products are the only appreciable sources of vitamin B_{12}; vegans should supplement with vitamin B_{12} • Vegans and vegetarians who do not consume dairy may need calcium and vitamin D
Infants, children, and adolescents	• Those who live in areas where municipal water is not fluoridated may need a fluoride supplement • The American Academy of Pediatrics recommends 400 IU of Vitamin D per day for all infants beginning shortly after birth, children, and adolescents
Pregnant women	• Pregnant women need 400 mcg folic acid from fortified foods, supplements, or prenatal vitamins • If iron status is low, iron supplementation may be indicated
Older adults	• Because of decreased gastric hydrochloric acid production and decreased intrinsic factor production (as well as reduced food intake), older adults may require supplemental vitamin B_{12} • Calcium and vitamin D may also need to be supplemented, depending upon intake, exercise level, and sunlight exposure
Darker-skinned people	• Darker-skinned people receive a smaller effective dose of ultraviolet radiation than do light-skinned people; depending upon sunlight exposure and intake levels, darker-skinned people may benefit from vitamin D supplementation
Cigarette smokers	• Vitamin C helps prevent cigarette smoke-induced oxidative damage • The DRI for vitamin C for smokers is 35 more per day compared to nonsmokers (males smokers age 19+ DRI is 125 mg vitamin C; female smokers age 19+ DRI is 100 mg vitamin D per day)
Chronic abusers of alcohol	• The metabolic effects of alcohol as a toxin coupled with poor dietary intake in chronic alcohol abuse may lead to deficiencies in vitamin status, particularly the B vitamins • Vitamin A can be toxic when combined with alcohol • See Table 9-1 for Nutrition Supplements Recommended for Chronic Abusers of Alcohol

Data from Academy of Nutrition and Dietetics, 2012; Wagner et al., 2008; Mead, 2008; Office of Dietary Supplements, 2011; Lieber, 2003; Institute of Medicine, 2000.

and DHA omega-3 fatty acid supplements may be recommended as secondary prevention (Evidence grade: Fair, Conditional).[61] However, no evidence exists to describe the relationship between consumption of omega-3 fatty acid supplements and the risk of CVD events in people who do not have CHD.[62]

Glucosamine and Chondroitin

On a global scale, joint health supplement sales now constitute an $800 million annual market. The primary product that people take is glucosamine, an amino-monosaccharide that is made in the body from glucose and glutamine by the cells that form cartilage (the chondrocytes).[34] Glucosamine supplements are derived from the exoskeleton of the crustacean chitin, and are often combined with chondroitin sulfate. Together, glucosamine and chondroitin are theorized to promote the production of collagen and other components in the joint matrix that attract water, producing an elastic layer that cushions and protects cartilage from mechanical stressors. Because these products are derived from shellfish, they may cause a reaction in those who are allergic to shellfish. Glucosamine sulfate with or without chondroitin has been shown to increase the effect of Coumadin, slowing down blood clotting rates even further. Glucosamine also negatively interacts with some cancer therapies and medications, including etoposide (VP16, VePesid), teniposide (VM26), and doxorubicin (Adriamycin).[63]

As mentioned earlier in the chapter, despite the booming sales of joint health products containing glucosamine and chondroitin, the majority of studies of these products on joint health have been largely negative. In 2006, the Glucosamine/Chondroitin Arthritis Intervention Trial (GAIT) found no clear benefit for most patients. In 2009, another randomized control trial found that glucosamine and chondroitin were no more effective than placebo in slowing cartilage damage from osteoarthritis. And in 2010, Norwegian researchers tested glucosamine for chronic lower back pain and degenerative lumbar osteoarthritis, finding no significant difference between glucosamine and placebo.[20-22] The Natural Medicines Comprehensive Database has ranked glucosamine sulfate as being likely effective for osteoarthritis, possibly effective for temporomandibular joint (TMJ) arthritis, and has found that no sufficient evidence exists to rate effectiveness for glaucoma and weight loss.[63]

Echinacea

The echinacea plant is indigenous to the United States and has been used by Native Americans to treat a variety of conditions and ailments. Today, individuals take echinacea, and the product is marketed for protection against the cold virus, upper respiratory infections, as well as other immune-enhancing functions. There are several species of the echinacea plant that are used to make medicine, from its leaves, flower, or root. Despite its North American origin, the majority of the clinical research that has been done on echinacea has been conducted in Germany, where the government's expert committee, the German Commission E, has approved echinacea as a supportive therapy for colds, chronic respiratory infections, and lower urinary tract infections.[34]

Oral echinacea is generally well tolerated, although long-term safety studies have not been conducted. There is a potential for hypersensitivity to the plant in individuals with asthma, atopy, or allergies to grass pollens. Echinacea is not advisable for those with autoimmune disorders including lupus, tuberculosis, multiple sclerosis, scleroderma, or HIV. Furthermore, preliminary animal studies suggest that high doses of the herb may lower male and female fertility, although this has not borne out in human studies. Echinacea may decrease the effectiveness of immune-suppressing drugs and may interact negatively with hepatotoxic medications (eg, anabolic steroids, amiodarone, methotrexate, and ketoconazole).[34]

Regarding its effectiveness, the Natural Medicines Comprehensive Database rates echinacea as being possibly effective for treatment of the common cold (although not prevention of the common cold) and vaginal yeast infections. It is ranked as being possibly ineffective for genital herpes, and there is insufficient evidence to determine its effectiveness for other conditions such as urinary tract infections, migraine headaches, chronic fatigue syndrome, flu, allergies, hay fever, ADHD, bee stings, and eczema.[64] The Cochrane Collaboration has published a systematic review on the herb, stating that there is some evidence that echinacea preparations that are derived from the aerial parts of *Echinacea purpurea* (the above-ground parts opposed to the roots) might be effective in early treatment of adult colds, although results are inconsistent. Other benefits of different echinacea preparations or those used for preventive purposes may exist, but have not been clearly demonstrated in the existing body of literature.[65]

Flaxseed and Flaxseed Oil

Flaxseed comes from the seed of the flax plant, and flaxseed oil comes from flaxseeds. The flax plant is thought to have originated in Egypt, and the seed has been used most commonly as a laxative, although it also has applications for hot flashes and breast pain. Flaxseed oil has been used to treat high cholesterol and it is thought by some to have cancer prevention properties. The high soluble fiber content is responsible for the laxative effect of flaxseed. If taken in high doses without adequate water, flaxseed can have the opposite of the desired effect, in that it makes constipation worse rather than promotes laxation. In rare cases, high intake without water can cause intestinal blockage. Some of the components in flaxseed are known to lower the body's absorptive capacity for certain oral medications. As such, flaxseed should be taken independent of prescription medication and/or other dietary supplements.

The most promising application of flaxseed is its impact on elevated total and LDL cholesterol levels. A meta-analysis published in 2009 evaluated at 28 studies that were designed to explore the role of flaxseed or its derivatives on adult lipid profiles. The study found that flaxseed significantly reduced circulating total and LDL-cholesterol concentrations, although the findings were dependent on the type of intervention, gender, and initial lipid profiles of the subjects. Results were most apparent in postmenopausal women, and in those who had high initial cholesterol concentrations.[66,67] At this point, there is no significant evidence to support the recommendation for use of flaxseed in cancer prevention, atherosclerosis, or other heart conditions.

Ginseng

Ginseng is a term that refers to a group of plants belonging to the genus *Panax*. The *Panax* plant contains bioactive compounds called saponins (or ginsenosides) that are located in the roots. Asian ginseng (*Panax ginseng*) is different from American ginseng (*Panax quinquefolius*) and Siberian ginseng (*Eleutherococcus senticosus*). Siberian ginseng, also called Russian ginseng, is not considered to be a true "ginseng" because it is not in the genus *Panax*, although it is sold alongside other *Panax ginseng* products.[34] The varying levels of saponins in different ginseng varieties exert inconsistent pharmacologic effects that may in turn explain conflicting results in published ginseng studies. Differences in time of harvest, lack of standardization of bioactive compounds, and differences in dosage, administration, and type of ginseng used may also contribute to inconsistent results.[34]

Much of the research that has been conducted on ginseng has been done in Asia, with few results having been translated into English, presenting a difficulty for certain analysis of the data. Other interpretive difficulties arise from the different ways in which Eastern and Western medicine look at the effects of ginseng. Traditional Eastern medicine practitioners suggest that the actions of opposing ginsenosides "adapt" to meet a person's individualized mental or physical state. This contrasts with the Western practitioners' approach, which assumes that the differing actions of the ginsenosides will instead neutralize each other. Existing research does not provide enough data to either fully support or refute either of these arguments.[34,68] As far as drug–supplement interactions are concerned, ginseng may interfere with phenelzine (an MAOI), corticosteroids, digoxin, estrogen therapy, and diabetes medications. Ginseng has been shown to increase bleeding time when taken along with other blood-thinning drugs or supplements. The increased use of ginseng in energy drinks has raised concern that ginseng, delivered along with caffeine, can increase hypertension. Because of its mild hormonal effects similar to those of estrogen, ginseng may interact with hormone replacement, oral contraception, or select estrogen receptor modulators. Ginseng use has been associated with cases of postmenopausal bleeding and premenopausal amenorrhea.[34,69]

The Natural Medicines Comprehensive Database rates American ginseng as being possibly effective for lowering postprandial blood sugar in people with type 2 diabetes and preventing respiratory tract infections such as the common cold or influenza in adults. Siberian ginseng has been ranked as being possibly effective for treating herpes simplex 2 (HSV-2) and relieving symptoms of the common cold, when used in combination with the herb called andrographis. *Panax ginseng* has been ranked as being possibly effective for aiding in thinking and memory, diabetes, male impotence, and premature ejaculation. The Cochrane Collaboration has published a review that cites a lack of convincing evidence that shows any cognitive enhancing effect of *Panax ginseng* in healthy people, and no high-quality evidence regarding its efficacy in patients with dementia.[70-73]

Ginkgo Biloba

Nobody wants to lose their mind, and the memory preservation supplement folks are well aware of this. Ginkgo is one of the top ten most commonly used dietary supplements, and sales of supplements that promise to prevent cognitive decline top $250 million per year in the United States alone.[9,74] The Ginkgo Evaluation of Memory (GEM) study is the largest clinical trial ever conducted to evaluate ginkgo's effect on memory and cognition.[75] The GEM trial was a randomized, double-blind, placebo-controlled trial of 3069 people aged 72–96 years. Participants in the study received twice-daily doses of 120 milligrams of ginkgo extract and showed no better results than placebo in slowing cognitive decline over a 6-year follow-up period in adults with normal cognition of mild cognitive impairment.[76] Another publication from the same study showed that *Ginkgo biloba* at 120 milligrams twice per day was not effective in reducing either the overall incidence rate of dementia or Alzheimer's disease incidence in elderly people with normal cognition or those with mild cognitive impairment.[77]

The Natural Medicines Comprehensive Database has rated ginkgo as being possibly effective for Alzheimer's disease and other forms of dementia, improving thinking problems caused by old age, improving thinking in young people, Raynaud's syndrome, claudication and peripheral vascular disease, vertigo and dizziness, premenstrual syndrome, and glaucoma, and improving color vision in people with diabetes. The database finds ginkgo to be possibly ineffective for tinnitus, winter depression in people with seasonal affective disorder, sexual difficulties related to antidepressant medicines, and mountain or altitude sickness in climbers. There is not enough evidence to determine whether ginkgo leaf extract has any effectiveness on anxiety, ADHD, stroke, hearing loss, fibromyalgia, radiation exposure, vitiligo, hypercholesterolemia, atherosclerosis, CHD, colorectal and ovarian cancers, chronic fatigue syndrome, or age-related macular degeneration.[78]

Side effects of ginkgo may include nausea, headache, GI distress, diarrhea, dizziness, or skin reactions. Ginkgo may also increase bleeding risk, and should be used with caution or not at all in those on anticoagulant therapies, those with bleeding disorders, or those who have upcoming surgeries. Ginkgo should not be taken with fluoxetine (Prozac), as it has been associated with hypomania. Ginkgo has also been shown to stimulate beta cell function in the pancreas, which may lead to hypoglycemia in those with diabetes, and particularly those on insulin therapy. For those taking thiazide diuretics for blood pressure control, ginkgo can reduce the efficacy of these drugs. Ginkgo is available as a tincture, capsule, tablet, or in infusion form. Raw ginkgo seeds contain a chemical called ginkgotoxin, which can cause seizures and death, although most commercial products and extracts contain very little ginkgotoxin and are safe if used orally and in small quantities.[34,79]

Garlic

While supplemental garlic is used widely, and is one of the best selling supplements in the United States, in Germany garlic supplements have been approved as a nonprescription medication to lower blood cholesterol and other heart disease risk factors. Garlic is the edible part of a plant bulb from the lily family. Allicin is the active ingredient in garlic, and is responsible for its distinctive smell. The method of preparation of garlic determines the amount of allicin in the end product. Allicin is highly unstable and changes chemical structure rather quickly, meaning that an aged garlic product, while less odorous, will also contain very little, if any, allicin. Crushing the clove releases more allicin, while other products include enteric coating to protect the allicin content from the acidic nature of the stomach.[80]

Besides causing bad breathe or a general garlicky odor, garlic is considered safe for most people when consumed by mouth, but possibly unsafe if used topically on the skin, as it can cause damage similar to a burn. Garlic affects the rate of metabolism of certain drugs, and it should be avoided if an individual is also taking Isoniazid (INH, Nydrazid), medications for HIV/AIDS (non-nucleoside reverse transcriptase inhibitors—NNRTIs), or Saquinavir (Fortovase, Invirase). Because both fish oil that contains eicosapentaenoic acid (EPA) and garlic slow blood clotting, the combination of these two supplements may increase the risk of bleeding in some individuals. Other herbs that increase the risk of bleeding, and should be avoided with garlic use, include angelica, clove, danshen, ginger, ginkgo, red clover, turmeric, vitamin E, willow, and others.[80]

The Natural Medicines Comprehensive Database rates garlic as being possibly effective for high blood pressure (reducing hypertension by as much as 7% or 8%), atherosclerosis, colon, rectal, and stomach cancer, as well as fungal infections of the skin. It is ranked as being possibly ineffective for diabetes, treating *H. pylori*, high cholesterol, breast and lung cancer, and peripheral arterial disease. There is insufficient evidence to rate garlic's effectiveness for BPH, common cold, corns on the feed, preeclampsia, prostate cancer, and warts.[80] The Cochrane Collaboration has published a number of reviews on garlic, finding that there is insufficient clinical trial evidence regarding the effectiveness of garlic in preventing or treating the common cold, insufficient evidence to determine the true impact of garlic on lowering blood pressure, and insufficient evidence to recommend increased garlic intake for preventing preeclampsia and its complications.[81-83]

In the event that an individual is taking garlic for the prevention of colon, rectal, and stomach cancer, the recommended dose is fresh or cooked garlic, 3.5–29 grams per week. For fungal skin infections (eg, ringworm, jock itch, and athlete's foot), garlic ingredient ajoene may be applied as a 0.4% cream, 0.6% gel, or 1% gel twice daily for one week. For the treatment of high blood pressure, recommended garlic doses are as follows:

1. Garlic extract 600–1200 milligrams divided and given 3 times daily
2. Standardized garlic powder extract containing 1.3% allicin content has been studied for this use
3. Fresh garlic 4 grams (approximately one clove) once daily has also been used; fresh garlic typically contains 1% allicin
4. Aged garlic extract 600 milligrams to 7.2 grams per day has also been used; aged garlic typically contains only 0.03% allicin.[80]

Coenzyme Q10

Coenzyme Q10 (Co-Q10, ubiquinone) is an electron and proton carrier that supports ATP synthesis in the lipid phase of the mitochondria membrane. The "Q" and the "10" refer to the quinone chemical group and the 10 isoprenyl chemical subunits that make up the chemical structure of Coenzyme Q10.[24] Coenzyme Q10 is synthesized endogenously in the intracellular environment through the body, particularly in the heart, liver, kidney, and pancreas.[34] Coenzyme Q10 levels are reduced with age, smoking, and statin use, and they are dependent on adequate vitamin B_6 status.[34] Because Coenzyme Q10 is not an essential nutrient, there is no RDA set. The supplement is sold in tablet form and in doses that range from 10 to 130 milligrams per capsule. Coenzyme Q10 has antioxidant properties, may mediate anticancer activity by its effect(s) on the immune system, and perhaps even suppress cancer growth directly.[24]

While no toxicity from Coenzyme Q10 has been reported in humans, higher than 100 mg/day doses may cause mild insomnia. Doses above 300 mg/day may cause increases in liver enzymes, although no liver toxicity has been reported. Other reported side effects from supplemental intake include rashes, nausea, epigastric pain, dizziness, photophobia, irritability, headache, heartburn, and fatigue. Coenzyme Q10 has the potential to reduce the body's response to warfarin, may decrease insulin requirements in those with diabetes, and may reduce the effectiveness or interfere with chemotherapeutic drugs that induce oxidative stress (eg, cyclophosphamide, cytoxan).[24,34]

With regards to its effect on hypertension, the Cochrane Collaboration conducted a systematic review and found that there is not enough reliable evidence to show whether or not Coenzyme Q10 can be useful as a medication to lower blood pressure.[84] For heart failure, the Academy of Nutrition and Dietetics Evidence Analysis Library found that there is Grade II (fair) evidence to state that patients with heart failure may benefit from using Coenzyme Q10. The use of Coenzyme Q10 is not supported for athletes, as it does not appear to enhance exercise performance, or reduce oxidative stress that is induced by exercise.[34]

Coenzyme Q10 and Cardiovascular Disease: What Does the Evidence Say?

The Academy of Nutrition and Dietetics' Evidence Analysis Library states that, "Not enough evidence exists to demonstrate the benefits or harm of supplemental Coenzyme Q10 and its use in CVD (Evidence Grade III – Limited)."[85]

Vitamin E

Vitamin E is a fat-soluble vitamin whose primary dietary sources are vegetable oils. Due to the generally adequate (or high) fat intake of the typical Western diet, vitamin E deficiency in a well-nourished population is rare. Vitamin E has antioxidant properties that may limit free-radical production and stop the production of reactive oxygen species that cause cellular damage. Vitamin E is of additional interest from a supplemental standpoint, due to its involvement in immune function. Despite many claims that have been made about vitamin E's potential to prevent and treat disease, a primary limitation to fully understanding its impact on health pertains to the lack of validated biomarkers for vitamin E status and intake that would otherwise help to serve as valid predictors of clinical outcomes.[45,57]

With regards to its effect on coronary heart disease, interest in vitamin E as a supplement spiked when it was demonstrated in some *in vitro* studies that the vitamin inhibits oxidation of LDL cholesterol (a crucial initial step in atherosclerosis). It is also thought that vitamin E helps prevent blood clot formations that could lead to heart attack or venous thromboembolism.[45,86]

Clinical trials have not supported widespread use of the supplement to prevent CHD. The Heart Outcomes Prevention Evaluation (HOPE) study followed nearly 10,000 people for 4.5 years who were at high risk of heart attack or stroke. The study found that those who took 400 IU/day of natural vitamin E did not have less CVD events or hospitalizations for heart failure or chest pain than did those on placebo. In the HOPE-TOO study, nearly 4000 of the original HOPE participants continued with vitamin E or placebo for another 2.5 years. HOPE-TOO demonstrated that after 7 years of treatment, not only did vitamin E provide no significant protection against heart attack, stroke, unstable angina, or death from heart disease or other causes, but those who took vitamin E were actually 13% more likely to experience, and 21% more likely to be hospitalized for heart failure.

Vitamin E and Cardiovascular Disease: What Does the Evidence Say?

The Academy of Nutrition and Dietetics' Evidence Analysis Project reports that, "Supplemental Vitamin E, given in both natural and synthetic forms, in doses between 30-600 mg/day or 400-800 IU/day, alone or in combination with other antioxidants, has not been shown to decrease the risk for all cause mortality, cardiovascular death, fatal or nonfatal MI. Doses at this level have not been shown to cause harm. (Evidence Grade II - Fair)."[87]

Diet Therapies as Complementary and Alternative Medicine

In addition to the use of dietary supplements, there are a number of diet therapies that may be considered as complementary or alternative therapies for conditions that have not been covered elsewhere in this book.

■ Autism

Autism is a behavioral syndrome that is defined as a group of behaviors associated with numerous genetic and acquired conditions that impact brain development. Autism is one of the most common developmental disabilities, and symptoms are typically apparent before 3 years of age. Currently, the CDC's Autism and Developmental Disabilities Monitoring (ADDM) Network estimates that about one in 88 children has been identified with an autism spectrum disorder (ASD).[88]

As a process, the act of eating may be highly dysregulated among people with ASD. Difficulties arise with impairments related to fine motor coordination, as well as aversion to certain food textures. What to others is considered to be normal visual and aural stimulation of the typical eating environment may be disturbing to those with ASD. Food avoidance or aversion can lead to limitations on foods in the diet and reduced quality of diet. Reduced energy intake can also be seen with disruptions during mealtime either from real or from imagined distractions. Limitations of self-feeding as a result of poor fine-motor coordination can further complicate the eating experience.[89]

Some individuals with ASD will exhibit urinary peptide abnormalities linked to intermediate peptides of gluten and casein metabolism. It has been theorized that some of the components of autism may be explained by excessive opioid activity associated with these peptides.[89,90] Reports are widespread of the use of a gluten-free, casein-free diet by parents as a CAM approach to treating children with autism. Despite these mostly anecdotal, and certainly convincing individual approaches, there is no overwhelming body of research-based evidence that supports the use of this therapeutic diet approach. One small study demonstrated significant reductions in autistic behavior among those following a gluten-free, casein-free diet for 1 year when compared to controls,[91] while another similarly small study showed no significant difference in outcome measures between the diet group and control group. In addition to the high cost and demand on parents' time and resources to construct a gluten- and casein-free diet, prolonged adherence to such a restrictive diet, especially during the crucial developmental periods of childhood, does raise concern for nutrient deficiencies. One study demonstrated that children with autism who were on restricted diets had an increased prevalence of essential amino acid deficiencies, as well as lower plasma levels of essential acids including the neurotransmitter precursors tyrosine and tryptophan, essentially a form of protein malnutrition[89,92]

■ Epilepsy

Although the mechanism is not entirely understood, it is generally accepted that starvation results in a decrease in seizure activity. Starvation causes acidosis, ketosis, dehydration, as well as hypoglycemia. The antiseizure diet, which is now referred to as ketogenic nutrition therapy, is designed of meals and formulas that restrict calories, protein, carbohydrate, and fluid in order to mimic the starved state.[93]

There are two variations of ketogenic nutrition therapy. The most well-known version is based on long-chain triglycerides (LCTs) obtained in the diet from whipping cream, butter, and other high-fat foods.[94] In this diet, 75% of estimated energy needs are given, and the calorie distribution is structured with three to five times as much fat as protein and carbohydrate combined. The second version of ketogenic nutrition therapy is based on medium-chain triglyceride (MCT) oil as the primary fat source. It appears that MCT oil is more ketogenic than LCT fats. In the MCT version of ketogenic nutrition therapy, 100% of the estimated energy requirements are given (allowing for more food) and the ratio is 3 grams fat to 1 gram protein plus carbohydrate.[95] Although the MCT diet allows for more food, it is considered to be less palatable than the LCT diet, and as such, LCT diet is more popular.[93]

The antiseizure ketogenic nutrition therapy book, *The Ketogenic Diet: A Treatment for Epilepsy* (3rd edition), recommends a systematic approach to initiating this diet.[96] The ideal hospitalization schedule outlined in the book is covered in Table 12–10.[76]

Regardless of which dietary approach is ultimately decided upon, GI adaptation to the high-fat content of the meal plan is required. It is imperative that a registered dietitian specializing in the ketogenic diet be involved in the creation and monitoring of this unique therapeutic dietary approach. Although ketogenic nutrition therapy is not considered a first-line treatment for epilepsy, it should be considered in children whose seizures are not well controlled on available medications.

Table 12–10. Suggested hospitalization schedule for initiation of the ketogenic diet.

Day 0	Child eats no carbohydrates at home and begins overnight fast at dinner
Day 1	Child is admitted to hospital; fasting continues
	Fluids are monitored and limited to 60-70 mL/kg body weight
	Nutrition consult with dietitian to obtain food preferences and begin assessment
	Baseline blood work ordered, antiepileptic medication levels monitored, IV started
	Intake and output monitored; seizure log maintained; and electrolytes, vitals, and activity monitored
Day 2	Monitor urine for ketones and finger-sticks for glucose to prevent hypoglycemia
	Vital signs monitored
	Dietitian begins calculating meal plans and starts to educate parents on how to plan and prepare diet
Day 3	Child is in ketosis and begins meals at 1/3 strength
	Antiepileptic drugs and electrolytes measured
	Weights, vitals, and finger-sticks continue
	Dietitian helps parents learn how to use scale and prepare meals
Day 4	Child progresses to 2/3 strength meals
	Dietitian completes basic meal plan and parents' diet education
Day 5	Child starts full diet and, if stable, is discharged home
	Follow-up appointments made prior to hospital discharge

Data from Freeman et al., 2000.

Side effects of the diet include profound hypoglycemia, acidotic dehydration, and/or hypokalemia. Later on in the diet's progression, kidney stones, hyperlipidemia, hyperuricemia, constipation, GERD, or pancreatitis may result.[97-100]

The ketogenic diet has been shown to be an effective approach for decreasing the frequency of seizures in patients refractory to antiepileptic medication.[95,101-104] The therapy is thought to be effective in at least half of the pediatric epilepsy patients who attempt it.[105] Some research also indicates that the ketogenic nutrition therapy may be as good, or perhaps even better than the new antiepileptic drugs available for the management of refractory seizures.[106]

- ## Muscle Cramps

Muscle cramps are experienced more regularly under certain conditions and in certain disease states. Muscle cramps during pregnancy are common, and are not fully understood. Athletes and those at risk for excessive sweat and dehydration are also predisposed to cramping.[107] Muscle cramps may be associated with dehydration, decreased chloride, and sodium, calcium, vitamin D, and/or magnesium deficiencies. A Cochrane Collaboration review found that it is unlikely that magnesium supplementation provides clinically meaningful cramp prophylaxis in older adults who experience skeletal muscle cramps. The effect of magnesium on alleviating pregnancy-associated rest cramps has not shown consistent effects in the literature.[108]

In hemodialysis, muscle cramps are thought to be related to shifts in electrolytes and fluids, indicating an early sign of ultrafiltration down to an individual's dry weight. Quinine may be used off-label for the treatment of leg cramps (although it should be avoided for routine use unless the cramps are disabling and do not respond to other approaches).[109] Supplemental vitamin E intake may also be beneficial for this condition, although no consensus exists regarding dosage. Acute relief may be provided by infusion of a hypertonic glucose solution (50 mL of 50% dextrose).[110] Muscle twitching, convulsions, or tetany may be linked to magnesium of vitamin B_6 excess or deficiency, calcium, vitamin D, and/or magnesium deficiencies.[48,49]

- ## Nausea and Vomiting

The underlying causes of and recommended standard diet therapy for nausea are covered in Chapter 7. This material pertains to the CAM treatments recommended for nausea management. The CAM therapies for which there is anecdotal evidence, although not much in the way of clinical trials, include the use of ginger, aromatherapy, and acupuncture.

Ginger has been used historically in Asian medicine to treat stomachache, nausea, and diarrhea. In ancient Greece, ginger was used to improve circulation, help with digestion, and alleviate nausea and other GI problems.[34] There are some studies that suggest that short-term use of ginger can safely mitigate pregnancy-related nausea and vomiting. In 2004, the American College of Obstetrics and Gynecologists endorsed ginger, stating, "treatment of nausea and vomiting of pregnancy with ginger has shown beneficial effects and can be considered as a nonpharmacologic option." Although no specific dosing recommendations exist, the ACOG review does cite a controlled trial that studied the efficacy of ginger in pregnancy-related nausea and vomiting using a dose of 350 milligrams of ginger taken three times per day.[34,111] Results are mixed on whether ginger is an effective treatment for nausea caused by motion, chemotherapy, or surgery.[112] Individuals on anticoagulant/antiplatelet therapies should take caution with ginger use, as theoretically it may have an additive effect.

For postoperative nausea and vomiting (PONV), aromatherapy is sometimes recommended, although there is insufficient evidence to say that it is an effective approach. A Cochrane Collaboration review found that isopropyl alcohol was more effective than saline placebo in reducing postoperative nausea and vomiting, although it was less effective than standard antiemetic drugs. The same review states that there is currently no reliable evidence for the use of peppermint oil.[113]

Another Cochrane review studied the role of acupuncture on postoperative nausea and vomiting, finding that electroacupuncture has shown a benefit for chemotherapy-induced acute vomiting, but adding that additional studies combining electroacupuncture with state-of-the-art antiemetics and in patients with refractory symptoms are recommended to determine true clinical relevance. Acupressure that is self-administered seems to have a protective effect against acute nausea, and can be easily taught to patients (although studies did not involve placebo control). The use of noninvasive electrostimulation seems unlikely to have a clinically relevant impact when patients are given current pharmacologic antiemetic therapy.[114]

■ Diabetes

In general, there is not much in the way of scientific evidence that points to substantial benefits recognized from dietary supplements for type 2 diabetes or its complications. While many dietary supplements have been studied with regards to their impact on glycemia, alpha-lipoic acid (ALA), chromium, omega-3 fatty acids, and polyphenols (antioxidants found in tea and dark chocolate) do not have overwhelming evidence to support their clinical use. Magnesium supplementation on blood sugar studies have yielded mixed results.[115] Cochrane Collaboration reviews have determined that:

1. There is no evidence to suggest the use of zinc supplementation in the prevention of type 2 diabetes.[116]
2. Omega-3 polyunsaturated fatty acid supplementation in type 2 diabetes does lower triglycerides and VLDL cholesterol (but may raise LDL) and has no statistically significant effect on glycemic control or fasting insulin.[117]
3. There is not sufficient evidence to support the use of cinnamon for type 1 or type 2 diabetes.[118]
4. Although some herbal mixtures may exhibit glucose-lowering effects, small sample sizes and methodological problems with study design cause an inability to make a determination about the use of ayurvedic treatments for diabetes.[119]
5. Some Chinese herbal medications do show hypoglycemic effects in type 2 diabetes; the results should be interpreted carefully though due to poor methodological quality, small sample sizes, and limited numbers of clinical trials; more high-quality studies are recommended to shed more light on the positive findings that do exist.[120]

Practitioner Resources

Interpreting existing data about CAM therapies is an important service that you as a professional can provide for your patients considering CAM. The following books and websites are valuable resources that contain evidence-based information about various CAM therapies and supplements.

- ■ Books

The Health Professionals Guide to Popular Dietary Supplements, 3rd ed. By Allison Sarubin Fragakis, MS, RD, with Cynthia A. Thomson, PhD, RD. American Dietetic Association, 2006. Available at: https://www.eatright.org/Shop/Product.aspx?id=4851

Tyler's Honest Herbal, 4th ed. By Steven Foster and Varro E. Tyler. Haworth Press, 1999. Available at: http://www.stevenfoster.com/publications/books/HH4.html

The ACP Evidence-Based Guide to Complementary and Alternative Medicine. By Bradly Jacobs, MD, MPH, and Katherine Gundling, MD, FACP. American College of Physicians, 2009. Available at: https://www.acponline.org/ebizatpro/ProductsandServices/Booksfrom ACPPress/ACPPressDetail/tabid/203/Default.aspx?ProductId=17185# .UQqvTOhYvFE

- ■ Websites

Government Sites

MedlinePlus, Herbs and Supplements: http://www.nlm.nih.gov/medlineplus/druginfo/herb_All.html

National Cancer Institute, Office of Cancer Complementary and Alternative Medicine: http://cam.cancer.gov/

NCCAM, CAM on PubMed Search: http://nccam.nih.gov/research/camonpubmed

NCCAM, CAM and Diabetes: http://nccam.nih.gov/health/diabetes/CAM-and-diabetes.htm

NCCAM, Hepatitis C: A Focus on Herbal Supplements: http://nccam.nih.gov/health/hepatitisc/hepatitiscfacts.htm

NCCAM, Resources for Health Care Providers: http://nccam.nih.gov/health/providers

Office of Dietary Supplements, National Institutes of Health: http://ods.od.nih.gov/

Education and Healthcare Institution Sites

The University of Arizona, Arizona Center for Integrative Medicine: http://integrativemedicine.arizona.edu/

University of Connecticut, Omega-3 Learning for Health & Medicine: http://www.omega3learning.uconn.edu/

Mayo Clinic, Alternative Medicine: http://www.mayoclinic.com/health/osteoarthritis/DS00019/DSECTION=alternative-medicine

Natural Medicines Comprehensive Database: http://naturaldatabase.therapeuticresearch.com/home.aspx?cs=&s=ND

Professional Associations

American Holistic Nurses Association: http://www.ahna.org/
Dietitians in Integrative and Functional Medicine: http://integrativerd.org/
The Institute for Functional Medicine: http://www.functionalmedicine.org/
The International Society of Nutrigenetics/Nutrigenomics: http://www.isnn.info/

References

1. Chiappelli F, Prolo P, Cajulis O. Evidence-based research in complementary and alternative medicine I: history. Evid Based Complement Alternat Med 2005;2(4):453–458.

2. Dossey B. Florence Nightingale and Holistic Nursing. National Student Nursing Association Imprint (2005, February/March):56–58.

3. Snyder M, Lindquist R. Issues in complementary therapies: how we got to where we are. Online J Issues Nurs 2001;6(2):1.

4. National Center for Complementary and Alternative Medicine. (2012, September 6). Appropriations History. Retrieved from January 26, 2013 NCCAM Funding: http://nccam.nih.gov/about/budget/appropriations.htm

5. National Center for Complementary and Alternative Medicine. (2012, April 10). NCCAM: Mission. Retrieved January 26, 2013 from The NIH Almanac: http://www.nih.gov/about/almanac/organization/NCCAM.htm

6. National Center for Complementary and Alternative Medicine. (2011, July). What is Complementary and Alternative Medicine. Retrieved January 25, 2013 from CAM Basics: http://nccam.nih.gov/health/whatiscam

7. National Center for Complementary and Alternative Medicine (NCCAM). (2012, January 3). Advance Research on CAM Natural Products. Retrieved January 25, 2013 from Strategic Objective 2: http://nccam.nih.gov/about/plans/2011/objective2.htm

8. National Center for Complementary and Alternative Medicine (NCCAM). (2012, January 16). Transcript. Retrieved from January 26, 2013 Q&A with NCCAM Director Dr. Josephine P. Briggs: http://nccam.nih.gov/video/briggs

9. US Department of Health and Human Services. Complementary and Alternative Medicine Use Among Adults and Children: United States, 2007. Centers for Disease Control and Prevention, National Center for Health Statistics; 2008.

10. US Department of Health and Human Services. Dietary supplement use in the United States has increased since the National Health and Nutrition Examination Survey (NHANES) III (1988–1994). NCHS Data Brief (2011, April);61:1–8.

11. US Department of Health and Human Services. Costs of Complementary and Alternative Medicine (CAM) and Frequency of Visits to CAM Practitioners: United States, 2007. Natl Health Stat Report (2009, July);1–14.

12. Packaged Facts. (2012, September 18). Solid Growth and Diverse Demographics for Vitamins and Supplements. Retrieved January 25, 2013 from Press Release: http://www.packagedfacts.com/about/release.asp?id=2997

13. Neutraceuticals World. (2013, January 1). Top 10 Trends for 2013. Retrieved January 25, 2013 from Neutraceuticals World Now: http://www.nutraceuticalsworld.com/issues/2013-01/view_editorials/top-10-trends-for-2013/

14. Nutrition Business Journal. (2012). NBJ's Global Supplement & Nutrition Industry Report 2012.

15. Tsouderos T. CAM: taxpayer money spent on studies with questionable scientific value. Chicago Tribune (2011, December 11); Tsouderos T. Federal center pays good money for suspect medicine. Chicago Tribune (2011, December 11).

16. Offit P. Studying complementary and alternative therapies. JAMA 2012;307(17):1803–1804.

17. American Medical Association. (2011, October 4). Demand drives more hospitals to offer alternative therapies. Retrieved January 26, 2013 from American Medical News: http://www.ama-assn.org/amednews/2011/10/03/prsd1004.htm

18. Shapiro R. Suckers: How Alternative Medicine Makes Fools of Us All. London, England: Random House; 2008.

19. Bausell R. Snake Oil Science: The Truth About Complementary and Alternative Medicine. Oxford University Press; 2009.

20. Clegg D, Reda D, Harris C, Klein M, O'Dell J, Hooper M, et al. Glucosamine, chondroitin sulfate, and the two in combination for painful knee osteoarthritis. J Engl J Med 2006;354(8):795–808.

21. Sawitzke A, Shi H, Finco M, Dunlop D, Bingham C, Harris C, et al. The effect of glucosamine and/or chondroitin sulfate on the progression of knee osteoarthritis: a report from the glucosamine/chondroitin arthritis intervention trial. Arthritis Rheum 2008;58(10):3183–3191.

22. Sawitzke A, Shi H, Finco M, Dunlop D, Harris C, Singer N, et al. Clinical efficacy and safety of glucosamine, chondroitin sulphate, their combination, celecoxib or placebo taken to treat osteoarthritis of the knee: 2-year results from GAIT. Ann Rheum Dis 2010;69(8):1459–1464.

23. Consumer Lab. (2012, May 8). Lead Contamination and Mislabeling in Joint Health Supplements with Glucosamine, Chondroitin, and MSM According to ConsumerLab.com. Retrieved January 25, 2013 from ConsumerLab.com: http://www.consumerlab.com/news/glucosamine_joint_supplements_reviewed/5_8_2012/

24. National Cancer Institute. (2012, November 9). CAM Definitions. Retrieved January 26, 2013 from Office of Cancer Complementary and Alternative Medicine: http://cam.cancer.gov/health_definitions.html; National Cancer Institute. (2012, August 10). Overview. Retrieved January 30, 2013 from Coenzyme Q10 (PDQ): http://www.cancer.gov/cancertopics/pdq/cam/coenzymeQ10/HealthProfessional; National Cancer Institute. (2012, July 20). Questions and Answers About Complementary and Alternative Medicine. Retrieved January 26, 2013 from Complementary and Alternative Medicine in Cancer Treatment (PDQ): http://www.cancer.gov/cancertopics/pdq/cam/cam-cancer-treatment/patient/page2#Reference2.3

25. Cox L. (2009, July 31). Why Do We Spend $34 Billion in Alternative Medicine? Retrieved January 26, 2013 from ABC World News with Diane Sawyer: http://abcnews.go.com/Health/WellnessNews/story?id= 8215703&page=1

26. National Center for Complementary and Alternative Medicine. (2011, July). Credentialing CAM Providers: Understanding CAM Education, Training, Regulation, and Licensing. Retrieved January 25, 2013 from CAM Basics: http://nccam.nih.gov/health/decisions/credentialing.htm

27. American Holistic Nurses Association. (2012). Mission Statement. Retrieved January 25, 2013 from About Us: http://www.ahna.org/AboutUs/MissionStatement/tabid/1931/Default.aspx

28. Eisenberg D, Cohen M, Hrbek A. Credentialing complementary and alternative medical providers. Ann Intern Med 2002;137(12):965–973.

29. Stein K, Kaw C, Crammer C, Gansler. The role of psychological functioning in the use of complementary and alternative methods among disease-free colorectal cancer survivors: a report from the American Cancer Society's studies of cancer survivors. Cancer (2009, September 15) 115(18 suppl):4397–4408.

30. Kelly K. Complementary and alternative medical therapies for children with cancer. Eur J Cancer 2004;40(14):2041–2046.

31. US Department of Health and Human Services. (2005, April). Retrieved January 26, 2013 from Thinking About Complementary & Alternative Medicine: A Guide for People with Cancer: https://pubs.cancer.gov/ncipl/detail.aspx?prodid=P042

32. Nutrition.gov. (2013, January 8). Questions to Ask Before Taking Vitamin and Mineral Supplements. Retrieved January 26, 2013 from Dietary Supplements: http://www.nutrition.gov/dietary-supplements/questions-ask-taking-vitamin-and-mineral-supplements

33. Nelms M, Sucher K. Pharmacology. In: Nelms M, Sucher K, Lacey K, Roth S, eds. Nutrition Therapy & Pathophysiology. 2nd ed. Belmont, CA: Wadsworth Cengage Learning; 2011.

34. Fragakis A, Thomson C. The Health Professional's Guide to Popular Dietary Supplements. 3rd ed. Chicago, IL: American Dietetic Association; 2007.

35. Burke P, Roche-Dudek M, Roche-Klemma K. Drug-Nutrient Resource Fifth Edition. Riverside, IL: Roche Dietitians, LLD; 2003.

36. Hall-Flavin D. (2013, January 17). MAOIs and Diet. Retrieved January 26, 2013 from Mayo Clinic: http://www.mayoclinic.com/health/maois/HQ01575

37. University of Pittsburgh Medical Center. (n.d.). MAOI Diet Facts. Retrieved January 26, 2013 from Patient Education Materials: http://www.upmc.com/patients-visitors/education/nutrition/pages/maoi-diet-facts.aspx

38. 103rd United States Congress. (1994, October 25). Dietary Supplement Health and Education Act of 1994. Pub. L. No. 103–417.

39. Office of Dietary Supplements. (2013, January 7). Multivitamin/mineral Supplements. Retrieved from January 26, 2013 Dietary Supplement Fact Sheet: http://ods.od.nih.gov/factsheets/MVMS-HealthProfessional/

40. Consumer Reports. (2012, June). The dangers of dietary supplements. Retrieved from January 26, 2013 Health: http://www.consumerreports .org/cro/2012/06/the-dangers-of-dietary-supplements/index.htm

41. Soller R, Bayne H, Shaheen C. The regulated dietary supplement industry: myths of an unregulated industry dispelled. American Botanical Council HerbalGram 2012;(93):42–57.

42. Cohen P. Assessing supplement safety—The FDA's controversial proposal. N Engl J Med 2012;366:389–391.

43. Skerrett P. (2012, February 2). FDA needs stronger rules to ensure the safety of dietary supplements. Retrieved January 26, 2013 from Harvard Health Blog: http://www.health.harvard.edu/blog/fda-needs-stronger-rules-to-ensure-the-safety-of-dietary-supplements-201202024182

44. Dennehy C. Dietary supplements & herbal medications. In: Katzung B, Masters S, Trevor S, eds. Basic & Clinical Pharmacology. 12th ed. New York, NY: McGraw-Hill; 2012 [chapter 64].

45. Office of Dietary Supplements. (2011, June 24). Dietary Supplements. Retrieved January 26, 2013 from Background Information: http://ods. od.nih.gov/factsheets/DietarySupplements-HealthProfessional/; Office of Dietary Supplements. (2011, June 24). Vitamin C. Retrieved January 30, 2013 from Dietary Supplement Fact Sheet: http://ods.od.nih.gov/ factsheets/VitaminC-HealthProfessional/

46. Blair K. Vitamin supplementation and megadoses. Nurse Pract 1986;11(7):19–26, 31–36.

47. Mayo Clinic. (2010, December 17). *Dietary supplements: skip megadoses*. Retrieved January 26, 2013 from Nutrition and healthy eating: http://www.mayoclinic.com/health/health-tip/HT00625/rss=6

48. Academy of Nutrition and Dietetics. Nutrient Supplementation for a Healthy Population: Tips for Choosing and Using Vitamin, Mineral and Other Nutrient Supplements. Academy of Nutrition and Dietetics, Evidence Analysis Library. Chicago, IL: Academy of Nutrition and Dietetics; 2012.

49. Academy of Nutrition and Dietetics. (2012). Physical Observations. Retrieved from January 30, 2013 Nutrition Care Manual: http://www. nutritioncaremanual.org

50. US Food and Drug Administration. (2002, January). Tips for the Savvy Supplement User: Making Informed Decisions and Evaluating Information. Retrieved January 26, 2013 from Dietary Supplements, Consumer Information: http://www.fda.gov/Food/DietarySupplements/ ConsumerInformation/ucm110567.htm

51. Izzo A, Ernst E. Interactions between herbal medicines and prescribed drugs: a systematic review. Drugs 2009;69(13):1777–1798.

52. Garrard J, Harms S, Eberly LE, Matiak A. Variations in product choices of frequently purchased herbs: caveat emptor. Arch Intern Med 2003;163(19):2290–2295.

53. US Food and Drug Administration. (2012, August 9). Avoiding Drug Interactions. Retrieved January 30, 2013 from Consumer Updates: http://www.fda.gov/forconsumers/consumerupdates/ucm096386.htm# supplements

54. Wagner C, Greer F. The Section on Breastfeeding and Committee on Nutrition. Prevention of rickets and vitamin D deficiency in infants, children, and adolescents. Pediatrics 2008;122(5):1142–1152.

55. Mead M. Benefits of sunlight: a bright spot for human health. Environ Health Perspect 2008;116(4):A160–A167.

56. Lieber C. Relationships between nutrition, alcohol use, and liver disease. Alcohol Res Health 2003;27(3):220–231.

57. Institute of Medicine. Dietary Reference Intakes: Vitamin C, Vitamin E, Selenium, and Carotenoids. Washington, DC: National Academies Press; 2000.

58. Schweitzer A. Dietary supplements during pregnancy. J Perinat Educ (2006, Fall);15(4):44–45.

59. Office of Dietary Supplements. (2005, October 28). Omega-3 Fatty Acids and Health. Retrieved January 30, 2013 from Dietary Supplement Fact Sheet: http://ods.od.nih.gov/factsheets/Omega3FattyAcidsandHealth-HealthProfessional/

60. Expert Panel on Detection, Evaluation, and Treatment of High Blood Cholesterol in Adults. Executive summary of the Third Report of the National Cholesterol Education Program (NCEP) Expert Panel on Detection, Evaluation, and Treatment of High Blood Cholesterol in Adults (Adult Treatment Panel III). JAMA 2001;285:2486–2497.

61. Academy of Nutrition and Dietetics. (2011). Disorders of Lipid Metabolism, Evidence-Based Nutrition Practice Guidelines, Executive Summary of Guidelines. Retrieved May 5, 2012 from Evidence Analysis Library: http://andevidencelibrary.com

62. Academy of Nutrition and Dietetics. (2007). Omega 3 Fatty Acids. Retrieved January 30, 2013 from Evidence Analysis Library: http://andevidencelibrary.com

63. US National Library of Medicine. (2011, December 9). Glucosamine sulfate. Retrieved January 30, 2013 from MedlinePlus: http://www.nlm.nih.gov/medlineplus/druginfo/natural/807.html

64. US National Library of Medicine. (2011, December 9). Echinacea. Retrieved January 30, 2013 from MedlinePlus: http://www.nlm.nih.gov/medlineplus/druginfo/natural/981.html

65. Linde K, Barrett B, Bauer R, Melchart D, Woelkart K. Echinacea for preventing and treating the common cold. Cochrane Databsae of Systematic Reviews (1) 2006.

66. Pan A, Yu D, Demark-Wahnefried W, Franco O, Lin, X. Meta-analysis of the effects of flaxseed interventions on blood lipids. Am J Clin Nutr 2009;90(2):288–297.

67. National Center for Complementary and Alternative Medicine. (2012, April). Flaxseed and Flaxseed Oil. Retrieved January 30, 2013 from Herbs at a Glance: http://nccam.nih.gov/health/flaxseed/ataglance.htm

68. Sonnenborn U, Proppert Y. Ginseng (Panax ginseng CA Meyer). Br J Phytother 1991;2:3–14.

69. Greenspan E. Ginseng and vaginal bleeding. JAMA 1983;249:2018.

70. US National Library of Medicine. (2011, February 28). American Ginseng. Retrieved January 30, 2013 from Medline Plus: http://www.nlm.nih.gov/medlineplus/druginfo/natural/967.html

71. US National Library of Medicine. (2012, October 8). Panax Ginseng. Retrieved January 30, 2013 from Medline Plus: http://www.nlm.nih.gov/medlineplus/druginfo/natural/1000.html

72. US National Library of Medicine. (2012, August 2). Siberian Ginseng. Retrieved January 30, 2013 from Medline Plus: http://www.nlm.nih.gov/medlineplus/druginfo/natural/985.html

73. Geng J, Dong J, Ni H, Lee M, Wu T, Jiang K, et al. Ginseng for cognition. Cochrane Database of Systematic Reviews (12) 2010.

74. Fiore, K. (2009, December 30). Ginkgo Doesn't Stop Cognitive Decline. Retrieved January 30, 2013 from ABC News: http://abcnews.go.com/Health/MindMoodNews/ginkgo-biloba-stop-cognitive-decline/story?id=9448315

75. National Center for Complementary and Alternative Medicine. (2012, January 3). The Ginkgo Evaluation of Memory (GEM) Study. Retrieved January 30, 2013 from Research: http://nccam.nih.gov/research/results/gems

76. Snitz B, O'Meara E, Carlson M, Arnold A, Ives D, Rapp S, et al. Ginkgo biloba for preventing cognitive decline in older adults: a randomized trial. JAMA 2009;302(24):2663–2670.

77. DeKosky S, Williamson J, Fitzpatrick A, Kronmal R, Ives D, Saxton J, et al. Ginkgo biloba for prevention of dementia: a randomized controlled trial. JAMA 2008;300(19):2253–2262.

78. US National Library of Medicine. (2012, October 8). Ginkgo. Retrieved January 30, 2013 from MedlinePlus: http://www.nlm.nih.gov/medlineplus/druginfo/natural/333.html

79. National Center for Complementary and Alternative Medicine. (2005, September). Ginkgo. Retrieved January 30, 2013 from Herbs at a glance: http://nccam.nih.gov/health/ginkgo/ataglance.htm

80. US National Library of Medicine. (2011, December 24). Garlic. Retrieved January 30, 2013 from Medline Plus: http://www.nlm.nih.gov/medlineplus/druginfo/natural/300.html

81. Lissiman E, Bhasale A, Cohen M. Garlic for the common cold. Cochrane Database of Systematic Reviews (3) 2012.

82. Stabler S, Tejani A, Huynh F, Fowkes C. Garlic for the prevention of cardiovascular morbidity and mortality in hypertensive patients. Cochrane Database of Systematic Reviews (8) 2012.

83. Meher S, Duley L. Garlic for preventing pre-eclampsia and its complications. Cochrane Database of Systematic Reviews (3) 2006.

84. Ho MJ; Bellusci A; Wright JM. Blood pressure lowering efficacy of coenzyme Q10 for primary hypertension. Cochrane Databse of Systematic Reviews (4) 2009, October 7.

85. Academy of Nutrition and Dietetics. (2004). What is the relationship between supplemental coenzyme Q10 and cardiovascular disease? Retrieved January 30, 2013 from Evidence Analysis Library: http://andevidencelibrary.com

86. Glynn R, Ridker P, Goldhaber S, Zee R, Buring J. Effects of random allocation to vitamin E supplementation on the occurrence of venous thromboembolism: report from the Women's Health Study. Circulation 2007;116:1497–1503.

87. Academy of Nutrition and Dietetics. (2004). What is the relationship between supplemental vitamin E and cardiovascular disease? Retrieved January 30, 2013 from Evidence Analysis Library: http://andevidencelibrary.com

88. Baio J. (2012, March 30). Prevalence of Autism Spectrum Disorders—Autism and Developmental Disabilities Monitoring Network, 14 Sites, United States, 2008. Morbidity and Mortality Weekly Report (MMWR), 61 (SS03), pp. 1–19.

89. Academy of Nutrition and Dietetics. (2012). Autism Spectrum Disorders. Retrieved from Nutrition Care Manual: http://www.nutritioncaremanual.org

90. Millward C, Ferriter M, Calver S, Connell-Jones G. Gluten- and casein-free diets for autistic spectrum disorder. Cochrane Database of Systematic Reviews (2) 2008.

91. Knivsberg A, Reichelt K, Hoien T, Nodland M. A randomised, controlled study of dietary intervention in autistic syndromes. Nutr Neurosci 2002;5(4):251–261.

92. Arnold G, Hyman S, Mooney R, Kirby R. Plasma amino acid profiles in children with autism: potential risk of nutritional deficiencies. J Autism Dev Disord 2003;33(4):449–454.

93. Academy of Nutrition and Dietetics. (2012). Epilepsy. Retrieved January 30, 2013 from Nutrition Care Manual: http://www.nutritioncaremanual.org

94. Livingston S, Pauli S, Pruce I. Ketogenic diet in the treatment of childhood epilepsy. Dev Med Child Neurol 1977;19:833–834.

95. Huttenlocher P, Wilbourn A, Signore J. Medium-chain triglycerides as a therapy for intractable epilepsy. Neurology 1971;21:1097–1103.

96. Freeman JM, Freeman JB, Kelly M. The Ketogenic Diet: A Treatment for Epilepsy. 3rd ed. New York, NY: Demos Publications; 2000.

97. Ballaban-Gil K, Callahan C, O'Dell C, Pappo M, Moshe S, Shinnar S. Complications of the ketogenic diet. Epilepsia 1998;39:744–748.

98. Erickson J, Jabbari B, Difazio M. Basal ganglia injury as a complication of the ketogenic diet. Mov Disord 2003;18:448–451.

99. Kang H, Chung D, Kim D, Kim H. Early- and late-onset complications of the ketogenic diet for intractable epilepsy. Epilepsia 2004;45(9): 1116–1123.

100. Vining E. Long-term health consequences of epilepsy diet treatments. Epilepsia 2008;49(suppl 8):27–29.

101. Schwartz R, Boyes S, Aynsley-Green A. Metabolic effects of three ketogenic diets in the treatment of severe epilepsy. Dev Med Child Neurol 1989;31:152–160.

102. Kinsman S, Vining E, Quaskey S, Mellits D, Freeman J. Efficacy of the ketogenic diet for intractable seizure disorders: review of 58 cases. Epilepsia 1992;33:1132–1136.

103. Thiele E. Assessing the efficacy of antiepileptic treatments: the ketogenic diet. Epilepsia 2003;44:26–29.

104. Levy R, Cooper P. Ketogenic diet for epilepsy. Cochrane Database Sys Rev (3) 2003.

105. Vining E. Clinical efficacy of the ketogenic diet. Epilepsy Res 1999;37:181–190.

106. LeFevre F, Aronson N. Ketogenic diet for the treatment of refractory epilepsy in children: a systematic review of efficacy. Pediatrics 2000;105(4):E46.

107. Ropper A, Samuels M. Disorders of muscle characterized by cramp, spasm, pain, and localized masses. In: Ropper A, Samuels M. Adam and Victor's Principles of Neurology. 9th ed. New York, NY: McGraw-Hill; 2009 [chapter 55].

108. Garrison S, Allan G, Sekhon R, Musini VK. Magnesium for skeletal muscle cramps. Cochrane Database of Systematic Reviews (9) 2012.

109. Greenberg D, Aminoff M, Simon R. Motor disorders. In: Greenberg D, Aminoff M, Simon R. Clinical Neurology. 8th ed. New York, NY: McGraw-Hill; 2012 [chapter 9].

110. Rocco M, Moossavi S. Hemodialysis. In: Lerma E, Berns J, Nissenson A, eds. CURRENT Diagnosis & Treatment: Nephrology & Hypertension. New York, NY: McGraw-Hill; 2009 [chapter 50].

111. American College of Obstetricians and Gynecologists. Practice Bulletin: nausea and vomiting of pregnancy. Obstet Gynecol 2004;103:803–814.

112. National Center for Complementary and Alternative Medicine. (2012, April). Ginger. Retrieved January 30, 2013 from Herbs at a glance: http://nccam.nih.gov/health/ginger

113. Hines S, Steels E, Chang A, Gibbons K. Aromatherapy for treatment of postoperative nausea and vomiting. Cochrane Database of Systematic Reviews (4) 2012.

114. Ezzo J, Richardson M, Vickrs A, Allen C, Dibble S, Issell B, et al. Acupuncture-point stimulation for chemotherapy-induced nausea or vomiting. Cochrane Database of Systematic Reviews (2) 2006.

115. National Center for Complementary and Alternative Medicine. (2008, June). Diabetes and CAM: A Focus on Dietary Supplements. Retrieved January 31, 2013 from Get the facts: http://nccam.nih.gov/health/diabetes/CAM-and-diabetes.htm

116. Beletate V, El Dib R, Atallah A. Zinc supplementation for the prevention of type 2 diabetes mellitus. Cochrane Database of Systematic Reviews (1) 2007.

117. Hartweg J, Perera R, Montori V, Dinneen S, Neil A, Farmer A. Omega-3 polyunsaturated fatty acids (PUFA) for type 2 diabetes mellitus. Cochrane Database of Systematic Reviews (1). 2008.

118. Leach M, Kumar S. Cinnamon for diabetes mellitus. Cochrane Database of Systematic Reviews (9) 2012.

119. Sridharan K, Mohan R, Ramaratnam S, Panneerselvam D. Ayurvedic treatments for diabetes mellitus. Cochrane Database of Systematic Reviews (12) 2011.

120. Liu J, Zhang M, Wang W, Grimsgaard S. Chinese herbal medicines for type 2 diabetes mellitus. Cochrane Database of Systematic Reviews (3) 2004.

Appendix A

Dietary Reference Intakes (DRIs): Estimated Average Requirements
Food and Nutrition Board, Institute of Medicine, National Academies

Life Stage Group	Calcium (mg/d)	CHO (g/kg/d)	Protein (g/d)	Vit A (µg/d)[a]	Vit C (mg/d)	Vit D (µg/d)	Vit E (mg/d)[b]	Thiamin (mg/d)	Riboflavin (mg/d)	Niacin (mg/d)[c]	Vit B6 (mg/d)	Folate (µg/d)[d]	Vit B12 (µg/d)	Copper (µg/d)	Iodine (µg/d)	Iron (mg/d)	Magnesium (mg/d)	Molybdenum (µg/d)	Phosphorus (mg/d)	Selenium (µg/d)	Zinc (mg/d)
Infants																					
0 to 6 mo																					
6 to 12 mo			1.0													6.9					2.5
Children																					
1–3 years	500	100	0.87	210	13	10	5	0.4	0.4	5	0.4	120	0.7	260	65	3.0	65	13	380	17	2.5
4–8 years	800	100	0.76	275	22	10	6	0.5	0.5	6	0.5	160	1.0	340	65	4.1	110	17	405	23	4.0
Males																					
9–13 years	1100	100	0.76	445	39	10	9	0.7	0.8	9	0.8	250	1.5	540	73	5.9	200	26	1055	35	7.0
14–18 years	1100	100	0.73	630	63	10	12	1.0	1.1	12	1.1	330	2.0	685	95	7.7	340	33	1055	45	8.5
19–30 years	800	100	0.66	625	75	10	12	1.0	1.1	12	1.1	320	2.0	700	95	6	330	34	580	45	9.4
31–50 years	800	100	0.66	625	75	10	12	1.0	1.1	12	1.1	320	2.0	700	95	6	350	34	580	45	9.4
51–70 years	800	100	0.66	625	75	10	12	1.0	1.1	12	1.4	320	2.0	700	95	6	350	34	580	45	9.4
>70 years	1000	100	0.66	625	75	10	12	1.0	1.1	12	1.4	320	2.0	700	95	6	350	34	580	45	9.4

Life Stage Group	Calcium (mg/d)	CHO (g/kg/d)	Protein (g/d)	Vit A (µg/d)[a]	Vit C (mg/d)	Vit D (µg/d)	Vit E (mg/d)[b]	Thiamin (mg/d)	Ribo-flavin (mg/d)	Niacin (mg/d)[c]	Vit B6 (mg/d)	Folate (µg/d)[d]	Vit B12 (µg/d)	Copper (µg/d)	Iodine (µg/d)	Iron (mg/d)	Magnes-ium (mg/d)	Molyb-denum (µg/d)	Phos-phorus (mg/d)	Selenium (µg/d)	Zinc (mg/d)
Females																					
9–13 years	1100	100	0.76	420	39	10	9	0.7	0.8	9	0.8	250	1.5	540	73	5.7	200	26	1055	35	7.0
14–18 years	1100	100	0.71	485	56	10	12	0.9	0.9	11	1.0	330	2.0	685	95	7.9	300	33	1055	45	7.3
19–30 years	800	100	0.66	500	60	10	12	0.9	0.9	11	1.1	320	2.0	700	95	8.1	255	34	580	45	6.8
31–50 years	800	100	0.66	500	60	10	12	0.9	0.9	11	1.1	320	2.0	700	95	8.1	265	34	580	45	6.8
51–70 years	1000	100	0.66	500	60	10	12	0.9	0.9	11	1.3	320	2.0	700	95	5	265	34	580	45	6.8
>70 years	1000	100	0.66	500	60	10	12	0.9	0.9	11	1.3	320	2.0	700	95	5	265	34	580	45	6.8
Pregnancy																					
14–18 years	1000	135	0.88	530	66	10	12	1.2	1.2	14	1.6	520	2.2	785	160	23	335	40	1055	49	10.5
19–30 years	800	135	0.88	550	70	10	12	1.2	1.2	14	1.6	520	2.2	800	160	22	290	40	580	49	9.5
31–50 years	800	135	0.88	550	70	10	12	1.2	1.2	14	1.6	520	2.2	800	160	22	300	40	580	49	9.5

(continued)

(*Continued*)

Life Stage Group	Calcium (mg/d)	CHO (g/kg/d)	Protein (g/d)	Vit A (µg/d)[a]	Vit C (mg/d)	Vit D (µg/d)	Vit E (mg/d)[b]	Thiamin (mg/d)	Riboflavin (mg/d)	Niacin (mg/d)[c]	Vit B$_6$ (mg/d)	Folate (µg/d)[d]	Vit B$_{12}$ (µg/d)	Copper (µg/d)	Iodine (µg/d)	Iron (mg/d)	Magnesium (mg/d)	Molybdenum (µg/d)	Phosphorus (mg/d)	Selenium (µg/d)	Zinc (mg/d)
Lactation																					
14–18 years	1000	160	1.05	885	96	10	16	1.2	1.3	13	1.7	450	2.4	985	209	7	300	35	1055	59	10.9
19–30 years	800	160	1.05	900	100	10	16	1.2	1.3	13	1.7	450	2.4	1000	209	6.5	255	36	580	59	10.4
31–50 years	800	160	1.05	900	100	10	16	1.2	1.3	13	1.7	450	2.4	1000	209	6.5	265	36	580	59	10.4

NOTE: An estimated average requirement (EAR) is the average daily nutrient intake level estimated to meet the requirements of half of the healthy individuals in a group. EARs have not been established for vitamin K, pantothenic acid, biotin, choline, chromium, fluoride, manganese, or other nutrients not yet evaluated via the DRI process.

[a] As retinol activity equivalents (RAEs). 1 RAE = 1 µg retinol, 12 µg β-carotene, 24 µg α-carotene, or 24 µg β-cryptoxanthin. The RAE for dietary provitamin A carotenoids is two-fold greater than retinol equivalents (RE), whereas the RAE for preformed vitamin A is the same as RE.

[b] As α-tocopherol. α-Tocopherol includes *RRR*-α-tocopherol, the only form of α-tocopherol that occurs naturally in foods, and the *2R*-stereoisomeric forms of α-tocopherol (*RRR*-, *RSR*-, *RRS*-, and *RSS*-α-tocopherol) that occur in fortified foods and supplements. It does not include the *2S*-stereoisomeric forms of α-tocopherol (*SRR*-, *SSR*-, *SRS*-, and *SSS*-α-tocopherol), also found in fortified foods and supplements.

[c] As niacin equivalents (NE). 1 mg of niacin = 60 mg of tryptophan.

[d] As dietary folate equivalents (DFE). 1 DFE = 1 µg food folate = 0.6 µg of folic acid from fortified food or as a supplement consumed with food = 0.5 µg of a supplement taken on an empty stomach.

SOURCES: Dietary Reference Intakes for Calcium, Phosphorous, Magnesium, Vitamin D, and Fluoride (1997); Dietary Reference Intakes for Thiamin, Riboflavin, Niacin, Vitamin B$_6$, Folate, Vitamin B$_{12}$, Pantothenic Acid, Biotin, and Choline (1998); Dietary Reference Intakes for Vitamin C, Vitamin E, Selenium, and Carotenoids (2000); Dietary Reference Intakes for Vitamin A, Vitamin K, Arsenic, Boron, Chromium, Copper, Iodine, Iron, Manganese, Molybdenum, Nickel, Silicon, Vanadium, and Zinc (2001); Dietary Reference Intakes for Energy, Carbohydrate, Fiber, Fat, Fatty Acids, Cholesterol, Protein, and Amino Acids (2002/2005); and Dietary Reference Intakes for Calcium and Vitamin D (2011). These reports may be accessed via www.nap.edu.

Dietary Reference Intakes (DRIs): Recommended Dietary Allowances and Adequate Intakes, Vitamins
Food and Nutrition Board, Institute of Medicine, National Academies

Life Stage Group	Vitamin A (µg/d)[a]	Vitamin C (mg/d)	Vitamin D (µg/d)[b,c]	Vitamin E (mg/d)[d]	Vitamin K (µg/d)	Thiamin (mg/d)	Riboflavin (mg/d)	Niacin (mg/d)[e]	Vitamin B6 (mg/d)	Folate (µg/d)[f]	Vitamin B12 (µg/d)	Pantothenic Acid (mg/d)	Biotin (µg/d)	Choline (mg/d)[g]
Infants														
0 to 6 mo	400*	40*	10	4*	2.0*	0.2*	0.3*	2*	0.1*	65*	0.4*	1.7*	5*	125*
6 to 12 mo	500*	50*	10	5*	2.5*	0.3*	0.4*	4*	0.3*	80*	0.5*	1.8*	6*	150*
Children														
1–3 years	300	15	15	6	30*	0.5	0.5	6	0.5	150	0.9	2*	8*	200*
4–8 years	400	25	15	7	55*	0.6	0.6	8	0.6	200	1.2	3*	12*	250*
Males														
9–13 years	600	45	15	11	60*	0.9	0.9	12	1.0	300	1.8	4*	20*	375*
14–18 years	900	75	15	15	75*	1.2	1.3	16	1.3	400	2.4	5*	25*	550*
19–30 years	900	90	15	15	120*	1.2	1.3	16	1.3	400	2.4	5*	30*	550*

(continued)

(continued)

Life Stage Group	Vitamin A (µg/d)a	Vitamin C (mg/d)	Vitamin D (µg/d)b,c	Vitamin E (mg/d)d	Vitamin K (µg/d)	Thiamin (mg/d)	Riboflavin (mg/d)	Niacin (mg/d)e	Vitamin B6 (mg/d)	Folate (µg/d)f	Vitamin B12 (µg/d)	Pantothenic Acid (mg/d)	Biotin (µg/d)	Choline (mg/d)g
31-50 years	900	90	15	15	120*	1.2	1.3	16	1.3	400	2.4	5*	30*	550*
51-70 years	900	90	15	15	120*	1.2	1.3	16	1.7	400	2.4h	5*	30*	550*
>70 years	900	90	20	15	120*	1.2	1.3	16	1.7	400	2.4h	5*	30*	550*
Females														
9-13 years	600	45	15	11	60*	0.9	0.9	12	1.0	300	1.8	4*	20*	375*
14-18 years	700	65	15	15	75*	1.0	1.0	14	1.2	400i	2.4	5*	25*	400*
19-30 years	700	75	15	15	90*	1.1	1.1	14	1.3	400i	2.4	5*	30*	425*
31-50 years	700	75	15	15	90*	1.1	1.1	14	1.3	400i	2.4	5*	30*	425*
51-70 years	700	75	15	15	90*	1.1	1.1	14	1.5	400	2.4h	5*	30*	425*
>70 years	700	75	20	15	90*	1.1	1.1	14	1.5	400	2.4h	5*	30*	425*

Appendix A 605

Life Stage Group	Vitamin A (µg/d)a	Vitamin C (mg/d)	Vitamin D (µg/d)b,c	Vitamin E (mg/d)d	Vitamin K (µg/d)	Thiamin (mg/d)	Riboflavin (mg/d)	Niacin (mg/d)e	Vitamin B6 (mg/d)	Folate (µg/d)f	Vitamin B12 (µg/d)	Pantothenic Acid (mg/d)	Biotin (µg/d)	Choline (mg/d)g
Pregnancy														
14–18 years	750	80	15	15	75*	1.4	1.4	18	1.9	600i	2.6	6*	30*	450*
19–30 years	770	85	15	15	90*	1.4	1.4	18	1.9	600i	2.6	6*	30*	450*
31–50 years	770	85	15	15	90*	1.4	1.4	18	1.9	600i	2.6	6*	30*	450*
Lactation														
14–18 years	1200	115	15	19	75*	1.4	1.6	17	2.0	500	2.8	7*	35*	550*
19–30 years	1300	120	15	19	90*	1.4	1.6	17	2.0	500	2.8	7*	35*	550*
31–50 years	1300	120	15	19	90*	1.4	1.6	17	2.0	500	2.8	7*	35*	550*

NOTE: This table (taken from the DRI reports, see www.nap.edu) presents recommended dietary allowances (RDAs) in **bold type** and adequate intakes (AIs) in ordinary type followed by an asterisk (*). An RDA is the average daily dietary intake level, sufficient to meet the nutrient requirements of nearly all (97–98 percent) healthy individuals in a group. It is calculated from an estimated average requirement (EAR). If sufficient scientific evidence is not available to establish an EAR, and thus calculate an RDA, an AI is usually developed. For healthy breastfed infants, an AI is the mean intake. The AI for other life stage and gender groups is believed to cover the needs of all healthy individuals in the groups, but lack of data or uncertainty in the data prevents being able to specify with confidence the percentage of individuals covered by this intake.

aAs retinol activity equivalents (RAEs). 1 RAE = 1 µg retinol, 12 µg β-carotene, 24 µg α-carotene, or 24 µg β-cryptoxanthin. The RAE for dietary provitamin A carotenoids is two-fold greater than retinol equivalents (RE), whereas the RAE for preformed vitamin A is the same as RE.

bAs cholecalciferol. 1 µg cholecalciferol = 40 IU vitamin D.

cUnder the assumption of minimal sunlight.

(continued)

(Continued)

[d]As α-tocopherol. α-Tocopherol includes *RRR*-α-tocopherol, the only form of α-tocopherol that occurs naturally in foods, and the *2R*-stereoisomeric forms of α-tocopherol (*RRR*-, *RSR*-, *RRS*-, and *RSS*-α-tocopherol), also found in fortified foods and supplements. It does not include the *2S*-stereoisomeric forms of a-tocopherol (*SRR*-, *SSR*-, *SRS*-, and *SSS*-a-tocopherol), also found in fortified foods and supplements.

[e]As niacin equivalents (NE). 1 mg of niacin = 60 mg of tryptophan; 0–6 months = preformed niacin (not NE).

[f]As dietary folate equivalents (DFE). 1 DFE = 1 μg food folate = 0.6 μg of folic acid from fortified food or as a supplement consumed with food = 0.5 μg of a supplement taken on an empty stomach.

[g]Although AIs have been set for choline, there are few data to assess whether a dietary supply of choline is needed at all stages of the life cycle, and it may be that the choline requirement can be met by endogenous synthesis at some of these stages.

[h]Because 10 to 30 percent of older people may malabsorb food-bound B_{12}, it is advisable for those older than 50 years to meet their RDA mainly by consuming foods fortified with B_{12} or a supplement containing B_{12}.

[i]In view of evidence linking folate intake with neural tube defects in the fetus, it is recommended that all women capable of becoming pregnant consume 400 μg from supplements or fortified foods in addition to intake of food folate from a varied diet.

[j]It is assumed that women will continue consuming 400 μg from supplements or fortified food until their pregnancy is confirmed and they enter prenatal care, which ordinarily occurs after the end of the periconceptional period—the critical time for formation of the neural tube.

SOURCES: Dietary Reference Intakes for Calcium, Phosphorus, Magnesium, Vitamin D, and Fluoride (1997); Dietary Reference Intakes for Thiamin, Riboflavin, Niacin, Vitamin B_6, Folate, Vitamin B_{12}, Pantothenic Acid, Biotin, and Choline (1998); Dietary Reference Intakes for Vitamin C, Vitamin E, Selenium, and Carotenoids (2000); Dietary Reference Intakes for Vitamin A, Vitamin K, Arsenic, Boron, Chromium, Copper, Iodine, Iron, Manganese, Molybdenum, Nickel, Silicon, Vanadium, and Zinc (2001); Dietary Reference Intakes for Calcium and Vitamin D (2005); and Dietary Reference Intakes for Water, Potassium, Sodium, Chloride, and Sulfate (2005); and Dietary Reference Intakes for Calcium and Vitamin D (2011). These reports may be accessed via www.nap.edu. (Reproduced with permission from the National Academy of Sciences, National Academies Press.)

Dietary Reference Intakes (DRIs): Recommended Dietary Allowances and Adequate Intakes, Elements
Food and Nutrition Board, Institute of Medicine, National Academies

Life Stage Group	Calcium (mg/d)	Chromium (µg/d)	Copper (µg/d)	Fluoride (mg/d)	Iodine (µg/d)	Iron (mg/d)	Magnesium (mg/d)	Manganese (mg/d)	Molybdenum (µg/d)	Phosphorus (mg/d)	Selenium (µg/d)	Zinc (mg/d)	Potassium (g/d)	Sodium (g/d)	Chloride (g/d)
Infants
0 to 6 mo	200*	0.2*	200*	0.01*	110*	0.27*	30*	0.003*	2*	100*	15*	2*	0.4*	0.12*	0.18*
6 to 12 mo	260*	5.5*	220*	0.5*	130*	11	75*	0.6*	3*	275*	20*	3	0.7*	0.37*	0.57*
Children
1-3 years	700	11*	340	0.7*	90	7	80	1.2*	17	460	20	3	3.0*	1.0*	1.5*
4-8 years	1000	15*	440	1*	90	10	130	1.5*	22	500	30	5	3.8*	1.2*	1.9*
Males
9-13 years	1300	25*	700	2*	120	8	240	1.9*	34	1250	40	8	4.5*	1.5*	2.3*
14-18 years	1300	35*	890	3*	150	11	410	2.2*	43	1250	55	11	4.7*	1.5*	2.3*

(continued)

(Continued)

Life stage Group	Calcium (mg/d)	Chromium (µg/d)	Copper (µg/d)	Fluoride (mg/d)	Iodine (µg/d)	Iron (mg/d)	Magnesium (mg/d)	Manganese (mg/d)	Molybdenum (µg/d)	Phosphorus (mg/d)	Selenium (µg/d)	Zinc (mg/d)	Potassium (g/d)	Sodium (g/d)	Chloride (g/d)
19–30 years	1000	35*	900	4*	150	8	400	2.3*	45	700	55	11	4.7*	1.5*	2.3*
31–50 years	1000	35*	900	4*	150	8	420	2.3*	45	700	55	11	4.7*	1.5*	2.3*
51–70 years	1000	30*	900	4*	150	8	420	2.3*	45	700	55	11	4.7*	1.3*	2.0*
>70 years	1200	30*	900	4*	150	8	420	2.3*	45	700	55	11	4.7*	1.2*	1.8*
Females															
9–13 years	1300	21*	700	2*	120	8	240	1.6*	34	1250	40	8	4.5*	1.5*	2.3*
14–18 years	1300	24*	890	3*	150	15	360	1.6*	43	1250	55	9	4.7*	1.5*	2.3*
19–30 years	1000	25*	900	3*	150	18	310	1.8*	45	700	55	8	4.7*	1.5*	2.3*
31–50 years	1000	25*	900	3*	150	18	320	1.8*	45	700	55	8	4.7*	1.5*	2.3*
51–70 years	1200	20*	900	3*	150	8	320	1.8*	45	700	55	8	4.7*	1.3*	2.0*
>70 years	1200	20*	900	3*	150	8	320	1.8*	45	700	55	8	4.7*	1.2*	1.8*

Life Stage Group	Calcium (mg/d)	Chromium (µg/d)	Copper (µg/d)	Fluoride (mg/d)	Iodine (µg/d)	Iron (mg/d)	Magnesium (mg/d)	Manganese (mg/d)	Molybdenum (µg/d)	Phosphorus (mg/d)	Selenium (µg/d)	Zinc (mg/d)	Potassium (g/d)	Sodium (g/d)	Chloride (g/d)
Pregnancy															
14-18 years	1300	29*	1000	3*	220	27	400	2.0*	50	1250	60	12	4.7*	1.5*	2.3*
19-30 years	1000	30*	1000	3*	220	27	350	2.0*	50	700	60	11	4.7*	1.5*	2.3*
31-50 years	1000	30*	1000	3*	220	27	360	2.0*	50	700	60	11	4.7*	1.5*	2.3*
Lactation															
14-18 years	1300	44*	1300	3*	290	10	360	2.6*	50	1250	70	13	5.1*	1.5*	2.3*
19-30 years	1000	45*	1300	3*	290	9	310	2.6*	50	700	70	12	5.1*	1.5*	2.3*
31-50 years	1000	45*	1300	3*	290	9	320	2.6*	50	700	70	12	5.1*	1.5*	2.3*

NOTE: This table (taken from the DRI reports, see www.nap.edu) presents recommended dietary allowances (RDAs) in **bold type** and adequate intakes (AIs) in ordinary type followed by an asterisk (*). An RDA is the average daily dietary intake level, sufficient to meet the nutrient requirements of nearly all (97–98 percent) healthy individuals in a group. It is calculated from an estimated average requirement (EAR). If sufficient scientific evidence is not available to establish an EAR, and thus calculate an RDA, an AI is usually developed. For healthy breastfed infants, an AI is the mean intake. The AI for other life stage and gender groups is believed to cover the needs of all healthy individuals in the groups, but lack of data or uncertainty in the data prevents being able to specify with confidence the percentage of individuals covered by this intake.

SOURCES: Dietary Reference Intakes for Calcium, Phosphorous, Magnesium, Vitamin D, and Fluoride (1997); Dietary Reference Intakes for Thiamin, Riboflavin, Niacin, Vitamin B₆, Folate, Vitamin B₁₂, Pantothenic Acid, Biotin, and Choline (1998); Dietary Reference Intakes for Vitamin C, Vitamin E, Selenium, and Carotenoids (2000); and Dietary Reference Intakes for Vitamin A, Vitamin K, Arsenic, Boron, Chromium, Copper, Iodine, Iron, Manganese, Molybdenum, Nickel, Silicon, Vanadium, and Zinc (2001); Dietary Reference Intakes for Water, Potassium, Sodium, Chloride, and Sulfate (2005); and Dietary Reference Intakes for Calcium and Vitamin D (2011). These reports may be accessed via www.nap.edu. (Reproduced with permission from the National Academy of Sciences, National Academies Press.)

Dietary Reference Intakes (DRIs): Recommended Dietary Allowances and Adequate Intakes, Total Water and Macronutrients

Food and Nutrition Board, Institute of Medicine, National Academies

Life Stage Group	Total Water[a] (L/d)	Carbohydrate (g/d)	Total Fiber (g/d)	Fat (g/d)	Linoleic Acid (g/d)	α-Linolenic Acid (g/d)	Protein[b] (g/d)
Infants							
0 to 6 mo	0.7*	60*	ND	31*	4.4*	0.5*	9.1*
6 to 12 mo	0.8*	95*	ND	30*	4.6*	0.5*	11.0
Children							
1-3 years	1.3*	130	19*	ND[c]	7*	0.7*	13
4-8 years	1.7*	130	25*	ND	10*	0.9*	19
Males							
9-13 years	2.4*	130	31*	ND	12*	1.2*	34
14-18 years	3.3*	130	38*	ND	16*	1.6*	52
19-30 years	3.7*	130	38*	ND	17*	1.6*	56
31-50 years	3.7*	130	38*	ND	17*	1.6*	56
51-70 years	3.7*	130	30*	ND	14*	1.6*	56
>70 years	3.7*	130	30*	ND	14*	1.6*	56
Females							
9-13 years	2.1*	130	26*	ND	10*	1.0*	34
14-18 years	2.3*	130	26*	ND	11*	1.1*	46
19-30 years	2.7*	130	25*	ND	12*	1.1*	46
31-50 years	2.7*	130	25*	ND	12*	1.1*	46
51-70 years	2.7*	130	21*	ND	11*	1.1*	46
>70 years	2.7*	130	21*	ND	11*	1.1*	46

(continued)

(Continued)

Life Stage Group	Total Water[a] (L/d)	Carbohydrate (g/d)	Total Fiber (g/d)	Fat (g/d)	Linoleic Acid (g/d)	α-Linolenic Acid (g/d)	Protein[b] (g/d)
Pregnancy							
14–18 years	3.0*	**175**	28*	ND	13*	1.4*	**71**
19–30 years	3.0*	**175**	28*	ND	13*	1.4*	**71**
Lactation							
14–18 years	3.8*	**210**	29*	ND	13*	1.3*	**71**
19–30 years	3.8*	**210**	29*	ND	13*	1.3*	**71**
31–50 years	3.8*	**210**	29*	ND	13*	1.3*	**71**

NOTE: This table (taken from the DRI reports, see www.nap.edu) presents recommended dietary allowances (RDA) in **bold type** and adequate intakes (AI) in ordinary type followed by an asterisk (*). An RDA is the average daily dietary intake level, sufficient to meet the nutrient requirements of nearly all (97–98 percent) healthy individuals in a group. It is calculated from an estimated average requirement (EAR). If sufficient scientific evidence is not available to establish an EAR, and thus calculate an RDA, an AI is usually developed. For healthy breastfed infants, an AI is the mean intake. The AI for other life stage and gender groups is believed to cover the needs of all healthy individuals in the groups, but lack of data or uncertainty in the data prevents being able to specify with confidence the percentage of individuals covered by this intake.

[a]Total water includes all water contained in food, beverages, and drinking water.
[b]Based on g protein per kg of body weight for the reference body weight, eg, for adults 0.8 g/kg body weight for the reference body weight.
[c]Not determined.

SOURCE: Dietary Reference Intakes for Energy, Carbohydrate, Fiber, Fat, Fatty Acids, Cholesterol, Protein, and Amino Acids (2002/2005) and Dietary Reference Intakes for Water, Potassium, Sodium, Chloride, and Sulfate (2005). The report may be accessed via www.nap.edu. (Reproduced with permission from the National Academy of Sciences, National Academies Press.)

Dietary Reference Intakes (DRIs): Acceptable Macronutrient Distribution Ranges
Food and Nutrition Board, Institute of Medicine, National Academies

Macronutrient	Range (Percent of Energy)		
	Children, 1–3 years	Children, 4–18 years	Adults
Fat	30–40	25–35	20–35
n-6 polyunsaturated fatty acids[a] (linoleic acid)	5–10	5–10	5–10
n-3 polyunsaturated fatty acids[a] (a-linolenic acid)	0.6–1.2	0.6–1.2	0.6–1.2
Carbohydrate	45–65	45–65	45–65
Protein	5–20	10–30	10–35

[a]Approximately 10 percent of the total can come from longer-chain n-3 or n-6 fatty acids.

SOURCE: Dietary Reference Intakes for Energy, Carbohydrate, Fiber, Fat, Fatty Acids, Cholesterol, Protein, and Amino Acids (2002/2005). The report may be accessed via www.nap.edu.

Dietary Reference Intakes (DRIs): Acceptable Macronutrient Distribution Ranges
Food and Nutrition Board, Institute of Medicine, National Academies

Macronutrient	Recommendation
Dietary cholesterol	As low as possible while consuming a nutritionally adequate diet
Trans fatty acids	As low as possible while consuming a nutritionally adequate diet
Saturated fatty acids	As low as possible while consuming a nutritionally adequate diet
Added sugars[a]	Limit to no more than 25% of total energy

[a]Not a recommended intake. A daily intake of added sugars that individuals should aim for to achieve a healthful diet was not set.

SOURCE: Dietary Reference Intakes for Energy, Carbohydrate, Fiber, Fat, Fatty Acids, Cholesterol, Protein, and Amino Acids (2002/2005). The report may be accessed via www.nap.edu.

Dietary Reference Intakes (DRIs): Tolerable Upper Intake Levels, Vitamins
Food and Nutrition Board, Institute of Medicine, National Academies

Life Stage Group	Vitamin A (μg/d)[a]	Vitamin C (mg/d)	Vitamin D (μg/d)	Vitamin E (mg/d)[b,c]	Vitamin K	Thiamin	Riboflavin	Niacin (mg/d)[c]	Vitamin B₆ (mg/d)	Folate (μg/d)[c]	Vitamin B₁₂	Pantothenic Acid	Biotin	Choline (g/d)	Carotenoids[d]
Infants															
0 to 6 mo	600	ND[e]	25	ND	ND	ND	ND	ND	ND	ND	ND	ND	ND	ND	ND
6 to 12 mo	600	ND	38	ND	ND	ND	ND	ND	ND	ND	ND	ND	ND	ND	ND
Children															
1–3 years	600	400	63	200	ND	ND	ND	10	30	300	ND	ND	ND	1.0	ND
4–8 years	900	650	75	300	ND	ND	ND	15	40	400	ND	ND	ND	1.0	ND
Males															
9–13 years	1700	1200	100	600	ND	ND	ND	20	60	600	ND	ND	ND	2.0	ND
14–18 years	2800	1800	100	800	ND	ND	ND	30	80	800	ND	ND	ND	3.0	ND
19–30 years	3000	2000	100	1000	ND	ND	ND	35	100	1000	ND	ND	ND	3.5	ND
31–50 years	3000	2000	100	1000	ND	ND	ND	35	100	1000	ND	ND	ND	3.5	ND

(continued)

(continued)

Life Stage Group	Vitamin A (µg/d)[a]	Vitamin C (mg/d)	Vitamin D (µg/d)	Vitamin E (mg/d)[b,c]	Vitamin K	Thiamin	Riboflavin	Niacin (mg/d)[c]	Vitamin B6 (mg/d)[c]	Folate (µg/d)[c]	Vitamin B12	Pantothenic Acid	Biotin	Choline (g/d)	Carotenoids[d]
51–70 years	3000	2000	100	1000	ND	ND	ND	35	100	1000	ND	ND	ND	3.5	ND
>70 years	3000	2000	100	1000	ND	ND	ND	35	100	1000	ND	ND	ND	3.5	ND
Females															
9–13 years	1700	1200	100	600	ND	ND	ND	20	60	600	ND	ND	ND	2.0	ND
14–18 years	2800	1800	100	800	ND	ND	ND	30	80	800	ND	ND	ND	3.0	ND
19–30 years	3000	2000	100	1000	ND	ND	ND	35	100	1000	ND	ND	ND	3.5	ND
31–50 years	3000	2000	100	1000	ND	ND	ND	35	100	1000	ND	ND	ND	3.5	ND
51–70 years	3000	2000	100	1000	ND	ND	ND	35	100	1000	ND	ND	ND	3.5	ND
>70 years	3000	2000	100	1000	ND	ND	ND	35	100	1000	ND	ND	ND	3.5	ND
Pregnancy															
14–18 years	2800	1800	100	800	ND	ND	ND	30	80	800	ND	ND	ND	3.0	ND
19–30 years	3000	2000	100	1000	ND	ND	ND	35	100	1000	ND	ND	ND	3.5	ND
31–50 years	3000	2000	100	1000	ND	ND	ND	35	100	1000	ND	ND	ND	3.5	ND

Life Stage Group	Vitamin A (μg/d)[a]	Vitamin C (mg/d)	Vitamin D (μg/d)	Vitamin E (mg/d)[b,c]	Vitamin K	Thia-min	Ribo-flavin	Niacin (mg/d)[c]	Vitamin B$_6$ (mg/d)	Folate (μg/d)[c]	Vitamin B$_{12}$	Panto-thenic Acid	Biotin	Choline (g/d)	Carote-noids[d]
Lactation															
14–18 years	2800	1800	100	800	ND	ND	ND	30	80	800	ND	ND	ND	3.0	ND
19–30 years	3000	2000	100	1000	ND	ND	ND	35	100	1000	ND	ND	ND	3.5	ND
31–50 years	3000	2000	100	1000	ND	ND	ND	35	100	1000	ND	ND	ND	3.5	ND

NOTE: A tolerable upper intake level (UL) is the highest level of daily nutrient intake that is likely to pose no risk of adverse health effects to almost all individuals in the general population. Unless otherwise specified, the UL represents total intake from food, water, and supplements. Due to a lack of suitable data, ULs could not be established for vitamin K, thiamin, riboflavin, vitamin B$_{12}$, pantothenic acid, biotin, and carotenoids. In the absence of a UL, extra caution may be warranted in consuming levels above recommended intakes. Members of the general population should be advised not to routinely exceed the UL. The UL is not meant to apply to individuals who are treated with the nutrient under medical supervision or to individuals with predisposing conditions that modify their sensitivity to the nutrient.

[a]As preformed vitamin A only.

[b]As α-tocopherol; applies to any form of supplemental α-tocopherol.

[c]The ULs for vitamin E, niacin, and folate apply to synthetic forms obtained from supplements, fortified foods, or a combination of the two.

[d]β-Carotene supplements are advised only to serve as a provitamin A source for individuals at risk of vitamin A deficiency.

[e]ND, Not determinable due to lack of data of adverse effects in this age group and concern with regard to lack of ability to handle excess amounts. Source of intake should be from food only to prevent high levels of intake.

SOURCES: Dietary Reference Intakes for Calcium, Phosphorus, Magnesium, Vitamin D, and Fluoride (1997); Dietary Reference Intakes for Thiamin, Riboflavin, Niacin, Vitamin B$_6$, Folate, Vitamin B$_{12}$, Pantothenic Acid, Biotin, and Choline (1998); Dietary Reference Intakes for Vitamin C, Vitamine E, Selenium, and Carotenoids (2000); Dietary Reference Intakes for Vitamin A, Vitamin K, Arsenic, Boron, Chromium, Copper, Iodine, Iron, Manganese, Molybdenum, Nickel, Silicon, Vanadium, and Zinc (2001); and Dietary Reference Intakes for Calcium and Vitamin D (2011). These reports may be accessed via www.nap.edu. (Reproduced with permission from the National Academy of Sciences, National Academies Press.)

Dietary Reference Intakes (DRIs): Tolerable Upper Intake Levels, Elements
Food and Nutrition Board, Institute of Medicine, National Academies

Life Stage Group	Arsenic^a	Boron (mg/d)	Calcium (mg/d)	Chromium	Copper (µg/d)	Fluoride (mg/d)	Iodine (µg/d)	Iron (mg/d)	Magnesium (mg/d)^b	Manganese (mg/d)	Molybdenum (µg/d)	Nickel (mg/d)	Phosphorus (g/d)	Selenium (µg/d)	Silicon^c	Vanadium (mg/d)^d	Zinc (mg/d)	Sodium (g/d)	Chloride (g/d)
Infants																			
0 to 6 mo	ND^e	ND	1000	ND	ND	0.7	ND	40	ND	ND	ND	ND	ND	45	ND	ND	4	ND	ND
6 to 12 mo	ND	ND	1500	ND	ND	0.9	ND	40	ND	ND	ND	ND	ND	60	ND	ND	5	ND	ND
Children																			
1–3 years	ND	3	2500	ND	1000	1.3	200	40	65	2	300	0.2	3	90	ND	ND	7	1.5	2.3
4–8 years	ND	6	2500	ND	3000	2.2	300	40	110	3	600	0.3	3	150	ND	ND	12	1.9	2.9
Males																			
9–13 years	ND	11	3000	ND	5000	10	600	40	350	6	1100	0.6	4	280	ND	ND	23	2.2	3.4
14–18 years	ND	17	3000	ND	8000	10	900	45	350	9	1700	1.0	4	400	ND	ND	34	2.3	3.6
19–30 years	ND	20	2500	ND	10000	10	1100	45	350	11	2000	1.0	4	400	ND	1.8	40	2.3	3.6
31–50 years	ND	20	2500	ND	10000	10	1100	45	350	11	2000	1.0	4	400	ND	1.8	40	2.3	3.6
51–70 years	ND	20	2000	ND	10000	10	1100	45	350	11	2000	1.0	4	400	ND	1.8	40	2.3	3.6
>70 years	ND	20	2000	ND	10000	10	1100	45	350	11	2000	1.0	3	400	ND	1.8	40	2.3	3.6

Life Stage Group	Arsenic[a]	Boron (mg/d)	Calcium (mg/d)	Chromium	Copper (µg/d)	Fluoride (mg/d)	Iodine (µg/d)	Iron (mg/d)	Magnesium (mg/d)[b]	Manganese (mg/d)	Molybdenum (µg/d)	Nickel (mg/d)	Phosphorus (g/d)	Selenium (µg/d)	Silicon[c]	Vanadium (mg/d)[d]	Zinc (mg/d)	Sodium (g/d)	Chloride (g/d)
Females																			
9–13 years	ND	11	3000	ND	5000	10	600	40	350	6	1100	0.6	4	280	ND	ND	23	2.2	3.4
14–18 years	ND	17	3000	ND	8000	10	900	45	350	9	1700	1.0	4	400	ND	ND	34	2.3	3.6
19–30 years	ND	20	2500	ND	10000	10	1100	45	350	11	2000	1.0	4	400	ND	1.8	40	2.3	3.6
31–50 years	ND	20	2500	ND	10000	10	1100	45	350	11	2000	1.0	4	400	ND	1.8	40	2.3	3.6
51–70 years	ND	20	2000	ND	10000	10	1100	45	350	11	2000	1.0	4	400	ND	1.8	40	2.3	3.6
>70 years	ND	20	2000	ND	10000	10	1100	45	350	11	2000	1.0	3	400	ND	1.8	40	2.3	3.6
Pregnancy																			
14–18 years	ND	17	3000	ND	8000	10	900	45	350	9	1700	1.0	3.5	400	ND	ND	34	2.3	3.6
19–30 years	ND	20	2500	ND	10000	10	1100	45	350	11	2000	1.0	3.5	400	ND	ND	40	2.3	3.6
31–50 years	ND	20	2500	ND	10000	10	1100	45	350	11	2000	1.0	3.5	400	ND	ND	40	2.3	3.6
Lactation																			
14–18 years	ND	17	3000	ND	8000	10	900	45	350	9	1700	1.0	4	400	ND	ND	34	2.3	3.6
19–30 years	ND	20	2500	ND	10000	10	1100	45	350	11	2000	1.0	4	400	ND	ND	40	2.3	3.6
31–50 years	ND	20	2500	ND	10000	10	1100	45	350	11	2000	1.0	4	400	ND	ND	40	2.3	3.6

(continued)

(Continued)

NOTE: A tolerable upper intake level (UL) is the highest level of daily nutrient intake that is likely to pose no risk of adverse health effects to almost all individuals in the general population. Unless otherwise specified, the UL represents total intake from food, water, and supplements. Due to a lack of suitable data, ULs could not be established for vitamin K, thiamin, riboflavin, vitamin B_{12}, pantothenic acid, biotin, and carotenoids. In the absence of a UL, extra caution may be warranted in consuming levels above recommended intakes. Members of the general population should be advised not to routinely exceed the UL. The UL is not meant to apply to individuals who are treated with the nutrient under medical supervision or to individuals with predisposing conditions that modify their sensitivity to the nutrient.

[a] Although the UL was not determined for arsenic, there is no justification for adding arsenic to food or supplements.

[b] The ULs for magnesium represent intake from a pharmacological agent only and do not include intake from food and water.

[c] Although silicon has not been shown to cause adverse effects in humans, there is no justification for adding silicon to supplements.

[d] Although vanadium in food has not been shown to cause adverse effects in humans, there is no justification for adding vanadium to food and vanadium supplements should be used with caution. The UL is based on adverse effects in laboratory animals and these data could be used to set a UL for adults but not children and adolescents.

[e] ND, Not determinable due to lack of data of adverse effects in this age group and concern with regard to lack of ability to handle excess amounts. Source of intake should be from food only to prevent high levels of intake.

SOURCES: Dietary Reference Intakes for Calcium, Phosphorous, Magnesium, Vitamin D, and Fluoride (1997); Dietary Reference Intakes for Thiamin, Riboflavin, Niacin, Vitamin B_6, Folate, Vitamin B_{12}, Pantothenic Acid, Biotin, and Choline (1998); Dietary Reference Intakes for Vitamin C, Vitamin E, Selenium, and Carotenoids (2000); Dietary Reference Intakes for Vitamin A, Vitamin K, Arsenic, Boron, Chromium, Copper, Iodine, Iron, Manganese, Molybdenum, Nickel, Silicon, Vanadium, and Zinc (2001); Dietary Reference Intakes for Water, Potassium, Sodium, Chloride, and Sulfate (2005); and Dietary Reference Intakes for Calcium and Vitamin D (2011). These reports may be accessed via www.nap.edu. (Reproduced with permission from the National Academy of Sciences, National Academies Press.)

Appendix B

USDA Food Patterns

The Food Patterns suggest amounts of food to consume from the basic food groups, subgroups, and oils to meet recommended nutrient intakes at 12 different calorie levels. Nutrient and energy contributions from each group are calculated according to the nutrient-dense forms of foods in each group (eg, lean meats and fat-free milk). The table also shows the number of calories from solid fats and added sugars (SoFAS) that can be accommodated within each calorie level, in addition to the suggested amounts of nutrient-dense forms of foods in each group.

Daily Amount of Food From Each Group

Calorie Level[1]	1000	1200	1400	1600	1800	2000	2200	2400	2600	2800	3000	3200
Fruits[2]	1 cup	1 cup	1½ cups	1½ cups	1½ cups	2 cups	2 cups	2 cups	2 cups	2½ cups	2½ cups	2½ cups
Vegetables[3]	1 cup	1½ cups	1½ cups	2 cups	2½ cups	2½ cups	3 cups	3 cups	3½ cups	3½ cups	4 cups	4 cups
Grains[4]	3 oz-eq	4 oz-eq	5 oz-eq	5 oz-eq	6 oz-eq	6 oz-eq	7 oz-eq	8 oz-eq	9 oz-eq	10 oz-eq	10 oz-eq	10 oz-eq
Protein foods[5]	2 oz-eq	3 oz-eq	4 oz-eq	5 oz-eq	5 oz-eq	5½ oz-eq	6 oz-eq	6½ oz-eq	6½ oz-eq	7 oz-eq	7 oz-eq	7 oz-eq
Dairy[6]	2 cups	2½ cups	2½ cups	3 cups	3 cups	3 cups	3 cups	3 cups	3 cups	3 cups	3 cups	3 cups
Oils[7]	15 g	17 g	17 g	22 g	24 g	27 g	29 g	31 g	34 g	36 g	44 g	51 g
Limit on calories from SoFAS[8]	137	121	121	121	161	258	266	330	362	395	459	596

1. **Calorie Levels** are set across a wide range to accommodate the needs of different individuals. The attached table "Estimated Daily Calorie Needs" can be used to help assign individuals to the food pattern at a particular calorie level.

2. **Fruit Group** includes all fresh, frozen, canned, and dried fruits and fruit juices. In general, 1 cup of fruit or 100% fruit juice, or ½ cup of dried fruit, can be considered as 1 cup from the fruit group.

3. **Vegetable Group** includes all fresh, frozen, canned, and dried vegetables and vegetable juices. In general, 1 cup of raw or cooked vegetables or vegetable juice, or 2 cups of raw leafy greens, can be considered as 1 cup from the vegetable group.

Vegetable Subgroup Amounts Per Week

Calorie Level	1000	1200	1400	1600	1800	2000	2200	2400	2600	2800	3000	3200
Dark-green vegetables	½ c/wk	1 c/wk	1 c/wk	1½ c/wk	1½ c/wk	1½ c/wk	2 c/wk	2 c/wk	2½ c/wk	2½ c/wk	2½ c/wk	2½ c/wk
Red and orange vegetables	2½ c/wk	3 c/wk	3 c/wk	4 c/wk	5½ c/wk	5½ c/wk	6 c/wk	6 c/wk	7 c/wk	7 c/wk	7½ c/wk	7½ c/wk
Beans and peas (eg, pintos, lentils, and split peas)	½ c/wk	½ c/wk	½ c/wk	1 c/wk	1½ c/wk	1½ c/wk	2 c/wk	2 c/wk	2½ c/wk	2½ c/wk	3 c/wk	3 c/wk
Starchy vegetables	2 c/wk	3½ c/wk	3½ c/wk	4 c/wk	5 c/wk	5 c/wk	6 c/wk	6 c/wk	7 c/wk	7 c/wk	8 c/wk	8 c/wk
Other vegetables	1½ c/wk	2½ c/wk	2½ c/wk	3½ c/wk	4 c/wk	4 c/wk	5 c/wk	5 c/wk	5½ c/wk	5½ c/wk	7 c/wk	7 c/wk

4. **Grains Group** includes all foods made from wheat, rice, oats, cornmeal, and barley, such as bread, pasta, oatmeal, breakfast cereals, tortillas, and grits. In general, 1 slice of bread, 1 cup of ready-to-eat cereal, or ½ cup of cooked rice, pasta, or cooked cereal can be considered as 1 ounce-equivalent from the grains group. **At least half of all grains consumed should be whole grains.**

5. **Protein Foods Group** includes meat, poultry, seafood, eggs, processed soy products, and nuts and seeds. In general, 1 ounce of lean meat, poultry, or seafood, 1 egg, 1 tablespoon peanut butter, or ½ ounce of nuts or seeds can be considered as 1 ounce-equivalent from the protein foods group. Also, ¼ cup of beans or peas may be counted as 1 ounce-equivalent in this group.

Protein Foods Subgroup Amounts Per Week

Calorie Level	1000	1200	1400	1600	1800	2000	2200	2400	2600	2800	3000	3200
Seafood	3 oz/wk	5 oz/wk	6 oz/wk	8 oz/wk	8 oz/wk	8 oz/wk	9 oz/wk	10 oz/wk	10 oz/wk	11 oz/wk	11 oz/wk	11 oz/wk
Meat, poultry, and eggs	10 oz/wk	14 oz/wk	19 oz/wk	24 oz/wk	24 oz/wk	26 oz/wk	29 oz/wk	31 oz/wk	31 oz/wk	34 oz/wk	34 oz/wk	34 oz/wk
Nuts, seeds, soy	1 oz/wk	2 oz/wk	3 oz/wk	4 oz/wk	4 oz/wk	4 oz/wk	4 oz/wk	5 oz/wk	5 oz/wk	5 oz/wk	5 oz/wk	5 oz/wk

6. **Dairy Group** includes all milks, including lactose-free products and fortified soymilk (soy beverage), and foods made from milk that retain their calcium content, such as yogurt and cheese. Foods made from milk that have little to no calcium, such as cream cheese, cream, and butter, are not part of the group. Most dairy group choices should be fat-free or low-fat. In general, 1 cup of milk or yogurt, 1½ ounces of natural cheese, or 2 ounces of processed cheese can be considered as 1 cup from the dairy group.

7. **Oils** include fats from many different plants and from fish that are liquid at room temperature, such as canola, corn, olive, soybean, and sunflower oil. Some foods are naturally high in oils, such as nuts, olives, some fish, and avocados. Foods that are mainly oil include mayonnaise, certain salad dressings, and soft margarine.

8. **SoFAS** are solid fats and added sugars. The limits for calories from SoFAS are the remaining amount of calories in each food pattern after selecting the specified amounts in each food group in nutrient-dense forms (forms that are fat-free or low-fat and with no added sugars).

- ## Estimated Daily Calorie Needs

To determine which food intake pattern to use for an individual, the following chart gives an estimate of individual calorie needs. The calorie range for each age/sex group is based on physical activity level, from sedentary to active.

	Calorie Range		
Children	**Sedentary**	⟶	**Active**
2–3 years	1000	⟶	1400
Females			
4–8 years	1200	⟶	1800
9–13 years	1600	⟶	2200
14–18 years	1800	⟶	2400
19–30 years	2000	⟶	2400
31–50 years	1800	⟶	2200
51+ years	1600	⟶	2200
Males			
4–8 years	1400	⟶	2000
9–13 years	1800	⟶	2600
14–18 years	2200	⟶	3200
19–30 years	2400	⟶	3000
31–50 years	2400	⟶	3000
51+ years	2200	⟶	2800

Sedentary means a lifestyle that includes only the light physical activity associated with typical day-to-day life.

Active means a lifestyle that includes physical activity equivalent to walking more than 3 miles per day at 3 to 4 miles per hour, in addition to light physical activity associated with typical day-to-day life.

Appendix C

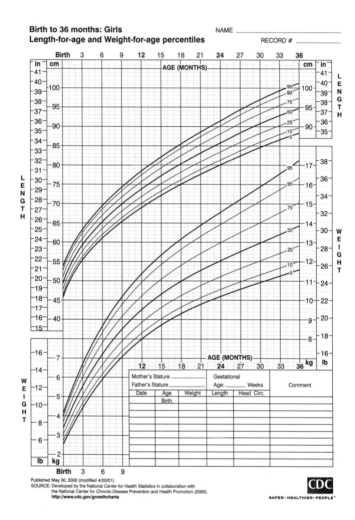

Birth to 36 months: Girls
Length-for-age and Weight-for-age percentiles

NAME _____

RECORD # _____

Published May 30, 2000 (modified 4/20/01).
SOURCE: Developed by the National Center for Health Statistics in collaboration with
the National Center for Chronic Disease Prevention and Health Promotion (2000).
http://www.cdc.gov/growthcharts

CDC

SAFER · HEALTHIER · PEOPLE™

Birth to 36 months: Boys
Length-for-age and Weight-for-age percentiles

NAME _____

RECORD # _____

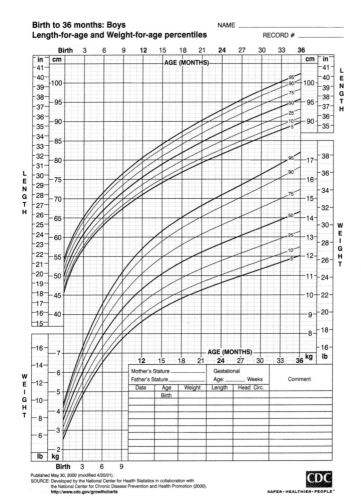

Published May 30, 2000 (modified 4/20/01).
SOURCE: Developed by the National Center for Health Statistics in collaboration with
the National Center for Chronic Disease Prevention and Health Promotion (2000).
http://www.cdc.gov/growthcharts

CDC
SAFER · HEALTHIER · PEOPLE™

Birth to 36 months: Girls
Head circumference-for-age and
Weight-for-length percentiles

NAME _____

RECORD # _____

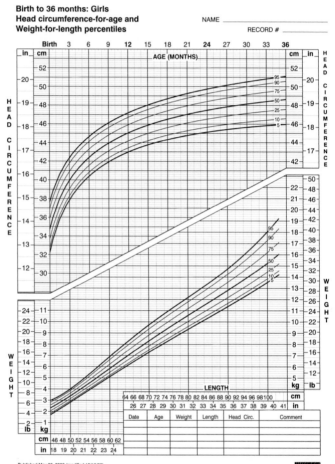

Published May 30, 2000 (modified 10/16/00).
SOURCE: Developed by the National Center for Health Statistics in collaboration with
the National Center for Chronic Disease Prevention and Health Promotion (2000).
http://www.cdc.gov/growthcharts

CDC
SAFER · HEALTHIER · PEOPLE™

Birth to 36 months: Boys
Head circumference-for-age and
Weight-for-length percentiles

NAME _____

RECORD # _____

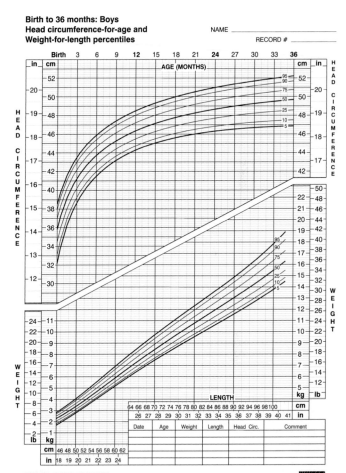

Published May 30, 2000 (modified 10/16/00).
SOURCE: Developed by the National Center for Health Statistics in collaboration with
the National Center for Chronic Disease Prevention and Health Promotion (2000).
http://www.cdc.gov/growthcharts

CDC

SAFER · HEALTHIER · PEOPLE™

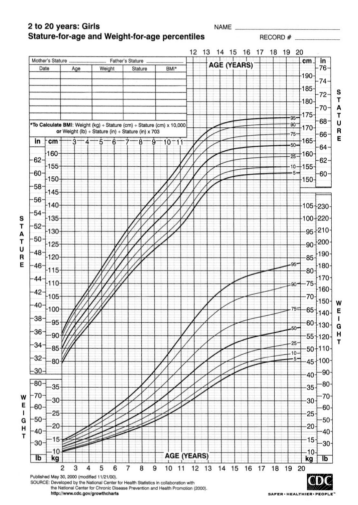

2 to 20 years: Girls
Stature-for-age and Weight-for-age percentiles

NAME _____

RECORD # _____

Published May 30, 2000 (modified 11/21/00).
SOURCE: Developed by the National Center for Health Statistics in collaboration with
the National Center for Chronic Disease Prevention and Health Promotion (2000).
http://www.cdc.gov/growthcharts

2 to 20 years: Boys
Stature-for-age and Weight-for-age percentiles

NAME _____

RECORD # _____

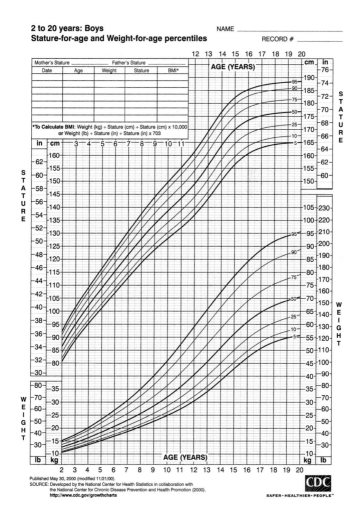

Published May 30, 2000 (modified 11/21/00).
SOURCE: Developed by the National Center for Health Statistics in collaboration with
the National Center for Chronic Disease Prevention and Health Promotion (2000).
http://www.cdc.gov/growthcharts

CDC
SAFER · HEALTHIER · PEOPLE™

2 to 20 years: Girls
Body mass index-for-age percentiles

NAME _____

RECORD # _____

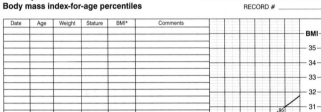

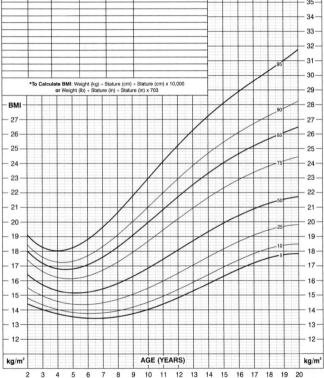

*To Calculate BMI: Weight (kg) ÷ Stature (cm) ÷ Stature (cm) x 10,000
or Weight (lb) ÷ Stature (in) ÷ Stature (in) x 703

Published May 30, 2000 (modified 10/16/00).
SOURCE: Developed by the National Center for Health Statistics in collaboration with
the National Center for Chronic Disease Prevention and Health Promotion (2000).
http://www.cdc.gov/growthcharts

SAFER · HEALTHIER · PEOPLE™

2 to 20 years: Boys
Body mass index-for-age percentiles

NAME _____

RECORD # _____

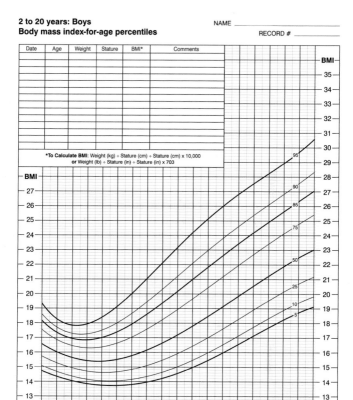

Date	Age	Weight	Stature	BMI*	Comments

*To Calculate BMI: Weight (kg) ÷ Stature (cm) ÷ Stature (cm) x 10,000
or Weight (lb) ÷ Stature (in) ÷ Stature (in) x 703

AGE (YEARS)

Published May 30, 2000 (modified 10/16/00).
SOURCE: Developed by the National Center for Health Statistics in collaboration with
the National Center for Chronic Disease Prevention and Health Promotion (2000).
http://www.cdc.gov/growthcharts

SAFER · HEALTHIER · PEOPLE

Appendix D

Useful Conversions for Nutrition

- English-Metric Conversions

Length

English (USA)	Metric
inch (in)	= 2.5 cm, 25.4 mm
foot (ft)	= 0.30 m, 30.48 cm
yard (yd)	= 0.91 m, 91.4 cm
mile (statute) (5280 ft)	= 1.61 km, 1609 m
mile (nautical) (6077 ft, 1.15 statute mi)	= 1.85 km, 1850 m

Metric	English (USA)
millimeter (mm)	= 0.039 in (thickness of a dime)
centimeter (cm)	= 0.39 in
meter (m)	= 3.28 ft, 39.4 in
kilometer (km)	= 0.62 mi, 1091 yd, 3273 ft

Weight

English (USA)	Metric
grain	= 64.80 mg
ounce (oz)	= 28.35 g
pound (lb)	= 453.60 g, 0.45 kg
ton (short- 2000 lb)	= 0.91 metric ton (907 kg)

Metric	English (USA)
milligram (mg)	= 0.002 grain (0.000035 oz)
kilogram (kg)	= 35.27 oz, 2.20 lb
metric ton (1000 kg)	= 1.10 tons

Volume

English (USA)	Metric
cubic inch	=16.39 mL
cubic foot	= 0.03 m3
cubic yard	= 0.765 m3
teaspoon (tsp)	= 5 mL
tablespoon (tbsp)	= 15 mL
fluid ounce	= 0.03 liter (30 mL)[a]
cup (c)	= 237 mL
pint (pt)	= 0.47 liter
quart (qt)	= 0.95 liter
gallon (gal)	= 3.79 liters
Metric	**English (USA)**
milliliter (mL)	= 0.03 oz
liter (L)	= 2.12 pt
liter	= 1.06 qt
liter	= 0.27 gal

1 liter ÷ 1000 = 1 milliliter or 1 cubic centimeter (10^{-3} liter).[a]
1 liter ÷ 1,000,000 = 1 microliter (10^{-6} liter).

[a] 1 mL = 1 cc.

Metric and Other Common Units

Unit/Abbreviation	Other Equivalent Measure
milligram/mg	1/1000 of a gram
microgram/μg	1/1,000,000 of a gram
deciliter/dl	1/10 of a liter (about ½ cup)
milliliter/mL	1/1000 of a liter (5 mL is about 1 tsp)
International Unit/IU	Crude measure of vitamin activity generally based on growth rate seen in animals

Household Units

3 teaspoons	= 1 tablespoon
4 tablespoons	= ¼ cup
5⅓ tablespoons	= ⅓ cup
8 tablespoons	= ½ cup
10⅔ tablespoons	= ⅔ cup
16 tablespoons	= 1 cup
1 tablespoon	= ½ fluid ounce
1 cup	= 8 fluid ounces
1 cup	= ½ pint
2 cups	= 1 pint
4 cups	= 1 quart
2 pints	= 1 quart
4 quarts	= 1 gallon

Index

Note: Page numbers followed with '*f*' and '*t*' represents figures and tables respectively.

A

Abbott nutrition, 481
Abdominal obesity, 264
Academy of Nutrition and Dietetics (AND), 101, 169, 289, 326, 386, 403, 435, 438, 531
Academy of Nutrition and Dietetics Evidence Analysis Library (EAL), 18–19, 200, 203, 269
  evidence-based guidelines of, 262
Acalculous cholecystitis (ACC), 549
Acanthosis nigricans, 75
Acceptable daily intake (ADI) level, 326
Acceptable macronutrient distribution ranges (AMDRs), 70
Activity energy expenditure (AEE), 146
Activity factor (AF), 68, 126–128
Activity levels
  definition of, 127*t*
  determination, 128*t*
  sources for, 127*t*
Acute kidney injury (AKI), 482–486
  nutrient recommendations, 484*t*
  nutrition prescription, 485*t*
  nutrition support, 485–486
  vitamin and mineral supplementation, 484*t*
Acute lung injury (ALI), 504
Acute-phase proteins, 62
Acute renal failure (ARF), 482
Acute respiratory distress syndrome (ARDS), 536
Adequate intake (AI), 9
  levels, 218
Adjustable gastric banding, 154*f*
Adjusted body weight (ABW), 69, 464
Administration on Aging (AOA), 243

Adolescents, 230
  calorie needs, 229–231
  dietary reference intakes (DRIs) for, 233*t*
  eating disorders, 235
  medical nutrition therapy for, 337–339
  nutrition for, 229–235
  protein, carbohydrate, and fat needs, 231–232
  type 1 diabetes, 337–339
    plasma blood glucose and HbA1c goals for, 338*t*
  type 2 diabetes, 339
  vitamin, mineral, fiber, and fluid needs, 232–235
Adult nutrition support
  adjunctive therapy
    antioxidant vitamins, 538
    arginine, 538–540
    glutamine, 538–540
    probiotics, 538
    soluble fiber, 540
    trace minerals, 538
  anti-inflammatory lipid profile EN formulas, 538
  appropriate formulas, selection of, 534
    elemental (hydrolyzed) formulas, 536
    specialized formulas, 536–537
    standard enteral formulas, 534–535
  energy assessment, 524–526
  energy, delivery of, 528–529
  enteral access, 527
    long-term, 528
    short-term, 527–528
  enteral feeds, timing, 528
  enteral *vs.* parenteral, 526–527

Adult nutrition support (*Cont.*):
fluid imbalance, 533
gastrointestinal side effects
constipation, 533
diarrhea, 532–533
hyperglycemia, 533
immune-modulating enteral
formulas, 537
populations and medical
conditions, 523–524
potential complications, 531
aspiration, 531–532
blue-dye use, 532
chlorhexidine mouthwash, 532
gastric *vs.* small bowel feeding
tube placement, 532
protein, delivery of, 529–530
refeeding syndrome, 533–534
tolerance to enteral feedings, 530
gastric residual volume
(GRV), 530
gut ischemia, 530–531
Advanced diabetes MNT resource
methods, 355*t*
Aging process, 236, 237
AIM-HIGH trial, 262
Air embolisms, 551
Albumin, 523
Albumin-to-creatinine ratio, 301
Alcohol, 350–351
definition, 269
primary prevention, 350
secondary prevention, 350–351
tertiary prevention, 351
Alcoholic liver disease
Academy of Nutrition and
Dietetics, 457
caffeine, 454
calorie needs, 454
chronic abuser of alcohol, 454
disorders, 454–457
fluids, 455
macronutrients, 454
meal patterning, 454
multivitamin, 454
nutrition, 454–457
supplements, 455*t*
support, 455, 456*t*
sugar, 454
Alcoholism, nutrition, 454–457
Alpha-glucosidase inhibitors
(AGI), 310
Alpha-lipoic acid (ALA), 589

Alzheimer's disease, 239
American Academy of Pediatrics,
195, 232, 432
iron recommendations, for infants
and toddlers, 219*t*
American College of Endocrinology
(ACE), 293
American College of Obstetricians
and Gynecologists, 186
American College of Sports
Medicine (ACSM), 186
American Congress of Obstetricians
and Gynecologists
(ACOG), 170
guidelines, 158
American Diabetes Association
(ADA), 50, 52, 289,
348, 368
diet group, 350
American Heart Association
(AHA), 241, 266
cholesterol guidelines, 253
lipid goal guidelines, 254*t*
American Institute for Cancer
Research (AICR), 509
American Society for Nutrition, 169
American Society for Parenteral
and Enteral Nutrition
(ASPEN), 38, 60
Amylin-mimetic, 311
Anaphylactic reactions, symptoms
of, 225–226
Anemia
L-carnitine for treatment of
anemia, 479*t*
vitamin C for treatment, 478*t*
Anhydrous dextrose, 542
Animal protein, 177
role of, 433
Anorexia, 511
Anthropometric parameters,
297–299
Anthropometry, 523
definition of, 41
Antibody tests, 395
Antidiabetes medications, 320
and MNT significance,
304*t*–308*t*
pharmacologic assessment and
monitoring of, 303–321
Antiendomysium antibodies
(EMA), 395
Antioxidants, 332–333

Antiseizure diet, 586
Antitissue transglutaminase
        antibodies (tTGA), 395
Appetite, 114
Arginine
    immune-enhancing qualities, 539
    supplementation, 501
Arm muscle circumference (AMC), 42
Artificial sweeteners, 182
Ascorbic acid. *See* Vitamin C
ASPEN guidelines, 533
Aspiration risk, 497, 511
Autism spectrum disorder (ASD), 585
Automated multiple-pass method
        (AMPM), 48

B
Baby-Friendly Hospital Initiative
        (BFHI), 201
    guidelines for baby-friendly
        designation, 202*t*
Balanced diet, 1, 19. *See also*
        Healthy meal plan
Bariatric surgery
    preoperative to postoperative
        nutrition interventions for,
        155*t*–156*t*
    types of, 151*t*
Basal analog insulin regimen,
        313–314
Basal-bolus analog insulin
        regimen, 313
Beano®, 389
Bean-zyme®, 389
Behavior modification theories, 97
Benign prostatic hypertrophy
        (BPH), 559
Biguanides, 309
Bile absorption, 412
Blood cell
    glucose levels effect of high- *vs.*
        low-GI foods on, 328*f*
    glucose targets in GDM
        pregnancy, 343*t*
    lipid goals, 300*t*
    values, 64*t*
Blood pressure, 191
Blood urea nitrogen (BUN), 513
Body mass index (BMI), 3, 34, 42,
        137, 157, 168, 170, 224, 297
    for-age percentile, 157*t*
    limitations to, 42
    tools, 151

Body weight
    equation, 69*t*
    measurements of, 115
Bone cells, types of, 422
Bone densitometry, 425
Bone mass measurement
        qualification criteria, 427*t*
Bone mineral density (BMD),
        423, 426
    testing, 425*t*
Bone-protecting hormonal
        factor, 422
Bowel diversion surgeries, diet
        therapy, 411
Boys
    body mass index-for-age
        percentiles, 631
    head circumference-for-
        age/weight-for-age
        percentiles, 627
    length-for-age/weight-for-age
        percentiles, 625
    stature-for-age/weight-for-age
        percentiles, 629
Breakfast, eating, 137–138
Breastfeeding, 201, 204
    breast milk, nutrient composition
        of, 194–196
    contraindications to, 201*t*
    encouraging and promoting,
        200–201
    exclusive, definition of, 194
    in infants, 344
    maternal diet and exercise,
        196–200
    nutrition for, 193–206
    supplement use, 200
Breast milk, 194, 207
    micronutrient profile of, 195
    nutrient profile comparison
        of, 197*t*
    production of, 196
Bulimia, 351
Burn patient
    energy needs, determining,
        498–499
    fluid needs, determining, 499–500
    nutrition assessment, 497–498
    nutrition needs for, 497
    nutrition support, 496–497,
        500–501
    protein needs, determining, 499
    supplements, 501

Burn patients
  estimating calorie needs, 498*t*
  nutrition and fluid
      recommendations, 503*t*
  protein
    fortified recipe, 500*t*
    tips for increasing, 499*t*
  shriners burn hospital micronutrient
      supplementation
      schedule, 501*t*

C
Caffeine, 200, 580
Calcium, 218, 232
  content, 429*t*, 430*t*
  dietary sources of, 428
  DRI values for, 427
  intake, 431*t*
  supplementation, 142, 431*t*
Calcium-containing products.
      See Dairy foods
Calcium-fortified soy milk, 14, 272
Calcium supplements, 472
Calculators, 55–59
Calories
  based meal plans, 181
  controlled meals, 18
  count, 160
  definition of, 1
  distribution guidelines, 517
  levels, USDA meal plan
      recommendations for, 181*t*
  needs, 69*t*, 238*t*, 508
Calories per kilogram method, 129
Calorimetry
  indirect, 495
  measurement, 124*t*
Canagliflozin monotherapy, 312
Cancer prevention guidelines, 511*t*
Cancer prevention/management,
      nutrition, 509–511
  energy needs, determining, 512
  nutrition-related treatment side
      effects
    diarrhea and constipation, 514
    dry mouth (xerostomia), 516
    mucositis and stomatitis,
        514–515
    nausea and vomiting, 513–514
    taste and smell alterations,
        515–516
  protein needs, determining, 512–513

Cancer-related mucositis, 515*t*
Cancer survivors, studies, 560
Carbohydrates (dextrose), 176,
      323–330, 542
  amount of, 293
  consistency, 343
  DRI for, 232
  fiber, 329
  fructose, 325
  for GDM meal pattern, sample
      distribution of, 343*t*
  glycemic index and glycemic load,
      327–329
  intake consistency, 323
  intolerance, 333
  medication dose adjustment,
      323–325
  nonnutritive sweeteners, 326
  nutritive sweeteners, 325
  polyols, 325–326
  recommended sources of, 177
  resistant starch and high-amylose
      foods, 326–327
  restriction, 142
  sample distribution of, 324*t*
  source of, 294, 325
Cardiovascular disease (CVD),
      292, 584, 585
  coronary artery bypass graft
      (CABG), 277–280
  heart disease prevention, 251–252
  heart failure, 281–283
  history of, 333
  hypercholesterolemia, 252–254
  hypertension, 267–277
  hypertriglyceridemia, 264–267
  interventions to lower LDL,
      254–260
  interventions to raise HDL,
      261–263
  lipid metabolism disorders, 252–267
  metabolic syndrome, 263–264
  nutrition and, 251–283
  patient education tools, 277–280
  risk of, 299, 315, 330
  therapeutic lifestyle change (TLC)
      diet, 260–261
Cardiovascular parameters, 299–301
Casein, 195
Casein-free diet, 586
Catabolic illness, nutritional
      needs, 523

Catheter-related blood stream infections (CRBSI), 552
Celecoxib, 559
Celiac disease, 19, 394–397
    gluten-free diet, 396–397
    nutritional implications of, 396
    progression of, 396
    symptoms of, 395
Center for Science in the Public Interest (CSPI), 96
Centers for Disease Control and Prevention (CDC), 434
    growth charts, 210
Central venous catheters (CVCs), 540
Certified diabetes educator (CDE), 104
Childhood obesity, 223
    rates of, 224
    root cause of, 224
Children
    medical nutrition therapy for, 337–339
    type 1 diabetes, 337–339
        medical nutrition therapy for, 337–339
        plasma blood glucose and HbA1c goals for, 338*t*
    type 2 diabetes, 339
        medical nutrition therapy for, 339
Chinese herbal medications, 589
Chlorhexidine mouthwash, 532
Cholesterol, 252, 258
    high levels, causes of, 252
Chondroitin, 559, 578
    use for osteoarthritis, 436
ChooseMyPlate.gov., 212*t*
    preschooler milestones from, 212*t*
Chronic abusers
    nutrition supplements, 455*t*
Chronic diseases, development/prevention of, 236
Chronic inflammatory illness, 493
Chronic kidney disease (CKD), 88, 330, 462–482
    calcium, 472
    dietetics' evidence analysis library, 476*t*
    energy needs, 463–464
    fish oil/omega-3 fatty acid, 480*t*
    goal of, 469
    high-phosphorus foods, 470*t*
    iron supplementation, 478*t*
    multivitamin supplementation, 480*t*

nondialysis, 463
nutrients, 472–481
nutrition and dietetics' evidence, 476*t*, 477*t*
nutrition referrals, 481–482
nutrition support, 481
overweight and underweight individuals, 466*t*
phosphate binder adjustments, 477*t*
phosphorus, 469–472
physical activity recommendations, 480*t*
potassium, 464–469, 481*t*
protein, 464
    recommendations, 475*t*
sodium, 479*t*
    and fluid, 472
stages of, 462*t*
vitamin B$_{12}$ and folic acid recommendations, 478*t*
vitamin C for treatment of anemia, 478*t*
Chronic obstructive pulmonary disease (COPD), 505, 536
    nutrition intervention strategies, 506*t*
Chylomicrons, 367
Cirrhosis, 454, 457
Clomid (clomiphene)
    use of, 556
Clostridium difficile, 532
Coenzyme Q10, 583–584
Cognitive behavioral therapy (CBT), 89
    practitioners of, 92
Cognitive dysfunction, 346
Colostomy, 412–414
    diet therapy for, 413, 413*t*
Colostrum, 195
Complementary and alternative medicine (CAM), 555
    classification, 556
    diet therapy, 564–566 (*See* Diet therapy)
    drug therapy, 564
    nutrition status, 564
    grapefruit, and drug interactions, 566
    monoamine oxidase inhibitor diet, 564–566

Complementary and alternative
    medicine (CAM) (*Cont.*):
  National Center for Complementary
      and Alternative Medicine
      (NCCAM), 556*t*
    definition of, 555
    nutrition, 555–556
    patients selection questions, 563*t*
    pharmacotherapy, 564–566
    practitioner resources
      books, 590
      professional associations, 591
      websites, 590
    practitioners, 563
      choosing tips, 560–564
      credentials, 560
      licensure of, 561*t*–562*t*
    tyramine, 564–566
    uses, 557–558
    vitamin supplementation, 560
    work, 558–560
Complete blood count (CBC),
    49, 548
Constipation, 381–389, 513
  additional approaches, 389
  cancer prevention/nutrition-related
      treatment side effects, 514
  diagnostic criteria, 384
  dietary fiber and, 384–386
  fluid intake, 387–388
  functional fibers, 386–387
  inactivity, 388–389
  nutrition diagnosis, 384*t*
  nutrition interventions for, 389
  Rome III consensus criteria
      for, 384*t*
Continuous glucose monitoring
      systems (CGMS),
      296, 297
Continuous renal replacement
      therapy (CRRT), 483
Continuous subcutaneous insulin
      infusion (CSII), 313
Copper deficiencies, 76
Co-Q10, ubiquinone. *See*
    Coenzyme Q10
Coronary artery diseases (CAD), 318
  risk of, 157
  screening for, 318
Coronary heart disease (CHD), 262
Cost-effective nutrition intervention
    programs, 221

Counseling tips and techniques,
    33–35, 77–88, 95–104, 99*t*
  acknowledge different learning
      styles, 99–100
  assign homework, 102–103
  avoid bias, 100
  characteristics of, 77–85
  cognitive behavioral therapy
      (CBT), 89–92
  empathy, 85–86
  evidence-based medicine,
      95–96
  health belief model (HBM), 88
  individualize your approach, 100
  know your ABC's, 97–99
  know your limits, 104
  motivational interviewing
      (MI), 93–94
  open-ended questions, 101
  plan for pitfalls, 104
  practice reflective listening,
      100–101
  set smart goals, 101–102
  stay current, 96–97
  supportiveness, 86–87
  theoretical approaches to, 88–94
  track outcomes besides weight,
      103–104
  transtheoretical model and stages
      of change, 88–89
  warmth, 87–88
C-reactive protein (CRP), 501
Crohn's disease (CD), 405
  complications of, 405
CV autonomic neuropathy
      (CAN), 318–319
Cystic fibrosis (CF), 506
Cystic fibrosis related diabetes
      (CFRD), 507
  nutrition recommendations, 508*t*

D
Daily calorie
  needs, estimation, 623
Dairy foods, 13–14, 429*t*
  USDA serving standard, 14
DASH. *See* Dietary approaches to
    stop hypertension
Deep breathing exercises, 557
Dehydration, 76
  risk, 371
Depression, 346

Diabetes
  diagnosis of, initial series of MNT
    encounters at, 290*t*
  diet therapy principles for, 339
  HbA1c correlation of, 295*t*
  long-term complications of
    physical activity, 317–318
  metabolic parameters to assess, 297*t*
  MNT goals for, 292
  MNT resource methods strategies,
    354*t*–355*t*
  National diabetes' groups glycemic
    control parameters, 293*t*
  nutrition and diet recommendations
    for control, 335*t*–336*t*
    complications, 337*t*
  overweight and obesity,
    classification of, 298*t*
  prevention, levels of, 289
Diabetes Control and Complications
  Trial (DCCT), 334
Diabetes mellitus
  medical nutrition therapy for,
    289–356
  alcohol, 350–351
  alpha-glucosidase inhibitors
    (AGI), 310
  amylin-mimetic, 311
  anthropometric parameters,
    297–299
  antidiabetic medications,
    pharmacologic assessment
    and monitoring of, 303–321
  assessment and monitoring
    parameter, 292–321
  basal analog insulin regimen,
    313–314
  basal-bolus analog insulin
    regimen, 313
  biguanides, 309
  cardiovascular parameters,
    299–301
  coronary artery diseases
    (CAD), 318
  CV autonomic neuropathy,
    318–319
  for diabetes mellitus, 289–356
  diet and genome interactions, 351
  dipeptidyl peptidase-IV
    inhibitors (DPP4i), 310
  dopamine receptor agonist, 311
  eating disorders, 352
  effectiveness of, 291–292
  fixed-dose insulin regimens, 312
  food intake assessment and
    monitoring, 292–293
  glucagon-like peptide-1
    receptor agonists, 310–311
  glycemic assessment and
    monitoring, 293–297
  goals of, 292
  HbA1c, 294
  insulin regimens, 312
  intermediate-acting insulin/
    rapid- or short-acting
    insulin regimens, 313
  meal planning tools and
    resources, 352–355
  metabolic assessment and
    monitoring, 297–299
  nephropathy and
    microalbuminuria, 319
  nonsulfonylureas, 309
  nutrient recommendations,
    321–336
  peripheral neuropathy, 318
  physical activity with
    general guidelines for,
    319–321
    gestational diabetes
      (GDM), 317
    long-term complications of
      diabetes, 317–318
    type 1 diabetes, 315–316
    type 2 diabetes, 316–317
  plant-based diets, 349–350
  renal parameters, 301–303
  retinopathy, 318
  secretagogues, 303
  self-monitoring blood glucose
    (SMBG), 294–296
  sensitizers, 309
  sodium–glucose cotransporter
    2 inhibitors, 311–312
  specific populations and
    circumstances, 336–349
  sulfonylureas, 303
  thiazolidinediones (TZDs),
    309–310
  wound healing, 351–352
Diabetes self-management education/
  training (DSME/T), 290
Diabetes self-management
  program, 87

Diabetes self-management support
(DSMS), 290
Diabetes-specific discharge
planning, 348
Diabetic diets, 321
Diagnostic and Statistical Manual
of Mental Disorders
(DSM), 162
Dialysis, 462–482
Diarrhea, 391–393
cancer prevention/nutrition-related
treatment side effects, 514
dietary recommendations for, 392t
etiology of, 532
foods not to consume, 393t
probiotics and prebiotics for
treatment, 391–393
Dietary allowances, 199t
Dietary approaches to stop
hypertension (DASH),
267, 273–277
diet, 268
nutrient goals, 274t
plan, 273, 274
eating pattern, 275t–276t
eating plan for different calorie
levels, 277t
style dietary, 301
Dietary assessment methods, 46, 72
Dietary data, 64–73
calorie counts, 72–73
energy needs estimation, 68–69
food frequency tools, 72
interactive DRI for healthcare
professionals, 73
macronutrient needs estimation,
70–72
supertracker, 73
Dietary fiber, 144, 234, 259–260, 381
dietary reference intake, 385t
estimation for, 386t
importance of, 408
list of, 387t
tips for, 387t
types of, 259
Dietary Guidelines Advisory
Committee (DGAC), 96
Dietary Guidelines for Americans
(DGAs), 2, 4–5, 96, 136,
206, 268
messages for consumers, 5t
recommendations for, 6t–7t

Dietary intake assessment
methods, 49
Dietary iron, sources of, 444
Dietary reference intakes (DRIs), 9,
70, 71t, 73, 142, 177, 406,
428t, 571
acceptable macronutrient
distribution ranges, 612
estimated average requirements,
600–602
nutrient pregnancy vs.
nonpregnancy, 181t
recommended dietary allowances,
603–606
adequate intakes, elements,
607–609
total water and macronutrients,
610–611
vitamins, 603–606
tolerable upper intake levels,
elements, 616–618
tolerable upper intake levels,
vitamins, 613–615
Dietary Supplement and Health
Education Act of 1994
(DSHEA), 566
Dietary supplements, 571
chondroitin, 578
coenzyme Q10, 583–584
echinacea plant, 578–579
efficacy/safety, 571
independent testing, 572–573
supplement interactions,
573–575
supplement needs, 575
toxicity, avoiding, 571–572
Federal law, 571
fish oil, 576–578
flaxseed/flaxseed oil, 579–580
garlic, 582–583
ginkgo biloba, 581–582
ginseng, 580–581
glucosamine, 578
health claims, 570
highlight/lowlights, 575–576
industry regulation, 566–570
information on, 573t
labels, 570–571
morphine, digitalis/digoxin, and
atropine, 573
safety tips for consumers, 572t
vitamin E, 584–585

Diet impact drug therapy, 564
Diet, side effects of, 587
Diet therapy, 132, 289, 368–379,
        379–416, 411, 564–566
    complementary/alternative
            medicine
        autism, 585–586
        diabetes, 589
        epilepsy, 586–587
        muscle cramps, 588
        nausea, 588–589
        vomiting, 588–589
    drug, 564
    nutrition status, 564
Digestion process, 361
Digestive disorders, 361
Digestive enzymes, secretion of, 381
Digestive system, anatomy of, 362f
Dipeptidyl peptidase-IV inhibitors
        (DPP4i), 310
Diverticular disease, 407–411
    low-residue diet, 410–411
    pathophysiology of, 411
Diverticulitis
    diet therapies for, 410t
    low-fiber foods for, 411t
Diverticulosis, diet therapies
        for, 410t
Division of Responsibility in Feeding
        approach, 211, 213
Dizziness, ginkgo, 581
Docosahexaenoic acid (DHA),
        265, 443
Dopamine receptor agonist, 311
Dose adjustment for normal eating
        (DAFNE), 313
Doxorubicin (Adriamycin), 578
Drug interactions, grapefruit, 566
Drug therapy, 148
Dry mouth, cancer prevention/
        nutrition-related treatment
        side effects, 516
Dual-energy x-ray absorptiometry
        (DEXA), 423
Dumping syndrome, 376–378
    management of, 378
Dysfunction, signs/symptoms, 85t
Dysgeusia, 513
Dyslipidemia, 299, 517
Dysphagia, 368–371, 370, 511
    diet food considerations, 370t
    liquid consistencies, 371t

national dysphagia diets, 368–370
    thickened liquids, 370–371

E
Early childhood, nutrition in,
        210–221
    calorie needs in, 213
    protein, carbohydrate, and fat
            needs in, 213–217
    toddler feeding practices,
            211–213
    USDA WIC program, 220–221
    vitamin, mineral, fiber, and fluid
            needs in, 217–220
Eating disorders, 235, 352
    diagnostic criteria for, 163t
    severity and type of, 162
    treatment of, 235
Eating frequency, 161
Echinacea plant, 577, 578–579
Echinacea purpurea, 579
Effective counselors, characteristics
        of, 85
Eicosapentaenoic acid (EPA), 265,
        443, 582
Eight food allergens, 226t
Elderly Nutrition Program
        (ENP), 243
Electrocardiogram (ECG), 317
Eleutherococcus senticosus, 580
Empathetic person, 86f
Empathetic person-centered
        counseling approach, 93
Empty calories, 24
End-stage renal disease
        (ESRD), 330
Energy balance concept, 130
Energy density, 20
    definition of, 22
Energy needs
    simplifying estimation of, 129
Energy-yielding macronutrients, 362
Epidemiology of Diabetes
        Interventions and
        Complications (EDIC)
        trial, 334
Erythromycin, 531
Esophagectomy, 541
Essential fatty acid deficiency
        (EFAD), 543
Estimated average glucose
        (eAG), 294

Estimated energy requirements
(EER), 174, 206, 213
for adolescents or adult
women, 175*t*
for age-specific boys and girls, 215*t*
equations, 129
for nonpregnant women, 174*t*
for pregnant women, 175*t*
Etoposide (VP16, VePesid), 578
Evidence Analysis Library (EAL), 50
Evidence Analysis project, 269
Evidence-based medicine (EBM),
validity of, 95
Evidence-based public health,
steps of, 95*t*
Exercise, 240–241

F
Fat, 330–332
dietary cholesterol, 332
labeling language, 279*t*
mediterranean diet, 331
omega-3 fatty acids, 331
plant sterol and stanol esters, 332
saturated fats, 332
trans fatty acid, 331–332
Fat-free milk, 619
Fat-soluble vitamins, deficiency/
toxicity, 78*t*–79*t*
Fat-soluble vitamin
supplementation, 507*t*
FDA-approved weight loss
medications, 147, 148
Federal Trade Commission (FTC), 566
Fiber. *See also* Dietary fiber
containing foods, 389
in food, 260*t*
Fibromyalgia, 439–442
Fick equations, 494
Finnish Diabetes Prevention Study
(DPS), 291
First law of thermodynamics, 113
Fish oil, 576–578
Fixed-dose insulin regimens, 312
Flavored milks, 14
Flaxseed, 579
Flaxseed/flaxseed oil, 579–580
Fluoride
schedule, 196*t*
supplementation, 196
FODMAPs, dietary sources of, 405
Folate, content of, 179*t*

Food allergens, 224–225
Food allergy, 224–227
diagnosis of, 226
reaction, 227*t*
*Food Allergy Research and
Education* (FARE), 227
Food and Drug Administration
(FDA), 325
Foodborne illness, 184
Food frequency questionnaire
(FFQ), 55, 72
Food intake
drug metabolism, 564
phytates, oxalates, and tannins, 564
Food intake assessment and
monitoring, 292–293
Food intolerances, 224
Food label, 9
Food models, 20
Fried foods, 513
Fructo-oligosaccharides (FOS), 405
Fruits, 14–16, 16*t*
importance, 15–16
juice, 15
Functional bowel disorder (FBD), 397
Fungal skin infections, 583

G
Gallbladder disease, risk factors, 460
Gallstones, 460–461
Gamma-linoleic acid (GLA), 538
Garlic, 582–583
heart disease risk factors, 582
rate of metabolism, 582
Gas, 389
by foods, 390*t*
by sugars, 390*t*
Gastric access, 496
Gastric residual volume (GRV), 530
risk of aspiration, 531
Gastric surgery, 376
procedures, 378*t*
diet tips and foods, 380*t*–381*t*
foods to avoid, 382*t*–383*t*
potential micronutrient
deficiencies, 380*t*
Gastroesophageal reflux disease
(GERD), 371–372, 372*f*
diet therapy for, 372, 373*t*
interventions for, 373
nutrition interventions and goals in
patients with, 373*t*

Gastrointestinal complications
    acalculous cholecystitis, 549
    metabolic bone disease, 549–550
    parenteral nutrition-associated
        liver disease, 549
Gastrointestinal disorders
    lower GI tract disorders
        celiac disease, 394–397
        constipation, 381–389
        diarrhea, 391–393
        diet therapy for, 379–416
        diverticular disease, 407–411
        ileostomy and colostomy,
            412–414
        inflammatory bowel disease
            (IBD), 405–407
        intestinal gas, 389–391
        intestinal surgery, 411–412
        irritable bowel syndrome (IBS),
            397–405
        malabsorption, 393–394
        short bowel syndrome (SBS),
            414–415
    nutrient absorption, 365–366
    nutrient digestion, 361–367
    nutrient transport, 366–367
    nutrition in, 361–416
    upper GI tract disorders
        diet therapy for, 368–379
        Dumping syndrome, 376–378
        dysphagia, 368–371
        gastric surgery, 376
        gastroesophageal reflux disease
            (GERD), 371–372
        hiatal hernia, 373–374
        peptic ulcer disease (PUD),
            374–376
        steatorrhea, 378–379
        xerostomia, 368
Gastrointestinal surgery, 541–542
Gastrointestinal tract, upset
    drugs, 565t
Gastrointestinal tubes, 548
Gastroparesis, 512
Generally recognized as safe
    (GRAS), 325
Geriatric PWD, 349
Gestational diabetes (GDM), 192
    diagnosis of, 317
    physical activity, 317
    screening, diagnosis, and
        treatment goals, 193t

GI function, 493
Ginkgo, 581
    side effects, 581
Ginkgo biloba, 574, 581–582
Ginkgo Evaluation of Memory
        (GEM), 581
Ginkgotoxin, 582
Ginseng, 580–581
Girls
    body mass index-for-age
        percentiles, 630
    head circumference-for-
        age/weight-for-age
        percentiles, 626
    length-for-age/weight-for-age
        percentiles, 624
    stature-for-age/weight-for-age
        percentiles, 628
Glomerular filtration rate
        (GFR), 301, 462
Glucagon-like peptide-
        1(GLP-1), 310
    receptor agonists, 310–311
Glucosamine, 557, 578
    use for osteoarthritis, 436
Glucosamine/chondroitin, 559
Glucosamine/Chondroitin Arthritis
        Intervention Trial (GAIT),
        436, 559, 578
Glucosamine sulfate, 578
Glucosamine supplements, 578
Glucose-lowering
        medications, 323
Glucose metabolism, 298
Glutamine, 538
Gluten, 395
Gluten-free diet, 398t–403t
Gluten-free grains, 396
Glycemic assessment and
        monitoring, 293–297
Glycemic control, benefits in, 316
Glycemic index (GI), 142, 328, 329
Glycemic load (GL), 328
Glycemic response, medications
        effect, 346t
Glycogen, 320
Gout, 438–439
    nutrition intervention for, 439
    nutrition interview
        considerations, 439t
    nutrition recommendations
        for, 441t

Grains, 11–13
  list of, 12t
  refined grains, 12
  USDA one-cup dairy serving
    sizes, 15t
  USDA-recommended intake
    levels, 13t
  whole grains, anatomy of, 12, 12f
Group counseling, 105
  sessions, 105t
Growth charts, 41

H
Hamwi equation, 45
Hamwi method, 494
Hand-held indirect calorimetry, 123
  RMR determination, 123
Harris-Benedict equation, 68, 498
HbA1c, 291, 294, 299
Health belief model (HBM), 88, 89t
Healthcare practitioner, 201
Healthcare professionals, 73
  tool, DRI for, 10
Healthcare spectrum, 36
Health checklist, 54f–55f
Healthy eating patterns
  parents role, 211
Healthy fats, 160
Healthy meal plan, 1–32
  calories consumed by kids, 25t
  dairy foods, 13–14
  empty calories food, 25t, 26t
  energy density, 24f
    lowering, tips for, 24t
  1992 food guide pyramid, 3f
  food label, daily values (DVs)
    used on, 11t
  fruit, 14–16, 16t
  good nutrition, government
    guidelines for, 1–10
    Dietary Guidelines for
      Americans, 2010, 4–5
    dietary reference intakes, 9–10
    food label, 9
    healthy people 2020, 5–8, 8t
    pyramids, plates, and portions, 1–4
  grains, 11–13
    anatomy of, 12f
    list of, 12t
    USDA one-cup dairy serving
      sizes, 15t
    USDA-recommended intake
      levels, 13t

menu planning, 10–27
  build food group foundations,
    11–18
  control portion size, 20–22
  food consumption, monitor
    frequency of, 18–19
  limit empty calories, 24–27
  promote variety in diet, 19–20
  reduce energy density, 22–24
MyPlate, 5f
MyPyramid, 4f
nutrition facts label, 10f
portion sizes, 23f
protein foods, 16–18, 17t
seafood guidelines for
  pregnant or breastfeeding
    women, 18t
tips to improve, 21t
tracking tools and guides,
  27–28
  ChooseMyPlate for Moms, 27
  ChooseMyPlate SuperTracker, 27
  NIH menu planner, 28
  Nutrihand, 28
  self-monitoring, 27–28
  USDA nutrient database,
    27–28
Healthy people, 5–8, 8t
  nutrition and weight status area of, 7
Heart disease, risk factors, 252t
Heart failure, 281–283, 534
  diet therapy for, 282t
  monitoring lab values, 283
  nutrition related lab values, 282t
Heart outcomes prevention
    evaluation (HOPE), 584
Hedonic system, 115
Helicobacter pylori infection, 374
Hematocrit, 64
Hemodialysis, 588
Hepatic diseases
  nutrient considerations/
    modifications, 456t
Hepatitis, 453
Herbs
  to use in home cooking, 271t
Herpes simplex 2 (HSV-2), 581
Hiatal hernia, 373–374
  in stomach, 374f
High biological value (HBV)
    protein, 466t
High-calcium diet, 142
High-calorie diet, 158

High-density lipoproteins (HDLs), 253, 300, 367
  alcohol, 262–263
  cholesterol, 332
  interventions to raise, 261–263
  niacin, 262
  physical activity, 262
High-energy-dense foods, 23
High-fat protein foods, 18
High-fiber diets, 321
High-fiber products, 329
High-fructose corn syrup (HFCS)
  component of, 16
High-glycemic index foods, 328
Highly active antiretroviral therapy
  (HAART) drugs, 516
High-monounsaturated fatty acid
  (MUFA), 331
High-phosphorus foods, 470*t*
High-potassium foods, 467*t*
High-potassium potatoes, 469*t*
High-protein digestibility-corrected
  amino acid score
  (PD-CAAS), 330
HIV/AIDS, nutrition, 516–518
Homeostatic system, 115
Hospitalized PWD
  special nutritional needs of, 348*t*
H. pylori, 582
Human insulin, key features of, 314*t*
Hunger. *See* Appetite
Hydrochloric acid (HCl)
  production, 376
Hypercholesterolemia, 252–254
  lipid goals, 253–254
Hyperemesis gravidarum.
  See Morning sickness
Hyperglycemia, 351, 479*t*, 546, 550
Hyperglycemia management, 458
Hyperglycemic hyperosmolar
  nonketotic coma
  (HHNK), 345
Hypericum perforatum, 574
Hyperkalemia, 483
Hyperlipidemia, in HIV
  infection, 517
Hyperphosphatemia, 483
Hypertension, 300
  dietary approaches to stop
    hypertension (DASH),
    273–277
  JNC 7 summary
    recommendations, 277

  lifestyle modifications to, 278*t*
  lower blood pressure approaches,
    267–273
Hypocaloric feeding, 494
Hypoglycemia, 323
  rates of, 312
  risk of, 316
  treatment, oral glucose
    supplementation
    effects, 347*t*
Hypotension, 74

I
ICD-9-CM criteria, 60
Ideal body weight (IBW), 45. *See
  also* Hamwi method
Ideal body weight range (IBWR), 45
Ileostomy, 412–414, 413
  diet therapy for, 413*t*
  nutrition considerations for, 414*t*
Immune-enhancing factors, 196
Immune function, 237
Immune-modulating enteral
  formulas, 537
  favorable *versus* less-favorable
    outcomes, 537*t*
Impaired fasting glucose (IFG), 291
Impaired glucose tolerance (IGT),
  291, 342
Indirect calorimetry measurement
  optimal conditions for, 524*t*, 526*t*
Infancy
  calorie needs, 206
  fat needs, 207
  introduction of solid foods, 208*t*
  nutrients and nonnutrients of, 207*t*
  nutrition during, 206–210
  protein needs, 206–207
  weaning foods, 207–208
Infant feeding, do's/don'ts, 209*t*
Inflammatory arthritis, types
  of, 438
Inflammatory bowel disease (IBD),
  405–407
  diet therapy in, 406
  high-oxalate foods to avoid, 408*t*
  nutrition concerns in, 406*t*
  nutrition interventions for, 404*t*
  recommended foods for, 409*t*
Inflammatory cytokines, activation
  of, 351
Injury and fever factor, 128*t*
Injury factor (IF), 68

Institute of Medicine (IOM), 157
  guidelines, 171
Insulin
  deficiency, 322
  regimens, 312
  resistance syndrome, 263
  secretagogue
    exercise precautions with, 321t
Insulin-like growth factor-1
    (IGF-1), 62
Insulin resistance syndrome, 263
Insulin-to-carbohydrate ratio (ICR),
    313, 323, 324t
Interdisciplinary team approach, 349
Intermediate-acting insulin
    injection, 313
Intermediate-acting insulin/rapid/short-
    acting insulin regimens, 313
Internal physiological systems, food
    intake in, 116t
International normalized ratio
    (INR), 548
Intestinal gas, 389–391
Intestinal surgery, 411–412
  ileocecal valve, 411–412
  sections and length of bowel
    remaining, 412
Intestinal villi, 365f
Intrauterine growth restriction
    (IUGR), 183
Iron
  absorption, 445, 445t
  containing foods, 446t
    for kids, 219t
  fortified cereals, 234
  fortified rice cereal, 208
  recommended dietary allowances
    for, 444t
Iron deficiency, 64, 218, 223
  anemia, 443–447
    dietary sources of iron,
      444–446
    iron supplements, 446–447
  symptoms of, 218
Irritable bowel syndrome (IBS),
    383, 397–405
  cause of, 397
  dietary management of, 404
  FODMAPs approach to
    management, 404–405
  probiotics and prebiotics use in
    treatment, 403–404
Isoniazid, 582

J
Jaundice, 549
Jejunum, 365
Joint National Committee on
    Prevention, Detection,
    Evaluation, and Treatment
    of High Blood Pressure
    (JNC7), 270, 277

K
Ketoacidosis, 346
Ketogenic diet, 587
Kidney disease, 473t–474t
Kidney Disease Outcomes Quality
    Initiative (K/DOQI)
    Nutrition Guidelines, 464
Kidney stones, 487–488, 587
Kidney transplantation, 473, 486–487

L
Laboratory data, 62–64
  iron status, 63
  serum proteins, 62–63
  vitamin and mineral status, 63–64
Lactase enzyme supplements, 391
Lactating women, fluid
    recommendations, 197
Lactation, 199
Lactose, 194
  intolerance, 180, 394
    calcium intake in, 395t
    exacerbation of, 394
Later childhood, nutrition in, 221–229
  childhood obesity, 223–224
  energy needs in, 221–222
  food allergy, 224–227
  National school lunch and breakfast
    programs, 228–229
  protein, carbohydrate, and fat
    needs in, 222
  vitamin, mineral, fiber, and fluid
    needs in, 222–223
Lean body mass, 345
Lipid emulsions, 543
Lipids, in food, 543
Lipodystrophy syndrome, 516, 517
Lipolysis, 493
Lipoproteins, 367t
Listeria monocytogenes, 184
Liver transplantation, 458–459
Long-chain triglycerides (LCTs), 586
Low-calorie diet (LCD), 135–136
  initiation, 136–137

Low-carbohydrate diets, 142–144, 143, 322, 536
Low-density lipoproteins (LDLs), 143, 251, 253, 367
 cholesterol, 310, 332
 dietary cholesterol, 258
 dietary fiber, 259–260
 interventions to, 254–260
 omega-3 fatty acids, 258–259
 particle size, 255
 saturated fat, 254–255
 saturated fat and LDL particle size, 255
 trans fat, 256–258
Lower blood pressure approaches, 267–273
 alcohol, 269–271
 calcium, 272–273
 magnesium, 272
 physical activity, 273
 potassium, 268–269
 sodium, 267–268
Lower gastrointestinal system, 379
Low-fat diet, 23
Low-fiber therapy, 410
Low-residue foods, 392
Low-residue refined grains, 392
Lupus, 442–443
 treatment of, 443

M
Macrocytic anemias, 443
Macronutrients, 321–323
 AMDR for, 70t
 consumption of, 323
 dietary carbohydrate, relative composition of, 322
 dietary fat, relative composition of, 322–323
 dietary protein, relative composition of, 322
 distribution of, 213–217
Macronutrient sources
 in elemental formulas, 536t
 standard enteral formula, 535t
Magnesium supplementation, on blood sugar, 589
Malabsorption, 393–394
 carbohydrate, 394
 fat, 394
 protein, 394
Malnutrition, diagnosis, 60–62, 61t–62t

Malnutrition screening tool (MST), 50
Malnutrition universal screening tool (MUST), 51, 51t
MAOI diet, 567t–569t
Massage therapy, 557
Maternal anemia, definition of, 180
Maternal glucose levels, 344
Maternal glycemia, 344
Meal planning tools and resources, 352–355
Meal replacements, 141
Medical nutrition therapy (MNT), 289, 290, 482
 alcohol, 350–351
  primary prevention, 350
  secondary prevention, 350–351
  tertiary prevention, 351
 alpha-glucosidase inhibitors (AGI), 310
 amylin-mimetic, 311
 anthropometric parameters, 297–299
 antidiabetic medications, pharmacologic assessment and monitoring of, 303–321
 basal analog insulin regimen, 313–314
 basal-bolus analog insulin regimen, 313
 biguanides, 309
 cardiovascular parameters, 299–301
 coronary artery diseases (CAD), 318
 CV autonomic neuropathy, 318–319
 for diabetes mellitus, 289–356
 diet and genome interactions, 351
 dipeptidyl peptidase-IV inhibitors (DPP4i), 310
 dopamine receptor agonist, 311
 eating disorders, 352
 effectiveness of, 291–292
 fixed-dose insulin regimens, 312
 food intake assessment and monitoring, 292–293
 glucagon-like peptide-1 receptor agonists, 310–311
 glycemic assessment and monitoring, 293–297
 goals of, 292
 HbA1c, 294
 insulin regimens, 312
 intermediate-acting insulin/rapid- or short-acting insulin regimens, 313

Medical nutrition therapy (MNT)
(*Cont.*):
  meal planning tools and resources,
    352–355
  metabolic assessment and
    monitoring, 297–299
  nephropathy and
    microalbuminuria, 319
  nonsulfonylureas, 309
  nutrient recommendations,
    321–336, 352
    carbohydrates, 323–330
    fat, 330–332
    macronutrients, carbohydrates,
      proteins, and fats,
      321–323
    micronutrients and antioxidants,
      332–333
    primary prevention, preventing
      diabetes, 333–334
    secondary prevention,
      controlling diabetes, 334
    tertiary prevention, controlling
      diabetes complications,
      334–336
  peripheral neuropathy, 318
  physical activity with
    general guidelines for, 319–321
    gestational diabetes
      (GDM), 317
    long-term complications of
      diabetes, 317–318
    type 1 diabetes, 315–316
    type 2 diabetes, 316–317
  plant-based diets, 349–350
  process, 292
  recommendations, 336
  renal parameters, 301–303
  retinopathy, 318
  secretagogues, 303
  self-monitoring blood glucose
    (SMBG), 294
    continuous glucose monitoring
      systems (CGMS), 296–297
    frequency and timing, 294–295
    interpreting results method,
      295–296
    for those with insulin
      dependence, 295
  sensitizers, 309
  sodium–glucose cotransporter
    2 inhibitors, 311–312

specific populations and
    circumstances, 336–349
  children and adolescents,
    337–339
  older adults, 345–349
  pregnancy, 340–344
  prepregnancy, 340
  sulfonylureas, 303
  thiazolidinediones (TZDs),
    309–310
  wound healing, 351–352
Medicare, 482
Meditation, 557
Mediterranean dietary pattern, 331
Medium-chain triglyceride (MCT),
    394, 456, 496, 517, 586
Megaloblastic anemias
  folate deficiency anemia, 448
  pernicious anemia, 447
  vitamin B_{12} deficiency, 448
Metabolic assessment and
    monitoring, 297–299
Metabolic bone disease, 549
Metabolic efficiency, definition
    of, 113
Metabolic energy consumption, 130*t*
Metabolic stressors, 129
Metabolic syndrome, 263–264
  apple-shaped fat patterning
    increases risk for, 265*f*
  clinical identification of, 264*t*
Methylmercury toxicity, potential
    harmful effects, 186
Meticulous glycemic control, 526
Metoclopramide, 531
Microalbuminuria, 319
Micronutrients, 332–333
Microvilli, 365
Midarm muscle circumferences
    (MAMC), 42
Mid upper arm circumference
    (MUAC), 42
Mifflin-St. Jeor equation, 68
Minerals
  deficiency/toxicity, 84*t*
  recommended dietary allowance
    (RDA), 571
Mini nutrition assessment (MNA®),
    52, 53*f*, 241
Monoamine oxidase (MAO), 564
Monoamine oxidase inhibitors
    (MAOIs) block, 564

Morning sickness, 190*t*
Motivational interviewing (MI),
    93, 134
    OARS of, 93*t*
    principles of, 94*t*
    strategies for, 94*t*
Mucositis, 514
Mucositis and stomatitis
    cancer prevention/nutrition-related
        treatment side effects,
        514–515
Multiorgan dysfunction syndrome
    (MODS), 540
Muscle cramps, 588
Muscle twitching, 588
MyPlate plan, 198*t*
MyPlate tool, 4, 5*f*
MyPyramid tool, 3, 4*f*

N
Nasojejunal (NJ) tubes, 527
National Center for Complementary
        and Alternative Medicine
        (NCCAM), 436, 555
National Cholesterol Education
        Program (NCEP), 253, 349
    cholesterol classifications, 253*t*
National Digestive Diseases
        Information, 384
National Dysphagia Diet (NDD), 368
National Health and Nutrition
        Examination Survey
        (NHANES), 43, 47, 72
    data, 230
National Health and Nutrition
        Examination Survey III
        (NHANES III), 421
National Health Interview Survey
        (NHIS), 557
    natural products, 557*t*
National Institute of Arthritis and
        Musculoskeletal and Skin
        Diseases (NIAMS), 436
National Institutes of Health Office of
        Dietary Supplements, 240
National Kidney Disease Education
        Program (NKDEP), 470
National Kidney Foundation, 462
National Osteoporosis Foundation,
        424, 434
National School Breakfast
        Program, 228

National Weight Control Registry
        (NWCR), 87, 132,
        135, 145
Natural products, 557*t*
Nausea, 513, 549
    nonpharmacologic treatments
        for, 190
Nausea and vomiting
    cancer prevention/nutrition-related
        treatment side effects,
        513–514
Nausea and vomiting in pregnancy
    (NVP), 189
Nephropathy, 301, 319
    annual screening for, 302*t*
Neural tube defects (NTDs),
    prevention of, 178
Neuroglycopenia, 346
Neuropathic joint disease, 318
The New American Plate, 510*f*
NHANES II weight table, 465*t*
Niacin/simvastatin, to lower
        cholesterol, 575
Nonalcoholic steatohepatitis
    (NASH), 454
Nondairy foods, 430*t*
Nonnutritive sweeteners (NNS),
    326, 327*t*
Nonpregnant women, EER for, 174*t*
Nonproliferative diabetic retinopathy
    (NPDR), 318
Nonsulfonylureas, 309
Nutrient absorption, drugs, 565*t*
Nutrient complications
    carnitine deficiency, 551
    essential fatty acid deficiency, 551
    hyperglycemia, 550–551
    refeeding syndrome, 550
Nutrihand, 28
Nutrition
    absorption
        primary sites of, 366*t*
    before and after surgery, 501–502
    application, 90*t*–91*t*
    assessment, 33–35, 59–60
        components of, 60*f*
        laboratory tests for, 65*t*–67*t*
    blood cell values, 64*t*
    body weight equation, 69*t*
    calculators, and tools, 55–59
    calorie needs, 69*t*
    care algorithm, 40*f*

Nutrition (*Cont.*):
  care process (*See* Nutrition care
      process (NCP))
  diagnosing malnutrition, 60–62,
      61*t*–62*t*
  DRIs for, 71*t*
  drugs, 565*t*
  dysfunction, signs and symptoms
      of, 85*t*
  education, 141
  empathetic person, 86*f*
  english-metric conversions, 632–634
  enteral *vs.* parenteral, 526–527
  evidence-based public health,
      steps of, 95*t*
  fat-soluble vitamins, deficiency
      and toxicity, 78*t*–79*t*
  group counseling, 105
    sessions, 105*t*
  health belief model, 89*t*
  health checklist, 54*f*–55*f*
  laboratory data, 62–64
    iron status, 63
    serum proteins, 62–63
    vitamin and mineral status, 63–64
  macronutrients, AMDR for, 70*t*
  malnutrition universal screening
      tool (MUST), 51*t*
  minerals, deficiency and
      toxicity, 84*t*
  mini nutritional assessment
      (MNA), 53*f*
  motivational interviewing,
      OARS of, 93*t*
  needs, 320*t*
  nutrition screen for, 50*t*
  obsolete therapeutic diets,
      examples of, 98*t*
  physical examination
      techniques, 74*t*
  poor foods, 20
  risk determination, 35–36, 37*t*, 41*t*
  short nutritional assessment
      questionnaire (SNAQ), 52*t*
  skin breakdown, risk for, 75*t*
  stages of change, 92*f*
  subjective global assessment
      form, 56*f*
  water-soluble vitamins, deficiency
      and toxicity, 80*t*–83*t*
  in wound care, 502–504
  writing smart goals and
      objectives, 102*t*

Nutritional assessment parameters,
    523–524
Nutritional needs, catabolic
    illness, 523
Nutrition assessment, 493
  energy needs, determining,
    494–495
  fluid needs, determining, 496
  protein needs, determining, 496
Nutrition care process (NCP),
    36–38, 38*f*
  steps, 37
Nutrition dietary data, 64–73
  calorie counts, 72–73
  energy needs estimation, 68–69
  food frequency tools, 72
  interactive DRI for healthcare
      professionals, 73
  macronutrient needs estimation, 70
  micronutrient needs estimation,
      70–72
  supertracker, 73
Nutrition facts panel, 386
  daily value (DV) on, 253
Nutrition-focused physical
    assessment (NFPA), 73–77
  body system alterations and
      nutrient status, 74–77
  vitamin- and mineral-specific
      clues, 77
Nutrition Labeling and Education
    Act of 1990 (NLEA), 9
Nutrition recommendations, 321–336
  carbohydrates, 323–330
  fat, 330–332
  macronutrients, carbohydrates,
      proteins, and fats, 321–323
  micronutrients and antioxidants,
      332–333
  primary prevention, preventing
      diabetes, 333–334
  secondary prevention, controlling
      diabetes, 334
  tertiary prevention, controlling
      diabetes complications,
      334–336
Nutrition-related medication, 323
Nutrition screeners, 41*t*
  determine nutrition checklist,
      52–53
  electronic, 55–59
  malnutrition screening tool
      (MST), 50

malnutrition universal screening tool (MUST), 51
mini nutrition assessment (MNA®), 52
short nutritional assessment questionnaire (SNAQ), 51–52
subjective global assessment (SGA), 54–55
web resource for, 57*t*–58*t*
Nutrition screening, 38–41
    with biochemical tests, 49
    BMI and body weight, 42, 42*t*
    equations and measurements, 42–44
    ideal body weight, 45*t*, 46–49
    multiple-pass method, 48*f*
    sample 24-hour recall form, 47*f*
    triceps skinfold measurements and MAMC, 43*t*
    using anthropometric data, 41–46, 44*t*
    vs. assessment, 59*t*
    weight change criteria, 46*t*
Nutrition support, goals, 524
Nutrition support teams (NSTs), 530
Nutrition therapy, 97
    goal of, 453

O

Obesity, 134, 168, 297, 529
    classification of, 133*t*, 298*t*
    classifying degree of, 133–134
    statistics, 33
Obsolete therapeutic diets, examples of, 98*t*
Office of alternative medicine (OAM), 555
Older adults, nutrition for, 157, 236–242
    assessing nutrition risk in, 241
    calorie needs for, 237
    carbohydrate, protein, and fat needs, 238
    exercise and aging, 240–241
    medical nutrition therapy for, 345–349
        acute care facilities, 348–349
        acute illness, 346–347
        hypoglycemia, 346, 347–348
        long-term care facilities, 349
        medications, 345–346
        nutrition, 345

physical activity, 345
        self-monitoring, 346
    MyPlate for, 242*t*
    nutrition assistance programs, 241–242
    physiological changes and nutrition impact, 236–237
    supplementation for, 239–240
    vitamin, mineral, fiber, and fluid needs for, 238–239
Omega-3 fatty acids, 258–259, 265
    fish oil, 576
    supplementation of, 342
"One-size-fits-all" approach, 77, 100
Optimal bone mineral density, 231
Oral echinacea, 579
Oral glucose tolerance test (OGTT), 192
Oral nutrition supplements, 515
Oropharyngeal secretions, 531
Osteoarthritis, 435–436
Osteomalacia, 432
Osteoporosis, 421–434
    conditions and medications, 424*t*
    diagnosis, 423–426, 426*t*
    nutritional management and mitigation of, 426–434
        calcium intake and recommendations, 427–428
        calcium supplements, 428–432
        protein and sodium, 433–434
        vitamin D intake and recommendations, 432
        vitamin D supplements, 432–433
    prevention of, 434
    related fractures, 421
    risk factors, 422–423, 423*t*
    summary recommendations, 434
Osteoporotic bone, 422*f*
"Out-of-the-bag" approach, 230
Overweight, 168, 297
    classification of, 133*t*, 298*t*
    classifying degree of, 133–134

P

P450 3A4 isoenzymes (3A4), 566
Panax ginseng, 580
Panax quinquefolius, 580
Pancreatectomy, 541
Pancreatitis, 461–462
Parathyroid hormone, 179

Parenteral nutrition (PN), 461, 497, 526
  adult maintenance mineral requirements, 547*t*
  assessment/monitoring parameters
    delivery of energy, 545–546
    delivery of protein, 546
    fluid/electrolytes, management of, 546–548
    laboratory data, evaluation of, 548–549
    physical findings, assessment of, 549
    tolerance to infusion, 546
  central venous catheters (CVCs), 540
  enteral feedings, transitioning, 552
  gastrointestinal complications
    acalculous cholecystitis, 549
    metabolic bone disease, 549–550
    parenteral nutrition-associated liver disease, 549
  gastrointestinal surgery, 541–542
  implanted port, 541
  inadequate enteral nutrition, 542
  initiation and timing, 541
  mechanical complications, 551–552
  nutrient complications
    carnitine deficiency, 551
    essential fatty acid deficiency, 551
    hyperglycemia, 550–551
    refeeding syndrome, 550
  patients' maintenance fluid requirements, 548*t*
  peripheral access, 541
  peripherally inserted central catheters (PICC), 540
  recommendation, 545*t*
  solution composition, 542
    carbohydrate (dextrose), 542
    electrolytes, 544
    fat (lipid), 543–544
    protein (amino acids), 542–543
    vitamins/trace minerals, 544–545
  solution, osmolarity of, 541
  tunneled catheters, 540–541
  vascular access, 540
Parenteral nutrition-associated liver disease, 549

Patient education tools, 277–280
  label reading, 278–279
  recipe resources, 279–280
  restaurant resources, 280
Pediatrics, 151–157
Peptic ulcer disease (PUD), 374–376, 374*f*, 375*t*
  foods not recommended, 377*t*
  nonmedication-related management of, 375
  treatment modality for, 374
Peripherally inserted central catheters (PICC), 540
Peripheral neuropathy, 317, 318
Person with diabetes (PWD), 289, 300
  benefits of physical activity, 315
  diaries of, 295
    substantial percentage of, 302
  vitamin and mineral needs of, 332
Pharmacological therapy, use of, 147
Phosphorus foods, high, 471
Phosphorus, needs, 547
Physical activity
  effects of, 145
  in elderly, risks and benefits of, 345*t*
  fluid consumption schedule for, 319*t*
  general guidelines for, 319–321
  gestational diabetes (GDM), 317
  long-term complications of diabetes, 317–318
  precautions, 145
  regimen, 145
  type 1 diabetes, 315–316
  type 2 diabetes, 316–317
  types of, 146
Physical activity level (PAL), 237
Physical examination techniques, 74*t*
Plant-based diets, 349–350
PN-associated liver disease (PNALD), 549
Polycystic ovarian syndrome (PCOS)
  risk of, 169
Polyols
  use of, 326
Portion control, 138–140
  strategies for, 140
Postgastric-surgery patient
  dietary interventions in, 379*t*
Postmenopausal women
  National Osteoporosis Foundation's clinician's recommendations for, 434*t*

Postoperative nausea and vomiting (PONV), 589
Potassium chloride, 269
Potassium foods
    high, 467t
    low, 468t
Potassium, needs, 547
Preconception diabetes care, 340
Preconception nutrition, 168–169
Predictive equations
    RMR determination, 123–124
Pregnancy, 157–158
    carbohydrate distribution, 194t
    contraindications to aerobic exercise, 188t, 189t
    exercises, 188t
    foods and substances to avoid, 183t
    medical nutrition therapy for
        gestational diabetes, 342–344
        lactation, 344
        pre-existing diabetes, 340–342
    nutrition during, 169–193
        calcium needs, 179–180
        calorie needs, 173–175
        carbohydrate needs, 176–177
        cravings and aversions, 190–191
        exercises, 186–188
        folate needs, 178–179
        food safety, 184–186
        foods to avoid, 182–184
        gestational diabetes, 192–193
        iron needs, 180
        listeriosis, 184
        macronutrient and micronutrient needs, 175–180
        meal planning, 180–182
        from merely surviving to absolutely thriving, 169–170
        methylmercury, 185–186
        nausea and vomiting, 189–190
        nutrition-related complications, 188–189
        pica, 191
        pregnancy-induced hypertension, 191–192
        protein needs, 177–178
        toxoplasmosis, 185
        weight gain guidelines for, 170–173
    potentially hazardous foods to avoid, 187t
    with pre-existing diabetes, optimal glycemic and blood pressure goals, 341t
    weight gain, components of, 173f
Prenatal nutrition risk screen form, 171t
Prepregnancy, 340
    medical nutrition therapy for gestational diabetes, 340
    type 1 and type 2 diabetes, 340
Preschoolers
    meal patterning for, 217t
    recommended calorie needs for, 216t
Primary care providers (PCPs), 34, 317
Professionals' Health Study, 298
Proliferative diabetic retinopathy (PDR), 318
Protein
    fortified recipe, 500t
    tips for increasing, 499t
Protein-calorie malnutrition, 541
Protein-calorie malnutrition (PCM), 463
Protein-energy malnutrition, 493, 523
Protein restrictions, 453
Proteins, 62–63, 159
    albumin, 62–63
    content of, 178t
    count, 160–161
    DRI recommendation for, 222
    foods, 11, 16–18, 17t
    healthy, 160
    intake and diabetic nephropathy, 330
    intake and normal renal function, 330
    prealbumin, 63, 63t
    role in, 231
    transferrin, 63
Proton pump inhibitor (PPI), 375
Psychotropic medications
    use of, 135
Public health organizations, 280
Pulmonary stress, nutrition
    acute respiratory distress syndrome, 504–505
    chronic obstructive pulmonary disease (COPD), 505–506
    cystic fibrosis, 506–509
Purines, 440t–441t

Q

Quantum theory, 44
Quinine, 588

R

Raynaud's syndrome, 581
Recommended dietary allowance
    (RDA), 2, 9, 217, 273
    for vitamin/mineral, 571
Reduced calorie diets, 135
Reflective listening, 100, 101
Registered dietitian (RD), 36, 169,
    226, 289
Regular meal pattern, 137
Renal parameters, 301–303
Respiratory quotient (RQ), 123
Resting energy expenditure (REE)
    measurement, 160
    reductions in, 145
    in sepsis, 494
Resting metabolic rate (RMR), 68, 115
Resting metabolic rate prediction
    equations, 125t–126t
Retinol-binding protein (RBP), 62
Retinopathy, 318
Rheumatic disease, 434–442
    fibromyalgia, 439–442
    gout, 438–439
    osteoarthritis, 435–436
    rheumatoid arthritis, 436–438
    Sjögren's syndrome, 442
Rheumatoid arthritis, 436–438
    diet therapy for, 438t
    nutrition interview questions, 437t
Risk determination, 35–36, 37t, 41t
Rome III Consensus Criteria, 384
Rosiglitazone, 310
Roux-en-Y gastric bypass, 153f
Russell's sign, 75

S

Sarcopenia, 236
Saturated fat, 254–255, 300
    NHANES top sources of, 256t
    substitution ideas for
        lowering, 257t
School health programs
    CDC guidelines for, 225t
Screeners, of nutrition, 41t
    determine nutrition checklist, 52–53
    electronic, 55–59
    malnutrition screening tool
        (MST), 50

malnutrition universal screening
        tool (MUST), 51
    mini nutrition assessment
        (MNA®), 52
    short nutritional assessment
        questionnaire (SNAQ),
        51–52
    subjective global assessment
        (SGA), 54–55
    types of, 39
    web resource for, 57t–58t
Screening, of nutrition, 38–41
    with biochemical tests, 49
    BMI and body weight, 42, 42t
    equations and measurements,
        42–44
    ideal body weight, 45t, 46–49
    multiple-pass method, 48f
    sample 24-hour recall form, 47f
    triceps skinfold measurements and
        MAMC, 43t
    using anthropometric data,
        41–46, 44t
    vs. assessment, 59t
    weight change criteria, 46t
Seafood, benefits of, 18
Seasoning foods, without
        salt, 270t
Secretagogues, 303
Segmentation, 362
Segment weight, ratio of, 122f
Self-feeding practices, 211
Self-kept records, 49
Self-monitoring, 147
Self-monitoring of blood glucose
        (SMBG), 294, 295, 303
    continuous glucose monitoring
        systems (CGMS),
        296–297
    frequency and timing,
        294–295
    interpretation of, 296
    interpreting results method,
        295–296
    records, 341
    for those with insulin
        dependence, 295
Self-monitoring tools, 27–28
Sensations, 114
Sensitizers, 309
Sepsis, 493
    resting energy expenditure
        (REE), 494

Serum triglycerides
American Heart Association
recommendations for, 266*t*
ATP III classification for, 266*t*
Set point, 113
Setting realistic physical activity
expectations, 145–146
Sex hormone-binding globulin, 168
Short bowel syndrome (SBS),
414–415
causes of, 414
diet therapy for, 416*t*
Short nutritional assessment
questionnaire (SNAQ),
51–52
Sickle cell disease (SCD), 449
potential micronutrient
deficiencies in, 449*t*
Sippy diet, 376
Sjögren's syndrome, 442
Sleeve gastrectomy, 154*f*
Small-bore feeding tubes, 528
Small intestine, 383*f*
S.M.A.R.T. goals, 353, 353*t*
Social distance, 100
Sodium
labeling language, 279*t*
sources of diet, 268*t*, 269*t*
tips to reduce, 271*t*
Sodium–glucose cotransporter
2 inhibitors, 311–312
Solid fats and added sugars
(SoFAS), 619
Sphincters, 364
ileocecal sphincter, 364
lower esophageal sphincter, 364
pyloric sphincter, 364
Spices
to use in lieu of salt for home
cooking, 271*t*
Spicy homemade salt-free herb
seasoning, 272*t*
Stages of change model,
88, 92
Stanols, 261
Steatorrhea, 378–379
Sterols, 261
Stimulus, control, 147
Stomach, 152*f*
hiatal hernia, 374*f*
lower esophageal and pyloric
sphincters, 364*f*
peristalsis and segmentation, 363*f*

Subjective global assessment
(SGA), 54–55
Subscapular skinfold thickness
(SSF), 43
Successful losers, characteristics of,
132, 132*t*
Sucrose-containing foods, 325
Sugar-sweetened beverages,
elimination of, 25
Sulfonylureas, 303
Syndrome X. *See* Insulin resistance
syndrome
Systematic inflammatory response
syndrome (SIRS), 523
Systemic catheter infections, 552
Systemic lupus erythematosus
(SLE), 442

T
Taste/smell alterations
cancer prevention/nutrition-related
treatment side effects,
515–516
Temporomandibular joint (TMJ)
arthritis, 578
Teniposide (VM26), 578
Therapeutic lifestyle changes
(TLC), 260, 261
components of, 261*t*
diet, 260–261
plant stanols and sterols, 261
recommendations, 281
Thiazolidinediones (TZDs),
309–310
Thyroid hormone, 423
Tolerable upper intake level (UL), 70
Total body surface area
(TBSA), 497
Total caloric expenditure, component
of, 123
Total energy expenditure (TEE), 115
determination, 126*t*
role in metabolism, components
of, 117*t*–118*t*
Total energy requirements, RMR
determination, 124–126
Total iron-binding capacity
(TIBC), 63
Total parenteral nutrition (TPN),
190, 407, 412, 415, 481
nutritional complications, 486
Toxoplasma gondii, 185
Trans fat, 256–258

Trans fatty acids, 331
Transplant recipients, 458*t*, 459*t*
Transtheoretical model, 88
Triceps skinfold thickness (TSF), 42
Triglyceridemia, 264
Triglycerides, 267
Tryptophan, 586
T-score, 424
Type 1 diabetes, 342
    physical activity, 315–316
Type 2 diabetes, 299
    etiology of, 339
    physical activity, 316–317
    risk factors for, 334
    therapy for, 303
Tyramine, 566, 567*t*–569*t*

U
Ulcerative colitis (UC), 405
Underweight
    definition of, 151
    reasons for, 159*t*
United Nations Children's Fund
        (UNICEF), 201
United States Department of
        Agriculture (USDA), 1
United States Department of Health
        and Human Services
        (DHHS), 2
Untreated dysphagia, nutritional
        consequences of, 369*t*
Upper intake levels (ULs), 9, 179, 571
Uremia, 472
Urolithiasis, 487
    high-oxalate foods, 488*t*
    high-sodium foods, 488*t*
USDA Food and Nutrition
        Services, 221
USDA food patterns
    daily amount of food, 620
    protein foods, 622
    vegetable, 621
USDA National School Lunch
        and Breakfast
        Programs, 229
USDA National School Lunch
        Program (NSLP), 228
USDA nutrient database, 27–28
USDA's Nutrition Evidence Library
        (NEL), 96
USDA's Special Supplemental
        Nutrition Program, 220

USDA's Supplemental Nutrition
        Assistance Program
        (SNAP), 241
US Diabetes Prevention Program
        (DPP), 291
US Food and Drug Administration
        (FDA), 9
US Public Health Service, 87
Usual body weight (UBW), 46

V
Vegetarian diet, 144
    therapeutic use of, 144
Vegetarian meal plan, 144
Vertigo, ginkgo, 581
Very low calorie diet (VLCD),
        135, 136
    complications and side effects,
        139*t*–140*t*
    requirements and
        contraindications, 138*t*
Very low density lipoproteins
        (VLDLs), 253, 367
Villi, 365
Vitamin
    recommended dietary allowance
        (RDA), 571
Vitamin B$_{12}$, 238–239
Vitamin C, 234, 446, 575
Vitamin D, 199, 232, 576
    content, 432*t*
    dietary reference intakes for, 433*t*
    monitoring, 472
    supplementation, 432
    synthesis, 237
Vitamin E, 574, 576, 584–585
    antioxidant properties, 584
Vitamin K, 544, 545
Vomiting, 513, 549

W
Waist circumference (WC), 133
Water-soluble dietary fiber-
        containing formulas, 533
Web-based meal planning tools, 27
Weight calculations, 119*t*
Weight gain
    components of, 173*t*
    during pregnancy, 171
    rate of, 172*t*
    for twins, 172*t*
Weight-loss diet, 143

Weight loss surgery (WLS), 148
    effectiveness of, 148
Weight loss therapy, 131
Weight maintenance program, 131
Weight management, 113–164
    body weight regulation, principles
        of, 113–115
        energy balance, 113–114
        energy expenditure factors, 115
        energy intake factors, 115
    disordered eating (DE), 162
    eating disorders (EDs), 162
    indicators for, 134
    overweight and obesity, medical
        nutrition therapy for,
        130–158
        assessment & monitoring
            parameters, 133–135
        behavioral interventions,
            146–147
        dietary interventions, 135–144
        FDA-approved medication
            interventions, 147–148
        physical activity interventions,
            144–146
        specific populations and
            circumstances, 151–158
        surgical interventions, 148–151
        weight management therapy,
            effectiveness of, 131–132
        weight management therapy,
            goals of, 130–131
    program, 138
        beneficial component, 141
    promoting weight gain, 158–162
        assessment and monitoring
            parameters, 159–160
        dietary interventions for,
            160–161
        effectiveness of, 159
        goals of, 158
        medication interventions,
            161–162
        physical activity
            interventions, 161
    quantifying body weight, 115–130
        amputation, accommodations
            for, 115–122

    amputation, energy and protein
        accommodations for, 130
    energy needs determination,
        123–129
    realistic weight goal setting, 115
    resources of, 162–164
    therapy, 134
Weight standards, 120t–121t
Well-balanced vegetarian diet, 232
Western medicine, 555
WHO DEXA T-score result
        diagnostic criteria, 425t
WIC Farmers' Market Nutrition
        Program, 220
WIC participation, health benefits
        of, 221t
WIC program, effectiveness of, 220
WIC services, 220
WOCN Guidelines, 503
World Cancer Research Fund
        (WCRF), 509
World Health Organization (WHO),
        201, 424
Wound care, nutrition
    energy needs, determining,
        502–503
    fluid needs, determining, 503
    protein needs, determining, 503
    vitamin and mineral
        supplementation, 503–504
Wound healing, 351–352

X
Xenical (orlistat) weight loss drug,
        149t–150t
Xerostomia, 368, 442. *See* Dry
        mouth
    nutrition recommendations
        for, 442t
    side effect of, 368
    treatment techniques, 369t

Y
Yoga, 557

Z
Zinc, 218
    supplementation, 508